Speech Motor Control

New developments in basic and applied research

Speech Motor Control

New developments in basic and applied research

Edited by

Ben Maassen

Pascal van Lieshout

OXFORD
UNIVERSITY PRESS

OXFORD
UNIVERSITY PRESS

Great Clarendon Street, Oxford OX2 6DP

Oxford University Press is a department of the University of Oxford.
It furthers the University's objective of excellence in research, scholarship,
and education by publishing worldwide in

Oxford New York

Auckland Cape Town Dar es Salaam Hong Kong Karachi
Kuala Lumpur Madrid Melbourne Mexico City Nairobi
New Delhi Shanghai Taipei Toronto

With offices in

Argentina Austria Brazil Chile Czech Republic France Greece
Guatemala Hungary Italy Japan Poland Portugal Singapore
South Korea Switzerland Thailand Turkey Ukraine Vietnam

Oxford is a registered trade mark of Oxford University Press
in the UK and in certain other countries

Published in the United States
by Oxford University Press Inc., New York

First published 2010

British Library Cataloguing in Publication Data
Data available

Library of Congress Cataloging in Publication Data
Speech motor control : new developments in basic and applied research / edited by Ben Maassen,
Pascal van Lieshout.
p. ; cm.
Includes bibliographical references.
ISBN 978–0–19–923579–7 (alk. paper)
1. Speech disorders. 2. Motor ability. 3. Apraxia. I. Maassen, Ben. II. Van Lieshout, Pascal H. H. M.
[DNLM: 1. Speech Disorders. 2. Psychomotor Disorders. 3. Speech—physiology. WL 340.2 S7423 2010]
RC423.S6396 2010
616.85'5—dc22

Typeset in Minion by Glyph International, India
Printed on acid free paper

ISBN 978–0–19–923579–7

Preface

The purpose of this book is to present recent and important theoretical developments in the area of research on speech motor control and to offer new insights by leaders in the field on the nature of speech disorders. In the past 5 years, research in these areas has shown tremendous progress due to new theory development that informs the design and interpretation of research and to a more advanced understanding of the complexities of brain functions related to speech production. Speech motor control is no longer considered an isolated process that can be studied completely independently from the other functions involved in speaking. New fundamental insights in speech motor control processes are emerging, showing a stronger embedding in general aspects of the origin, development and maintenance of cognitive, linguistic and motor processes as well as demonstrating its unique properties as part of the human genetic make-up. Clearly, this highly complex system defies the notion of a simple modular hierarchy. Parallel to this, one of the major developments in the area of speech motor research is a stronger interdisciplinary collaboration. Integration seems to be the key-concept: integration of principles and models of perception-action relations in general and speech as an audio-visual-speech-motor performance in particular; biomechanical and neurobiological aspects of motor control in general, and the biomechanics and neurological control mechanisms of speech in particular; the genetics of motor learning (automation) and of language disorders in general, and of speech motor learning and phonology in particular. The research and views that will be presented in this book will testify to the complex nature of speaking, highlighting the need to move away from traditional paradigms and associated interpretations, both in normal and disordered speech. Obviously, many of these views are in need of further experimental verification, but in the end they serve the important function of driving new research in the near and perhaps more distant future. In this sense, the current book is as much a reflection on what is currently the state-of-the art in speech motor research as a guide to what needs to be done in order to move our field further forward. As in every other research area, speech motor research benefits from the expertise of other experts in neuroscience, psychology, linguistics, psychoacoustics and general motor control. The chapters presented in this book are written by scholars who reflect this wide variety of expertise and interest in speech motor control and bring their unique viewpoints to our attention.

The basis for this volume was created at the 5th International Conference on Speech Motor Control, which was held in Nijmegen, June 7–10, 2006. The contents of both this volume and the conference are a natural sequel to the preceding volume (2004) and conference (2001) taking advantage of the developments mentioned above and adding specific emphasis to state-of-the-art research in recent years. A special focus in the current volume is on brain plasticity in relation to development and learning. This volume also puts more emphasis on clinical applications in the area of speech motor disorders. In recent years, we have witnessed various new approaches in diagnosis and treatment. To recognize such contributions, this book includes clinical research papers that bear a direct relationship to the more basic science chapters. Thus, there is a special section labelled 'clinical impact' in which recent controversies in dysarthria and Childhood Apraxia of Speech (CAS) are addressed. This section in particular expresses the impact recent research developments have on clinical practice.

The scope of this volume will reflect state-of-the art research in the area of modelling, genetics, brain imaging, behavioural experimentation and clinical applications. As editors of this book, we are particularly pleased to present you as a reader with these exciting and (as we hope) stimulating papers on a variety of topics that will be of interest to basic scientists, clinical scientists and clinicians, as well as students in these areas. The volume is divided in six sections: Modelling, Genetics and Neurology, Development, Fluency Disorders, Clinical Impact, and Methods. Following is a brief characterization of these sections and the individual chapters.

The *first section* has a strong emphasis on the nature of motor/phonetic representations in speech production and the role of different feedback sources (auditory and somatosensory) on the control of articulation in speech. In chapter 1, Wolfram Ziegler discusses the role of syllables in apraxic error generation and based on his review proposes a non-linear architecture of phonetic representations that include gestural, syllabic and metrical tiers. In chapter 2, Bernd Kröger, Peter Birkholz, Anja Lowit, and Christiane Neuschaefer-Rube present a new action-based neurocomputational model of speech production (called ACT) which includes sensory (i.e. somatosensory and auditory), motor, phonetic, and phonemic neural representations. Details of this model, its capabilities and how it compares to other current models are presented. In chapter 3, Sazzad Nasir and David Ostry review the evidence that somatosensory precision in speech is important to the nervous system, even in absence of effects on speech acoustics, and appears to be achieved through impedance or stiffness control. Recent data from their lab are presented to support their hypothesis. In chapter 4, Mark Tiede, Suzanne Boyce, Carol Espy-Wilson, and Vincent Gracco discuss the role of auditory representations in speech and present data from a recent study in which they used an articificial palate to study its impact on motor equivalence and formant patterns in the production of /r/ sounds.

The *second section* focuses on the genetic and neural basis of speech production mechanisms and the potential consequences of impairments in these areas. In chapter 5, Soo-Eun Chang and Christy Ludlow provide a detailed overview of brain imaging studies in children using techniques once thought to be challenging for application in infants and children. Focusing on fluency disorders, the authors discuss findings that point on the one hand to trait-related deficits in adults and children forming the basis of developmental stuttering, and on the other hand to differences between adults and children that may represent changes in brain structure and function as a consequence of a lifetime of stuttering. In chapter 6, Angela Morgan, Frédérique Liégeois, and Faraneh Vargha-Khadem present an overview of motor speech characteristics of children with congenital or acquired brain damage, in particular related to mutations on the FOXP2 gene, and damage to brain structures due to surgical interventions. They discuss the role of bilateral versus unilateral neuropathology, and the involvement of the fronto-striatal and fronto-cerebellar loops in dyspraxia and dysarthria. In chapter 7, Hermann Ackermann and Axel Riecker review recent findings from functional imaging studies that point towards a 'minimal brain network' of motor aspects of speech production. They argue that the functional imaging techniques are providing new insights into the pathomechanisms of various dysarthric deficits and their relationship to the underlying neural substrate.

The *third section* provides new insights in the various aspects of speech motor development in relation to both motor and language factors. In chapter 8, Lisa Goffman reports on empirical findings detailing complex interactions between language and motor domains in normally developing and language disordered learners, emphasizing that speech motor variability may serve as an index of learning. In chapter 9, Aude Noiray, Marie-Agnès Cathiard, Lucie Ménard, and Christian Abry discuss recent experimental work on anticipatory coarticulation in lip rounding with both adults and children in support of their Movement Expansion Model (MEM), and are thereby able to link this effectively to the larger topic of acquisition of speech motor skills that support fluency in a language. In chapter 10, Jordan Green and Ignatius Nip present an overview of their recent work on speech motor development, highlighting the dynamic and nonlinear nature of these processes over time. A conceptual framework is unfolded for studying early speech motor development, which guides current and future lines of their research.

The *fourth section* is dedicated to new theoretical and empirical approaches towards understanding the speech motor problems in people who stutter. In chapter 11, Pascal van Lieshout and Aravind Namasivayam discuss the concept of variability in articulation and the problems with current measures to assess its impact and characteristics. They propose a different approach based on dynamical systems theory and present data on a small group of persons who stutter and matched controls to illustrate these measures. In chapter 12, Peter Howell, Andrew Anderson, and Jorge Lucero discuss the use of functional data analysis (FDA) techniques to analyze spatio-temporal variability in articulator movements and acoustic signals. They illustrate the use of such measures with recent data from their lab.

The *fifth section* presents a variety of papers on theoretical and experimental approaches towards the classification and interpretation of speech symptoms in childhood dysarthria and apraxia of speech and other speech motor disorders. In chapter 13, Gary Weismer and Yungjung Kim present a historical overview of the Mayo Clinic perspective on motor speech disorders, and argue that this perspective should be abandoned in favour of a different approach in which the focus is on speech related commonalities as core phenomena of motor speech disorders. In chapter 14, Ben Maassen, Lian Nijland and Hayo Terband discuss different developmental models of childhood apraxia of speech and based on the divergent approaches and results to characterize CAS, challenge the modular view on the cognitive architecture of the infant speech production system. An alternative approach for clinical classification and research is suggested based on developmental trajectories and computational simulation studies. In chapter 15, Lawrence Shriberg argues in favour of a neurodevelopmental framework for research in Childhood Apraxia of Speech (CAS) that is motivated by the notion that the core speech processing features of idiopathic CAS and its clinical signs remain unknown to date. The rational and methods for such a framework are discussed and illustrated with findings from studies on CAS related to genetically-based disorders. In chapter 16, Joseph Duffy addresses the important relationship between the differential diagnosis of acquired motor speech disorders and the localization and diagnosis of neurologic diseases using examples from selected clinical cases. In chapter 17, Christopher Dromey describes data from three speech disorders to illustrate how changes in articulation may arise in the context of treatment that is solely focused on the larynx. These interactions between different parts of the speech production system are further discussed with respect to the implications for our understanding of disordered speech motor control as well as for intervention strategies in these populations. In chapter 18, Elina Tripoliti and Patricia Limousin present an overview of stereotactic surgery and electrical stimulation of deep brain structures in patients with Parkinson's disease to discuss the role of basal ganglia in speech motor control, noting the variable outcome of these interventions and the need for further research into ways speech is affected by deep brain stimulation.

In the *sixth section*, several recent state-of-the-art methodologies are presented that will provide important information on various aspects of articulation processes in speech. Chapter 19 by Bruce Murdoch discusses advantages and disadvantages of 3D electromagnetic articulography (EMA), 3D electropalatography (EPG) and a pressure-sensing EPG, and their potential applications in assessing articulation in normal and disordered speakers. In chapter 20, Phil Hoole and Andreas Zierdt discuss current developments in the use of five-dimensional electromagnetic articulography for speech research. They detail some of the drawbacks, but also highlight how the specific features of this system allows for particularly succinct and robust characterizations of tongue configurations, provides more natural speaking conditions and permits longer recording sessions. In chapter 21, Tim Bressmann discusses recent developments in 2D and 3D ultrasound imaging of the tongue in normal populations and glossectomy patients, demonstrating effects on motor control in the form of compensatory post-operative increases of tongue velocity and height. In addition, exciting possibilities of 4D imaging with the newest generation of ultrasound transducers are discussed.

As editors of this book, we are very pleased and grateful that we were able to get the commitment of all the authors in this book to share their knowledge on recent developments in theoretical, experimental and technological aspects of speech motor research in normal and disordered speech. We are convinced that anyone who has a scientific or clinical interest in speech motor control will be thrilled by the quality of the chapters that are presented in the various sections. This volume is a worthy successor of the previous book on speech motor control and we expect to witness how the ideas, suggestions and questions presented in this volume find solid ground in the various exciting and innovative new studies that will be initiated in the very near future and beyond.

Acknowledgements

The editors of this book would like to acknowledge the generous financial and/or administrative support from the Dutch Royal Academy of Science (KNAW), the National Institute on Deafness and Other Communication Disorders (National Institutes of Health), the Hendrix Foundation, the Departments of Medical Psychology, Paediatric Neurology and ENT of the Radboud University Nijmegen Medical Centre, and the Centre for Neuroscience and Centre for Cognition of the Donders Institute for Brain, Cognition and Behaviour of the Radboud University Nijmegen in the planning and implementation of the 5th International Conference on Speech Motor Control, including the editorial support to publish this book. We also wish to pay special tribute to Hayo Terband for all his hard work on coordinating important aspects of the review process and contributing many useful ideas and solutions during this time. Furthermore, we wish to acknowledge the contributions of all our reviewers, including our special consultants, Raymond D. Kent and Wouter Hulstijn, who provided valuable feedback to earlier versions of the manuscripts. Their efforts are highly appreciated.

Ben Maassen
Pascal van Lieshout
Nijmegen/Toronto, August 2009

Contents

List of contributors

Christian Abry – Université Stendhal, Grenoble, France.

Hermann Ackermann – Department of General Neurology, Hertie Institute for Clinical Brain Research, University of Tübingen, Tübingen, Germany.

Ingrid Aichert – EKN – Clinical Neuropsychology Research Group, Bogenhausen Hospital, München, Germany.

Andrew Anderson – Division of Psychology and Language Sciences, University College London, London, UK.

Peter Birkholz – Department of Phoniatrics, Pedaudiology, and Communication Disorders, University Hospital Aachen and RWTH Aachen University, Aachen, Germany.

Suzanne E. Boyce – Department of Communication Sciences & Disorders, University of Cincinnati, Cincinnati, OH, USA.

Tim Bressmann – Department of Speech-Language Pathology, University of Toronto, Toronto, Canada.

Marie-Agnès Cathiard – Université Stendhal, Grenoble, France.

Soo-Eun Chang – Department of Communicative Sciences and Disorders & Department of Radiology, College of communication arts and sciences, Michigan State University, East Lansing, MI, USA.

Christopher Dromey – Department of Communication Disorders, Brigham Young University, Provo, UT, USA.

Joseph R. Duffy – Division of Speech Pathology, Department of Neurology, Mayo Clinic & Mayo Medical School, Rochester, MN, USA.

Carol Y. Espy-Wilson – Speech Communication Laboratory, Institute of Systems Research, and Department of Electrical and Computer Engineering, University of Maryland, College Park, MD, USA.

Vincent L. Gracco – School of Communication Sciences and Disorders, McGill University & Centre for Research on Language, Mind and Brain, Montreal, QC, Canada & Haskins Laboratories, New Haven, CT, USA.

Jordan R. Green – Department of Special Education and Communication Disorders, University of Nebraska – Lincoln, Lincoln, NE, USA.

Lisa Goffman – Speech, Language, & Hearing Sciences, Purdue University, West Lafayette, IN, USA.

Phil Hoole – Institute of Phonetics and Speech Processing, Munich University, München, Germany.

Peter Howell – Division of Psychology and Language Sciences, University College London, London, UK.

Yunjung Kim – Department of Communication Sciences & Disorders, Louisiana State University, Baton Rouge, LA, USA.

Bernd J. Kröger – Department of Phoniatrics, Pedaudiology, and Communication Disorders, University Hospital Aachen and RWTH Aachen University, Aachen, Germany.

Frédérique Liégeois – Institute of Child Health, University College London, London, UK.

Patricia Limousin – Sobell Department, Unit of Functional Neurosurgery, Institute of Neurology, University College London, London, UK.

Anja Lowit – Speech and Language Therapy Division, Department of Educational and Professional Studies, University of Strathclyde, Glasgow, UK.

Jorge Lucero – Department of Mathematics, University of Brasilia, Brasilia, Brasil.

Christy L. Ludlow – Laboratory on Neural Bases of Communication and Swallowing HHS, James Madison University Harrisonburg, Harrisonburg VA, USA.

Ben Maassen – Center for Language and Cognition Groningen (CLCG) & University Medical Centre, University of Groningen, Groningen, The Netherlands & Medical Psychology/Pediatric Neurology, Radboud University Nijmegen Medical Centre, Nijmegen, The Netherlands.

Lucie Ménard – Département de linguistique et de didactique des langues, l'Université du Québec à Montréal, Montreal, QC, Canada.

Angela Morgan – Murdoch Childrens Research Institute, Royal Childrens Hospital, University of Melbourne, Melbourne, Australia.

Bruce E. Murdoch – Motor Speech Research Centre, School of Health and Rehabilitation Sciences, The University of Queensland, Brisbane, Australia.

Aravind K. Namasivayam – Oral Dynamics Lab, Department of Speech-Language Pathology, University of Toronto and Toronto Rehabilitation Institute, Toronto, ON, Canada.

Sazzad M. Nasir – Department of Psychology, McGill University, Montreal, QC, Canada.

Christiane Neuschaefer-Rube – Department of Phoniatrics, Pedaudiology, and Communication Disorders, University Hospital Aachen and RWTH Aachen University, Aachen, Germany

Ignatius S. B. Nip – School of Speech, Language, and Hearing Sciences, San Diego State University, San Diego, CA, USA.

Lian Nijland – Medical Psychology/ENT, Radboud University Nijmegen Medical Centre, Nijmegen, The Netherlands.

Aude Noiray – Haskins Laboratories, New Haven CT, USA & GIPSA-Lab, Université Stendhal-INPG, Grenoble, France.

David J. Ostry – Department of Psychology, McGill University, Montreal, QC, Canada & Haskins Laboratories, New Haven, CT, USA.

Axel Riecker – Department of Neurology, Medical Center, University of Ulm, Ulm, Germany.

Lawrence D. Shriberg – Waisman Center, University of Wisconsin-Madison, Madison, WI, USA.

Anja Staiger – EKN – Clinical Neuropsychology Research Group, Bogenhausen Hospital, München, Germany.

Hayo Terband – Medical Psychology/Pediatric Neurology/ENT, Radboud University Nijmegen Medical Centre, Nijmegen, The Netherlands.

Mark K. Tiede – Haskins Laboratories, New Haven CT, USA.

Elina Tripoliti – Sobell Department, Unit of Functional Neurosurgery, Institute of Neurology, University College London, London, UK.

Pascal van Lieshout – Oral Dynamics Lab, Department of Speech-Language Pathology & Institute of Biomaterials and Biomedical Engineering & Department of Psychology, University of Toronto and Toronto Rehabilitation Institute, Toronto, ON, Canada.

Faraneh Vargha-Khadem – Institute of Cognitive Neuroscience & Institute of Child Health, University College London, London, UK.

Gary Weismer – Department of Communicative Disorders, Waisman Center, University of Wisconsin-Madison, Madison, WI, USA.

Wolfram Ziegler – EKN – Clinical Neuropsychology Research Group, Bogenhausen Hospital, München, Germany.

Andreas Zierdt – Institute of Phonetics and Speech Processing, Munich University, München, Germany.

Section 1

Modelling of speech production

Chapter 1

Apraxia of speech: what the deconstruction of phonetic plans tells us about the construction of articulate language

Wolfram Ziegler, Anja Staiger, and Ingrid Aichert

Abstract

Apraxia of speech is considered as a speech motor planning impairment. Apraxic speech errors may therefore inform us about the structure of phonetic plans. Recent studies have suggested that syllabic motor integration mechanisms play a role in apraxic error generation, which contradicts earlier views of a segment-by-segment planning process. However, learning experiments in apraxic speakers have revealed that syllables should not be viewed as indivisible motor primitives. Moreover, supra-syllabic (metrical) mechanisms can also be shown to play an important role in the genesis of apraxic errors. We therefore propose a non-linear architecture of phonetic representations which embraces gestural, syllabic, and metrical tiers.

1.1 Introduction

1.1.1 Syllables and phonemes in phonetic encoding

Speech is probably one of the most complex and most intensively exercised motor skills of humans. All normally developing individuals learn it from birth on and exercise speech motor behaviour day by day, over their whole lifetime.

How can we describe the processes or representations that are constituted through speech motor learning? What are the core features of this highly automated skill that are established during its acquisition? The theory developed by Levelt and coworkers (Levelt et al., 1999) gives a clear answer to this question: It postulates that during speech motor learning we acquire motor programmes for frequently occurring syllables and store them in a 'mental syllabary'.

Experimental evidence for the existence of a mental syllabary comes from reaction time data showing that, in naming tasks, the production of high-frequency syllables involves shorter latencies than the production of syllables with lower frequencies (Carreiras and Perea 2004; Cholin 2008; Cholin et al., 2005, 2006; Laganaro and Alario 2006; Levelt and Wheeldon 1994). Over and above such experimental evidence there is a further important reason why syllables might be considered major building blocks of speech motor planning: we need only several hundreds of them to construct more than 80% of the words we produce every day, hence this small number of units comes over our lips thousands of times when we learn to speak. Take the syllable [di:], which – according to the CELEX database (Baayen et al., 1995) – occurs more than 40,000 times in a million words, and consider further that a three-year-old child may perhaps produce 5,000 words per day, i.e., 1.8 million words per year.[1] On her 10th birthday this child will have produced the motor pattern for [di:] about 500,000 times. According to Levelt's theory, such a frequent use of always the same bundle of lingual, labial, mandibular, velar, and laryngeal gestures participating in the construction of [di:] transforms the recurring motor pattern into a stable, overlearned movement programme and burns it onto the premotor-cortical hard-disk that houses the child's phonetic lexicon. From there it can be accessed rapidly and safely whenever the syllable occurs in an utterance. The only thing the motor system then needs to do is unpack the gestural scores encapsulated in the plan and unfold the speech movements prescribed by these scores (Levelt et al., 1999).

If frequency is the core argument, why don't we consider *phonemes* to be the relevant units in speech motor planning? Phoneme programmes would have an even stronger generative power, since little more than 40 of them suffice to produce any German word. And, as a consequence, phonemes are even more frequent than syllables – the phoneme [d], for instance, is used in more than 570 different German syllables and occurs more than four times as often as the syllable [di:] (Aichert et al., 2005). What hinders us to assume that phoneme-sized motor programmes are acquired through frequent repetition and stored to form the building blocks of speech motor plans? Levelt's theory has a clear answer to this question as well: if it were phonemes, the process of accessing such a small inventory would cost almost nothing, but a powerful machinery would be needed to coarticulate these small units and integrate them into a smoothly flowing stream of syllables, words, and phrases. Hence, a phonetic planning theory based on phonemes alone would leave large parts of the motor organization of speaking unexplained. Taking syllables as the building blocks of phonetic encoding, on the contrary, all the coarticulation processes within syllables are considered part of the learned motor routines, and only little coarticulatory smoothing is still to be done by the *Articulator* to transform strings of syllables into a coherent stream of connected speech (Levelt et al., 1999).

Yet, if smoothness is the relevant issue, why then should phonetic encoding be limited to syllables and not go for motor programmes of a still larger grain size, e.g., words? Whole-word phonetic representations would have the advantage that they also contain movement information relating to the metrical properties of a word and to between-syllable transitions, and would therefore generate perfectly smooth and fluent articulations. The argument against this view is that a lexicon of word-sized motor programmes would be huge, and, still more important, would not be sufficiently generative. Whenever a new word comes up in our language, considerable speech motor learning effort would be needed before we are able to produce it, and any derived or inflected form of a word or any cliticization would require a new motor programme. Levelt's syllable-based theory resolves these problems a lot more parsimoniously.

However, the concept of a syllabary containing a limited number of overlearned motor programmes leaves a similar gap with respect to the generativity and plasticity of our speech motor system: when we speak, we sometimes also encounter *infrequent* or even new syllables, which,

[1] Mehl et al. (2007) reported that adult speakers produce more than 15,000 words per day. We consider three-to-ten-year-old speakers to probably produce less than this – 5,000 appears to be a rather conservative guess. For a similar estimate cf. also Levelt (2001), p. 13468.

according to a strictly syllable-based phonetic planning theory, would be beyond our speech motor skills. These syllables would, if no other representation of articulatory skills exists, have to be learned from scratch, in an infant-like manner. This is definitely not the case, as the anecdote of a small polar bear from the Berlin zoo, named 'Knut' [knu:t], demonstrates. In 2007, *Knut* became popular all over the country within a few days, due to his unfortunate fate and his cute appearance, and everybody in the country was talking about the little bear. Notably, the syllable [knu:t] was very infrequent beforehand,[2] hence speakers of German could not have a motor programme for it, but nonetheless there was no nationwide dyslalic distortion and no stuttering or trial-and-error groping on Knut's name during the first days of his public life. By contrast, everybody in the country was able to pronounce Knut's zero-frequency name accurately and fluently, without any prior practice.

Levelt's model offers a tentative explanation for this observation, proposing that in such cases speakers revert to an auxiliary encoding route by assembling a phonetic plan for the new syllable from smaller building blocks, such as segments. A major implicit assumption of this theory is that speakers dispose of stored motor programmes not only for frequent syllables, but also for such smaller units, e.g., for phonemes. Another strong assumption is that the articulatory machinery is flexible enough to deal with gestural input of both syllabic and segmental size, and that it is capable of generating a smooth and co-articulated stream of speech movements from a patchwork string of syllabic and segmental motor plans. Furthermore, the sub-syllabic encoding route, if it exists, must be almost as efficient as the syllabic route, since no audible degradation of accuracy or fluency has ever been reported for infrequent, phonotactically well-formed syllables. In fact, only a very small reaction-time disadvantage of low-frequency syllables (around 10 ms) was observed under highly artificial experimental conditions (Cholin et al., 2006; Levelt and Wheeldon 1994). This leaves us with the question of which units definitely play a role in the programming of speech movements, and how these units are composed to phonetic plans for the production of words and phrases.

1.1.2 **Apraxia of speech: a clinical model for the deconstruction of phonetic plans**

In the present chapter we address the issue of how phonetic plans are constructed from the perspective of impaired speech motor programming in apraxia of speech (AOS). Apraxia of speech is an acquired speech disorder in adults, resulting from lesions to left anterior peri- or sub-sylvian cortex, mostly after infarction of the left middle cerebral artery. The disorder is characterized by a frequent occurrence of phonetic sound distortions and phonemic errors, and by dysfluent and dysprosodic speech. The impairment is distinguished from *dysarthria*, since its symptoms cannot be explained by motor pathomechanisms such as paresis, hypokinesia, ataxia, dyskinesia, tremor, etc. For instance, the observation that articulatory aberrations in apraxic speakers are highly inconsistent and that patients may occasionally even produce symptom-free speech is not compatible with our common understanding of dysarthric pathomechanisms. AOS is also distinguished from aphasic *phonological impairment*, on the basis of the obvious motor nature of the problem, which is evidenced, for instance, by the occurrence of phonetically ill-formed utterances. Although the theoretical underpinnings of the distinction between phonological encoding, phonetic planning, and motor execution processes are still debated, there is widespread conviction among clinicians that AOS patients constitute an identifiable clinical population

[2] Knut is an infrequent German male first name. The syllable [knu:t] is not in the CELEX-syllable lexicon of German spoken or written word forms (Aichert et al., 2005), hence its token frequency is formally zero.

requiring special therapeutic management. There is also high agreement that the impairment must be located to a stage where more abstract phonological representations are transformed into motor commands for the movements of the speech organs, i.e., to the phonetic encoding stage of spoken language production (for references see McNeil et al., 1997; Ziegler, 2008).

Since AOS is considered to interfere with the process of generating phonetic plans for speaking, the speech patterns that are characteristic of this syndrome may tell us something about the phonetic encoding process itself or about the make-up of phonetic representations. More specifically, analyses of the error patterns of apraxic speakers may inform us about the sites of fracture of phonetic plans in this specific condition and thereby allow us to delineate the architecture of the phonetic planning process.

The present chapter reviews several lines of research which followed this agenda: it reports on experiments probing the status of phonemes and syllables in AOS, explicates evidence challenging the assumption of holistic syllable programmes, and sketches recent observations characterizing the role of supra-syllabic metrical structures in this syndrome. In the end, a non-linear model of phonetic plans is proposed which integrates multiple hierarchic layers into a unitary concept of how phonetic plans are constructed.

1.2 The status of the syllable in apraxia of speech

Levelt's phonetic encoding theory directs the focus of apraxic error analysis on the syllable as the core unit of phonetic encoding. More specifically, Levelt (2001) suggested that overlearned motor actions like those related to high frequency syllables 'typically get stored in the premotor cortex' (Levelt 2001, p. 13469). The lesion sites that are presumed to be associated with AOS are not far from left inferior premotor cortex (for a review cf. Ziegler 2008), hence an obvious expectation might be that the syllabic motor programmes are no longer accessible in patients with this syndrome. This is the hypothesis postulated in a review article by Varley and Whiteside (2001), who made the additional assumption that apraxic speakers are forced to revert to the sub-syllabic route of phonetic encoding postulated in Levelt's dual-route model. In their example, phonetic encoding of the word 'cat' in apraxic speakers involves a sequential access to motor routines for [k], [æ], and [t], while healthy adult speakers would simply access, on a direct route, the motor routine for the whole syllable [kæt]. In Varley and Whiteside's theory, the cumbersome segment-by-segment encoding process 'may present the speaker with AOS with an insurmountable computational task' and thereby make apraxic speech so laborious and error-prone (Varley and Whiteside 2001, p. 44).

1.2.1 Syllable frequency effects

A prediction following from the assumption that apraxic speakers have no access to the mental syllabary is that syllable frequency has no effect on their speech accuracy, because patients are postulated to always use the same sub-syllabic programming mechanism, irrespective of the specific properties of a syllable to be produced. This prediction was tested in a word repetition experiment by Aichert and Ziegler (2004). In this experiment, two-syllabic words were controlled for the structure and frequency of their first (stressed) syllables. Four frequency groups were formed, with the subgroup of most frequent syllables ranking below 250, and the least frequent ones above 1,000. When the error rates of ten patients with AOS were pooled for each of the four frequency groups, accuracy turned out to be significantly higher in the syllables with the highest frequencies (70% of all syllables correct) as compared to all other freqency groups (56–59% correct). A similar effect was found in three French-speaking apraxic patients examined by Laganaro (2008).

Staiger and Ziegler (2008) extended this research from word repetition to spontaneous speech. They examined large samples of spontaneous speech (> 1000 syllables per participant) in three patients and pooled speech errors according to the frequency and the complexity of syllables. Each patient had a significant effect of syllable frequency on error rate, and when syllable complexity was controlled for, this advantage was still significant in two of them, with a non-significant trend in the third patient. A frequency effect has meanwhile also been described in two further apraxic patients (Staiger 2008). Summarizing these data, the hypothesis that apraxic speakers are insensitive to syllabic properties like syllable frequency cannot be maintained. The finding that syllables with very high frequencies are particularly resistant to apraxic degeneration is consistent with the assumption that phonetic planning aspects are consolidated through frequent repetitions of always the same syllabic motor patterns. The more consolidated a syllable is, the less is it vulnerable to apraxic failure.

One of the questions that still remain to be answered is how specific the syllable frequency effect is for the syndrome of AOS. Although Wilshire and Nespoulous (2003) failed to detect a syllable frequency effect in two patients with aphasic phonological impairment, Laganaro (2005) found such an effect in patients with conduction aphasia, and Stenneken et al. (2005, 2008) found frequency-dependent distribution effects in the spontaneous speech of a patient with Wernicke's aphasia. This leaves us with the problem of whether there are still other pathomechanisms of spoken language production that may be sensitive to syllable frequency (cf. Laganaro 2008).

1.2.2 **Syllable boundary effects**

The influence of the syllabic decomposition of words on apraxic error patterns was confirmed by another experiment reported in Aichert and Ziegler (2004), which expanded on the role of consonant clusters in AOS. Take, as an example, the word 'fragment' (Fig. 1.1). In this word, there are three positions in which abutting consonants occur: initial, medial, and final. Yet, while in the initial and the final cluster the two consonants pertain to the same syllable constituent, the two abutting consonants of the medial cluster pertain to two different syllables, i.e., [frag] and [mənt]. If apraxic encoding were purely segment-based, one would not expect to obtain different error patterns on within- vs. cross-syllabic clusters, since the encoding mechanism would not recognize

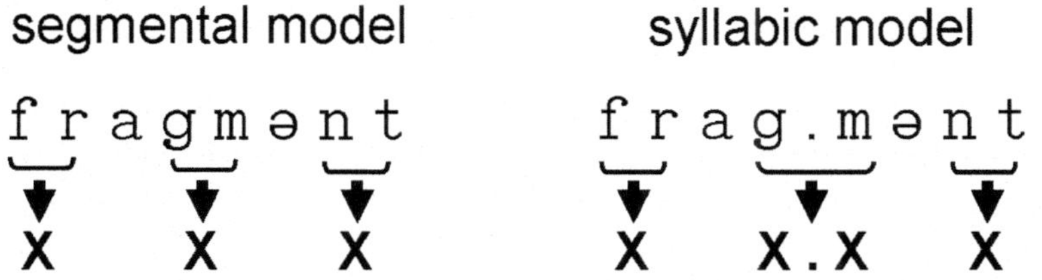

Fig. 1.1 Consonant cluster reduction in a segmental (left) and a syllabic model of stepwise phonetic encoding (right). Reduction errors are symbolized by arrows pointing from two target consonants to a single error segment X. The syllable boundary (right) is indicated by a dot. In the segmental model, the syllable boundary between [g] and [m] in [fragmənt] is not visible at the phonetic level, hence the cluster [gm] underlies similar error mechanisms as [fr] and [nt]. In the syllabic model, [g] and [m] pertain to different encoding units and are therefore not engaged in a common error mechanism such as cluster reduction. Empirical data support the model on the right (Aichert and Ziegler 2004).

syllable boundaries.[3] However, in a comparison of words with initial, medial, and final clusters the patients reported by Aichert and Ziegler (2004) made entirely different types of errors on within-syllable vs. across-syllable clusters: when an error occurred in one of the within-syllable positions, clusters were very frequently reduced to single consonants, e.g., [frag] to [fag] or [mənt] to [mən] (74% and 54% of onset- and coda-clusters, respectively), whereas this was rarely so for consonants abutting across syllable boundaries (9%). Hence, the error mechanism in the apraxic speakers examined in this study was obviously sensitive to syllable boundaries, implying that consonant sequences such as [g], [m] in 'fragment' were not involved in reduction errors.

The experimental finding of preserved syllabicity in adult apraxic speech is also consistent with clinical observations according to which apraxic speakers tend to segregate syllables (Kent and Rosenbek 1983), and with earlier findings of decreased between-syllable coarticulation (Ziegler and Cramon 1985). It suggests that syllabicity is visible at the surface of apraxic speech, although it does not explain how syllable boundary information might penetrate into the phonetic representations of apraxic speakers. With view to the syllable frequency effects reviewed above, the most parsimonious explanation would be in terms of a syllabic encoding mechanism.

1.2.3 **Phonemes vs. syllables in the re-construction of phonetic plans**

The status of the phonetic encoding unit in AOS is also an important issue when it comes to treatment, i.e., to the re-construction of lost motor skills in apraxic patients. If, as proposed in Darley's original definition of this syndrome, AOS is an impairment of movement programming 'for the volitional production of *phonemes*' (Darley 1968), a major goal of apraxia treatment should be the remediation of segmental movement plans, as described by Rosenbek (1985). A segmental approach was also proposed by Varley and Whiteside (2001, p. 47), with the aim of strengthening the compensatory use of the indirect, segment-by-segment assembly of words postulated by these authors. Clinically, segmental treatment approaches play an important role and have widely been used by speech therapists (Wambaugh 2002). Dabul and Bollier (1976), for instance, reported on a training of isolated segments with subsequent exercises focussing on the sequencing of learned phonemes. They encountered sequencing difficulties still after the training, which they ascribed to persisting fundamental problems of the patients to produce the trained phonemes in isolation.

Theories advocating a role of larger units in phonetic encoding and a partial preservation of motor routines at higher integration levels in AOS would, on the contrary, explicitly reject a training of isolated segments, since such an approach misses the level of organization of phonetic gestures in speech motor programming (Aichert & Ziegler 2004; Odell 2002; Ziegler and Jaeger 1993). Such considerations have motivated treatment approaches based on larger units. A method proposed by Wambaugh et al.(1996), for instance, focused on a training of segments by embedding them into minimally contrastive mono- and disyllabic words. Other approaches based on exercises focussing on syllabic or even suprasyllabic units were proposed, for instance, by Jaeger and Ziegler (1993) or by Brendel and Ziegler (2008).

Overall, the issue of which units should be addressed in the treatment of AOS is still controversial. Aichert (2008) therefore tackled this issue directly by comparing, in four patients with severe AOS, the effects of an intensive segment-based training with an equally intensive training of syllables. In a baseline-assessment, the six most severely impaired segments and syllables,

[3] A similar approach was chosen in a study of developmental apraxia of speech by Maassen et al. (2001).

respectively, were identified in each patient individually. Three segments and three syllables were selected as treatment targets, the remaining three items from each unit served as untreated controls. The target phonemes / syllables were trained over periods of 45 minutes, respectively.

After the *segmental* learning, only one out of four patients had decreased error rates and decreased reaction times on isolated productions of the target phonemes. The other three patients did not improve during the 45-minutes learning. Moreover, none of the patients improved in a transfer-condition, i.e., when the trained consonants were embedded in syllables. After the *syllable* learning, on the contrary, three out of four patients improved specifically on the target syllables. Two of them also showed transfer-effects, i.e., improved on two-syllabic words containing the trained syllables (Aichert 2008).

These results suggest that syllables can more easily be learned than segments, hence they may constitute more natural units of phonetic encoding. Production of consonants isolated from their context is a rather artificial condition which rarely occurs in conversation and may be disproportionately impaired in apraxic speakers (cf. Dabul and Bollier 1976). It also plays no role in speech motor learning during language development. Moreover, as Aichert (2008) demonstrated, there is no straightforward transfer from isolated production of consonants to a syllabic context, even in cases of limited segmental learning, suggesting that the composition of syllables from phonemes is a process that needs to be learned separately. This is consistent with the view that within-syllable coarticulation is part of the phonetic code (Levelt et al., 1999). Syllables, on the contrary, turned out to be re-learnable for apraxic speakers, even during very short training periods. Moreover, as soon as they had been learned, syllables proved to be generative in the sense that they could be used in a larger context, without any extra training of the composition process.

1.3 **Are phonetic plans for syllables holistic entities?**

The data reported in the preceding section provide strong evidence for a specific role of syllables in the phonetic encoding process in apraxic speakers. This supports theories postulating syllable-based phonetic plans (Levelt et al., 1999) and suggests that apraxic speakers are still capable of accessing phonetic representations of this size.

The original idea of a mental lexicon of overlearned motor plans for syllables implies that the entries in such a lexicon are opaque, holistic units. As soon as a syllable has acquired the status of an overlearned motor pattern and become a member of the mental syllabary, its gestural components unfold in a highly automated manner, irrespective of the internal structure of a syllable. For the errors made by apraxic speakers one would predict from these assumptions that – at least in the more frequent syllables – syllable structure has no effect on error rates.

1.3.1 **Syllable complexity effects**

At first sight, a number of observations in apraxic speakers appear inconsistent with this prediction. Many descriptions of apraxic error patterns have pointed out that patients make errors especially on phonologically complex units, with a tendency to systematically replace them by less complex ones, e.g., consonant clusters by singletons (e.g. Rosenbek et al., 1984). As mentioned above, Aichert and Ziegler (2004) found that consonant clusters in the onset- and coda-positions of syllables are particularly often reduced to single consonants. In several other experimental studies, the complexity of syllable structure has been emphasized as an important factor influencing the occurrence of errors in patients with AOS or Broca's aphasia (e.g. Romani and Calabrese 1998; Romani and Galluzzi 2005; Nickels and Howard 2004). In a recent analysis of three patients with AOS, Staiger and Ziegler (2008) found a significant effect of syllable complexity (defined as the occurrence of at least one consonant cluster) on the rate of syllable errors also in *spontaneous speech*. The number of errors was more than 50% higher in syllables with clusters than in syllables without clusters. Together with the findings from earlier word repetition studies this seems to be suggestive of a sub-syllabic error mechanism and to contradict the holistic nature of overlearned syllables.

However, the complexity effect in apraxic speakers may be confined to syllables for which the assumption of a holistic representation cannot be made, since they are not accessible in the patient's mental syllabary. To resolve this issue, Staiger and Ziegler (2008) examined the influence of complexity for high-frequency and low-frequency syllables, separately. In all three patients included in this study, the complexity effect remained present only in the low-frequency syllable group. On an average the patients made 54% more errors on complex as compared to simple low-frequency syllables. In contrast, no complexity effect was seen on syllables with very high frequencies. As an interpretation of this result, sub-syllabic encoding mechanisms apparently play a minor role in AOS as long as a syllable is sufficiently frequent, i.e., its motor pattern is overlearned to a sufficiently high degree. Beyond a certain frequency threshold, the bonds of syllabic motor integration appear to become weaker and sub-syllabic mechanisms become more important in the creation of apraxic speech errors. This reconciles observations of complexity effects in apraxic speech with the assumption that a selected repertoire of holistic speech motor programming units may still exist in which these effects are absent.

In the study reviewed here the high-frequency threshold had been set to a syllable frequency rank of 250, in a syllable repertoire containing approximately 12,000 entries. Hence, a very small sub-section from a large inventory of syllables, i.e., only the 250 most frequent ones, was identified to be relatively preserved irrespective of syllable complexity. Several problems remain to be resolved with this result. First, the syllabary account offers no readily identifiable way of proving that the syllables considered part of a subject's mental syllabary and those which are insensitive to a complexity effect are actually the same. Second, since error rates were generally lower on the high-frequency syllables, a potential influence of complexity may have been obscured by a ceiling effect. Third, even the most frequent syllables cannot be considered entirely error-free in AOS, i.e., the vulnerability of a syllable to apraxic failure is not all-or-nothing. Hence, if we accept the mental syllabary concept we have to concede that although the entries in the syllable lexicon may still be accessible to apraxic patients their gestural contents can partially be disrupted. Strong additional assumptions would be needed to reconcile this result with the idea of a repertoire of holistic speech motor programmes.

1.3.2 **Re-constructing syllables from their parts**

Another approach towards the issue of a holistic nature of syllabic motor representations is through a syllable learning approach. In the theory referred to above, the property of a syllable to be part of the mental syllabary is considered to depend on syllable frequency, with the idea that frequent repetition of always the same articulations turns a syllable into an overlearned motor pattern, which can then be retrieved as a ready-made motor representation. This entails that an automated syllabic motor programme can only be acquired by practicing this very same syllable, while a training of any other, structurally related syllable would have no effect. For instance, [knast] (engl.: jail) is a low-frequency syllable (rank 6,100) which is probably not a part of the syllable lexicon, whereas one of its close neighbours, i.e., the syllable [nat], is among the top 250 syllables of German (rank 238) and must therefore be considered highly overlearned. However, even though the motor patterns of the two syllables are closely related, there are no theoretical grounds to assume that the phonetic encoding of [knast] might benefit from the many instances of articulating the syllable [nat]. By virtue of the holistic, amorphous nature of [nat], the syllable [knast] inherits not even the smallest portion of the motor skill embodied in its close relative. On the basis of these considerations it may be revealing to know how syllables are re-learned in AOS. Consider an apraxic patient who has lost the ability of producing the syllable [knast]. If, in speech therapy, the phonetic plan for this syllable is to be re-constructed through motor learning, the learning theory implicit to the holistic syllable concept would predict that improvement can only be achieved by practicing [knast], whereas exercises based on structurally related syllables such as [nas], [kas], [nat], etc. would have no direct effect unless some other learning mechanism is postulated.

This prediction was tested in a recent study by Aichert and Ziegler (2008). Four patients with mild to moderate apraxic impairment underwent a massed practice treatment of 24 monosyllabic target words. Each syllable contained a consonant cluster both in the onset and the coda, with two or three consonants per cluster. Word frequency and syllable frequency were low. For each target syllable, a set of 15 training syllables was derived by deleting one or two consonants in the onset or coda clusters, which resulted in less complex, although formally related training syllables. Figure 1.2 contains a selection of training syllables for the target syllable [knast].

The training was based on a massed practicing of the 15 training cognates of a target syllable within a short training block. The target syllable itself was not included in the training trials. Immediate transfer effects were measured by presenting, before and after each training block, the respective target word for auditory repetition.

In this experiment, error rates on the transfer syllables decreased from more than 50% pre-training to 27% post-training. Two of the patients also showed a significant, training-related increase in speaking rate, as measured by target word durations. Specific improvements of the transfer syllables could still be demonstrated in a delayed administration of all target syllables at the end of a training session (Aichert and Ziegler 2008). The outcome of this experiment has meanwhile been confirmed in another four apraxic patients (Aichert 2008). Furthermore, in a follow-up experiment we were able to demonstrate that the transfer effect between syllables is position-true, i.e., that a transfer can for instance not be achieved between onset consonants in the trained syllables and coda consonants in the target syllables, or vice-versa (Schoor et al. in preparation).

By conclusion, these data demonstrate that apraxic speakers are able to re-construct the motor pattern of a complex syllable by practicing syllables which are made-up of substructures of the

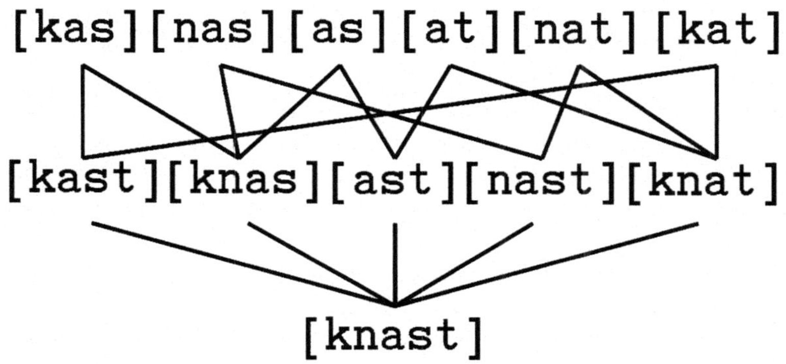

Fig. 1.2 Learning the complex syllable [knast] from its less complex parts. Massed practice training of the syllables in the upper two rows leads to an improvement of the target syllable in the bottom row (Aichert and Ziegler 2008).

target syllable's skeleton. This suggests that speech motor learning does not necessarily require practice of always exactly the same speech fragment. In contrast, practice-effects appear to spread from one syllabic pattern to other, structurally related patterns.

1.4 **Linear string models of phonetic encoding**

The preceding sections were related to theories based on the assumption that phonetic plans consist of 'primitives' prescribing the movements of the speech muscles for some circumscribed fragment of an utterance, e.g., a phoneme or a syllable. If an utterance consists of several such fragments, several phonetic plans have to be accessed in a row and transformed into speech movements. The unfolding of the gestural scores encapsulated in each single phonetic plan is part of a motor implementation process downstream the phonetic encoder (Levelt et al., 1999). Moreover, in theories strictly based on isolated encoding units, the linking of the movements triggered by each single phonetic plan and their integration into a smooth stream is also not an integral part of the phonetic encoding component.[4] In this sense, phonetic plans for words are linear strings of phonetic plans for sub-lexical units.

Such a theory entails strong predictions regarding the error rates in conditions where the phonetic encoder fails, i.e., in AOS. Apraxic impairment would cause a disruption of the access to or the integrity of phonetic plans in a certain proportion of cases, depending on the degree of severity of a patient's impairment. In mild cases the rate of failure may amount to only a small percentage of the phonetic encoding units of an utterance, whereas in severe cases almost every unit may be affected by the apraxic patho-mechanism. The number of distorted units (phonemes, syllables, or other primitives) in a given utterance and a given speaker will then depend only on the total number of such units and the severity of the speaker's impairment. It will, in particular, not depend on the internal properties of these units (e.g., if a syllable is simple or complex), since phonetic plans are considered holistic, and it will also not depend on how the phonetic units combine to larger linguistic units (e.g., syllables to metrical feet) as long as these mechanisms are not considered part of the phonetic encoding process. Figure 1.3 illustrates the proportionate error assumption for the example of a strictly phoneme-based linear model.

In a recent study we formally tested this assumption in ten patients with AOS (Ziegler et al., 2008). The patients were examined in a word repetition test based on 72 words and nonwords of different lengths and complexities, with syllable numbers varying from one to four and phoneme numbers from two to 14, including syllables with high and low complexities, and words with different metrical patterns (cf. Liepold et al., 2003).

Five 'error source models' were tested, differing in their assumptions on which phonological unit constitutes the core unit of phonetic encoding: (i) the phoneme, (ii) the syllable constituent (i.e., onset, nucleus, and coda), (iii) the syllable, (iv) the metrical foot, or (v) the word. For each of these models, a proportionate error score was computed for each of the 72 words and each of the 10 patients. As an example, if a patient made 4 phoneme errors in a word consisting of 12 phonemes, as illustrated in Fig. 1.3, the proportionate error score of this word in the phoneme-model was .33. Or, if a patient made an error on 1 of 2 syllables of a word, the respective error score in the syllable-model was .5.

For further calculations, the error scores of the 10 patients were averaged for every word, and since the materials consisted of 36 pairs of structurally equivalent words and nonwords, the error scores of the 2 cognates of a word–nonword pair were also averaged. As a result, each of

[4] In a short side note, Levelt et al. (1999, p. 5) acknowledge that mechanisms of 'phonetic composition' might also exist at the level of phonetic encoding, but this idea is not elaborated any further in their theory.

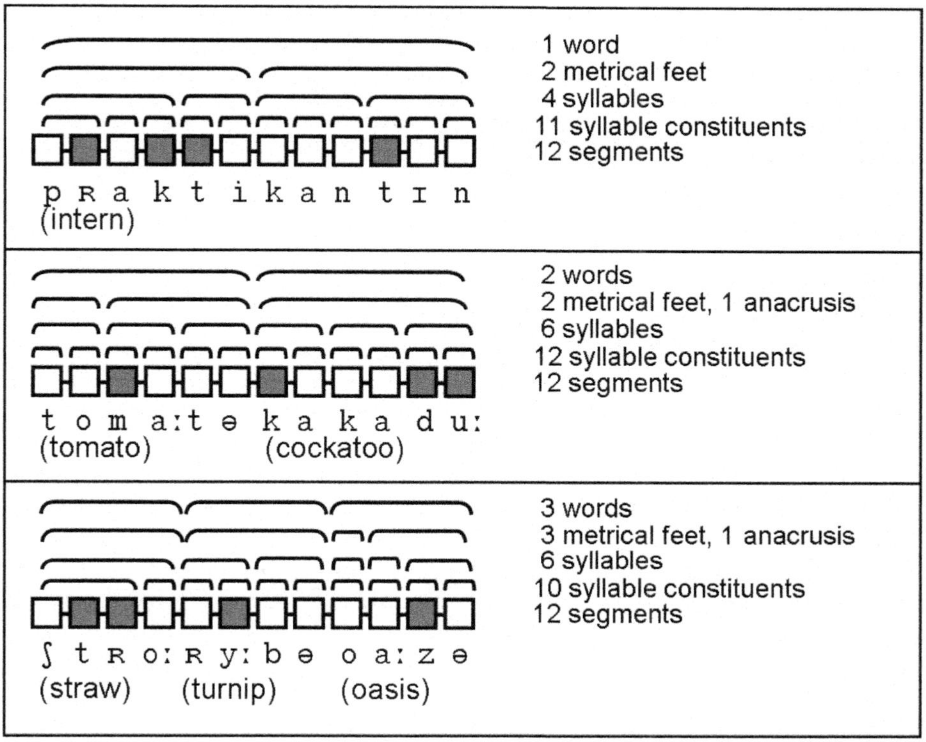

Fig. 1.3 Proportionate error model (segment-type). The model is based on the assumption that segments are the core units of phonetic encoding and that words are linear strings of segments. Impaired phonetic encoding then leads to distortions of a fixed proportion of the phonemes of an utterance, depending only on the severity of impairment. Three speech samples are presented with 12 segments each (squares), but with different metrical structures (indicated by horizontal brackets). The hypothetical case of an apraxic patient is illustrated, who fails on every third encoding unit, on the average (grey squares). The proportionate error model predicts that error rate is independent of other structural factors characterizing the three speech samples (cf. Ziegler et al., 2008).

36 structurally different items was characterized by an average proportionate error score for each of 5 different error count models (for details cf. Ziegler et al., 2008).

On the assumption that apraxic error rates are proportionate to the number of encoding units, the prediction was now that the most appropriate error source model would yield relative error rates which are evenly distributed over the 36 different phonological templates. More specifically, the error counts of the appropriate model should not systematically be influenced by other structural properties of the test words. If, as an example, a purely syllable-based phonetic encoding mechanism was postulated, syllable-based error counts should not depend on the metrical properties of a word or on the average number of phonemes or constituents in the syllables of a word.

This prediction was tested for each of the five models by a linear regression analysis, with the respective error score as dependent variable and four mutually independent form factors as regressors: (1) the average number of phonemes per syllable constituent (a measure of the occurrence of consonant clusters), (2) the average number of syllable constituents per syllable (a measure of the occurrence of onsets and codas in the syllables of a word), (3) the average number of syllables in a metrical foot (a measure of the complexity of metrical feet), and (4) the number of feet (including degenerate feet) in a word (a measure of the metrical complexity of a word).

Table 1.1 Results of multiple linear regression analyses for five different error source models (columns). In each cell of a column, '+' or '–' indicate whether or not the corresponding structural factor (rows) had a significant influence on error counts ($p < .05$; cf. Ziegler et al., 2008)

Error source Regressor	PHO*	ONC*	SYL*	MFT*	WRD*
Metrical feet per word	+	+	+	–	+
Syllables per metrical foot	–	–	–	+	+
Constituents per syllable	–	–	–	+	+
Segments per constituent	–	+	+	+	+

* *Errors counted by:* PHO – phonemes, ONC – syllable constituents (onset, nucleus, coda) SYL – syllables, MFT – metrical feet, WRD – whole words. For explanations see text.

As a major result of this study, the prediction of an even distribution of relative error scores across words of different phonological structures could not be verified for any of the five error source models. It turned out, for example, that the relative number of phoneme errors was higher in monosyllabic as compared to disyllabic (trochaic) words. Hence, if a given number of phonemes distributes over two syllables (e.g., five phonemes in [blu:mə], engl. *flower*), the number of phoneme errors is smaller than when the same number of phonemes crowds in a monosyllabic word (e.g., in [knɛçt], engl. *farm labourer*). On the contrary, the proportion of distorted phonemes increased significantly in words comprising more than one foot (like ['pʀaktɪ'kantɪn][6] or [to'ma:tə])[5] relative to words comprising only a single metrical foot (e.g. ['ʀy:bə][6] or ['kakadu:][6]).

Similar influences were seen in the regression analyses of all of the five error source models. Table 1.1 contains an overview of the factors which had a significant influence on the different error counts.

The matrix in Table 1.1 illustrates that error counts based on large units, such as whole words or metrical feet, were influenced by properties characterizing the finer grains of phonological structure, whereas models assuming small primitives of phonetic encoding, i.e., segments, revealed influences from higher structural levels. In models postulating phonetic primitives in-between these extremes, e.g., in the syllable model, influences from both lower and higher levels were seen (Ziegler et al., 2008).

On the whole, these results suggest that the proportionate error assumption, which is based on the idea that speech motor programmes are linear strings of phonetic primitives, cannot easily be maintained. One might add that the patterns of influencing factors seen in Fig. 1.3 and in Table 1.1 also cannot be explained on the assumption that phonetic plans for words are made-up from a mixture of syllabic and segmental plans. Alternatively, phonetic plans might be conceived of as being organized in a hierarchical fashion, with motor routines for small, local fragments of spoken utterances being embedded, in a stepwise fashion, into routines for successively larger sections. Such a view, however, cannot easily be reconciled with the concept of a mental store where ready-made speech motor programmes for phonetic primitives, like phonemes or syllables, are retrieved.

1.5 A non-linear architecture of phonetic plans for words

The idea that phonetic plans integrate motor information from several levels of phonological structure has recently been cast in a non-linear model of word production in AOS (Ziegler 2005;

[5] For the words mentioned as examples in this paragraph see Fig. 1.3.

2009). In this model, a recursion of probabilistic relationships between successive phonological tiers was used to predict the accuracy of apraxic word production.

1.5.1 **Probabilities of local accuracy**

The model is based on the consideration that a fragment U of an utterance, which consists of two smaller fragments, u1 and u2, is accurate if and only if each of the two sub-units is produced accurately. If u1 and u2 are independent phonetic primitives, comparable to the units of the model sketched in Fig. 1.3, the probability p(U) of U being accurate can be computed as

$$p(U) = p(u1) * p(u2), \tag{1}$$

where p(u1) and p(u2) denote the probabilities of u1 and u2 being accurate.

Following the segmental encoding hypothesis sketched above, for instance, an apraxic patient's speech problem may amount to making an error on every fourth phonetic encoding unit, i.e., she/he would be accurate on three of four phonemes, on the average. This patient's probability of being accurate on a two-phoneme word, such as [ku:] (engl.: cow), would then be

$$p([ku:]) = p([k]) * p([u:]) = 0.75 * 0.75 = 0.56. \tag{2}$$

If, however, construction of a phonetic plan for [ku:] implies more than only two independent encoding steps, since, for instance, the two phonemes must be glued together by some phonetic composition process (coarticulation), the probability that [ku:] is produced without an error would be lower than .56, because the composition process itself is an additional source of potential failure. An alternative possibility is that construction of a phonetic plan for [ku:] is less expensive than 0.56. This may occur, for instance, when [k] and [u:] need not be encoded as entirely independent primitives, but are integrated into some overarching (e.g. syllabic) motor routine. These two opposing alternatives can be modelled by introducing, in equation (2), a constant factor c, yielding

$$p([ku:]) = p([k]) * p([u:]) * c = 0.56 * c. \tag{3}$$

The value of c, if it can be determined, allows us to decide between the alternative hypotheses mentioned above: if the segmental encoding hypothesis is valid, c will turn out to be close to 1. If additional phonetic processing is required to combine two phoneme plans, c will assume a value < 1. If, as a third alternative, phonemes are integrated into larger phonetic representations, c will assume a value > 1.

Similar considerations can also be made for units other than the phoneme, e.g., for syllables and the composition of two syllables to a metrical foot, or for articulatory gestures and their combinations. Equation (1) above can therefore be generalized to

$$p(U) = p(u1) * p(u2) * c, \tag{4}$$

to describe the probability of accurate production of a complex unit U as a function of the probabilities that its sub-units u1 and u2 are accurate.

1.5.2 **A hierarchy of stepwise phonetic integration**

The method sketched in the preceding section can be applied recursively within a hierarchy of increasingly complex phonological structures. In Ziegler (2005), a model of word production accuracy was proposed which was based on such a hierarchic embedding, taking phonemes as a starting point. An extension of this model to phonetic gestures as the basic modelling tier was presented more recently (Ziegler, 2009).

This model, which is illustrated in Fig. 1.4, assumes that inaccuracy in AOS may start at a gestural level. Taking loans from *feature geometry* (Clements 1985), three gestural tiers were distinguished, i.e., oral gestures (including lip, tongue-tip, and tongue-back gestures), velar gestures (velar raising or lowering), and glottal gestures (glottal opening or closing). Gestures were defined as the transitions between the phonetic features of two adjacent phonemes. For instance, the transition from a voiceless to a voiced segment involves a glottal (closing) gesture, the transition from a tongue-tip fricative to a tongue-tip plosive involves a tongue-tip gesture etc.

To simplify matters it was postulated that the probability that a gesture is performed accurately is the same for all of these gestures. When a word is spoken, a series of gestures has to be planned, and the probability of accurate production of the whole word is a function of the probabilities of all gestures being accurate, as exemplified in equation (4) of the preceding paragraph. Since these gestures are considered part of a tree-like hierarchy of motor integration, their combination to increasingly complex patterns implies modifications of their expected accuracy by multiplicative factors. At the bottom end of the hierarchy, to begin with, two gestures can be combined to a coalition of two synchronous (e.g. oral and glottal) gestures. Further-on, such combinations of gestures may connect two segments within a syllable constituent to form a consonant cluster,

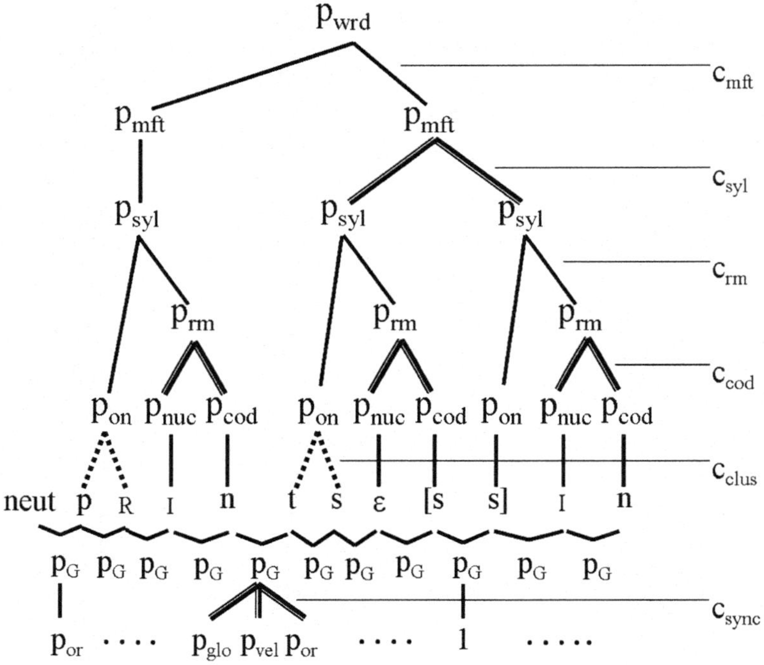

Fig. 1.4 Non-linear model of phonetic encoding of the word *Prinzessin* (engl. *princess*). The *p*-variables on each tier represent probabilities of accurate production of the units corresponding to the respective nodes. The c-variables on the right represent weighting coefficients correcting for an increase or a decrease of the likelihood of accurate production relative to a purely combinatorial function of sub-ordinate probabilities. Double lines indicate particularly strong, dotted lines particularly weak connectivities (Ziegler 2005; 2009).

Note or: oral gesture; glo: glottal gesture; vel: velar gesture; G: combined gesture; on: onset; nuc: nucleus; cod: coda; rm: rime; syl: syllable; mft: metrical foot; neut: neutral speech onset configuration; sync: synchronization; clus: cluster formation.

link a coda-constituent to a syllable nucleus to form a rime, glue a rime to an onset constituent to form a syllable, connect two syllables to generate a metrical foot, and combine a metrical foot with another foot or with an unparsed syllable to form a word (see Fig. 1.4 for an example). On each of these steps, a new factor is introduced in the model which modifies the probability of accuracy of the respective node as a function of the probabilities of its subjacent units, according to the relationship described by equation (4).

On the whole, a model results which predicts the probability of a word to be produced accurately by a multiplicative term, including a base variable representing the probability of gestural accuracy and six coefficients weighting the stepwise combination of gestures to words. For more details describing this approach see Ziegler (2005) and Ziegler (2009).

1.5.3 Testing the model with data from apraxic speakers

The model sketched above was tested empirically with data from a word repetition test (Liepold et al., 2003). Since this test has been used for clinical purposes over a period of many years, a substantial data base including a total of 120 test administrations to apraxic patients was available. From the test materials, a selection of 72 items was chosen which covered a broad range of word lengths (one to four syllables) and syllable structures. Each word was described by a metrical tree structure, similar to the example of Fig. 1.4. Furthermore, an estimate of the likelihood of each word to be accurate was derived from the empirical data set by calculating the proportion of patients in the sample who had produced the word without an error. In the case of the word *prinzessin* (engl. *princess*) depicted in Fig. 1.4, 38 out of 120 trials were correct, hence the estimate for p_{wrd} in this case was 38/120 = 0.317. Overall, a vector of 72 such probabilities was to be predicted, in a non-linear multiple regression analysis, by seven regression variables, i.e., by a probability value for accurate gestures (the *p*-values at the basis of the tree structure of Fig. 1.4) and six correction parameters (the c-values in the right column of Fig. 1.4).[6]

The non-linear regression model accounted for more than 84% of the variability in the 72 accuracy scores, suggesting that accuracy of apraxic word production is to a large extent influenced by only the structural factors depicted in Fig. 1.4. The resulting likelihood of a single gesture to be correct was .89. A major question asked in the modelling trial was if the c-coefficients on each of the structural layers would signal particularly strong or particularly weak bonds within the phonetic architecture of a word. Particularly strong bonds were found between the syllables of a metrical foot ($c_{syl} > 1$ in Fig. 1.4), suggesting that the combination of two syllables to a trochaic foot causes significantly lower phonetic planning costs than one would predict on purely combinatorial grounds. This was consistent with the findings obtained in the linear modelling approaches described in an earlier section of this chapter. Furthermore, low phonetic planning demands were also revealed at the point where a coda constituent is attached to a vocalic nucleus, i.e., in rime formation (Ziegler, 2005). Particularly weak connectivities, on the contrary, were found between the consonants of onset- or coda clusters ($c_{clus} < 1$ in Fig. 1.4). At this point in the model, the likelihood of accurate production was significantly decreased relative to other locations in the tree structure of a word. This is consistent with what was said earlier in this chapter regarding the influence of syllable complexity on accuracy in AOS.

One of the unexpected results of the study reviewed here was that the synchronous production of two gestures was boosted by a facilitating coefficient ($c_{sync} > 1$ in Fig. 1.4). On the basis of earlier findings indicating coarticulation problems in apraxic speakers (e.g. Ziegler and von

[6] Since the materials used in this analysis consisted of words and nonwords, a further regressor was introduced to account for lexicality. This aspect will not be described in any further detail here.

Cramon 1985) we had expected to obtain the opposite, i.e., a decrease in accuracy when two gestures have to be performed in synchrony. A rather straightforward explanation of this unexpected finding may be that many of the instances in which gestural synchrony played a role in the test materials were highly predictable. For instance, co-occurrence of velar lowering with glottal adduction is obligatory in German, since nasal consonants are always voiced. Furthermore, since vowels are always voiced, the glottal gestures left or right to the nucleus of a syllable are highly predictable. Another obligatory pattern in German phonology is that obstruents in the coda position are always voiceless. Hence, the fact that the gestural synchrony coefficient c_{sync} assumed a value >1 may simply reflect the fact that synchrony in the examples mentioned above is a highly overlearned pattern, which, as a motor-synergy, may resist the phonetic disintegration processes underlying AOS. As a matter of fact, voiced final obstruents, voiceless vowels, or voiceless nasal consonants are rarely, if ever, encountered in apraxic speech (cf. Ziegler, 2009).

The model discussed here starts at a level of abstract phonetic gestures, such as lip closing, velar lowering, glottal opening, and so on. These units by themselves represent rather complex motor events, i.e., patterned activities of distributed ensembles of speech muscles. In the case of lip closure, for instance, muscles of the upper and lower lip interact with mandibular muscles to achieve the motor goal of bilabial closure (Gracco and Abbs 1985). This basic level of speech motor organization was beyond the scope of the auditory-based approach considered here. Yet, speech motor planning in apraxic speakers may go astray already at such an early level of speech motor organization, preventing patients from achieving even the basic articulatory goals at the bottom-end of the model depicted in Fig. 1.4. This may be the case in patients with more severe apraxic impairment and may even lead to complete muteness. In less severe cases, apraxic impairment interferes with how these gestures are assembled to increasingly complex patterns. The sites of fracture in this disintegration process are not arbitrary, but are rather determined by the connection strengths within a word's phonetic skeleton.

1.6 **Conclusion**

In this chapter we have reviewed recent studies of error production in AOS, claiming that the results of these studies inform us about the construction of phonetic plans for speaking. Phonetic or phonological impairments in patients with brain lesions have the property of cracking spoken words and phrases into smaller pieces, which provides compelling evidence against the view that spoken language is entirely formulaic, i.e., composed of indivisible fragments (words, phrases) representing meaningful concepts. It suggests that articulate language is *constructed* through some generative process by which smaller units are combined to form a potentially infinite number of spoken words or phrases. At the level of speech movement planning, the theory proposed by Levelt et al. (1999) postulates that *syllables* are the major building blocks of such a re-combination process. The studies reviewed in the first part of this chapter are largely consistent with this view, and they also contradict the assumption that the motor programmes of apraxic speakers are disintegrated to the level of phonemes. Nonetheless, syllabic motor plans seem to be less opaque and holistic than psycholinguistic theory postulates. In the second part of this chapter we have reviewed evidence that syllables need not be learned *holistically* – they can also be learned from their parts. This suggests that speech motor primitives, if they exist, may emanate from a variegated learning process. As a consequence, when they are transformed into fully learned motor routines they may still treasure the footprints of their learning process and, in this sense, not be holistic.

On the basis of such considerations, the last two sections of this chapter presented modelling accounts of the error patterns in patients with AOS. We first demonstrated that the phonetic plans of spoken words cannot be conceived of as linear strings of phonetic primitives, and then introduced a non-linear model of phonetic encoding, in which the accuracy of word production in AOS was predicted by recursive computations of the likelihood of accurate production of increasingly larger units. This model successfully predicted empirical data from a large number of apraxic speakers. The shape of the resulting model suggests that phonetic plans for words are hierarchical structures, in which certain connectivities, e.g., between the phonemes of a syllabic rime or between the syllables of a metrical foot, are particularly strong, whereas others, for instance the bonds between the consonants of a syllable cluster, are weaker (Fig. 1.4).

Non-linear architectures of this kind differ from phoneme- or syllable-based theories of phonetic encoding in several ways. The major difference is that the non-linear model proposed here dispenses with the notion of a store of ready-made building blocks emerging from massed motor practice. What we learn during the long period of speech acquisition may rather be characterized as some implicit knowledge of how we can orchestrate our vocal tract muscles to produce the sound patterns that characterize our native language. This knowledge extends from very basic muscular synergisms to the prosodic structures at the level of metrical feet. New words or new syllables pose no problem to this system, as long as they correspond to the sound pattern of a speaker's language. The effect of frequency of occurrence, in this view, is not confined to crystallized units like the syllable [di:]. It rather spreads over all tiers of a hierarchical motor organization, from gestures to metrical feet, and characterizes structural relationships rather than ready-made particles.

How can such a view be reconciled with the syllable frequency effect found in normal and apraxic speech? The assumption that phonetic plans are hierarchically nested structures still leaves the option that particularly frequent patterns of co-occurring gestures crystallize to highly integrated nodes, e.g., syllabic rimes, whole syllables, or even larger formulaic patterns. The fact that these units can be retrieved faster and more securely than others need not be explained by a lexical-store account. It may simply reflect the principle that frequent repetitions of exactly the same gestural pattern may create particularly strong connections in the structural representation of a phonetic plan. A major advantage of non-linear, hierarchical phonetic representations for the understanding of such effects is that they circumvent the problem of a still unknown number of different encoding units (syllables, phonemes, etc.), and that they also avoid the untractable difficulty of telling, for any given unit, whether or not it is part of a supposed lexicon of motor programmes. Moreover, structural models as the one proposed here offer a parsimonious explanation of observations of incomplete deconstruction or gradual re-construction of phonetic plans in apraxic speakers.

As a conclusion, we are left with a dichotomy between two opposing accounts of phonetic encoding: one based on ready-made motor primitives that are retrieved from a mental store, the other based on hierarchical structures representing implicit knowledge of how articulate language is constructed, from the gestural to the metrical level. Investigations of speech production in healthy speakers are needed to supplement the evidence presented here and decide between the two theoretical accounts.

Acknowledgment

The studies reviewed in this chapter were supported by DFG-grants Zi 469 4-1 / 4-2 / 6-1 / 6-2 / 8-1 / 8-2 / 9-1 / 10-1.

References

Aichert, I. (2008). *Die Bausteine der phonetischen Enkodierung: Untersuchungen zum sprechmotorischen Lernen bei Sprechapraxie.* Lübeck: Der Andere Verlag.

Aichert, I., Marquardt, Ch. & Ziegler, W. (2005). Frequenzen sublexikalischer Einheiten des Deutschen: CELEX-basierte Datenbanken. *Neurolinguistik, 19*, 5–31.

Aichert, I. & Ziegler, W. (2004). Syllable frequency and syllable structure in apraxia of speech. *Brain and Language, 88*, 148–59.

—— (2008). Learning a syllable from its parts: Cross-syllabic generalisation effects in patients with apraxia of speech. *Aphasiology*, 22, 1216–29.

Baayen, R. H., Piepenbrock, R., & Gulikers, L. (1995). *The CELEX lexical database (CD-ROM).* Linguistic Data Consortium, University of Pennsylvania, PA, Philadelphia.

Brendel, B. & Ziegler, W. (2008). Effectiveness of metrical pacing in the treatment of apraxia of speech. *Aphasiology, 22*, 77–102.

Carreiras, M. & Perea, M. (2004). Naming pseudowords in Spanish: Effects of syllable frequency. *Brain and Language, 90*, 393–400.

Cholin, J. (2008). The mental syllabary in speech production: An integration of different approaches and domains. *Aphasiology, 22*, 1127–41.

Cholin, J., Levelt, W. J., & Schiller, N. O. (2006). Effects of syllable frequency in speech production. *Cognition, 99*, 205–35.

Cholin, J., Schiller, N. O., & Levelt, W. J. M. (2005). The preparation of syllables in speech production. *Journal of Memory and Language, 50*, 47–61.

Clements, G. N. (1985). The geometry of phonological features. *Phonology Yearbook, 2*, 225–52.

Dabul, B. & Bollier, B. (1976). Therapeutic approaches to apraxia. *Journal of Speech and Hearing Disorders, 41*, 268–76.

Darley, F. L. (1968). Apraxia of speech: 107 years of terminological confusion. *Paper presented at the Annual Convention of the ASHA.*

Gracco, V. L. & Abbs, J. H. (1985). Dynamic control of the perioral system during speech: Kinematic analyses of autogenic and nonautogenic sensorimotor processes. *Journal of Neurophysiology, 54*, 418–32.

Jaeger, M. & Ziegler, W. (1993). Der metrische Übungsansatz in der Sprechapraxiebehandlung: Ein Fallbericht. *Neurolinguistik, 7*, 31–41.

Kent, R. D. & Rosenbek, J. C. (1983). Acoustic patterns of apraxia of speech. *Journal of Speech and Hearing Research, 26*, 231–49.

Laganaro, M. (2005). Syllable frequency effect in speech production: Evidence from aphasia. *Journal of Neurolinguistics, 18*, 221–35.

—— (2008). Is there a syllable frequency effect in aphasia or in apraxia of speech or both? *Aphasiology, 22*, 1191–200.

Laganaro, M. & Alario, F. X. (2006). On the locus of syllable frequency effect. *Journal of Memory and Language*, 55, 178–96.

Levelt, W. J. M. (2001). Spoken word production: A theory of lexical access. *Proceedings of the National Academy of Sciences of the USA, 98*, 13464–71.

Levelt, W. J. M., Roelofs, A., & Meyer, A. S. (1999). A theory of lexical access in speech production. *Behavioral and Brain Sciences, 22*, 1–38.

Levelt, W. J. M. & Wheeldon, L. R. (1994). Do speakers have access to a mental syllabary? *Cognition, 50*, 239–69.

Liepold, M., Ziegler, W., & Brendel, B. (2003). Hierarchische Wortlisten. Ein Nachsprechtest für die Sprechapraxiediagnostik. Dortmund, Borgmann.

Maassen, B., Nijland, L., & Van der Meulen, S. (2001). Coarticulation within and between syllables by children with developmental apraxia of speech. *Clinical Linguistics and Phonetics, 15*, 145–50.

McNeil, M. R., Robin, D. A., & Schmidt, R. A. (1997). Apraxia of speech: Definition, differentiation, and treatment. In M. R. McNeil (ed.), *Clinical Management of Sensorimotor Speech Disorders* (pp. 311–44). New York – Stuttgart: Thieme.

Mehl, M.R., Vazire, S., Ramírez-Esparza, N., Slatcher, R.B., & Pennebaker, J. W. (2007). Are women really more talkative than men? *Science, 317*, 82.

Nickels, L. & Howard, D. (2004). Dissociating effects of number of phonemes, number of syllables, and syllabic complexity on word production in aphasia: It's the number of phonemes that counts. *Cognitive Neuropsychology, 21*, 57–78.

Odell, K. H. (2002). Considerations in target selection in apraxia of speech treatment. *Seminars in Speech and Language*, 23, 309–24.

Romani, C. & Calabrese, A. (1998). Syllabic constraints in the phonological errors of an aphasic patient. *Brain and Language, 64*, 83–121.

Romani, C. & Galluzzi, C. (2005). Effects of syllabic complexity in predicting accuracy of repetition and direction of errors in patients with articulatory and phonological difficulties. *Cognitive Neuropsychology, 22*, 817–50.

Rosenbek, J. C. (1985). Treating apraxia of speech. In D. F.Johns (ed.), *Clinical Management of Neurogenic Communicative Disorders* (pp. 267–312). Boston: Little, Brown & Co.

Rosenbek, J. C., Kent, R. D., & Lapointe, L. L. (1984). Apraxia of speech: An overview and some perspectives. In J. C. Rosenbek, M. R. McNeil, & A. E. Aronson (eds), *Apraxia of Speech: Physiology, Acoustics, Linguistics, Management* (pp. 1–72). San Diego: College-Hill Press.

Schoor, A., Aichert, I., & Ziegler, W. (in preparation). Learning syllables in apraxia of speech: Are there systematic subsyllabic transfer effects?

Staiger, A. (2008). *Frequenz und Struktur sublexikalischer Einheiten in der Spontansprachebei Sprechapraxie.* Doctoral Dissertation. LMU München.

Staiger, A. & Ziegler, W. (2008). Syllable frequency and syllable structure in the spontaneous speech production of patients with apraxia of speech. *Aphasiology, 22*, 1201–15.

Stenneken, P., Bastiaanse, R., Huber, W., & Jacobs, A. M. (2005). Syllable structure and sonority in language inventory and aphasic neologisms. *Brain and Language, 95*, 221–22.

Stenneken, P., Hofmann, M., & Jacobs, A. M. (2008). Sublexical units in aphasic jargon and in the standard language. Comparative analyses of neologisms in connected speech. *Aphasiology, 22*, 1142–56.

Varley, R. & Whiteside, S. P. (2001). What is the underlying impairment in acquired apraxia of speech? *Aphasiology, 15*, 39–49.

Wambaugh, J. L. (2002). A summary of treatments for apraxia of speech and review of replicated approaches. *Seminars in Speech and Language, 23*, 293–308.

Wambaugh, J. L., Doyle, P. J., Kalinyak-Fliszar, M. M., & West, J. E. (1996). A minimal contrast treatment for apraxia of speech. *Clinical Aphasiology, 24*, 97–108.

Wilshire, C. E. & Nespoulous, J. -L. (2003). Syllables as units in speech production: Data from aphasia. *Brain and Language, 84*, 424–47.

Ziegler, W. (2005). A nonlinear model of word length effects in apraxia of speech. *Cognitive Neuropsychology, 22*, 603–23.

—— (2008). Apraxia of speech. In G. Goldenberg & B. Miller (eds), *Handbook of Clinical Neurology* (pp. 269–85). London: Elsevier.

—— (2009). Modelling the architecture of phonetic plans: Evidence from apraxia of speech. *Language and Cognitive Processes, 24*, 631–61.

Ziegler, W. & Cramon, D. Y. v. (1985). Anticipatory coarticulation in a patient with apraxia of speech. *Brain and Language, 26*, 117–30.

Ziegler, W. & Jaeger, M. (1993). Aufgabenhierarchien in der Sprechapraxie-Therapie und der 'metrische' Übungsansatz. *Neurolinguistik, 7*, 17–29.

Ziegler, W., Thelen, A. K., Staiger, A., & Liepold, M. (2008). The domain of phonetic encoding in apraxia of speech: Which sub-lexical units count? *Aphasiology, 22*, 1230–47.

Chapter 2

Phonemic, sensory, and motor representations in an action-based neurocomputational model of speech production

Bernd J. Kröger, Peter Birkholz, Anja Lowit, and Christiane Neuschaefer-Rube

Abstract

Neural models of speech production are highly valuable for our understanding of normal as well as of disordered speech production processes. However, only few quantitative neural models of speech production are available. This paper introduces an action-based neurocomputational model of speech production (called ACT) comprising a high-quality articulatory-acoustic speech synthesizer as a front-end module. Some basic features of ACT are (i) the use of sensory information in motor control of speech production including feed-forward and feedback processing, (ii) a separation of motor planning and motor execution, which can be attained from using the concept of ACTion (concept of vocal tract action units or articulatory gestures), and (iii) the inclusion of principles of self-organization for the buildup of neural mappings for speech production during speech acquisition. The organization of ACT including sensory (i.e., somatosensory and auditory), motor, phonetic, and phonemic neural representations and the gathering of knowledge during learning or training stages of speech acquisition is described in this paper. Currently ACT is capable of producing speech items of a 'model language' comprising a set of 65 CV- and CCV-syllables where C stands for voiced or voiceless plosives, nasals, or the apical lateral.

2.1 Introduction

Neural models of speech production describe (i) the *neurolinguistic processes* from conceptualization to phonological encoding and (ii) the *neurophonetic processes*, i.e., phonetic encoding, sensorimotor control, and the articulatory-acoustic realization of speech items. Within neurolinguistic models of speech production (e.g., Dell 1999; Levelt 1999), many neurophonetic aspects of speech production are not addressed in detail. A promising comprehensive quantitative neurophonetic model of speech production has been proposed by Guenther (Directions Into Velocities of Articulators [DIVA] model, see Guenther 2006; Guenther et al. 2006). In DIVA, feed-forward and feedback control is separated. *Feed-forward control* starts with the activation of a phonemic state within the speech sound map for a speech item (i.e., sound, syllable, word, or utterance), subsequently activating virtual motor commands at the level of the articulatory velocity and position map. These motor commands directly control an articulatory-acoustic model, which is capable of producing simulations of articulatory speech movements and acoustic speech signals. In DIVA, *feedback control* starts with the calculation of sensory (i.e., auditory and somatosensory) feedback signals on the basis of the articulatory-acoustic output of the articulatory-acoustic model. These sensory feedback signals are compared with stored sensory states for the speech item under production and in the case of noticeable differences between stored and current sensory signals appropriate error signals are calculated and corrective motor commands are issued to the articulators (Guenther et al. 2006).

The organization of the speech production model ACT introduced in this chapter is based on DIVA. However, it emphasizes three aspects: (i) The basic unit of sensorimotor control of speech articulation is the *vocal tract action unit* or *articulatory gesture* (Goldstein et al. 2006, 2007 Kröger et al. accepted). Consequently a planning and execution stage can be separated for vocal tract movements, leading to two motor representations: on the one hand a *primary motor representation* directly defines activations of functional groups of muscles for each time instant and directly controls the execution of articulation, and on the other hand a *motor plan representation* defines motor plans for speech items (here: speech sounds, syllables, words, or short utterances) by specifying vocal tract action scores or gestural scores (Goldstein et al. 2006; Kröger and Birkholz 2007) on the planning level of the model. (ii) The phonemic to motor state and the phonemic to sensory state mappings introduced in the DIVA model are implemented in our model by using *self-organizing maps* (Kohonen 2001). Thus the phonemic to motor as well as the phonemic to sensory mappings are implemented by including a self-organizing map as central neural layer of these mappings. This central neural layer is called *phonetic map* in our approach. (iii) Since the phonemic to motor state mapping including the phonetic map implies the storage of motor states for each speech item, this neural processing path is assumed to represent the processing of *frequent* speech items (cf. concept of mental syllablary, Levelt and Wheeldon 1994; Levelt et al. 1999). In addition, infrequent speech items can be generated in ACT by using an alternative neural pathway via a *motor planning module.*

2.2 Neural representations

ACT differentiates neural maps, neural mappings (also called neural associations), and neural processing modules. *Neural processing modules* (see boxes without black outline in Fig. 2.1) are complex units that themselves comprise maps and mappings that currently are not specified in detail. It is the task of processing modules to transform *neural states* or *neural activation patterns* of one neural representation into states or activation patterns of other neural representations. *Neural maps* (indicated by black outlined boxes in Fig. 2.1) are ensembles of (virtual) neurons coding phonemic, phonetic, sensory, or motor states of speech items. *Neural mappings* (indicated by arrows in Fig. 2.1) represent ensembles of synaptic links between neurons in different neural maps. Within these mappings each neuron of one map is connected with each neuron of the other map (Kröger et al. 2006a, 2006b). The degree of connectivity per link is called *link weight* or *synaptic weight* and ranges from fully excitatory connection (synaptic link weight value = 1) to fully inhibitory connection (synaptic link weight value = −1). Link weights or synaptic weights are adjusted during the learning or training stages, i.e., during the babbling and the imitation stage of speech acquisition in the current model. ACT comprises self-organizing maps and mappings and makes use of non-supervised learning (Kohonen 2001), which models early phases of speech acquisition, i.e., babbling and imitation training (see Section 2.2.3).

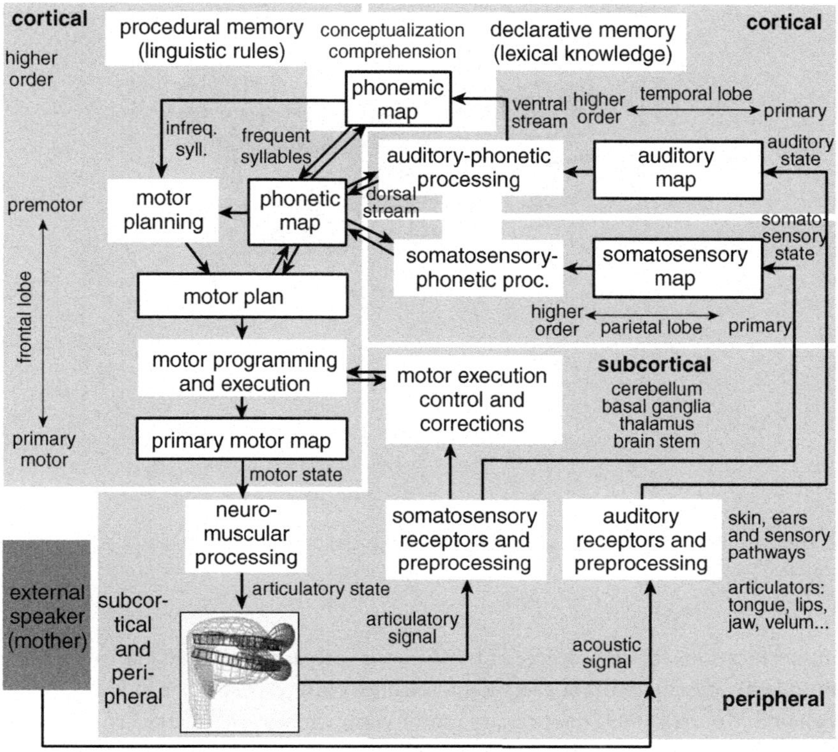

Fig. 2.1 Organization of the quantitative computer-implemented neural model of speech production. Boxes with black outline: neural maps; boxes without black outline: neural processing units comprising neural maps and mappings not specified in detail; arrows: neural mappings, associations, or projections. The associations of the phonemic map, sensory maps, and motor programme map via the phonetic map are bidirectional, leading to a multidirectional activation of phonemic, sensory, and motor plan states.

2.2.1 **Primary motor state representation and articulatory state representation**

The three-dimensional articulatory-acoustic vocal tract model VTM; Fig. 2.2, Birkholz et al. 2006; Birkholz and Kröger 2006, 2007) is controlled for each time instant by a set of *articulatory parameters*. These parameters define the location of articulators relative to other articulators, i.e. the location of lower lips relative to jaw, the location of tongue body relative to jaw, and the location of tongue tip relative to tongue body (Kröger et al. 2006b, 2006c). The set of model articulators in our three-dimensional VTM are lower jaw, tongue body, tongue tip, velum, lips, hyoid, and glottis. Hyoid position directly defines the vertical position of the larynx and the vertical and horizontal position of the tongue root. Phonatory parameters (i.e. arytenoid lateral position for controlling glottal aperture and lung volume for controlling subglottal pressure) are part of this set of articulatory parameters. While the position of velum and lower jaw are controlled by one parameter (one degree of freedom: vertical displacement), all other articulators are controlled by two parameters reflecting two degrees of freedom for displacement of the articulator relative to other articulators. The articulators are controlled in our model by a set of *primary motor parameters*. These primary motor parameters transform articulatory parameters into velocity and

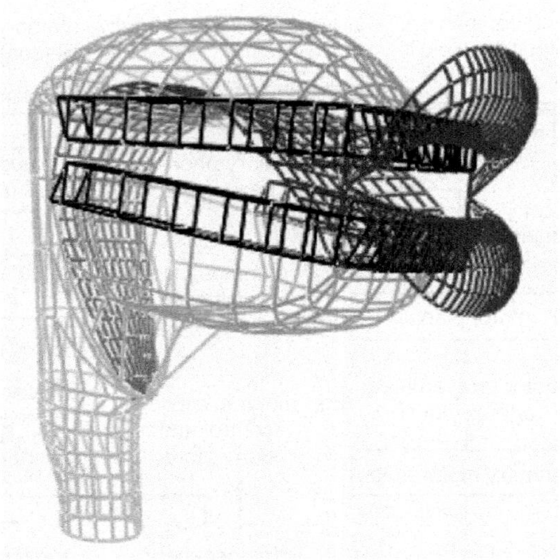

Fig. 2.2 The geometrical grid-representation of the three-dimensional articulatory-acoustic vocal tract model (VTM).

position specifications for each degree of freedom for each articulator by specifying a neural primary motor activation pattern for each point-in-time. With respect to the task dynamics concept (Saltzman and Munhall 1989) the primary motor parameters as well as the articulatory parameters are related to the task dynamics body articulator space while task-space specific parameters are represented at the motor plan level in ACT (see below).

2.2.2 Sensory state representations

Somatosensory information is gained from the articulator positions and from the contact areas quantified by the VTM. The somatosensory neural activation pattern (or somatosensory state) on the level of the *somatosensory map* (Fig. 2.1) represents the proprioceptive and tactile feedback state at the current point-in-time. A proprioceptive state is characterized by the specification of all proprioceptive model parameters, i.e., by the neural specification of the absolute position of all articulators with respect to the craniofacial reference system (i.e., with respect to the scull or hard palate, Kröger et al. 2006b). The absolute positioning of articulators is comparable to tract variable or task space information in terms of the task dynamics approach (Saltzman and Muhnall 1989) and can be calculated in our approach from the set of articulatory parameters for each point-in-time. A tactile state is characterized by the specification of a set of tactile model parameters, e.g., contact area of articulators (e.g., lips, tongue tip, tongue body) and contact area of vocal tract walls (e.g., alveolar ridge, hard palate, soft palate, Kröger et al. 2006a, 2006b). This contact area can be specified for each point-in-time directly within the VTM.

The auditory neural activation pattern is calculated from the acoustic transfer function of the VTM. The resulting frequency values of the first three formants F1, F2, and F3 are extracted from the transfer function by using a peak picking algorithm. The resulting formant values are bark-scaled and forwarded in steps of 10 ms towards the *auditory map* (Fig. 2.1).

The sensory (somatosensory and auditory) states represent the feedback sensation (or the auditory sensation of external speech signals) at the current point-in-time at the level of the somatosensory and auditory maps (Fig. 2.1). These point-in-time sensory states are then stored in a short-term memory in syllable-sized chunks at the level of the sensory-phonetic processing modules (Fig. 2.1). Thus point-in-time and period-in-time sensory states are differentiated in ACT.

2.2.3 **Phonemic state representation**

At the level of the *phonemic map* each neuron represents a phoneme (single sound neurons) or a frequent syllable (syllable neurons) of the *model language*, i.e., the language that is trained by ACT. The model language comprises 5 vowel phonemes (/i/, /e/, /a/, /o/, and /u/), 45 CV-syllables (with C = /b/, /d/, /g/, /p/, /t/, /k/, /m/, /n/, and /l/), and 20 CCV-syllables (with C1 = /b/, /g/, /p/, /k/ and C2 = /l/, i.e., with consonant clusters /bl/, /gl/, /pl/, and /kl/). Thus the model language comprises 65 phonemic representations for syllables in total. Two of these 65 syllables (i.e., /lo/ and /ble/) are defined to be infrequent in our model language and thus are not trained during the imitation training phase of speech acquisition. During the production of a speech item, the neural activation occurring within the phonemic map causes an activation of motor plans via the phonetic map for frequent syllables (neural pathway for frequent syllables). Thus, in the case of frequent syllables, the activation of a syllable neuron within the phonemic map initiates the activation of the corresponding motor plan. In the case of infrequent syllables, the activation pattern within the phonemic map (activation of one to three single sound neurons) leads to the co-activation of neurons within the phonetic map that represent phonetically similar syllables. For example, in the case of /le/, all neurons within the phonetic map that represent /lV/-syllables are activated. In addition the co-activation of gesture neurons within the gesture map (a co-activation that is initiated by the single sound neurons of the phonemic map) directly specifies the set of gestures that is needed for assembling the motor plan of the syllable on the level of the motor planning module. The detailed specification of inter-gestural timing is then gained from the motor plans of the phonetically similar syllables, which are activated at the level of the phonetic map (see arrow between phonetic map and motor planning module in Fig. 2.1).

2.2.4 **Motor plan state representation**

The motor plan state for each speech item needs (i) the specification of a set of vocalic, consonantal, velopharyngeal, and glottal vocal tract action units, assembling the speech item and (ii) the specification of all spatial and temporal characteristics for each action unit, i.e., end-articulator, target, gestural rapidity, duration of gesture, and inter-gestural temporal coordination (see Kröger and Birkholz 2007). ACT uses vocal tract action units in a bivalent way (i) as sensorimotor control units and (ii) as phonological units. Browman and Goldstein (1989, 1992) described gestures as phonological units and as units of dynamically defined control regimes. The concept of actions as sensorimotor control units is based on Bernstein (1967) and adapted for speech movements by Saltzman and Kelso (1983), Saltzman (1985), Kelso et al. (1986), and Saltzman and Munhall (1989). It is very important to note that the goal of actions in general is *functional* (Bernstein 1967). A functional goal in the case of speech gestures is to produce perceptual relevant distinct cues for discriminating and identifying phonological units. This elucidates the phonological character of vocal tract actions and is thus in agreement with Browman and Goldstein's notion of gestures. For a current characterization of vocal tract action units or articulatory gestures see also Goldstein et al. (2006, 2007).

The *motor plan map* is an ensemble of neurons that specifies the motor plan or vocal tract action score (also called gestural score) of a speech item. The *vocal tract action score* or *gestural score* not only specifies the set of vocal tract actions or gestures needed for the production of a speech item, but also specifies all *intra-gestural parameters* and the *parameters for inter-gestural temporal coordination* (*inter-gestural timing parameters*). A vocal tract action or gesture defines a

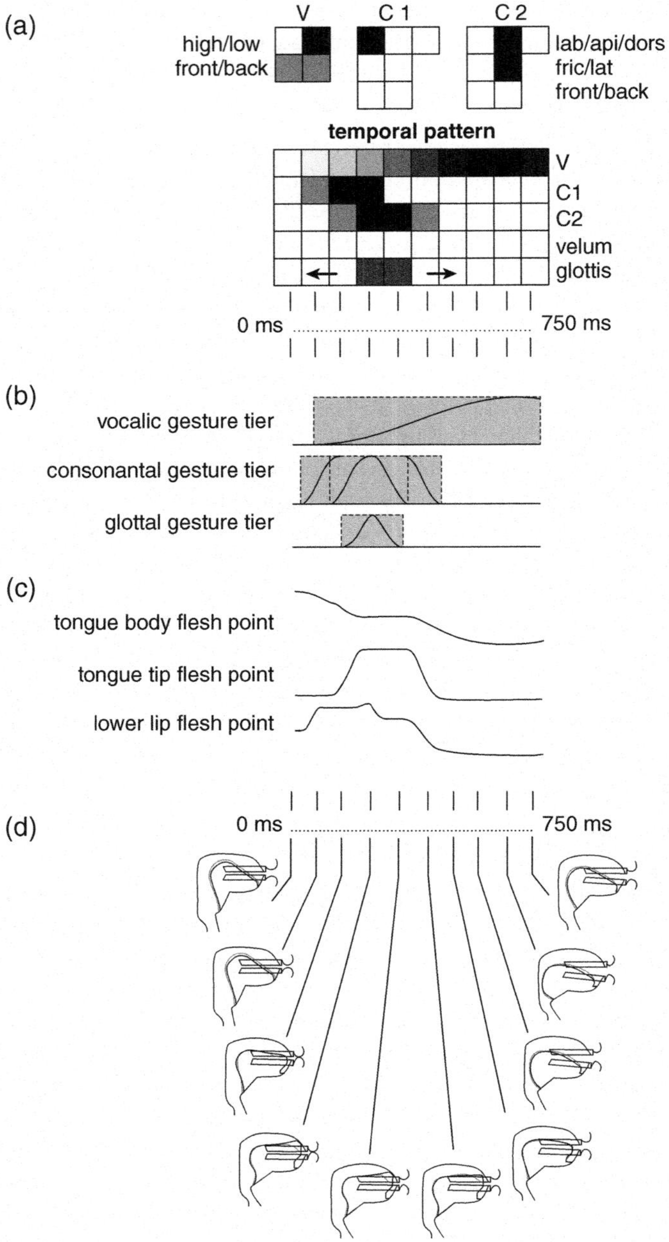

Fig. 2.3 Realization of the syllable /pla/: (a) neural activation pattern of motor plan, (b) plot of degree of realization for gestures ordered with respect to three gestural tiers, (c) plot of vertical displacement of model articulator flesh points, and (d) temporal sequence of 10 vocal tract states for a realization of the syllable /pla/. The *neural activation pattern* comprises four neuron clusters, i.e., a cluster representing the *temporal pattern* for the speech item (V-, CV-, or CCV-item) and three neuron clusters representing the vocalic and the two consonantal gestures (V, C1, C2). Each box within a neuron cluster represents a neuron. Each neuron can be activated on a scale from no activation (white) to full activation (black). The neuron cluster for the temporal pattern comprises

Fig. 2.3 (*Cont.*) rows representing the mean degree of realization for the vocalic (V), consonantal (C1, C2), velopharyngeal, and glottal gestures within distinct time intervals. The columns represent a time series of 75 ms intervals (here 750 ms in total). Arrows within the temporal pattern indicate directions for possible variations of intergestural temporal coordination and for possible variation of gestural length (exemplified here for the glottal opening gesture). The neuron cluster representing the vocalic gesture comprises four neurons representing the vocalic target dimensions high/low and front/back. The remaining neuron clusters for the consonants represent the gesture performing vocal tract organ (labial, apical, dorsal), the type of closure (fricative or lateral), and in the case of the fricatives the exact place of articulation (front or back). The degree of realization for all gestures displayed in the temporal pattern (a) is identical with the curves for degree of realization for each gesture displayed in (b) but the temporal resolution is better in (b). The flesh-point displacements shown in (c) indicate the resulting gestural movement patterns generated for different model end-articulators. The temporal succession of 10 vocal tract states in (d) represents the model vocal tract configuration in the middle of time intervals represented by the ten columns of the temporal pattern (see vertical lines in (a) and (d)).

goal-directed movement of an ensemble of articulators (e.g., lower jaw, lower lips, and upper lips in the case of a labial closing gesture, cf. Saltzman and Munhall 1989; Browman and Goldstein 1989, 1992; Goldstein et al. 2006, 2007). This action goal is functionally defined leading to discrete categories such as 'produce a bilabial closure'. In addition, the functionally defined goal includes temporal aspects, e.g., 'produce a closure for a voiced plosive realization with appropriate rapidity (i.e., not too slow in order to separate it from an approximant realization)' or 'produce the bilabial closure for a voiced plosive realization with appropriate duration of closure (i.e., not too long in order to separate it sufficiently from a voiceless plosive realization)'. (Intra-)gestural parameters or vocal tract action parameters that must be specified for each gesture or vocal tract action are the gesture performing vocal tract organ (or gesture performing end-articulator), gestural target, gestural rapidity, and gestural duration. Gestural rapidity together with current gestural duration specifies the current degree of realization of a gesture (Kröger and Birkholz 2007). In addition, parameters for inter-gestural temporal coordination specify the temporal start and ending of each gesture with respect to the temporal location of each other gesture. An example of a *neural motor plan activation pattern* is presented in Fig. 2.3. A neuron's activation level within the *temporal pattern* specifies the degree of realization for the gesture represented by that neuron at that particular time instant. Thus, the temporal pattern displays the points in time for the start and ending of gestures as well as the degree of realization in between.

Gestures are organized on *rows* with respect to the type of gesture, i.e., on the vocalic (tract shaping), consonantal, velopharyngeal, and glottal row (Goldstein and Fowler 2003). Intergestural coordination can be specified by phasing rules in articulatory phonology (Browman and Goldstein 1992) or by using coupling graphs (Goldstein et al. 2006). It should be noted that the temporal coordination is not specified by rules in ACT but results from neural learning or training during the imitation phase of speech acquisition. After neural learning or training the resulting neural motor plan activation patterns (such as that in Fig. 2.3) are stored for each frequent syllable by the link weights of the phonetic to motor plan mapping.

2.2.5 **Phonetic state representation**

The *phonetic map* (Fig. 2.1) is a neural self-organizing map as defined by Kohonen (2001). Each neuron of this map represents a phonetic state by linking a sensory and motor plan state. Some phonetic states are linked with phonemic states in order to tag phonetic realizations of phonemic states (i.e., vowels or frequent syllables). The detailed organization of the phonetic map emerges during babbling and imitation training (see below). The phonetic map is defined here typically as a neural map comprising 25 × 25 (= 625) neurons. The size of the map has been varied between 10 × 10 to 30 × 30 maps without indicating substantial changes with respect to the organization and to the phonetic features of the map. Thus we used a map size that on the one hand is able to include sufficient phonetic detail but on the other hand constraints computational processing time within practicable limits (i.e., lower than 2 hours for processing a specific set of training data). The feature of phonetotopy occurring in phonetic maps is discussed in detail in Kröger et al. (2008).

2.3 **Training the model: modelling early stages of speech acquisition – babbling and imitation**

The main goal of training is to enable the model to produce speech items of a (simple) 'model language' comprising V(owel)-items and one- or two-syllabic words composed of CV- and CCV-syllables, with C(onsonant) as defined in Section 2.2.3. Training comprises *frequent syllables*, which are therefore also labelled as 'well practiced', or 'overlearned'. *Infrequent syllables* are defined to be produced without training. Other syllable structures such as CVC can be produced as well by using ACT but are not included in this chapter. While the structure of the maps is defined a priori in our model, training leads to a specification of all link weights quantifying a neural mapping. This specification of link weights allows the association of neural states of different maps connected by a mapping.

2.3.1 **Babbling training**

Method: It is assumed that a set of pre-linguistic proto-speech items (proto-vowels and proto-syllables) can be produced by ACT directly at the beginning of speech acquisition training. This set of proto-gestures used for babbling training comprises (i) proto vocalic (labial and tongue body) vocal tract forming gestures, e.g., a labial rounding or spreading gesture, or a tongue body front raising, back raising or lowering gesture; (ii) proto consonantal (labial, tongue body, or tongue tip) vocal tract closing gestures; (iii) proto glottal opening and closing gestures for devoicing and voicing; (iv) proto velopharyngeal opening and closing gestures for production of nasality or no nasality; and (v) proto pulmonary gestures for providing the vocal tract system with sufficient subglottal pressure and airflow for speech-like phonation. Length and temporal coordination of proto-gestures is varied, leading to a training set comprising round about 1300 babbling training items (see Table 2.1). Training is performed by taking training items (motor plan states) from this training set in random order, calculating the appropriate sensory states. If the succession of motor plan state and appropriate sensory states are activated at the level of the motor plan map and sensory maps, the link weights of the appropriate mappings connecting the motor plan map and the sensory map with the phonetic map, i.e., the link weights of the sensory to phonetic and motor plan to phonetic mapping are continuously adjusted. The mathematical procedure for adjusting link weights for these mapping in each training step (i.e., with each training item) and thus the self-organization of the phonetic map is described in Kröger et al. (2009) for a smaller model language comprising only CV-syllables where C are voiced plosives.

Results: About 2,600,000 training steps were sufficient in order to reproduce motor plan states from a specific sensory state with a mean error below 2%. This performance value was calculated by comparing the neural motor plan state calculated from the sensory to motor plan mapping with the initial motor plan state chosen for testing the performance of the network. On the level of the phonetic map the self-organization of phonetic states, resulting from unsupervised learning, indicates that all proto speech items defining the babbling training set are ordered with respect

Table 2.1 Organization of the babbling training set

Subset	variation #1	variation #2	sum
proto-V (1)	Target of vocalic gesture within [i]-[a]-[u]-continuum (150 × 1 = **150**)		**150**
proto-CV with C = voiced proto-plosives (lab, api, dors) or lateral (4)	Target of vocalic gesture within [i]-[a]-[u]-continuum (50 × 4 = **200**)	Length of consonantal closing gesture and temporal coordination of vocalic and consonantal gesture (15 × 4 = **60**)	**260**
proto-CV with C = proto- nasals (lab, api) (2)	Target of vocalic gesture within [i]-[a]-[u]-continuum (50 × 2 = **100**)	Length of consonantal closing gesture and temporal coordination of consonantal closing and velopharyngeal gesture (15 × 2 = **30**)	**130**
proto-CV with C = voiceless proto-plosives (lab, api, dors) (3)	Target of vocalic gesture within [i]-[a]-[u]-continuum (50 × 3 = **150**)	Length of consonantal closing gesture and temporal coordination of consonantal closing and glottal gesture (15 × 3 = **45**)	**195**
proto-CCV with C1 = voiced proto-plosives (lab, dors), C2 = /l/ (2)	Target of vocalic gesture within [i]-[a]-[u]-continuum (50 × 2 = **100**)	Length of both consonantal closing gesture and temporal coordination of both consonantal closing gestures (81 × 2 = **162**)	**262**
proto-CCV with C1 = voiceless proto-plosives (lab, dors), C2 = /l/ (2)	Target of vocalic gesture within [i]-[a]-[u]-continuum (50 × 2 = **100**)	Length of both consonantal closing gesture and temporal coordination of both consonantal closing and glottal gesture (90 × 2 = **180**)	**280**
Total	**800**	**477**	**1277**

This training set comprises five subsets that each are organized with respect to up to two criteria of variation. The number in brackets indicates the number of subset items (column 1) or the number of training items per variation (bold) = (number of variations) × (number or subset times). The sum of all training items per subset (covering all variations) is listed in the last column. Abbreviations: lab = labial; api = apical; dors = dorsal.

to three main groups: proto V items, proto CV items, and proto CCV items. Moreover, proto CV and proto CCV items form subgroups with respect to manner, place, and voicing of initial consonant. The phonetic map at this stage of babbling comprises phonetic states with gestural targets representing the whole [i]-[a]-[u]-continuum in the case of vocalic gestures, a continuum of closure duration in the case of consonantal gestures, and a continuum of inter-gestural timing relations for all proto [V], proto [CV], and proto [CCV] items. This 'grossness', 'roughness', or 'non-distinctiveness' in spatial and temporal specification during babbling is the basis for training language-specific gestures and language-specific speech items. After babbling, the intra-gestural parameters of proto gestures and the inter-gestural temporal coordination of proto speech items become 'fine-tuned' during imitation training due to the demands of a specific language.

2.3.2 **Imitation training**

The driving force for babbling training is to play around with one's own vocal tract organs, to perceive the occurring articulatory and acoustic results produced by this vocal tract and to make associations between articulation (motor plan states) and sensation (auditory and somatosensory states). The driving force of imitation training is to reproduce language-specific external speech items (e.g., words produced by an external speaker) perceived by the model. During babbling training the model already developed knowledge for sensorimotor relations and is thus capable of using its knowledge for activating motor plans for imitating an externally produced auditory state. The model then fine-tunes this motor plan during a series of trial and error productions of the speech item in order to enable the reproduction of the external speech item satisfactorily.

Method: The set of imitation training speech items comprised 3 realizations for each of the 68 frequent speech items, i.e., for the 5 vowels, for the 44 CV syllables (/lo/ is defined to be infrequent, see Section 2.2.3), and for the 19 CCV syllables (/ble/ is defined to be infrequent, see Section 2.2.3) introduced above. The imitation training set thus comprised 204 training items, produced by a male speaker of Standard German. It should be noted that imitation training also included the notion of the phonemic state of the external speech items since all speech items trained during imitation were language-specific.

Results: In total 10 cycles of training leading to 2040 training steps were sufficient in order to obtain link weights for each neuron of the phonemic map to at least one neuron within the phonetic map indicating a strong neural association (i.e., a link weight values > 0.8). Each training item comprised a motor plan, a sensory, and a phonemic state. Imitation training started with the already trained phonetic map resulting from babbling training. The ordering of phonetic states within the (self-organizing) phonetic map already established during babbling training remains stable during imitation training. Thus the model is now capable of producing each frequent V-item, CV-item, and CCV-item of the model language.

2.4 **The functional processes and the organization of ACT**

Following the DIVA model (Guenther 2006; Guenther et al. 2006), ACT comprises feed-forward and feedback control (Fig. 2.1). *Feed-forward control* in ACT starts with the phonological representation of a speech item under production (e.g., vowel, syllable, word, or utterance) activating a single or a succession of specific phonemic states at the level of the *phonemic map*. Each syllable within the model language that is defined as frequent (see Section 2.3.3), is represented by a single 'neuron' at the level of the phonemic map. The activation of a syllable on the level of the phonemic map is called phonemic state or phonemic activation pattern within the phonemic map and leads to a co-activation of an appropriate motor plan state, auditory state, and somatosensory state (see Section 2.2). The motor plan and sensory states for frequent syllables are trained or learned during babbling and imitation training (see Section 2.3) and are stored by an ensemble of link weights quantifying the phonetic to phonemic, phonetic to motor plan, and the phonetic to sensory neural associations (and vice versa), i.e., the mappings between the *phonemic map*, the *motor plan map*, and the *sensory maps* (*auditory and somatosensory map*) via the *phonetic map* (Fig. 2.1). The motor plan of infrequent syllables is assembled via the *motor planning module* (Fig. 2.1) by adapting specifications for gestures and for the inter-gestural temporal coordination from phonetically similar frequent syllables.

The execution (or programming and execution) of each vocal tract action unit by articulators is defined by the motor programming and motor execution module. Programming and execution depends on the context of vocal tract actions, i.e., on the specification of preceding, following, and temporal overlapping actions, since actions share common articulators (e.g., the jaw in the case of overlapping vocalic and consonantal labial, apical, or dorsal actions) and thus often influence each other (Kröger et al. 2006c). Programming and execution of the motor plan of a speech item leads to an activation of a time series of *primary motor states* and subsequently to a time series of *articulatory* (including phonatory) *states* – i.e., a specification of articulatory movements for all model articulators carrying out the appropriate speech item. Thus feed-forward control starts with the discrete phonemic state and proceeds via motor planning to motor programming and motor execution.

A time series (or temporal succession) of *articulatory states* is input to the VTM, which generates an articulatory and acoustic speech signal. The articulatory signal comprises the three-dimensional surface of all model articulators (lips, lower jaw, tongue, velum, Birkholz et al. 2006). The acoustic signal results from simulation of the vocal tract acoustics in the time-domain by using a transmission line circuit analog (Birkholz et al. 2007). Both signals are used for calculating somatosensory and auditory feedback signals in the *somatosensory and auditory preprocessing modules* (Fig. 2.1).

Feedback control in ACT starts with somatosensory (proprioceptive and tactile) and auditory signals. Proprioceptive muscle-related signals are processed by the *motor execution control* and *correction module* (Fig. 2.1). Furthermore somatosensory (proprioceptive and tactile) and auditory information is processed by the *somatosensory-phonetic* and *auditory-phonetic processing modules* (Fig. 2.1). For the duration of the syllable under production the time course of somatosensory information is stored in short-term memory (part of the somatosensory-phonetic processing module) and subsequently this information can be compared with the learned somatosensory state of the syllable. In parallel, the acoustic signal produced by the VTM is transformed into an auditory activation pattern for each time instant at the level of the *auditory map* by the *auditory preprocessing module* (Fig. 2.1). Furthermore, this time course of the auditory activation pattern (in the auditory map) is stored in short-term memory on the level of the auditory-phonetic processing module. If current sensory (i.e., auditory and somatosensory) states of the speech item (feedback sensory states) deviate from the sensory state for this speech item activated via the phonetic to sensory mappings (i.e., sensory states activated during feed-forward control), an error signal is generated within the auditory-phonetic or somatosensory-phonetic processing module. This error signal is projected to the phonetic map for generating corrective motor plan information (cf. Guenther 2006; Guenther et al. 2006).

Acoustic information of external speakers is processed via the same auditory signal pathway as is used for feedback control (Fig. 2.1). It is also possible to compare auditory activation patterns produced by external signals with learned auditory states of syllables, e.g., in order to tune motor plans of these syllables during imitation training (see Section 2.3.2).

2.5 **Discussion**

This chapter outlines a quantitative computer-implemented action-based neural model of speech production, called ACT. The chapter in addition describes training the model for a model language comprising a specific set of vowels CV-, and CCV-syllables. This training represents early stages of model-based speech acquisition (babbling and imitation stage). The model mainly focuses on the sensorimotor control part of speech production starting from a phonological description of the speech item under production. Following Guenther (2006) and Guenther et al. (2006) the model described here comprises feed-forward and feedback control subsystems. In addition a separation of motor planning and motor execution occurs in ACT as a result of introducing the *concept of action* in speech production, which has been suggested as a control concept for speech production (e.g., Kelso et al. 1986; Saltzman and Munhall 1989; Goldstein et al. 2006, 2007). Furthermore, a dual route concept for separating the planning of frequent and infrequent syllables as was suggested, e.g., by Levelt et al. (1999), is part of this model.

During the babbling stage (Oller et al. 1999), the sensory to phonetic and the phonetic to motor plan mappings are trained on a variety of proto-speech items, comprising a continuum of proto-vocalic and proto-syllabic states. Each neuron within the phonetic map represents a realization of these proto-speech items. Self-organization (Kohonen 2001) causes these proto-speech items to be ordered with respect to phonetic features such as low-high, front-back in the case of proto-vowels, and with respect to phonetic features such as place and manner of articulation in the case of proto-CV-syllables and with respect to different types of proto-syllables (CV vs. CCV). After babbling training, ACT is capable of generating motor plans for these proto-speech items from auditory and/or somatosensory information.

While babbling training is based on self-productions, imitation training is driven by externally produced speech items (speech items produced by mother or caregiver). The goal of babbling training was to associate sensory and motor plan states from self-productions. The goal of imitation training is to imitate external meaningful speech items (such as words) or parts of these items (such as syllables) as good as possible in order to associate phonemic, sensory, and motor plan states. Babbling training is an important precursor of imitation training since the model speaker after babbling training already is capable of activating motor plans from sensory states since sensory-to-motor-inversion knowledge and thus auditory-to-articulation-inversion knowledge is available. This capability is required during imitation training since only the auditory states of external speech items are available. During imitation training, in addition, neural associations arise between the phonetic and the phonemic map. Thus after imitation training, phonetic realizations of frequent language specific speech items (e.g., syllables) are each represented by a subgroup of neurons within the phonetic map.

In the case of this modelling study 1,300 babbling training items and 204 imitation training items representing 68 frequent speech items (V, CV, and CCV), forming the basis of a so-called model language were trained. The high amount of 2,600,000 babbling training steps results from the fact that all temporal and spatial combinations of proto-gesture were trained. It is more realistic to introduce imitation training already in parallel to babbling training (cf. Oller et al. 1999) in order to reduce the amount of babbling training items and to focus on important subsets or sub-dimensions of temporal coordination of actions occurring in the model language under acquisition. This on the one hand leads to a reduction of babbling training steps but on the other hand leads to an increase in imitation training trials since imitation may be imperfect if babbling knowledge (i.e., auditory-to-articulatory inversion knowledge) is incomplete.

The separation of motor planning on the one hand and motor programming and execution on the other hand results from the concept of vocal tract actions, which have to be arranged in vocal tract action scores. This separation is very advantageous for the modelling of motor speech disorders such as apraxia of speech (AOS) or dysarthria, as well as fluency disorders (Van Lieshout et al. 1996). While motor planning is a central concept in ACT, motor programming and motor execution are not differentiated in our model.

A dual neural pathway approach (Levelt et al. 1999; Varley and Whiteside 2001) is assumed for generating motor plans for frequent and infrequent syllables in ACT. The pathway for frequent syllables accesses the *mental syllabary* in Levelt's approach (Levelt and Wheeldon 1994; Levelt et al. 1999; Indefrey and Levelt 2004) or the phonetic map in ACT, respectively. In parallel to the Levelt approach, in ACT motor plans of frequent syllables are stored as a whole in the phonetic to motor plan mapping. The pathway for infrequent syllables, also called *subsyllabic encoding route* (Levelt et al. 1999; Varley and Whiteside 2001), is assumed to assemble motor plans from smaller subsyllabic units. While these subsyllabic units are assumed to be segmental in the approaches of Levelt et al. (1999) and Varley and Whiteside (2001), ACT assumes a subsyllabic assembly by vocal tract action units. It should be noted that infrequent syllables are assembled in the motor planning module of ACT by looking for phonetically similar frequent syllables from the phonetic map (see also Section 2.3.3 of this chapter). In contrast to Varley and Whiteside (2001), ACT does *not* assume an independence of frequent and infrequent pathways (see arrow from phonetic map to motor planning map in Fig. 2.1). A quantitative spell-out of the motor programming module and the production of frequent and infrequent syllables are topics of our current research activities.

Acknowledgment

This work was supported in part by the German Research Council DFG Grant Nr. Kr 1439/13-1.

References

Bernstein N (1967) *The Coordination and Regulation of Movement.* (Pergamon, London)

Birkholz P, Jackel D, Kröger BJ (2006) Development and control of a 3D vocal tract model. Proceedings of the IEEE International conference on Acoustics, Speech, and Signal Processing, ICASSP 2006 (Toulouse, France), pp. 873–6

Birkholz P, Jackel D, Kröger BJ (2007) Simulation of losses due to turbulence in the time-varying vocal system. IEEE Transactions on Audio, Speech, and Language Processing 15: 1218–25

Birkholz P, Kröger BJ (2006) Vocal tract model adaptation using magnetic resonance imaging. Proceedings of the 7th International Seminar on Speech Production. (Belo Horizonte), Brazil, pp. 493–500

Birkholz P, Kröger BJ (2007) Simulation of vocal tract growth for articulatory speech synthesis. Proceedings of the International Congress of Phonetic Sciences (Saarbrücken, Germany)

Browman C, Goldstein L (1989) Articulatory gestures as phonological units. *Phonology* 6: 201–51

Browman CP, Goldstein L (1992) Articulatory phonology: an overview. *Phonetica* 49: 155–80

Dell GS, Chang F, Griffin ZM (1999) Connectionist models of language production: lexical access and grammatical encoding. *Cognitive Science* 23: 517–41

Goldstein L, Fowler CA (2003) Articulatory phonology: a phonology for public language use. In: Schiller NO, Meyer AS (eds) *Phonetics and Phonology in Language Comprehension and Production.* (Mouton de Gruyter, Berlin, NewYork), pp. 159–207

Goldstein L, Byrd D, Saltzman E (2006) The role of vocal tract action units in understanding the evolution of phonology. In: Arbib MA (ed.) *Action to Language via the Mirror Neuron System.* (Cambridge University Press, Cambridge), pp. 215–49

Goldstein L, Pouplier M, Chen L, Saltzman L, Byrd D (2007) Dynamic action units slip in speech production errors. *Cognition* 103: 386–412

Guenther FH (2006) Cortical interaction underlying the production of speech sounds. *Journal of Communication Disorders* 39: 350–65

Guenther FH, Ghosh SS, Tourville JA (2006) Neural modeling and imaging of the cortical interactions underlying syllable production. *Brain and Language* 96: 280–301

Indefrey P, Levelt WJM (2004) The spatial and temporal signatures of word production components. *Cognition* 92: 101–44

Kelso J, Saltzman E, Tuller B (1986) The dynamical perspective on speech production: data and theory. *Journal of Phonetics* 14: 29–59

Kohonen T (2001) *Self-organizing Maps.* (Springer, Berlin, New York)

Kröger BJ, Birkholz P, Kannampuzha J, Neuschaefer-Rube C (2006a) Modeling sensory-to-motor mappings using neural nets and a 3D articulatory speech synthesizer. Proceedings of the 9th International Conference on Spoken Language Processing (Interspeech 2006 – ICSLP), pp. 565–8

Kröger BJ, Birkholz P, Kannampuzha J, Neuschaefer-Rube C (2006b) Learning to associate speech-like sensory and motor states during babbling. Proceedings of the 7th International Seminar on Speech Production (Belo Horizonte, Brazil), pp. 67–74

Kröger BJ, Birkholz P, Kannampuzha J, Neuschaefer-Rube C (2006c) Spatial-to-joint coordinate mapping in a neural model of speech production. DAGA-Proceedings of the Annual Meeting of the German Acoustical Society (DEGA, Braunschweig, Germany), pp. 561–2 (or see http://www.speechtrainer.eu)

Kröger BJ, Birkholz P (2007) A gesture-based concept for speech movement control in articulatory speech synthesis. In: Esposito A, Faundez-Zanuy M, Keller E, Marinaro M (eds) *Verbal and Nonverbal Communication Behaviours, LNAI 4775* (Springer Verlag, Berlin, Heidelberg), pp. 174–89. http://dx.doi.org/10.1007/978-3-540-76442-7_16

Kröger BJ, Kannampuzha J, Lowit A, Neuschaefer-Rube C (2008) Phonetotopy within a neuro-computational model of speech production and speech acquisition. In: Fuchs S, Loevenbruck H, Pape D, Perrier P (eds) *Some Aspects of Speech and the Brain.* (Peter Lang, Berlin), pp. 59–90

Kröger BJ , Kannampuzha J, Neuschaefer-Rube C (2009) Towards a neurocomputational model of speech production and perception. *Speech Communication* 51: 793-809.

Kröger BJ, Kopp S, Lowit A (accepted) A model for production, perception, and acquisition of actions in face-to-face communication. *Cognitive Processing.* DOI: 10.1007/s10339-009-0351-2

Levelt WJM, Wheeldon L (1994) Do speakers have access to a mental syllabary? *Cognition* 50: 239–69

Levelt WJM, Roelofs A, Meyer A (1999) A theory of lexical access in speech production. *Behavioral and Brain Sciences* 22: 1–75

Van Lieshout PHHM, Hulstijn W, Peters HFM (1996) From planning to articulation in speech production: what differentiates a person who stutters from a person who does not stutter? *Journal of Speech, Language, and Hearing Research* 39: 546–64

Oller DK, Eilers RE, Neal AR, Schwartz HK (1999) Precursors to speech in infancy: the prediction of speech and language disorders. *Journal of Communication Disorders* 32: 223–45

Saltzman EL (1985) Task dynamic coordination of the speech articulators: a preliminary model. Haskins Laboratories Status Report on Speech Research SR-84: 1–18

Saltzman EL, Kelso JAS (1983) Skilled actions: a task dynamic approach. Haskins Laboratories Status Report on Speech Research SR-76: 3–50

Saltzman EL, Munhall KG (1989) A dynamic approach to gestural patterning in speech production. *Ecological Psychology* 1: 333–82

Varley R, Whiteside S (2001) What is the underlying impairment in acquired apraxia of speech? *Aphasiology* 15: 39–49

Chapter 3

Control of movement precision in speech production

Sazzad M. Nasir and David J. Ostry

Abstract

Interest to date in precision in speech production has focused on kinematic adjustments related to auditory information. In this paper we review evidence that somatosensory precision in speech is also important to the nervous system and appears to be achieved through impedance or stiffness control. We used a robotic device to apply lateral loads to the jaw that altered the motion path and hence somatosensory feedback without affecting speech acoustics. The loads were designed to maximally affect the consonant or vowel-related portion of an utterance. We found that with training subjects corrected for both vowel and consonant-related loads, such that the motion path and presumably the associated somatosensory input returned to that normally experienced under no-load conditions. A control study was run in which subjects first trained with vowel-related loads and then following adaptation the direction of load was reversed unexpectedly. The reversal of the load resulted in deflections that were comparable in magnitude to those observed at the end of adaptation. Our findings indicate that even in the absence of any effect on speech acoustics, somatosensory precision is equally important for vowel-related movements and for consonants. We further conclude that the adaptation observed here was achieved by impedance control (since impedance control produces resistance in all directions). The results are thus consistent with the idea that impedance control is used in attaining the precision requirements of orofacial movement in speech.

3.1 Introduction

3.1.1 Some issues in speech motor control

Why are the speech movements the way they are? What is special about them? Like limb movement, speech acquisition involves a sensorimotor learning task. Both auditory and somatosensory feedback contribute to speech production. Presumably, speech is dominated by auditory goals, much as limb movement is guided principally by vision. However, like any motor function, somatosensory input, mediated by the muscle and skin receptors, plays a crucial role in the control of speech movements. It is interesting to entertain the possibility that the integration of different sensory inputs gives rise to the characteristic pattern of each movement that we see.

The differences that exist between speech and other movements may be attributed very generally to this process of multisensory integration. However it should be noted that differences between limbs and speech articulators and the different physiological properties of the muscles that innervate these two types of articulators may also contribute to differences between limb and speech movements. A related issue, that is the source of considerable debate, is the extent to which speech is special: is there anything at all that non-speech movements can teach us about speech? The documented commonalities between speech and limb movement, suggest that it would be worthwhile to consider the extent to which principles of motor control gleaned through the studies of non-speech movements could be applied to speech production. Before moving on further, a few characteristics of speech production should be noted that bear not only on speech control but may more broadly shed light on how sensorimotor regulation of movement is achieved by the nervous system.

Among healthy normal adults, speech movements occur predominantly in the sagittal plane. They involve very little lateral motion, which is unlike chewing movements that occur mainly in the frontal plane. Figure 3.1 shows a frontal view of jaw movements in speech and chewing – two types of orofacial motions with different movement kinematics. Jaw movement was recorded during repetitions of the utterance, *straw* (/stɹɔ/) and during repeated chewing of a piece of gum. Notice that during speech, jaw position hardly deviates from the mid-sagittal plane. One therefore wonders out of the many possibilities for sound production that could have been used for speech, why it mostly frequently involves two-dimensional planar motion, and indeed why off midline movements such as those of the tongue are generally symmetrical about the sagittal plane? The problem is reminiscent of Bernstein's formulation of the degrees of freedom problem in motor control: to make a reaching movement in three spatial dimensions, the nervous system opts for a particular reaching trajectory generated from a very selective combination of muscle forces out of infinitely many choices (Bernstein 1967). It is likely that mid-sagittal symmetry, along with the geometrically symmetric arrangement in the positions of the articulators, naturally facilitates speech movements in the sagittal plane, for example, perhaps by providing effective constriction-based airway channelling. Presumably, the nervous system takes into account the

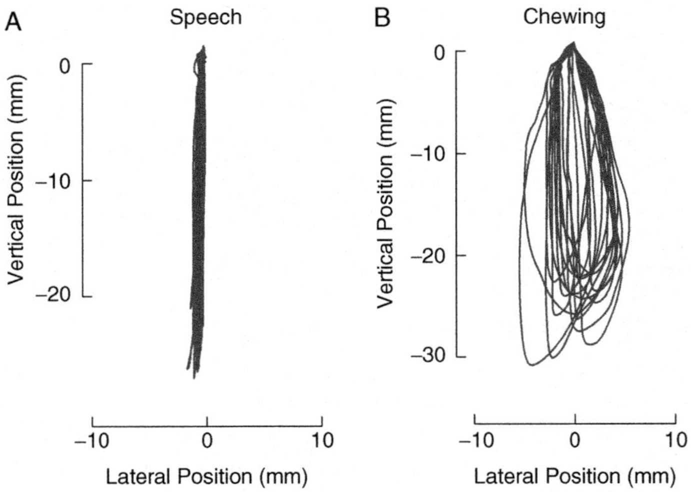

Fig. 3.1 Frontal view of jaw position during speech (A) and chewing (B). Notice that jaw position during speech deviates little from the mid-sagittal plane.

peripheral arrangement of the vocal apparatus to produce speech. However, it is less clear whether the nervous system is largely oblivious to this restriction of movement to the sagittal plane or whether instead it actively limits lateral movements in general during speech? If, for example, a speech movement were deflected laterally, would the nervous system make any corrections for such a perturbation?

Speech movements can require fairly precise positioning of the articulators with a high degree of coordination among them. For example, during production of the fricative consonant, s, (/s/) the jaw has to be raised and maintained in a rather precise elevated position in order to generate the turbulent airflow that gives rise to the /s/ sound. On the other hand, there appears to be greater latitude in the position of the jaw for the production of the vowel, a (/æ/). This then poses the question whether, with regard to the complexity of articulator positioning or the degree of their coordination, if all speech movements are created equal. It may not be surprising to see that the role of the articulators shifts to maintain varying degrees of precision depending on the classes of speech sounds produced. One may think of analogous examples in reaching movement where the position accuracy of the limb may vary from one part of the movement to the other. The precision requirement near the target is presumably the highest. A question thus arises as to what extent is the varying degree of precision that is required within a single goal-directed movement centrally planned and to what extent can this be attributed to mechanical or kinetic properties of the limb or articulator at the periphery executing that movement?

Even when producing similar sounds, precision requirements may differ along different spatial dimensions. Figure 3.2A shows the formant frequencies during production of the vowels and dipthongs of the words *saw* (/sɔ/), *say* (/seɪ/), *sas* (/sæs/), and *sane* (/seɪn/). Figure 3.2B gives the corresponding position of the jaw in the sagittal plane – protrusion and elevation. As can be seen, jaw position is less variable in the protrusion–retraction direction than in the raising–lowering direction (even though the full range of forward–backward motion is on the order of 10 mm). Overall, kinematic measures with larger amplitudes are more variable in general. This seemingly innocuous fact does not have to be true *apriori*, but reveals a deeper fact that noise in biological signal scales with amplitude. One of the beautiful elucidations of this principle is Fitt's law that was formulated in the context of reaching movements to targets of varying sizes (Fitt 1954; Harris and Wolpert 1998). This law at its core embodies the idea that reaching to a smaller target requires more time. A pertinent question is whether the fundamentals of speech movements are subject to these same principles of motor control and whether a great deal about speech production can be

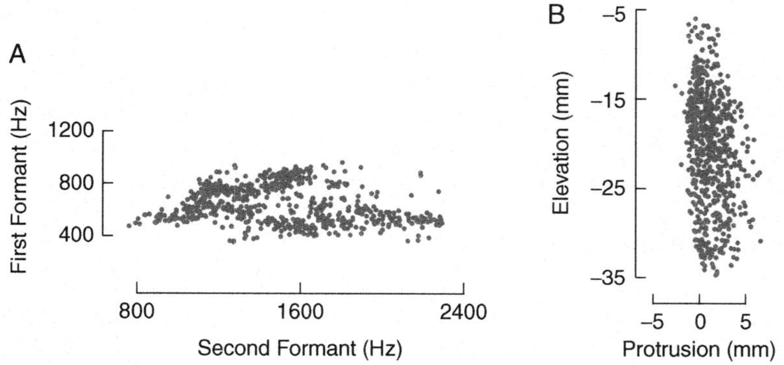

Fig. 3.2 Example of acoustical precision (A) and variabillity (B) during speech. The kinematic precision of the jaw in the horizontal direction is different from that in the vertical direction. Variability differences in formant frequencies can likewise be noted.

learnt from the general rules of motor control. It should be noted that although the tongue plays a primary role in the production of speech sounds, nevertheless the jaw plays an important part to help achieve a stable position for the tongue. Understanding the role of individual articulators may enable us to understand the role of the other articulators in speech production.

3.1.2 Role of somatosensory input in speech control

Speech production is heavily influenced by acoustical feedback, but like any other motor act it is also driven by somatosensory input and, hence, also has somatosensory goals (Nasir and Ostry 2008; Tremblay et al., 2003). It is of interest to determine how these two sensory goals interact in speech motor control and, more specifically, what role somatosensory input plays in guiding speech movement. The prevalent use of robotic devices in recent years has found wide-ranging applications in studies of limb and postural control that bears on the role of somatosensory feedback (see, e.g., Shadmehr and Mussa-Ivaldi 1994). In particular, with the use of these devices, one now has better insights into different limb control mechanisms, consolidation of motor memories, and the basis of variability, to mention just a few. A robotic device enables one to design loads that can be used to perturb the limb in a specific manner, such as subjecting the limb to a predictable force-field during learning, to assess the input–output properties of the nervous system through the response of the limb to such perturbations. Although mechanical perturbations have been used for many years to study properties of oral cavity function, the use of computer-controlled robotic devices to understand speech movements is a fairly recent development. Indeed, it was perturbation of the jaw's movement path while talking that remarkably demonstrated an independent somatosensory goal in speech (Tremblay et al., 2003). This was done by dissociating auditory and somatosensory feedback as the robot deflected the jaw and, hence, proprioception, without affecting speech acoustics. Similar techniques have been used here to answer some of the questions of speech motor control that we raised above (Nasir and Ostry 2006). In the experiments to be reviewed in this chapter, the loads were designed to target either the consonant or vowel-related portion of an utterance, since these are the major sound categories in speech, and were applied in a lateral direction to address the question of whether the lateral position of the jaw is actively regulated. In this way we wanted to determine somatosensory precision requirements for both classes of speech sounds. In addition, we wanted to gather experimental evidence on the mechanism that provides for somatosensory precision in speech production. It should be noted that though the loads were applied to the jaw during speech, our findings may help to understand orofacial control in other goal-directed tasks, such as chewing.

Altering sensory feedback and looking at the motor consequences is a time-honoured method for gauging how the nervous system controls movements (Abbs and Gracco 1983, for an application in speech). There are also studies that look at the effect on speech movements as auditory feedback is altered (Houde and Jordan 1998; Jones and Munhall 2005). Here, we elaborate on a similar theme, where during speech the altered sensory feedback is proprioception.

3.1.3 Role of impedance control

In a typical force-field learning task two types of learning strategies are called for to understand the response of the nervous system to the load. In one control strategy, termed feed-forward mapping, a precise mapping of the force-field is learned. In this case, muscles generate force that compensate exactly the applied load. Alternatively, a mechanism based on impedance control may be used, as a means to deal with a field that interferes with the stability of the limb. In cases where maintaining a precise limb position is required or the nature of the force is uncertain, impedance control offers the best strategy. On the other hand a predictable force-field is probably best dealt with using a feed-forward approach. Both of these strategies may of course contribute together to varying degrees in any given movement.

For limb movements, impedance control – resistance to movement – has been invoked as a potential means to aid in the achievement of precision (Burdet et al., 2001; Hogan 1985). Impedance control is achieved by coactivating antagonist muscles to increase the stiffness of the limb. Anything that resists movement contributes to the impedance of limb. Inertia, viscous damping of the limb and stiffness, which gives rise to spring-like properties of the limb, all are components of impedance. Impedance control is thought to provide for an effective mechanism to attain precision in limb movement.

According to the Hooke's law the stiffness (spring constant), K, of an ideal spring (no inertia and no damping) is defined as:

$$F_{ext} = Kx,$$

where the spring is displaced by an amount x by an external perturbation F_{ext} and K denotes the resistance to displacement. If the spring system is also given damping and inertia, then the previous equation reads:

$$F_{ext} = Kx + b\frac{dx}{dt} + m\frac{d^2x}{dt^2},$$

where b and m are the damping coefficient and the inertia, respectively, and dx/dt and d^2x/dt^2 are velocity and acceleration. Transformed into Fourier space, Hooke's law is written as:

$$\tilde{F}(\omega)_{ext} = Z(\omega)x,$$

where impedance, Z, is defined as:

$$Z(\omega) = K + i\omega - \omega^2 m.$$

Notice that when written as above impedance contains in it the stiffness term. In general for any dynamical system a generalized Hooke's law can be defined with a suitable definition of impedance.

For a biological articulator, impedance can be actively modulated by the nervous system. This aspect of active impedance control provides a plausible biological basis to achieve stable positioning of articulators. If an ideal spring has infinite stiffness then from Hooke's law, for any finite perturbation, the resulting displacement is zero. Thus increasing the stiffness, or impedance in general, enables the nervous system to achieve a stable articulator position. In doing so the nervous system may endeavour to increase impedance globally or can change it only to the extent necessary to offset the perturbation. For example, consider a moving limb, which is being pushed off the plane by an external force. The nervous system can choose to resist the perturbation by increasing the limb impedance in all directions. Or it can offset the perturbation by increasing impedance in the direction to which the perturbation is applied. The capacity for directional change in stiffness lets the nervous system maintain stable articulator positioning only in the dimensions demanded by the task.

Plausibly, impedance control could play a prominent role during certain phases of speech, due to different requirements for stability, and hence, for various degrees of precision. By looking at the response of speech articulators to perturbations that are delivered in conjunction with either vowel or consonant-related movement, one may hope to gain insights into the control mechanism underlying speech movements.

In this chapter we will review experiments aimed at addressing the problems noted above (see Nasir and Ostry 2006 for more details). The organization of the chapter is as follows. It starts off with a description of the experimental protocol using a robot to perturb speech movements. This is followed by a presentation of the main findings illustrating adaptation in a force-field learning task and acoustical effects that may arise due to learning. The patterns of kinematic variability of jaw movements in the production of consonants and vowels are then discussed. The role of impedance control in achieving precision in speech production is presented afterwards. The chapter closes with discussion and a brief conclusion.

3.2 Experimental paradigm

We assessed the strategies involved in the achievement of precision in speech using the following experimental setup. The subject was seated comfortably in a chair resting the head against a cushion. The subject wore a custom-made acrylic-metal dental appliance (Fig. 3.3A). The subject's head

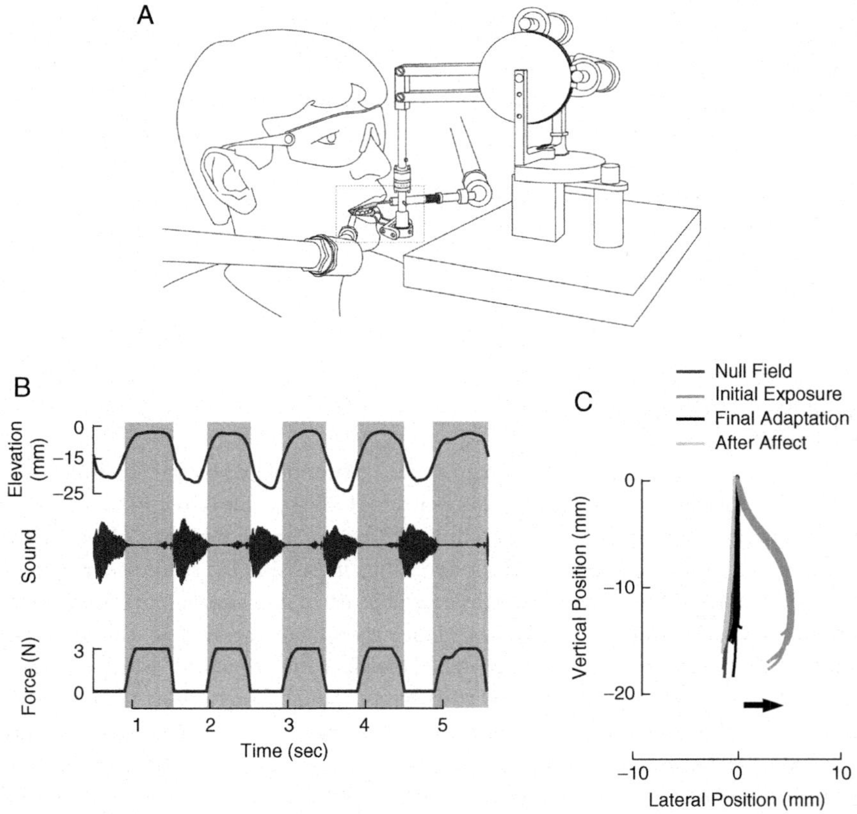

Fig. 3.3 Schematic of experimental methods and typical patterns of adaptation. A. A robotic device was used to deliver loads to the jaw. B. A lateral force was used that scaled with the elevation of the jaw. C. An example of adaptation, where the jaw path is deflected upon the load's introduction (light grey), but returns to the baseline level at the end of training (black).

was restrained during the experiment by connecting a second dental appliance, which was glued to the maxillary teeth, to an external frame consisting of a set of articulated metal arms. A computer controlled robotic device was connected to the lower appliance and was used to deliver a load to the jaw. A force/torque sensor was mounted at the tip of the robotic device to measure the restoring force applied by the subject in opposition to the load. Three-dimensional jaw movements were recorded by encoders in the robot arm. The subject's voice was recorded using a directional microphone (Nasir and Ostry 2006; 2008; Tremblay et al., 2003).

The robotic device applied a lateral load to the jaw while the subject repeatedly produced a test utterance. The goal of the manipulation was to perturb the jaw in a systematic manner and to assess the response of the nervous system in such a learning task. As previously noted, an analogous paradigm where the limb is subject to a force-field, has been used widely to study properties of limb movement control (Shadmehr and Mussa-Ivaldi 1994).

The loads were applied during production of the vowel or consonant part of a test-utterance and were, thus, able to perturb the somatosensory feedback during these phases of movement. Figure 3.3B shows an example of force application during consonant production. The top panel shows the vertical position of the jaw during repetitions of the test utterance straw. The second panel shows the raw speech waveform. The bottom panel shows the commanded force to the jaw. Lateral loads were applied to the jaw either during the closing or opening phase of the movement (shaded part in Fig. 3.3B shows an example of load applied during the closing phase of the movement). For a closing-related load, the load came on at the mid-point of jaw closing phase and stayed on until the mid-point of jaw lowering. For opening-related loads, the load came on midway through jaw opening and stayed on until mid-way through jaw closing. The load pushed the jaw laterally in proportion to jaw elevation such that the load was at its peak when the jaw was either fully closed or fully open. The loads thus had a destabilizing effect on the movements of the jaw and served to reduce positioning accuracy in speech movements.

The experiment was carried out in blocks and each block consisted of 15 repetitions of the test utterance. No load was applied during the first three blocks which constituted the 'null-field' condition of the experiment and provided a baseline pattern of jaw movement in the absence of any applied load. The subject was subsequently trained with the load on for the next twenty to twenty-five 'training' blocks, consisting of approximately 300 repetitions of the test utterance. Following training, the load was unexpectedly turned off. In this 'after-effect' block, 'catch' trials were recorded in the absence of load. The after-effect block gives clues to the kind of control mechanism employed by the nervous system to learn the force-field task.

The test utterance for consonant-related perturbations was chosen to have a consonant or consonant-cluster at the beginning and a vowel at the end. The consonant-cluster in *straw* was chosen with the goal of achieving a level of movement complexity that was sufficient to prompt adaptation to the load. The vowel ending in the test utterance was chosen to provide for large amplitude movement of the jaw. It should be noted that the consonant part of the test utterances corresponds to a jaw position near to closure, whereas the vowel part of the word corresponds to maximum jaw opening. Thus the consonant and vowel sounds were largely confined to the two movement extremes, where, possibly, a high degree of movement precision is required by virtue of the jaw having to maintain a relatively stable position.

Subjects were divided into a vowel group, a consonant group, and one impedance control group. Each subject experienced either vowel- or consonant-related loads. The vowel group subjects (seven in total) experienced the load during jaw opening; the consonant group subjects (four in total) experienced the load during closing. In a separate impedance control group (four subjects in total), where a vowel-related load was applied, the after-effect block was replaced by an unexpected 180° switch in the direction of load and no after-effect block was recorded.

3.3 **Results**

3.3.1 **Adaptation patterns**

How does the load affect the movement path of the jaw? The load initially affects the curvature of the jaw path, but with training subjects adapt to the load by reducing the curvature. The maximum perpendicular distance from the movement path to a straight line from movement start to end was taken as a measure of curvature. The curvature was computed for each repetition of the test utterance. The raising segment, which began with the jaw fully open and ended with the jaw fully closed, was used for the analyses. The start and end of the movement were scored at 20% of peak vertical velocity. Adaptation was assessed by computing the mean curvature for the first 35% and the last 35% of the force-field training trials. Null-field performance was based on curvature measured during the three null-field familiarization blocks.

A frontal plane view of jaw movement is shown in Fig. 3.3C. During null-field trials, movements are initially straight (grey). With the load's onset the path is deflected laterally (light grey); with training the curvature decreases as the nervous system responds to the movement error introduced by the load (black); following unexpected removal of load there is no after-effect (pale grey). Subjects differed in their degree of adaptation. Figure 3.3C shows an example of complete adaptation, however more typically, there is a significant decrease of curvature relative to the beginning of training but performance never returns to baseline levels (Nasir and Ostry 2006).

Adaptation was observed for vowel- and consonant-related loads (Fig. 3.4). As shown, the null-field curvatures are indicated in grey. As the load is introduced the jaw deviates significantly (light grey). After-training there was a reduction in curvature (black). For vowel-related loads, six of seven subjects showed adaptation (Fig. 3.4A), as indicated by a significant decrease in curvature over the course of training ($p < 0.01$). For consonant-related loads all four subjects tested showed significant adaptation (Fig. 3.4B).

The amount of adaptation was further assessed on a per subject basis by computing the reduction in curvature over the course of training as a proportion of the curvature due to the introduction of load. A value of 1.0 indicates complete adaptation. For vowel-related loads, the amount of adaptation averaged across subjects was 0.46 ± 0.09 (mean ± SE). For consonants, the mean

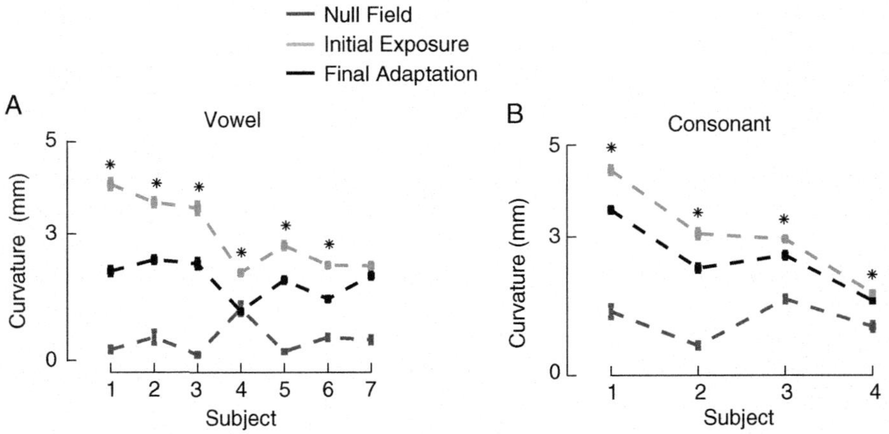

Fig. 3.4 Observed adaptation patterns for consonants and vowels. Curvature increases with the introduction of load (light grey) relative to no load conditions (grey). Adaptation is observed following training (black). Stars designate significant adaptation ($p < 0.01$).

adaptation was 0.35 ± 0.05. Thus there was comparable adaptation when loads coincided with either vowel or consonant production ($p > 0.5$). This suggests that precision requirements are similar for both kinds of speech movements.

3.3.2 Acoustical effects

What role does the somatosensory input play in mediating the adaptation? Clearly, the load affects the movement path of the jaw and, thus, directly alters somatosensory input. The load may also affect the acoustics by altering the vocal tract shape. Any systematic changes in the acoustics due to the load would suggest a role for auditory input in mediating the observed adaptation.

Acoustical effects were assessed by computing spectral measures related to the application of the load. For the consonant-related loads, we manually selected a window that contained the /s/ in *straw*. For the vowel, the selected window contained the /a/ in *straw*. The spectral measures were the first and second formant frequencies for vowels and the centroid frequency for /s/ (Fig. 3.5). Notice that the first two formants correspond to the elevation and protrusion dimensions of the oral cavity. The spectral measures in the null-field condition are indicated in white, the introduction of load is in light grey, and after-training is in black. Across subjects, there were no differences found in any of the acoustical measures due to the introduction of load ($p > 0.05$). Moreover, there were no differences in the acoustics from the start to end of training ($p > 0.05$) (Nasir and Ostry 2006). The absence of any measurable acoustical effect suggests that somatosensory input is the primary drive in mediating the adaptation observed in these experiments.

3.3.3 Kinematic variability

It was an intriguing finding that subjects showed comparable adaptation during vowel and consonant related loads, whereas the movements associated with their production had, on the surface, different variability patterns. If error tolerance of a goal-directed movement is reflected in its variability, then movements with greater variability may lead to a lesser degree of adaptation in a force-field learning task, because for those movements subjects would have to correct less for movement errors. The production of the fricative consonant /s/ presumably requires more precise positioning of the articulators than the production of vowel-like sounds such as /a/ and,

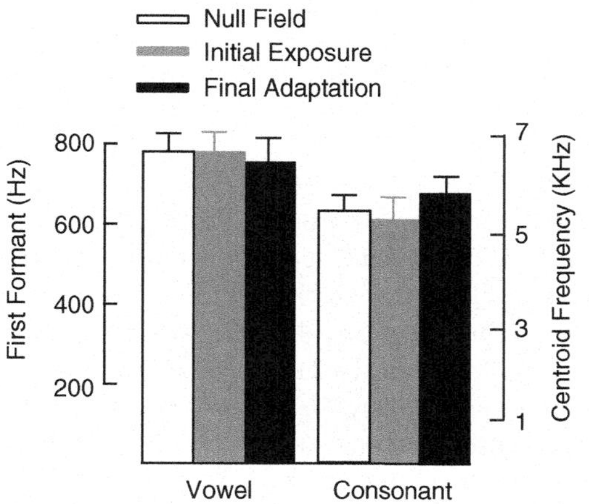

Fig. 3.5 Effect on the acoustics. The first and second formants of vowels, and the centroid frequency for /s/ were computed under no load conditions (white), at the introduction of the load (light grey) and at the end of training (black).

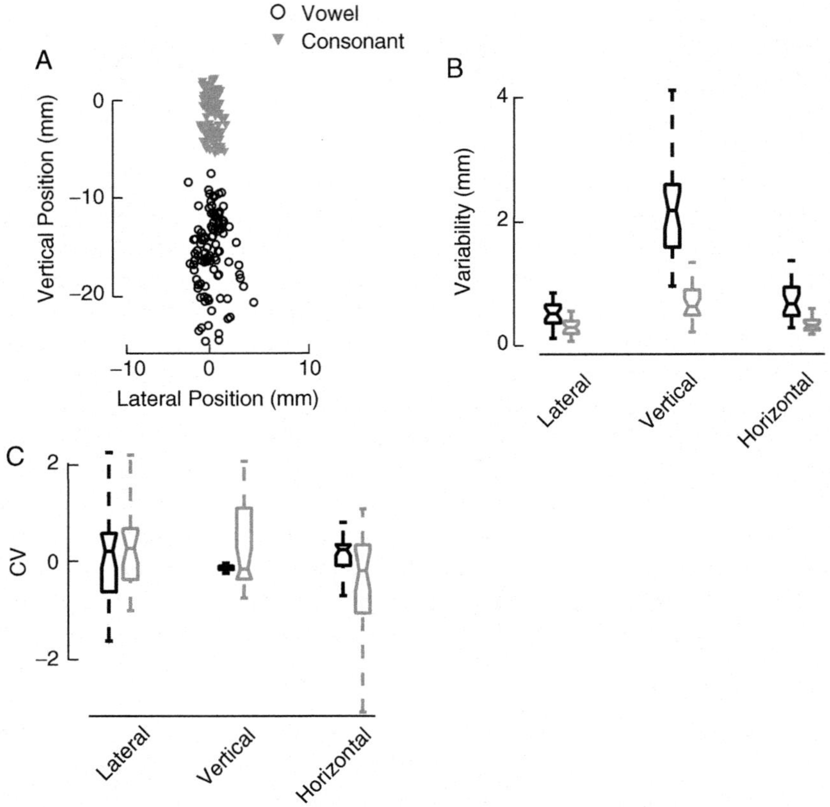

Fig. 3.6 Precision of jaw position during vowel and consonant production. A. Frontal plane view of jaw position during consonants (filled grey triangles) and vowels (black circles) for the utterance *straw*. B. Variability in jaw position across subjects. C. CV for consonants and vowels. CV is a measure of normalized variation. Once differences in variability due to differences in movement amplitude are accounted for, differences in kinematic variability are eliminated.

hence, may show greater sensitivity to error in a learning task. If this is the case, then consonant-related movements associated with /s/ should have resulted in more adaptation. As this clearly was not the case, we wanted to determine whether the kinematic precision of vowel and consonant movements are indeed different.

Figure 3.6 shows a representative sample of jaw positions in the frontal plane during repetitions of the word *straw* (Fig. 3.6A). The movement extremes during opening or closing were used to obtain estimates of the variability of the vowel or consonant-related utterance. The figure gives jaw position during both consonant and vowel production. As can be seen, jaw positions during the consonant phase are more tightly clustered than during vowel production, suggesting a greater kinematic precision for consonants. Figure 3.6 further summarizes in box-plots the variability of jaw position across subjects during consonant and vowel productions for the same utterance.

The precision of the jaw position was computed using two measures of jaw variability, which were calculated on a per subject basis: the first was variability relative to the mean jaw position at maximum opening or maximum closing, the second was the coefficient of variation (CV), which is the standard deviation of jaw position divided by the mean jaw position. The rationale for using this measure is, as we have already noted, that in many biological signals variability is proportional to amplitude. That is, larger values are naturally more variable. The CV normalizes variability with respect to amplitude and hence enables one to test whether there are differences in variability in vowels and consonants once differences in movement amplitude are factored out. Figures 3.6B and 3.6C show in box-plots the variability and CV of the jaw position during consonant and vowel production for the test utterances. Reliable differences in variability of jaw position in the vertical direction were observed between vowels and consonants for both test words ($p < 0.01$), whereas the two other spatial directions, protrusion and lateral, did not show any differences. When we tested for differences using the CV, no reliable differences in variability were found in any of the three spatial directions between vowels and consonant for either of the test words. Note that the CV provides normalization in that variability is simply linearly adjusted for differences in amplitude. This simple correction, nevertheless, can account for differences in kinematic precision between vowel and consonants.

Notice that comparable kinematic precision was observed in the lateral position of the jaw during the vowel and consonant production. On the basis of this one may expect to see no difference in the adaptation patterns for consonants and vowels for a lateral load, as was the case in the present study. Therefore, it is not surprising that both consonant- and vowel-related movements showed similar adaptation for they did not have different precision requirements, as measured by the CV, to begin with. It should be recalled, however, that the adaptation measure was computed with reference to the jaw trajectory in three dimensions and, hence, compensation to a lateral load as measured by this 3D measure presumably reflects compensation in all three dimensions. This, taken together with the finding of comparable patterns of normalized variation for consonant- and vowel-related movements, points to the conclusion that the nervous system assigns equal weight in controlling their precision.

3.3.4 **Impedance control**

We explored the way in which subjects achieved adaptation in the present force-field learning task that involved destabilizing loads, with their maximum at movement ends. What kind of control strategy could be employed by the nervous system in order to achieve the observed adaptation? We will provide several lines of evidence to suggest that impedance control was chiefly used to achieve the adaptation in the present studies.

One signature that distinguishes impedance control and feed-forward control is the response to catch trials, when the force-field is turned off unexpectedly following learning. If a feed-forward strategy has been employed to compensate for the applied force, then during a catch trial the kinematic response should mirror that observed at the load's introduction, producing what has been termed as after-effect. On the other hand, for impedance learning, there is no after-effect during the catch trials and the absence of after-effect is a defining characteristic of this control strategy. If the jaw were to behave like a spring with infinite stiffness, then according to Hooke's law any finite external perturbation would produce zero displacement. Therefore, increasing the value of stiffness is a good control strategy for the nervous system in order to offset sudden and uncertain external perturbations. In such a case, during the catch trials, the trajectory would be no different than the trajectory at the end of a force-field learning task since muscle coactivation, which changes impedance, results in no change to net torque and hence no change in movement. Figure 3.3C shows examples of after-effect trials recorded at the end of training (pale grey). In this case the movement path is no different from that observed under null-field conditions (grey). As noted before, had adaptation involved a feed-forward control strategy to offset the external load, one would have expected a negative after-effect with a curvature approaching that of initial-exposure trials.

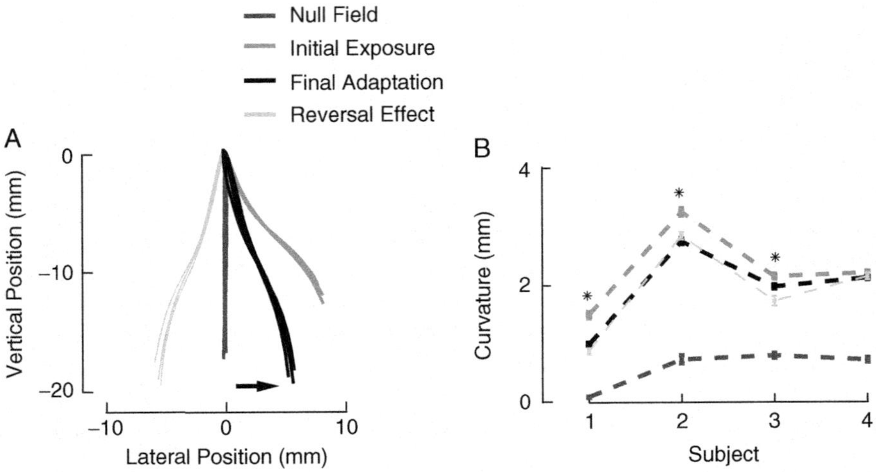

Fig. 3.7 Control of jaw impedance. A. Frontal view of the movement path under conditions of force-field reversal. When the direction of the load was reversed unexpectedly after training, the movement path (thin light grey) was the mirror image of the path at the end of training (black). The black arrow indicates the direction of the training load. B. All but one subject showed adaptation in the reversal experiment.

We directly tested the idea that subjects use impedance control to achieve precision at movement endpoints. We ran four new subjects for whom, following adaptation, the direction of the force-field was reversed unexpectedly rather than switched off completely as in the case of catch trials. On the basis of the analogy to a highly stiff spring, we reasoned that if an impedance-based control strategy was being employed to achieve adaptation then subjects' performance following force-field reversal would not differ from that observed at the end of training. Figure 3.7A shows a frontal view of performance in the force-field reversal study. The test word was *straw* and the load was applied during the vowel. Null-field conditions are in grey. A large lateral deflection is observed with the introduction of load (light grey); substantial adaptation occurs following training (black). When the direction of the load is unexpectedly reversed, the movement path is a mirror image of that observed at the end of training (thin light grey). Figure 3.7B shows significant adaptation to load by all but one subject ($p < 0.01$). Light grey denotes curvature at the introduction of load and black denotes curvature after training. When the load is reversed, curvature (thin light grey) does not differ from that observed at the end of training. Consistent with the idea that adaptation under these conditions is based on impedance control, movement curvature during the force-field reversal trials did not differ from that observed at the end of training ($p > 0.05$ for all subjects).

We further quantified impedance over the course of learning for each of our subjects and for both test-utterances. This was done to assess quantitatively whether subjects indeed increased their impedance over the course of learning. For this, a coefficient of impedance was computed by subdividing each movement into two parts, one in which commanded force was zero and the other in which force increased as a result of displacement of the jaw. We recorded a 3D sensed force vector for each of the two segments and took the magnitude of the vector difference as the measure of force change. The curvature of the movement path was taken as a measure of position change. The impedance coefficient was defined as the ratio between the difference in force and the difference in curvature. This measure captures information about impedance that is suitable for the assessment of impedance change over learning.

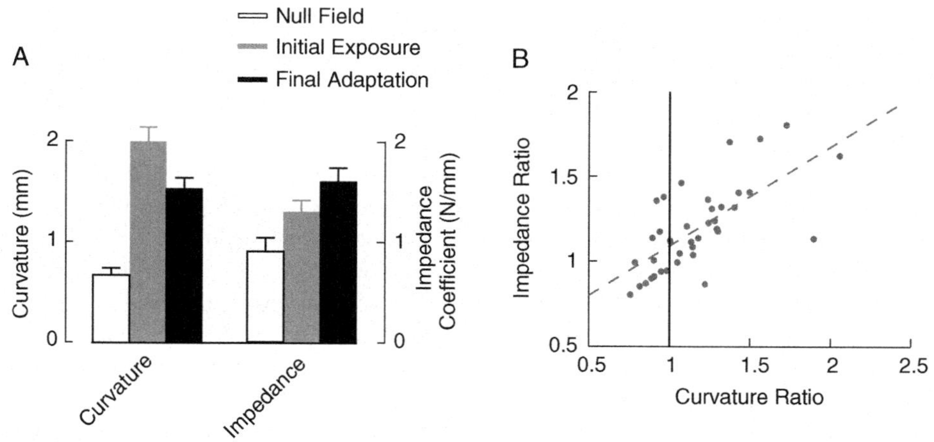

Fig. 3.8 Quantification of impedance. A. Impedance progressively increases over the course of training while curvature decreases with adaptation. B. A linear relation is observed between impedance and curvature. Subjects with greater amounts of adaptation show greater impedance.

Figure 3.8A shows patterns of impedance and associated movement curvature pooled over subjects, test words, and vowel- versus consonant-related loads. Movement curvature is low under null-field conditions (white), increases following the introduction of load (light grey) and decreases significantly with adaptation (black) ($p < 0.01$). In contrast, jaw impedance shows a steadily increasing pattern such that impedance coefficient is low initially and progressively increases with learning to result in a significantly higher impedance coefficient at the end of training ($p < 0.01$). This suggests that subjects achieved adaptation by increasing impedance to help reduce movement curvature.

The relationship between impedance and movement curvature was also assessed quantitatively by computing impedance change and curvature change on a per subject basis over the course of learning. Figure 3.8B shows data for all participants. The abscissa shows the ratio between curvature during initial force-field exposure and curvature at the end of training. Values greater than 1.0 indicate adaptation whereas values less than 1.0 denote lack of adaptation. Larger values indicate greater curvature reduction. The ordinate of the plot shows the ratio of the impedance coefficient at the end of training to that observed with the initial introduction of load. As can be seen, the impedance ratio correlates well with the amount of adaptation ($r = 0.8$) (Nasir and Ostry 2006). Thus, as expected, subjects that had greater impedance at the end of training showed greater adaptation.

In short, subjects in the present study compensate for destabilizing loads at the extremes of speech movements by increasing impedance to reduce displacement of the jaw. These results are in line with other demonstrations that impedance control plays a significant role in speech production (Shiller et al., 2002; 2005). Moreover, they are consistent with observed changes in impedance in comparable situations of human limb movement.

3.4 **Discussion**

Some aspects of the observed adaptation are somewhat surprising when compared to what is observed in studies oflimb movement. In speech tasks, not all subjects adapt to the load. Moreover, for adapted subjects, the adaptation is seldom complete, as opposed to the near complete adaptation typically observed in limb control studies. This may point to a larger tolerance of error in speech movements. Below we elucidate further on the difference between the adaptation patterns of speech and limb movements.

In response to the application of load, subjects typically showed two trends. Most subjects adapted, but some did not. Subjects tested with altered auditory feedback show a comparable trend, where approximately 15% of subjects show no sign of adaptation (Purcell and Munhall 2006). It would be worthwhile to determine whether these two failures are related. It can be envisaged that individuals who fail to adapt to altered mechanical environments may be more sensitive to auditory than to somatosensory feedback and those who fail with auditory perturbations may rely more heavily on proprioception. In contrast, in force-field learning tasks involving limb movements, typically all subjects show adaptation. Another intriguing difference between adaptation studies with limb and jaw movement is that adaptation is hardly complete in speech. It could be that multisensory integration involving proprioceptive and auditory feedback is conducive to providing an increased tolerance to movement error. However, incomplete adaptation may also reflect a broader target range in speech production and hence greater ease in bringing movements within the target zone without full adaptation.

It is unknown the extent to which the phenomena reported here are restricted to speech movements per se. Indeed, the phenomena perhaps more generally characterize orofacial motor learning and are not restricted to speech. The presence of compensation for loads in a lateral direction that is thought to play a limited role in speech production may indicate that impedance control, and presumably the observed adaptation as well, is a general feature of orofacial movement. Nevertheless, these compensations are observed here in the presence of speech movements, suggesting that the nervous system actively regulates the lateral position of the jaw in speech production. A restriction on motion out of the sagittal plane in combination with peripheral geometrical preference for midsagittal plane movement provides for a solution to Bernstein's problem in the context of speech production. Moreover, we can recall at this point that speech movement hardly deviates from the sagittal plane as compared to chewing motion. A priori it could have been the case that speech movements have little lateral deviation and accordingly there is little need for correction by the nervous system. Alternatively, an active control mechanism, such as suggested by our study, keeps speech movement within the sagittal plane. Note also that for both vowels and consonants, the CV is no different in the lateral direction than for movements in the sagittal plane. This implies that precision requirements in the lateral direction are as great as those in the sagittal plane.

3.5 **Conclusion**

In summary, we have assessed sensorimotor adaptation in speech production, by using mechanical loads to perturb the movement path of the jaw during consonant or vowel production. The load initially produced a lateral deviation of the jaw. With training, for those subjects that adapted to the load, the deviation was reduced. The extent of adaptation was comparable for vowel- and consonant-related loads. Likewise, variability of jaw position, as measured by the CV, was comparable for the vowel and consonant portion of the movements. This would suggest that the two classes of speech sounds – vowels and consonants – have similar precision requirements for jaw positioning. The loads were small enough not to have any noticeable acoustical effects, thereby assigning a prominent role for somatosensory input in mediating the observed adaptation. As the movement extremes of the jaw were perturbed, impedance control, as expected, was found to be the primary means by which the nervous system achieves stability.

To conclude, application of robotic devices to speech motor control helps to elucidate any commonality or difference between speech production and the control of limb movement. Whether the same neural principles of motor control underlie movement in both systems is yet to be determined. Indeed, multisensory integration may produce different movement outcomes in speech or limb movement despite the fact that common neural principles underlie the two. For example, the sensitivity to movement error may be dictated by tolerance for sensory errors that control the movement. Movements of the limb that are principally guided by vision may have different precision requirements than those principally guided by audition. It is likely that speech control system will prove to be a fertile ground not only for purposes of understanding the speech motor production per se, but also to uncover general principles of motor control that underlie any movement.

References

Abbs, J.H. and Gracco, V.L. (1983). Sensorimotor actions in the control of multi-movement speech gestures. Trends. Neurosci. 6, 391–5.

Bernstein, N.A. (1967). *The coordination and regulation of movements.* Pergamon, London.

Burdet, E., Osu, R., Franklin, D.W., Milner, T.E., and Kawato, M. (2001). The central nervous system stabilizes unstable dynamics by learning optimal impedance. Nature 414, 446–9.

Fitts, P.M. (1954). The information capacity of the human motor system in controlling the amplitude of movement. J. Exp. Psychol. 47, 381–91.

Harris, C.M. and Wolpert, D.M. (1998). Signal-dependent noise determines motor planning. Nature. 394, 780–4.

Hogan, N. (1985). The mechanics of multi-joint posture and movement control. Biol. Cyber. 52, 315–51.

Houde, J.F. and Jordan, M.I. (1998). Sensorimotor adaptation in speech production. Science. 279, 1213–16.

Jones, J.A. and Munhall, K.G. (2005). Remapping auditory-motor representations in voice production. Curr. Biol. 15, 1768–72.

Nasir, S.M. and Ostry, D.J. (2006). Somatosensory precision in speech production. Curr. Biol. 16, 1918–23.

Nasir, S.M. and Ostry, D.J. (2008). Speech motor learning in profoundly deaf adults. Nat. Neurosci. 11, 1217–22.

Purcell, D.W. and Munhall, K.G. (2006). Adaptive control of vowel formant frequency: Evidence from real-time formant manipulation. J. Acoust. Soc. Am. 120, 966–77.

Shadmehr, R. and Mussa-Ivaldi, F.A. (1994). Adaptive representation of dynamics during learning of a motor task. J. Neurosci. 14, 3208–24.

Shiller, D.M., Ostry, D.J., and Laboissiere, R. (2002). The relationship between jaw stiffness and kinematic variability in speech. J. Neurophysiol. 88, 2329–40.

Shiller, D.M., Houle, G., and Ostry, D.J. (2005). Voluntary control of human jaw stiffness. J. Neurophysiol. 94, 2207–17.

Tremblay, S., Shiller, D.M., and Ostry, D.J. (2003). Somatosensory basis of speech production. Nature. 423, 866–9.

Chapter 4

Variability of North American English /r/ production in response to palatal perturbation

Mark K. Tiede, Suzanne E. Boyce,
Carol Y. Espy-Wilson, and Vincent L. Gracco

Abstract

It is well established that the lowered third formant constituting the primary acoustic percept of American English /r/ can be achieved with different tongue shapes in production, which may be broadly grouped into 'bunched' and 'retroflex' production strategies. There is also evidence showing that some speakers select one or the other of these production strategies depending on the coproduction context, thus suggesting that the two are motorically equivalent. The research question pursued in this work is whether such motor equivalence in /r/ production is a generally accessible property of fluency in American English. While the vocal tract morphology of a given speaker may lead her to prefer one tongue shape uniformly, introduction of a perturbation interfering with normal articulation habits may potentially induce that speaker to explore the use of an alternative shape. To investigate this possibility, subjects in this study were fitted with a custom palatal prosthesis incorporating a protrusion along the alveolar ridge, and observed during /r/ production with and without the prosthesis using electromagnetometry. Results show that a majority of subjects responded to the artificial palate by alternating between tongue shapes. Regardless of tongue shape, no subjects showed significant differences across condition in formant patterns for /r/. All subjects showed a pattern of motor equivalence between tongue constriction location and corresponding lip protrusion, as displaced by the palate or as an aftereffect of wearing it. These results are consistent with the primacy of acoustic goals in the production of /r/.

4.1 Introduction

Human speakers have a remarkable aptitude for producing intelligible speech when confronted with constraints on normal articulation. Ventriloquists, for instance, speak effectively without moving their lips; surgical patients who have undergone resection of the tongue, lips, or other articulators find means of compensating for loss of function to recover adequate speech facility.

How speakers do this, how quickly and under what conditions, has been a matter of much scientific fascination.

One persistent question is whether such compensation is immediate, or whether speakers require a period of trial and error to reorganize their articulation effectively. In a pioneering bite-block study, Lindblom et al. (1979) established that speakers succeeded in producing near-normal vowel formants despite the constraint on mandible position, and were able to do so from the first glottal cycle. Studies in which the effects of unexpected perturbation of jaw position during bilabials were evaluated with respect to lip compensation (including Folkins and Abbs 1975; Gomi et al., 2002; Kelso et al., 1984) have shown that the time course of such compensation is both rapid (e.g. 15–35 ms in OOI reported by Kelso et al.) and complete (the lips achieve closure). However, studies investigating adaptation to prostheses affecting oral tract morphology have shown that such adaptation takes place gradually (though at subject-specific rates), and that learned modifications to normal production can persist as after-effects following removal (Baum and McFarland 1997; Jones and Munhall 2003; Hamlet and Stone 1978; Savariaux et al., 1995). Compensation has also been shown for cases where equivalent acoustic effects are produced by mechanically uncoupled articulators. For instance, insertion of a bite block limiting lip rounding did not prevent speakers from producing the rounded vowel /y/ in a study by Riordan (1977). Instead, and without practice, speakers immediately lowered their larynx to extend the length of the vocal tract, producing the formants characteristic of /y/ using this alternative strategy.

Another issue of interest is the degree to which such mechanisms of compensation resemble the coproduction effects of normal speech. A number of investigators have reported variation in the way articulator movements combine to produce acoustic output for particular segments: Perkell and colleagues (Perkell et al., 1993) have reported small but consistent 'trading relations' between lip rounding and tongue-body raising for /u/, and between lip rounding, backing of constriction along the palate, and palatal constriction degree for /r/ (Guenther et al., 1999). For /u/, lip rounding and tongue-body raising have the effect of lowering F2; in the Perkell et al. study, a greater degree of tongue-body raising was more likely to be accompanied by less lip rounding, and vice versa. For /r/, a more posterior constriction along the palate, lip rounding, and narrower constriction via tongue raising all serve to lower F3; again, the Guenther et al. study showed that more reliance on one of these articulatory maneuvers was accompanied by less of another, and vice versa. Clearly, alternative methods for achieving the same acoustic result occur during ordinary speech, even in the absence of gross perturbations such as bite blocks.

However, the motor equivalence demonstrated by trading relations among articulators for /u/ and /r/ is different in kind from the qualitatively different articulatory variants associated with production of North American English (AE) [ɹ]. Speakers of this family of dialects may use one of several tongue configuration types to produce acoustically similar patterns for F1, F2, and F3 (Delattre and Freeman 1968; Mielke et al., in press; Westbury et al., 1998). Broadly speaking, phonetic descriptions of AE /r/ group the observed variants into 'retroflex' (with the tongue tip raised and the dorsum lowered) and 'bunched' (with the tongue tip lowered and the dorsum raised) varieties. Although these tongue configurations are similar in that they divide the vocal tract into three cavities, with constrictions at the lips, palate, and pharynx, they use different articulators for the primary constriction (tongue tip vs. tongue dorsum). From an articulatory perspective they are thus qualitatively different in the same way that, say, tip-up /s/ (made with a raised tongue tip and blade) is different from /ʃ/ (made with a bunched tongue blade and dorsum). Unlike the sibilant contrast, however, in /r/ production the first three formants resulting from these different tongue configurations are indistinguishable (Delattre and Freeman 1968; Westbury et al., 1998; Zhou et al., 2008). AE /r/ is thus an unusual case of articulatory heterogenous homophony (Fig. 4.1).

At present there are no known dialectal or anatomical factors that predict which configuration a speaker prefers (Delattre and Freeman 1968; Westbury et al., 1998). The different tongue

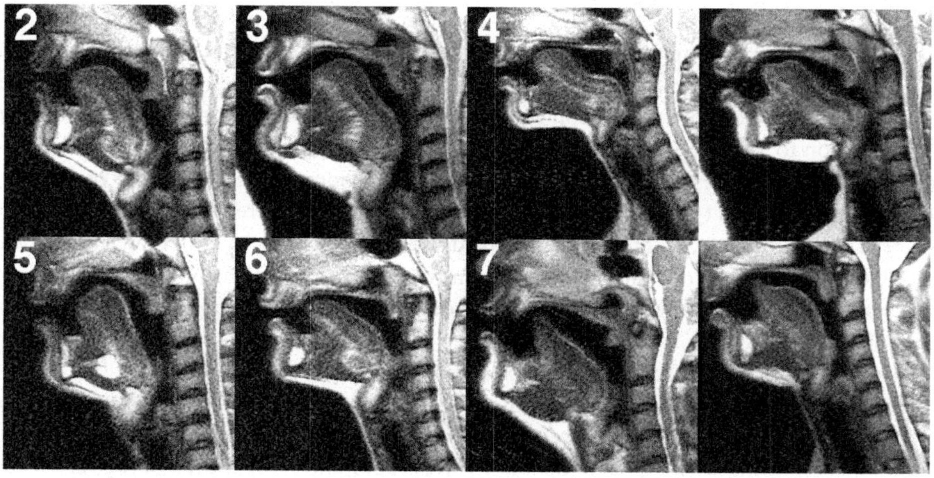

Fig. 4.1 Native speakers of North American English producing sustained /r/ as in 'pour'. Data from Tiede et al. (2004). The numbers correspond to the tongue shapes distinguished by Delattre and Freeman (1968); the additional two images without numbers show shapes not encountered by them.

configurations of North American English have been proposed as an example of 'covert allophony' (Mielke et al., in press) – that is, since any of the various configurations are equivalent for linguistic purposes, the choice of which configuration to use is in linguistic free variation. Since the articulatory configuration used by a speaker cannot be deduced by the listener from acoustic information, the choice is insensitive to sociolinguistic variables (like dialect) that might cause production to coalesce behind a particular production strategy. In other words, the choice of which configuration to use is peculiarly individual to the speaker. Moreover, although some speakers appear to produce /r/ with consistent tongue shape, certain other speakers seem to switch between configurations according to phonetic context (Delattre and Freeman 1968; Guenther et al., 1999; Secord et al., 2007). Figure 4.2 provides an example of a subject whose typical tongue configuration for /r/ is retroflex, but who switches to a more bunched configuration for /r/ when

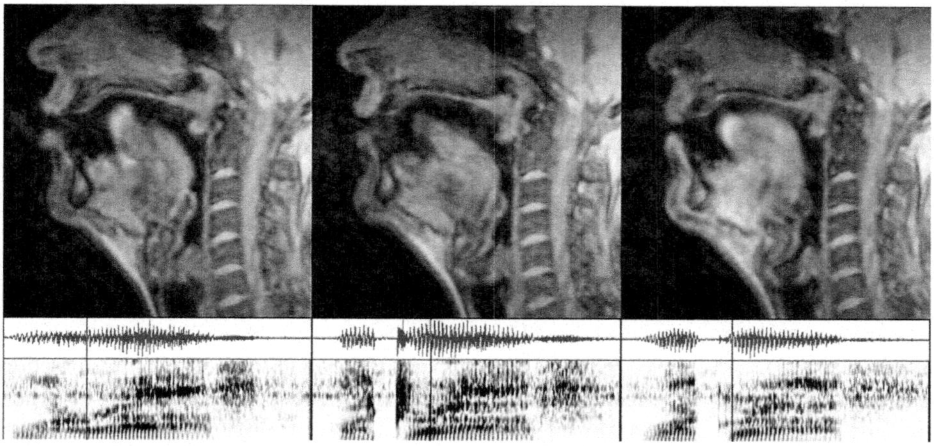

Fig. 4.2 Cine-MRI of the sequences (left to right) 'warav', 'wadrav', and 'wagrav', showing frames corresponding to /r/ midpoints. Collected by K. Honda and M. Tiede at ATR in Kyoto, Japan, using a synchronized sampling method (Masaki et al., 1999).

the preceding segment is velar. A study of 32 American English speakers by Mielke et al. (in press) found that speakers fall into three groups according to how they use alternative tongue configurations for /r/. Some speakers maintain two or more production strategies, and alternate between them freely in certain contexts. A second group also maintains two or more strategies, but adapts their selection to specific production contexts. Finally, a third group uses a single configuration consistently for all contexts in normal speech. Similar behaviour has been noted for real words by Delattre and Freeman (1968) and Kent (personal communication regarding data discussed in Shriberg and Kent 1995), and for nonsense words by Guenther et al. (1999). It appears to be the case that speakers work out individual solutions both to the problems of producing /r/ given personal vocal tract morphology, and of accommodating /r/ production to coarticulatory and prosodic demands.

Given that /r/ is an articulatorily complex sound, requiring three constrictions along the vocal tract in addition to precise positioning of the lateral edges of the tongue, it is unsurprisingly one of the last to be mastered in language acquisition (Smit 1993). Presumably, some portion of the developmental trajectory for /r/ production involves exploration by children of the various possible vocal tract configurations that produce appropriate acoustics, followed by solidification of strategies for dealing with coarticulatory demands (Hoffman et al., 1980). It is suggestive that speech pathologists make use of palatal perturbation as a means of facilitating /r/ production in school-age children with persistent /r/ production difficulties. For example, a study reported by Clark et al.(1993) found that those treated with a prosthesis incorporating mid-palatal thickening made significant improvements relative to a control group in all aspects of /r/ production. It seems likely that the children who improved in this study were encouraged by the perturbation to explore alternative methods for producing /r/, perhaps by switching from one production variant to another. Having learned to use a particular method successfully under perturbed conditions, they were then able to exploit the new skill in normal speech production.

Depending on the speaker, the developmental period may thus conclude with a single, preferred tongue configuration for /r/ and suppression of alternative production strategies, or a mix of active strategies that depend on production context. But even for those speakers adopting a single strategy, retention of a previously practiced alternative would be potentially advantageous in maintaining intelligible speech when facing unanticipated or unusual articulatory constraints. Some evidence for such a 'fallback' strategy is provided by an X-ray study conducted by Putnam and Ringel (1976), in which pre- and post-production articulations were contrasted for subjects undergoing a trigeminal nerve block intended to eliminate somatosensory feedback from oral structures (including the anterior two-thirds of the tongue): they report that although neither subject used retroflex tongue shapes consistently in the control condition, in the nerve-block condition both subjects increased tongue bunching and retracted the location of their primary tongue constrictions, with acoustic changes described as minor and 'primarily nonphonemic' in nature (p. 247). Their results suggest that when confronted with loss of afferent feedback necessary for appropriate control of the tongue tip, these subjects were able to make use of a secondary production strategy relying less on tongue body/tip differentiation.

To summarize: fluent speakers of North American English produce /r/ with one or more qualitatively different tongue configurations; tune these configurations as needed via trading relations among articulators; and adapt readily to perturbation, sometimes by switching between configurations. In this work, we explore the ability of adult speakers to adjust their production of /r/ in reaction to a form of palatal perturbation likely to interfere with well-established articulatory habits. We anticipate the following range of responses: First, speakers may not compensate at all but instead continue to use their habitual patterns of articulation, though this would likely produce distinct differences in the acoustic output. Second, speakers may compensate through small 'trading relations' made to their preferred tongue configuration for /r/. For instance, they may move a retroflex tongue shape backwards along the palate, or use a more extreme form of lip rounding, thus maintaining a formant structure equivalent to their pre-perturbation production. A third possibility is that speakers may maintain equivalent acoustic patterns under perturbation by switching between alternative tongue configurations for /r/; in other words, behaviour similar to that shown for one speaker in Guenther et al. (1999), and for a number of speakers in Mielke et al. (in press), in which qualitatively different tongue configurations selected for articulatory efficiency in coproduction resulted in equivalent acoustic output. We hypothesize that all subjects may use trading relations, but those subjects who do switch configurations in their normal speech will also make use of these alternative postures when their normal articulatory habits are disrupted.

4.2 **Methods**

4.2.1 **Subjects**

Four adult native speakers of North American English participated in this study, two males and two females, with normal hearing and no apparent speech deficits. All spoke rhotic dialects with substantial third formant lowering in all /r/ contexts. Each subject participated in a speech production experiment in which their speech and articulatory movements were recorded.

4.2.2 **Materials**

Subjects were asked to produce the nonsense words 'ara' (/ara/), 'eeree' (/iri/), and 'ooroo' (/uru/) in isolation. For three of the subjects (F1, F2, M1) these were elicited in a randomized order within a larger study observing obstruents in VCV contexts (Shiller et al., 2006). The fourth subject (M2) was asked to produce randomly permuted stimuli drawn from these templates: VrV, VCrV, VrCV; where V was one of /a/, /i/, or /u/, and C was one of /b/, /d/, or /g/.

4.2.3 **Production conditions**

Each of these utterances was repeated ten times within four separate blocks (in the final block only five repetitions were elicited), with each block corresponding to a distinct perturbation/adaptation condition. In two blocks, subjects wore a custom-fitted palatal prosthesis with retaining ball clasps that followed the design of Baum and McFarland (1997): a buildup of dental acrylic was used to centre a perturbation over the alveolar ridge, measuring 6 mm at maximum, tapering to 1 mm in parallel with the premolar teeth (see Fig. 4.3). Three subjects wore prostheses constructed for an earlier study (Aasland et al., 2006); that worn by M2 was fabricated to the same specifications.

The experiments proceeded as follows:

Block 1: pre-perturbation, pre-adaptation (BASE)

Block 2: perturbed, pre-adaptation (PERT)

Block 3: perturbed, adapted (ADAPT)

Block 4: prosthesis removed, adapted (POST)

An intervening 20-min adaptation period during which subjects read aloud with prosthesis in place was interpolated between Blocks 2 and 3.

4.2.4 **Recordings**

An electromagnetic midsagittal articulometer (EMMA) system was used to transduce the movement of sensors attached to each subject's speech articulators (see Fig. 4.4). Three subjects were recorded using an AG200 system (Carstens Medizinelektronik); M2 was recorded using the

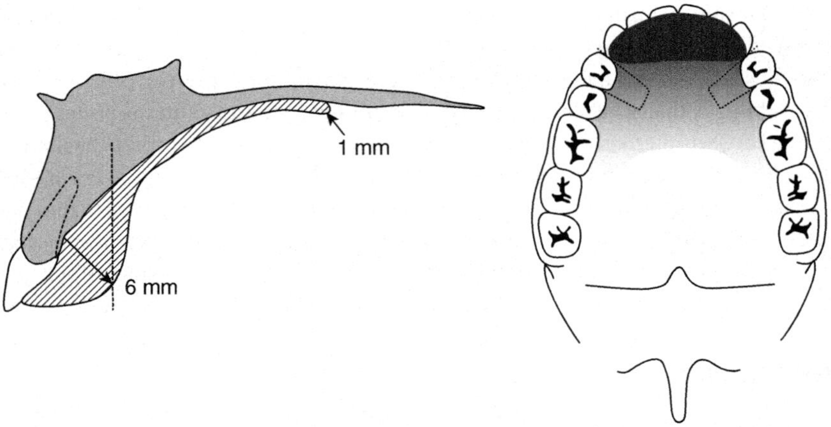

Fig. 4.3 Midsagittal and inferior views of palatal prosthesis (reproduced with permission from Baum and McFarland 1997; copyright 1997 Acoustical Society of America).

system of Perkell et al. (1992). Subject M2 had an especially large tongue, and so four sensors were placed in his case to maintain the approximate 12-mm separation between sensors used for the other subjects. Movement data were recorded at 200 Hz, and concurrently recorded audio at 16 kHz.

4.2.5 **Data analysis**

Raw EMMA voltage signals were first converted to positions over time on the midsagittal plane, and the reference sensors (N, I) were used to translate and rotate each position signal to a consistent maxillary frame of reference. For each token, a temporal measurement offset was determined by

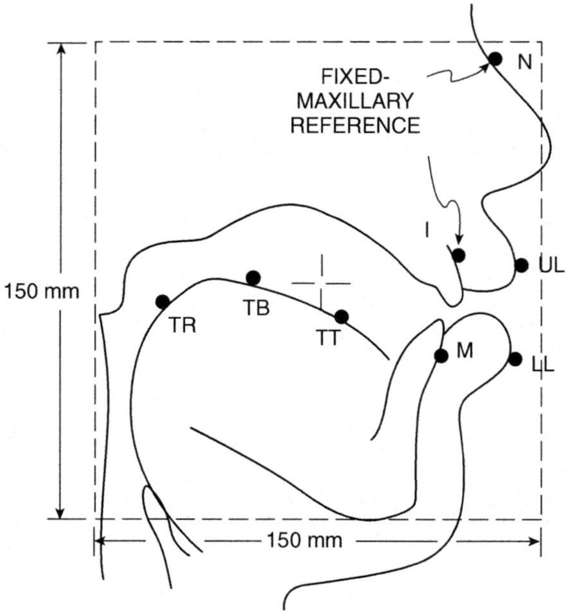

Fig. 4.4 EMMA sensor arrangement (adapted, with permission, from Perkell et al., 1992; copyright 1992 Acoustical Society of America).

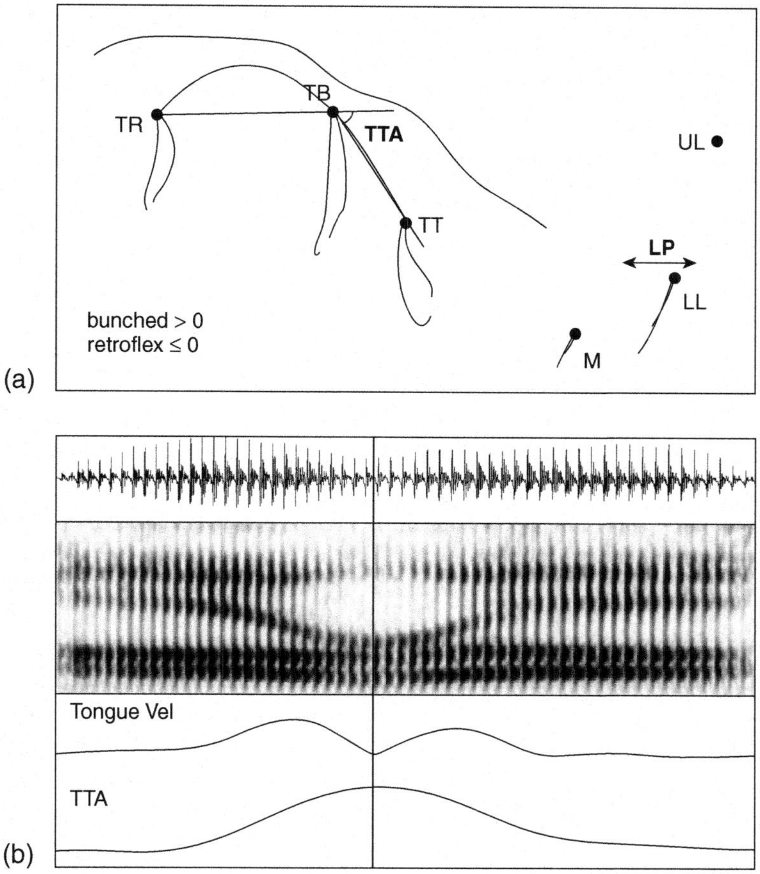

Fig. 4.5 A. Example token of unperturbed bunched shape /ara/ produced by subject M1 showing tongue tip angle measure (TTA) as defined on EMMA sensor measurements. Lip protrusion (LP) is characterized using horizontal position of lower lip. The tongue sensors are connected with a cubic spline, and the upper line shows a palatal trace. B. Corresponding temporal plot showing minimum tongue velocity measurement offset corresponding to /r/.

the point of minimum tongue velocity corresponding to /r/, with that velocity computed (as central-differenced Euclidean speed) across all tongue sensors (see Fig. 4.5).

Tongue configuration at that offset was characterized by the tongue tip angle (TTA), subtended by lines between sensors TR:TB and TB:TT (for subject M2, the midpoint between the two central sensors was used as 'TB'). By convention, negative TTA values were characterized as 'retroflex'; positive values as 'bunched.' Negative angles indicate that the TT sensor is raised towards the alveolar ridge relative to tongue body position (as captured by the TB and TR sensors). Conversely, if the angle formed by the line segments is positive, then the TT sensor is lowered relative to TB and TR, indicating a bunched tongue shape. Figure 4.6 shows examples of both tongue 'polarities' from a subject switching between configurations.

An additional measure of lip protrusion (LP) was obtained using the horizontal position of the lower lip sensor at the measurement offset, relative to the coordinate sensor I (upper incisor). Larger values for LP indicate greater lip protrusion. Formant values were evaluated using order-20 LPC evaluated on a 25-ms Hamming-filtered window centred on the measurement offset.

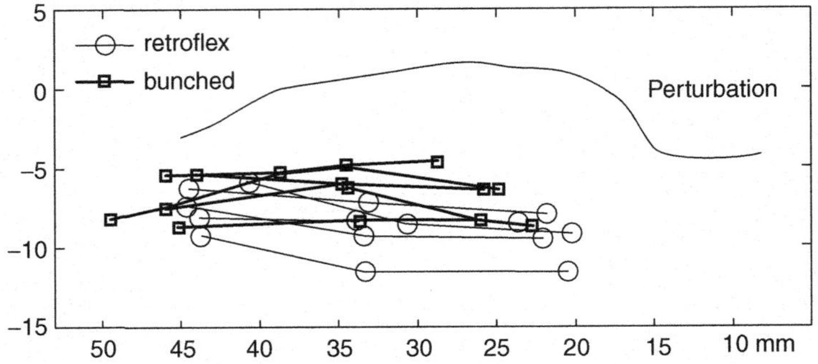

Fig. 4.6 Line segments connecting tongue sensors measured at velocity minimum associated with /r/ for individual tokens of subject F1 producing /uru/ (ADAPT block: perturbation in place and post-adaptation). The upper line shows a palatal trace.

The resulting measures obtained for each token were thus TTA (measured in degrees), LP (measured in mm), and F3 (measured in Hz).

4.3 **Results**

4.3.1 **Articulation**

As a first step in understanding subject response to perturbation, consider Fig. 4.7, which shows the distribution of TTA measures by vowel context, subject, and condition. The mean value is shown with 95% confidence intervals. In those instances where a subject produced both bunched and retroflex examples for the same stimulus (e.g., M1 PERT), distributions for each have been computed separately.

It is immediately apparent that /r/ production is idiosyncratic. As noted above, cross-speaker differences in tongue configurations for /r/ are well documented. It has also been reported that while a speaker's preferred tongue shape is typically consistent for a given phonetic context, many speakers alternate between different configurations depending on context. Data obtained from these subjects in the pre-perturbation BASE condition support both observations. Speaker F1, for instance, uses a retroflex tongue configuration for the /ara/ vowel context (median TTA = −6.8°), a strongly bunched configuration for /iri/ (29.2), and a less strongly bunched configuration in the /uru/ context (9.8). Speaker F2 uses a bunched configuration for all of the vowel conditions, although the degree of bunching is much more strongly marked for the /iri/ context (63.5 vs. 38.1, 47.5 for the other vowels). Speaker M1 also prefers a bunched configuration for all vowel contexts, but he reserves the greatest amount of bunching for /ara/ (49.1 vs. 42.9, 35.6). Speaker M2 however is highly consistent, using approximately the same degree of bunching for all vowel contexts (median values between 33° and 35° for all vowels).

Whatever their preferred pattern, all of the subjects are consistent in their use of either retroflex or bunched tongue configuration across the ten repetitions of the BASE condition. The only exception to that generalization comes from subjects F1 and M1, who each produce nine bunched and one retroflex productions in the /uru/ context. It is notable that for each the single retroflex production came within the first few trials after placement of the sensors, when subjects were presumably still adapting to their presence (itself a form of perturbation).

Responses to perturbation (PERT condition) were also idiosyncratic. Two subjects (F2, M1) show a mix of productions including retroflexion despite their initial preference for

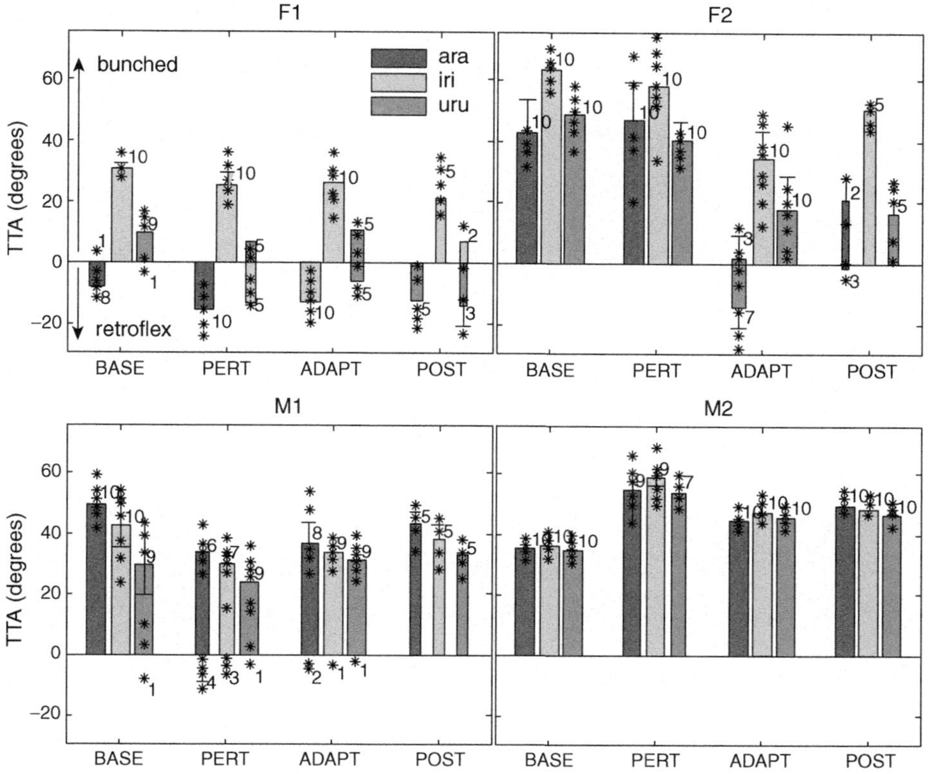

Fig. 4.7 Distribution of TTA results, by vowel context, subject, and condition, showing 95% C.I.s. Separate confidence intervals were computed for 'retroflex' (TTA< = 0) distributions where appropriate. Individual values plotted as asterisks. The width of each bar is proportional to the number of repetitions for that condition.

bunched configurations. Subjects F1 and M2 react to the loss of oral tract volume by moving the tongue tip away from the alveolar perturbation, which has the effect of enhancing their preferred production strategy by either increasing retroflexion (F1) or degree of bunching (M2). In all cases the general trend was towards increased variability. A non-parametric Friedman's test for column effects (BASE vs. PERT conditions) adjusting for possible row (vowel, subject) effects confirms a significant response ($p < 0.05$) to the perturbation measured on TTA (see Table 4.1).

Table 4.1 Friedman's test for column effects (BASE vs. PERT conditions) adjusting for possible row (vowel, subject) effects on TTA. The null hypothesis is that the palatal perturbation has no effect on TTA, rejected here with $p < 0.05$

Source	**SS**	**df**	**MS**	**Chi-square**	**p > Chi-sq**
Columns	147.3	1	147.3	4.209	0.040
Interaction	3303.9	11	300.4	–	–
Error	4526.8	216	20.1	–	–
Total	7978.0	239	–	–	–

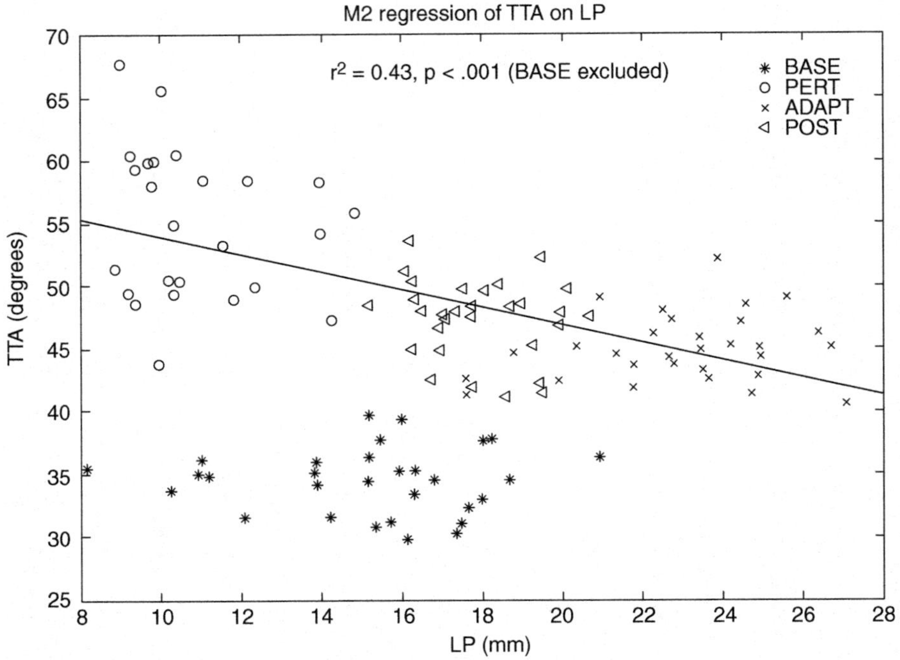

Fig. 4.8 Regression of TTA on LP for subject M2. Excluding the initial uncorrelated BASE condition, TTA and LP show a significant trading relation following the introduction of the perturbation.

Clear patterns of adaptation (ADAPT condition) were suggested only in the responses of M2. After increasing his overall degree of bunchiness and variability in the PERT condition, both declined after adaptation, though not to the initial baseline values, and remained higher in the final POST perturbation condition. LP for this subject, initially uncorrelated with TTA, showed a significant ($r^2 = 0.43$, $p < .001$) trading relation with degree of bunching following introduction of the perturbation (see Fig. 4.8). F2 showed reduced TTA overall in the ADAPT condition, including retroflex productions for the first time.

4.3.2 **Acoustics**

As noted above, previous studies have failed to find any consistent differences in formant patterns across the different tongue configurations for /r/. Of interest here is the extent to which subjects control their acoustic productions for /r/ in response to a perturbation that disrupts their habitual articulatory production, particularly when they show a mix of qualitatively different tongue configurations in response. Figure 4.9 shows F3 for /r/ scatterplotted against the TTA of the tongue configuration that produced it, superimposed on a histogram of TTA values.

The first point to be noted is the lack of correlation between F3 values and tongue configuration types. Certainly different speakers produce F3 values in different parts of the formant space, and Hagiwara (1995) has shown that productions of F3 may vary by 500 Hz or more. However, these different minimum F3 values are equally likely to occur for retroflex or bunched tongue configuration patterns: acoustically, the two are indistinguishable. This was confirmed by a repeated measures ANOVA, which showed no significance on the possible effects of Tongue Polarity (TTA grouped into retroflex/bunched levels) on measured F3 values (see Table 4.2).

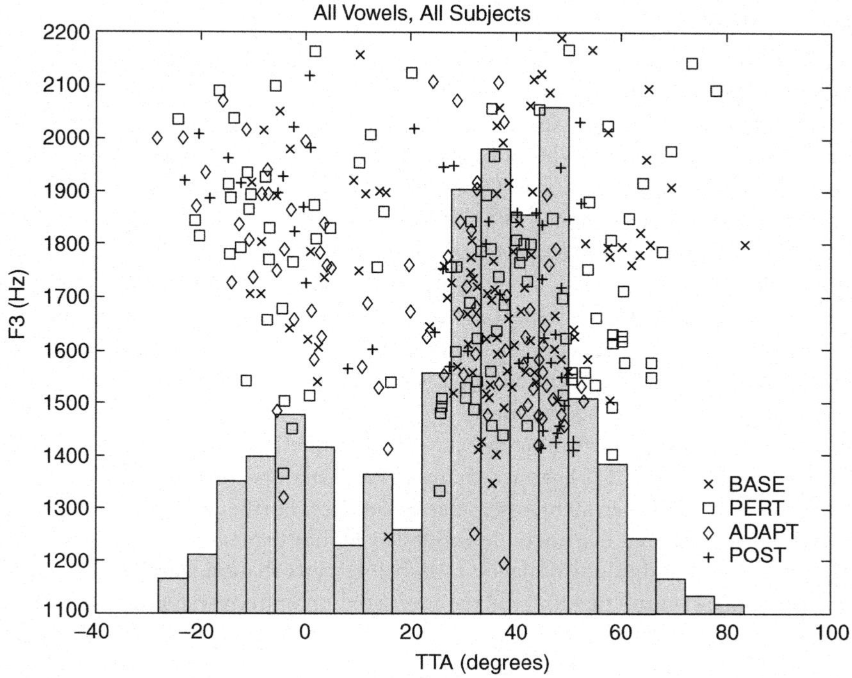

Fig. 4.9 Scatterplot of TTA with corresponding F3, superimposed on a histogram of TTA values, showing no effect of tongue configuration on acoustics. Note the bimodal distribution of TTA.

Table 4.2 Repeated measures one-way ANOVA testing for an effect of independent variable Tongue Polarity [retroflex,bunched] classification on observed F3 measures. The percentage of variability in F3 associated with Polarity (eta squared) is 8.54; the null hypothesis (that tongue configuration has no effect on F3) is sustained

Source	SS	df	MS	F	P
Subjects	3703392.0	3	1234464.0	0.922	0.5262
Polarity	374875.2	1	374875.2	0.280	0.633
Error	4017062.0	3	1339020.7	–	–
Total	8095329.2	203		–	–

These results confirm for within-subject data the results of previous work on between-subject data, namely, that the perceptually salient third formant values for /r/ produced using retroflex and bunched tongue shapes are indistinguishable.

Secondly, Fig. 4.9 illustrates that there is a clear bimodal distribution in tongue tip angle. This indicates that subjects are not using the full continuum of possible tongue configurations between bunched and retroflexed postures. Rather, the results show that subjects select *either* a bunched or a retroflex configuration, with variations for tuning purposes within those categories presumably subject to the kinds of trading relations illustrated in Fig. 4.8.

4.4 Discussion

The results from this chapter point to several conclusions. First, it appears that subjects react to palatal perturbation differently in different vowel contexts. For subjects who switched between tongue configuration types, one subject (F1) showed the most extreme behaviour for /uru/, another subject (F2) showed the most extreme behaviour for /ara/, and a third subject (M1) switched between configuration types for all three vowel contexts. As noted above, previous observations (Delattre and Freeman 1968; Westbury et al., 1998; Mielke et al., in press) have shown that normal speakers of North American English produce /r/ using a variety of tongue configurations. The subjects in this study appear to be a typical sample; in the BASE condition, only subjects F2 and M2 show the same tongue configuration for all vowel contexts, while subject F1 shows retroflex only for /ara/ and M1 shows retroflex only for /uru/. Given this level of variability across subjects in the BASE condition, it is not surprising that subjects in this study would show idiosyncratic patterns of adaptation.

Second, different subjects have different patterns of adaptation to the presence of the prosthesis; some subjects (F1, M1, M2) show a change in articulatory behaviour immediately while others react later in the experiment, after adaptation (F2). Further, when they did react to the prosthesis, subjects showed considerable variability within context and condition. Given our data from the BASE condition, we suggest that, before perturbation, subject F1 belongs to the Mielke et al. (in press) group that uses tongue configuration in free variation, subjects F2 and M1 belong to the group that uses different configurations in different phonetic contexts, while subject M2 belongs to the group that uses a single configuration in all contexts. (Note that their BASE data show that subjects F2 and M1 have patterns of switching according to vowel context.)

Of the four subjects, only three (F1, F2, and M1) switched between retroflex and bunched configurations for at least one condition and one vowel context. It is notable that these are the same subjects who showed signs of using both configurations in the BASE condition. Only one subject, M2, was consistent in terms of tongue configuration under all conditions and vowel contexts; however, he did increase the amount of bunching under perturbation. It may not be a coincidence that of the three subjects who switched, two were female and one was an average-sized male. In contrast, subject M2 had the largest vocal tract of all the subjects (as well as the largest tongue). Because the prosthesis was made to the same dimensions for each subject, it presumably took up more of the available room, and represented a greater disruption, in the vocal tracts of the smaller subjects. It is possible that these subjects reacted by switching because the proportionately greater disruption forced them into using a secondary strategy. In contrast, subject M2 was able to maintain a consistent tongue configuration (while adjusting his TTA somewhat in the direction of greater bunching) because the prosthesis to him represented a smaller disruption.

The amount of individual variation in subject behaviour found in this study across context and conditions, although considerable, is consistent with previous findings in studies using a palatal prosthesis (Baum and McFarland 2000). In general, subjects showed a greater degree of switching behaviour as a result of perturbation. Two of the three subjects who switched configurations showed more of that behaviour in the early perturbation conditions, PERT and ADAPT. In contrast, subject F2 changed her degree of tongue bunching in the two prosthesis conditions, PERT and ADAPT, but switched from bunched to retroflex only for /ara/ in the ADAPT condition. Additionally, for any one context/condition combination subjects used a retroflex configuration for some trials and a bunched configuration for other trials. In other words, when subjects switched between retroflex and bunched configurations, they did so inconsistently.

These results show that the presence of a prosthesis does affect subject articulatory behaviour. In fact, the generalization seems to be that subject behaviour becomes more variable – that is, more labile – under perturbation. Subjects appear to be experimenting with alternate methods of producing /r/, and this experimental behaviour appears to continue for some subjects into the ADAPT and POST conditions, though for these subjects it may be the case that insufficient time and practice were available for effective adaptation. At the same time, the alternative tongue configurations used by the subjects do not cover the articulatory space between retroflex and bunched configurations in a continuous fashion. Instead, there is a bimodal distribution of tongue tip angle (TTA), such that most tongue configurations occur with a tongue tip angle over 20° or under 5°. These results confirm the hypothesis that subjects have two distinct strategies for tongue configuration while producing /r/.

An additional point concerns the lack of an effect of tongue configuration on the produced F3 minimum. As noted above, investigators have consistently reported that the different tongue configurations used by speakers for North American /r/ show indistinguishable acoustic profiles, at least for the first three formants. Further, as Guenther et al. report, the formant values at F3 minima during /r/ are consistently maintained over different phonetic contexts by a complex combination of adjustments to lip position, constriction size, and constriction location. Our data show a similar picture; even in the PERT and ADAPT conditions, when subjects appear to be experimenting with alternative tongue configurations, there is no corresponding bimodal distribution of F3 minima to match the bimodal distribution of TTA. A notable aspect of the Guenther et al.'s (1999) paper was the finding that the F3 minimum value remained consistent between retroflex and bunched configurations. However, in the said paper, only one subject appeared to switch tongue configuration, and in only one phonetic context. Our data include a wider variety of subjects producing a wider variety of tongue configurations in a wider variety of phonetic contexts. Thus, our results provide strong support for the notion that speakers (1) have a repertoire of articulatory strategies for /r/ (including the use of qualitatively different tongue configurations) that produce equivalent acoustics in normal speech, and (2) call on these strategies in the face of articulatory perturbations.

What might be the nature of these articulatory strategies, and how would they develop? On the one hand, studies of trading relations show that speakers readily make small, mutually offsetting adjustments as needed when tuning a basic production plan to resolve competing demands on the articulators. However, given the articulatory complexity of /r/, it may be that the possible range of such adjustments for some speakers is insufficient to comfortably adapt to all contexts. Instead, such speakers prefer to make a wholesale change to the basic plan when that alternative can be more readily adapted to a particular production context. We suggest that speakers normally acquire such alternative production strategies during the exploratory period associated with childhood, and that a likely pathway is through learning to coproduce /r/ in clusters. As an

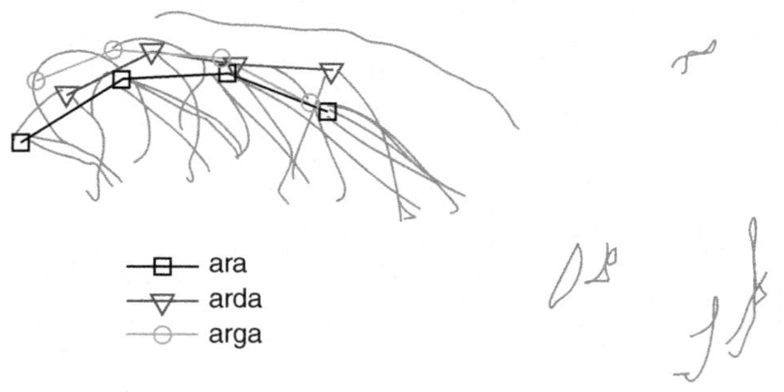

Fig. 4.10 Subject M2 productions of /ar(C)a/. The upper line shows a palatal trace. Note the tendency towards retroflexion in the 'arda' context.

example, Fig. 10.10 shows sensor positions at the F3 minimum associated with /r/ contrasting representative examples of /ara/, /arda/, and /arga/ productions from subject M2. Although this subject did not switch from his preferred bunched tongue configuration in the VCV productions of his experiment, he nonetheless shows clear signs of retroflexion in his production of /arda/.

Coarticulatory experiences of this sort may be the mechanism whereby subjects learn to produce and continue to maintain alternate tongue configurations for /r/, although (as noted above, and as we found in the BASE condition), speakers may or may not choose to incorporate both sets of allophones into their normal articulatory habits. We propose, however, that the option of using an alternative tongue configuration remains 'in storage' and available for use when changes in the articulatory environment disrupt normal speaking habits. In this view, when the presence of a perturbation leads speakers to explore a new set of articulatory habits, the ability to revisit alternative production strategies for /r/ makes the task of adaptation both easier and, on 'least effort' principles, more efficient.

References

Aasland, WA, Baum, SR and McFarland, DH (2006). Electropalatographic, acoustic, and perceptual data on adaptation to a palatal perturbation. *Journal of the Acoustical Society of America,* 119(4), 2372–81.

Baum, SR and McFarland, DH (1997). The development of speech adaptation to an artificial palate. *Journal of the Acoustical Society of America,* 102(4), 2353–59.

Baum, SR and McFarland, DH (2000). Individual differences in speech adaptation to an artificial palate. *Journal of the Acoustical Society of America,* 107(6), 3572–5.

Clark, CE, Schwarz, IE and Blakeley, RW (1993). The removable R-appliance as a practice device to facilitate correct production of /r/. *American Journal of Speech-Language Pathology,* 2, 84–92.

Delattre, P and Freeman, D (1968). A dialect study of American R's by X-ray motion picture. *Linguistics,* 44, 29–68.

Folkins, JW and Abbs, JH (1975). Lip and jaw motor control during speech: responses to resistive loading of the jaw. *Journal of Speech and Hearing Research,* 18(1), 207–19.

Gomi, H, Honda, M, Ito, T and Murano, EZ (2002). Compensatory articulation during bilabial fricative production by regulating muscle stiffness. *Journal of Phonetics,* 30, 261–79.

Guenther, FH, Espy-Wilson, CY, Boyce, SE, Matthies, ML, Zandipour, M and Perkell, JS (1999). Articulatory tradeoffs reduce acoustic variability during American English /r/ production. *Journal of the Acoustical Society of America,* 105(5), 2854–65.

Hagiwara, R (1995). Acoustic realizations of American English /r/ as produced by women and men. *UCLA Working Papers in Phonetics,* 90, 1–187.

Hamlet, S and Stone, M (1978). Compensatory alveolar production induced by wearing a dental prosthesis. *Journal of Phonetics,* 6, 227–48.

Hoffman, PR, Schuckers, GH and Daniloff, RG (1980). Developmental trends in correct /r/ articulation as a function of allophone type. *Journal of Speech and Hearing Research,* 23(4), 746–56.

Jones, JA and Munhall, KG (2003). Learning to produce speech with an altered vocal tract: the role of auditory feedback. *Journal of the Acoustical Society of America,* 113(1), 532–43.

Kelso, JA, Tuller, B, Vatikiotis-Bateson, E and Fowler, CA (1984). Functionally specific articulatory cooperation following jaw perturbations during speech: evidence for coordinative structures. *Journal of Experimental Psychology,* 10(6), 812–32.

Lindblom, B, Lubker, J and Gay, T (1979). Formant frequencies of some fixed-mandible vowels and a model of speech motor programming by predictive simulation. *Journal of Phonetics,* 7, 147–61.

Masaki, S, Tiede, MK, Honda, K, Shimada, Y, Fujimoto, I, Nakamura, Y and Ninomiya, N (1999). MRI-based speech production study using a synchronized sampling method. *Journal of the Acoustical Society of Japan (E),* 20(5), 375–9.

Mielke, J, Baker, A and Archangeli, D (in press). Variability and homogeneity in American English /r/ allophony and /s/ retraction. In C. Fougeron, B. Kühnert, M. D'Imperio and N. Vallée (eds.), *Variation, Detail, and Representation (LabPhon 10)*. Mouton de Gruyter, Berlin.

Perkell, JS, Cohen, MH, Svirsky, MA, Matthies, ML, Garabieta, I and Jackson, MT (1992). Electromagnetic midsagittal articulometer systems for transducing speech articulatory movements. *Journal of the Acoustical Society of America*, 92(6), 3078–96.

Perkell, JS, Matthies, ML, Svirsky, MA and Jordan, MI (1993). Trading relations between tongue-body raising and lip rounding in production of the vowel /u/: a pilot 'motor equivalence' study. *Journal of the Acoustical Society of America*, 93(5), 2948–61.

Putnam, A and Ringel, R (1976). A cineradiographic study of articulation in two talkers with temporarily induced oral sensory deprivation. *Journal of Speech and Hearing Research*, 19, 247–66.

Riordan, CJ (1977). Control of vocal-tract length in speech. *Journal of the Acoustical Society of America*, 62(4), 998–1002.

Savariaux, C, Perrier, P and Orliaguet, JP (1995). Compensation strategies for the perturbation of the rounded vowel [u] using a lip tube: a study of the control space in speech production. *Journal of the Acoustical Society of America*, 98(5), 2428–42.

Secord, WA, Boyce, SE, Donohue, JS, Fox, RA and Shine, RE (2007). *Eliciting Sounds, Techniques and Strategies for Clinicians*. Singular, New York.

Shiller, DM, Tiede, MK and Gracco, VL (2006). Adaptation of speech production to palatal perturbation: kinematic analysis using electromagnetometry. *Journal of the Acoustical Society of America*, 119(5), 3302 (A).

Shriberg, LD and Kent, RD (1995). *Clinical Phonetics*. Allyn & Bacon, Boston.

Smit, AB (1993). Phonologic error distributions in the Iowa-Nebraska Articulation Norms Project: consonant singletons. *Journal of Speech and Hearing Research*, 36(3), 533–47.

Tiede, MK, Boyce, SE, Holland, CK and Choe, KA (2004). A new taxonomy of American English /r/ using MRI and ultrasound. *Journal of the Acoustical Society of America*, 115(5), 2633 (A).

Westbury, J, Hashi, M and Lindstom, M (1998). Differences among speakers in lingual articulation for American English /r/. *Speech Communication*, 26, 203–26.

Zhou, X, Espy-Wilson, CY, Boyce, S, Tiede, M, Holland, C and Choe, A (2008). A magnetic resonance imaging-based articulatory and acoustic study of 'retroflex' and 'bunched' American English /r/. *Journal of the Acoustical Society of America*, 123(6), 4466–81.

Section 2

Genetics and neurology

Chapter 5

Brain imaging in children

Soo-Eun Chang and Christy L. Ludlow

Abstract

During the past decade, many studies have been conducted on normal and disordered pediatric populations using brain imaging techniques once thought to be challenging for application in infants and children. In this chapter, we review the potential and shortcomings of techniques used to study brain anatomy and function in young children, focusing on new knowledge regarding the brain basis for normal speech and language development, as well as developmental speech disorders such as stuttering. We discuss the current understanding to date based on these studies, and emphasize the need to examine young children when considering developmental disorders.

Recently published functional and structural MRI studies on children and adolescents who stutter replicate some of the findings reported from adult studies, pointing to trait-related deficits that may relate to the basis of developing stuttering. On the other hand, other deficits found in adults have not been replicated in children, indicating that some differences may represent changes in brain structure and function as a consequence of a lifetime of stuttering. These studies provide several new hypotheses for structural and functional deficits relating to stuttering. Research in younger children closer to stuttering onset is needed to address these hypotheses.

5.1 **Introduction**

The past decade has seen rapid growth in the use of noninvasive neuroimaging techniques applied to examine infants and children. These techniques can capture structural and functional brain development *in vivo*, and have the potential for elucidating neurological correlates of typical and atypical speech, language, and cognitive development during early life. Despite the multitude of practical and technical challenges to neuroimaging research in children, such research is crucial. The adult brain represents the end result of the complex interplay among genetics, environment, behaviour, and development. Hence, functional and structural brain organization of speech and language skills may well differ between adults and children. That is, findings in adults may not be directly applicable to children.

One obvious example is the difficulty in trying to understand the basis of a developmental speech disorder by studying adults. In such cases, interpretations of findings are confounded, as adults who have lived with a disorder throughout life may have altered brain function and/or anatomy as a result. Namely, brain structural and functional differences may be due to compensatory behaviour in reaction to the disorder as much as due to the disorder itself. To clarify this issue, and better understand differences in functional and structural development between typically and atypically developing children, it is best to study children as close to the onset of symptom presentation as possible, and follow them longitudinally, gathering both behavioural and neuroimaging data to better understand the basis of the disorder.

In this chapter we selectively review noninvasive neuroimaging techniques that have been applied to paediatric research, with a focus on magnetic resonance imaging (MRI). Although positron emission tomography (PET) is another neuroimaging technique that has been widely used in adults, it involves measuring brain activity by injecting radioactive tracers into the bloodstream and examining its flow, metabolism, or receptor binding. PET is not further discussed here, as it involves exposure to ionizing radiation, and so its use in paediatric research is limited to cases with life-threatening disorders.

This is not an exhaustive review of the techniques or of brain development itself, as such reviews are already available (Paterson et al., 2006; Paus et al., 2001; Sowell et al., 2004a; Sowell et al. 2004b; Thompson et al., 2005; Toga et al., Thompson, and Sowell 2006). Rather we focus on structural MRI and functional magnetic resonance imaging (fMRI), that are increasingly being used to examine brain structure and function in children with typical and atypical speech and language development. Notably, we focus on MRI techniques but not on EEG and ERP methods, although the latter are much more established techniques that have been widely used to study infants and children (Benasich et al., 2006; Bernal et al., 2000; Davies et al., 2004; Licht et al., 1988; Rivera-Gaxiola et al., 2007; Sanders et al., 2006; Shafer et al., 1998; Silva-Pereyra et al., 2005). Application of structural MRI and fMRI in paediatric research, however, have begun much more recently and will likely continue to provide spatially detailed information on neural bases of normal and disordered speech and language development during childhood. We highlight findings from some of these studies and address the potential for their further use in studying children with developmental speech-language disorders. Finally, we summarize recent MRI findings on children who stutter, which suggest that structural and functional differences found in adults who stutter may be the result of both the effect of stuttering and the brain basis for the disorder.

5.2 Methods for studying the structural development of the brain

5.2.1 Structural MRI

Structural MRI has been used extensively to study infants and children. Principles of MRI and the basis of its signals can be found elsewhere (Paus et al., 2001). For structural MRI, scanning sequences that allow maximum contrast between white and grey matter are used to allow for separate quantification of white and grey matter tissue volumes in the brain.

The smallest volume element of a structural MRI image is a voxel, a box-shaped volume on a three-dimensional grid. Methods of analyses are either manual or automated; such as manual tracing of selective regions of interest (ROIs); automated voxel-wise analysis on a whole-brain basis, referred to as voxel-based morphometry (VBM); or computational anatomical methods that measure gyral/sulcal complexity or cortical thickness across individuals and time (Sowell et al., 2002, 2004a; Thompson et al., 2005).

In manual tracing, high-resolution MRI scans of each individual are taken without warping or stretching brain images to a standard template, so that measurements can be made from individuals' original brain images. Pre-selected ROIs are traced in each brain, and measurements such as length, area, and volume are collected and compared between individuals or groups (Fig. 5.1).

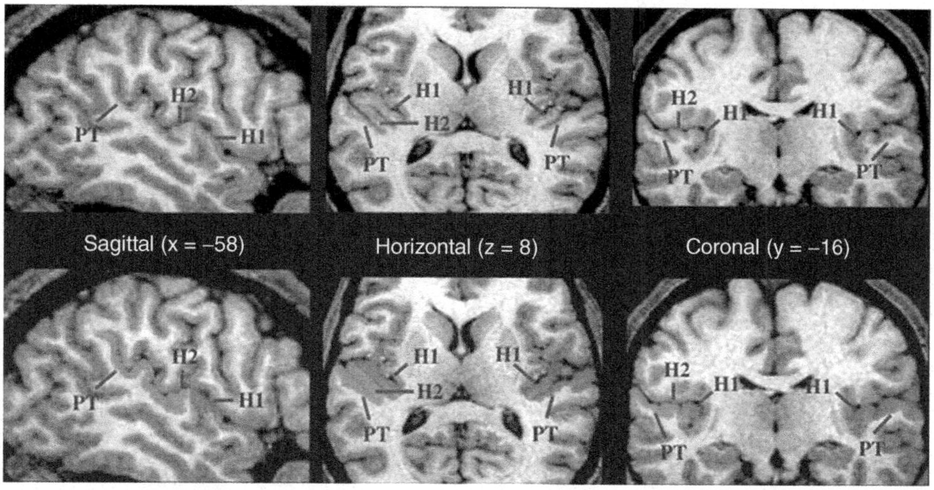

Fig. 5.1 Manual identification and labelling of auditory regions Heschl's gyrus (HG) and planum temporale (PT) (Dorsaint-Pierre et al., 2006. Figure reprinted here with permission).

Manual tracing is clearly beneficial in cases where regional anatomy is highly variable across individuals. Although there is structural variability among adults, variability within the same age range may be greater in children's brains. Manual measures, however, can be affected by subjective bias, requiring inter- and/or intra-reliability checks between skilled neuroanatomists. In addition, by focusing on only a few regions of interest, other regions that may be important could be missed. When studies examine only few brain regions, it is challenging to compare results across studies. Despite these challenges, manual tracing remains a powerful technique, and can be used in conjunction with more automated, whole-brain-based methods that complement each other (Dorsaint-Pierre 2006).

Whole-brain image processing methods include the following steps: acquiring a high-resolution MRI scan (Fig. 5.2A), stripping off the skull from the image to extract the brain (Fig. 5.2B), registration or warping of an individual brain to a standard template so that each brain is put into a common space (Fig. 5.2C), segmentation of tissues into grey matter, white matter, and cerebrospinal fluid (CSF) (Fig. 5.2D), spatial smoothing (Fig. 5.2E), and voxel-wise statistical analysis using a general linear model (Fig. 5.2F). Each step is achieved using automated algorithms provided by freely available imaging analysis software such as FSL (http://www.fmrib.ox.ac.uk/fsl/) or SPM (http://www.fil.ion.ucl.ac.uk/spm/).

Voxel-based morphometry is an automated whole-brain analysis method that provides unbiased, objective whole-brain group comparisons of grey and white matter on a voxel-by-voxel basis. When studying paediatric brains, it is preferable to either use a study-specific template based on the study participants, or a paediatric template (Wilke et al., 2002) based on subjects with comparable ages rather than an adult-based template, in order to minimize possible errors in normalization. The normalization step can further be optimized by separately normalizing segmented grey matter and white matter to their respective templates (Fig. 5.3B) rather than just doing a normalization on the whole brain (Fig. 5.3A). This is incorporated in the optimized version of VBM, which may be beneficial when studying younger brains. Adding a 'modulation' step corrects for any changes in absolute volume due to spatial normalization. During normalization, smaller or bigger brains undergo different degrees of stretching and shrinking in different regions (i.e., smaller areas could be stretched to two times their original volume after normalization),

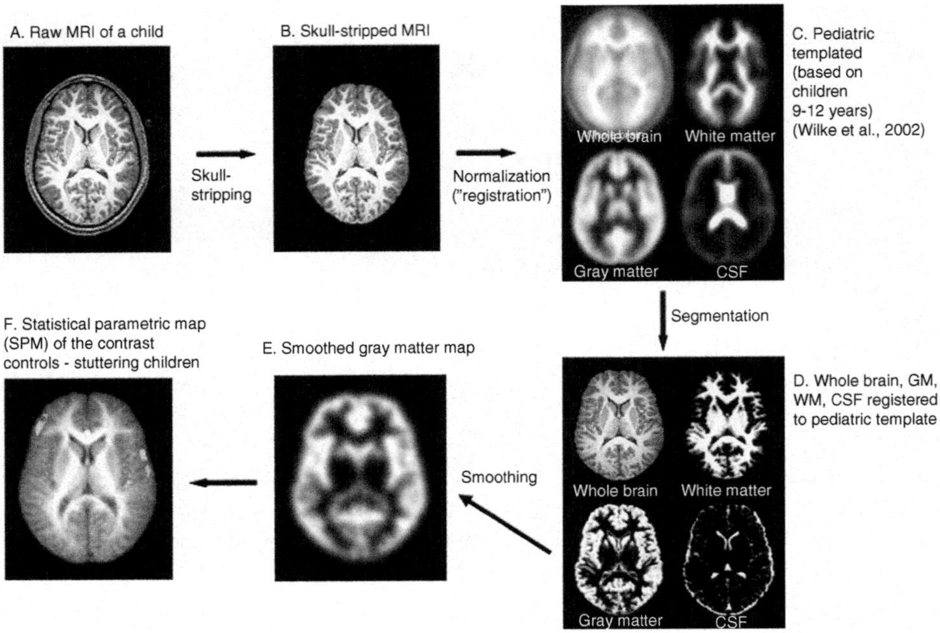

Fig. 5.2 Processing pipeline for automated, whole-brain structural brain analysis. A high-resolution structural scan acquired from an individual ('raw' image) (A) undergoes skull stripping using an automated algorithm (Smith 2002) (B), followed by a normalization step that involves a robust and automated linear (affine) registration onto a standard template (Jenkinson and Smith 2001). Here, a whole-brain paediatric template and segmented grey matter (GM), white matter (WM), and cerebrospinal fluid (CSF) template maps are shown (Wilke et al., 2002; Wilke et al., 2003) (C). In standard VBM processing, raw images are normalized to the whole-brain template, followed by segmentation into the three tissue types. In the case of optimized VBM analysis, raw images are first segmented and then normalized onto their respective tissue templates (see Fig. 5.3) (D). Spatial smoothing with a Gaussian linear filter (typically 6–12 mm), which transforms the grey (or white) matter segmented output to represent 'gray matter density' (proportion of GM to non-GM) (in the case of non-modulated data), and also alleviates possible effects of misregistration (E). Voxel-wise statistical analysis can involve the general linear model (GLM), which models group membership, using any relevant covariates (i.e., age, handedness), with appropriate contrasts set up to compare the groups. Here, the contrast between controls and children who stutter (control-stutter) in grey matter volume are shown overlaid on an average brain based on all subjects' normalized brains (F) (from Chang et al., 2008).

which can distort the original volume information. Multiplying the normalized images by their relative volume before and after spatial normalization compensates for this distortion and restores volume information. Hence, grey or white matter differences detected using unmodulated VBM data represent regional differences in grey or white matter density, or concentration. However, differences found through modulated VBM reflect differences in absolute volume (Ashburner and Friston 2000; Good et al., 2001; Mechelli et al., 2005).

One comparison of manual and automated methods found comparable results when using either method (Maguire et al., 2003). Others, however, found differences between the two; the manual method was better able to detect volumetric differences in regions with large anatomical variability, while whole-brain automated methods were better able to detect differences in more

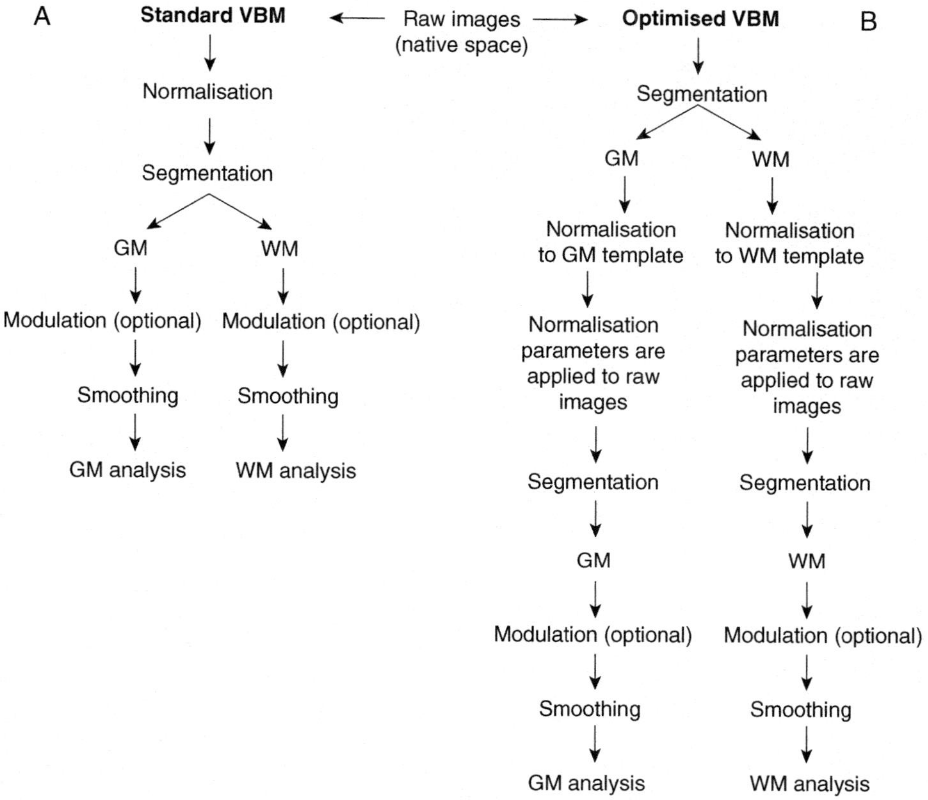

Fig. 5.3 Diagram of standard (A) and optimized (B) versions of voxel-based morphometry (Mechelli et al., 2005. Figure reprinted here with permission). See text and Fig. 5.2.

homogeneous structures (Eckert et al., 2005; Tisserand et al., 2004). Manual and automated methods provide complementary information, and the choice between the two will depend on the purpose of the study. If there are no clear hypotheses regarding a specific region of the brain, more automated methods such as VBM can provide an initial screen for group differences. On the other hand, if a specific structure is of interest, manual tracing may be more suitable, although it is much more labour intensive and cannot be used in studies involving large numbers of subjects.

Computational anatomy presents as a solution for studying larger populations without sacrificing information on anatomical variability (Thompson et al., 2004). To examine differences in the cortex associated with development, aging, disease, and heritability, advanced mathematical methods that model the structural variability of the brain are applied to large populations. This involves creating a three-dimensional cortical surface model for each individual, which represents their cortical surface anatomy in detail. Each individual's brain is then put into a coordinate frame for comparing structural measures across individuals. This is followed by cortical pattern matching, to ensure that anatomical landmarks such as cortical sulci will occur in the same coordinate across subjects. Cortical pattern matching involves manually defining each subject's major sulcal curves and using these as anchor points when warping one brain to another, matching sulcal features exactly. In this way, an average brain can be created to serve as a group template, which retains anatomical features that are common to individuals in a group. Relative to this average brain, individual anatomical differences in gyral patterns, cortical complexity,

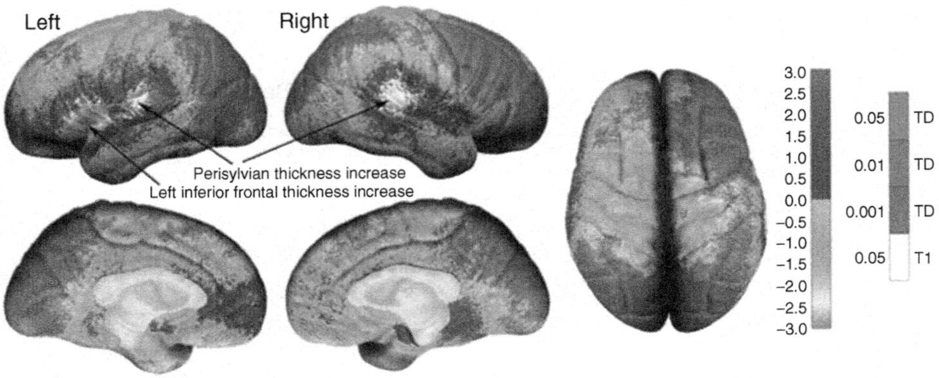

Fig. 5.4 Longitudinal mapping of cortical thickness changes in children between 5 years and 11 years of age. Colour bar to the left shows colour coding corresponding to *t* values at each cortical surface point, and significance values are overlaid in shades of red (significant thickness decreases [TD] and increases [TI]) represented in the colour bar to the right (Sowell et al., 2004. Figure reprinted with permission). (See Plate section).

cortical pattern asymmetry, cortical thickness, and cortical density can be computed. Correlations are then computed between these measures and age, and/or clinical symptoms, etc. (Fig. 5.4) (for more detail on this analysis technique, see Thompson et al., 2004).

In the practical sense, structural MRI imaging is conducted while the child is at rest using procedures to put the child at ease, such as showing favourite videos during scanning. When measures are used to minimize head movement, it is possible to acquire high quality data. In any neuroimaging procedure, sufficient preparation steps are critical to ensure that the child is comfortable about participation. This may require several visits to the MRI facility during which both the child and parent could be exposed to the sights and sounds of the scanner, and if available, using a mock scanner for practice sessions. Several research groups have successfully scanned large groups of young children with such training, with over a 50% success rate in healthy children as young as five years of age, and higher success in older children (Wilke et al., 2003).

5.2.2 Diffusion tensor imaging (DTI) and white matter tractography

Diffusion tensor imaging uses an imaging sequence that is sensitized to the movement of water molecules (Stejskal and Tanner 1965). This sequence tags water molecules and follows their movement in three-dimensional space, which is useful for imaging white matter structure. This is because water moves preferentially in a direction parallel to fatty substances such as myelin and axonal membranes (Fig. 5.5A). By acquiring multiple images sensitized to the movement of water in different directions, the magnitude and directionality of water movement in three-dimensional space can be quantified to examine white matter at a microstructural scale across the whole brain (Le Bihan 2003). The main parameters derived from diffusion weighted images are fractional anisotropy (FA) (Fig. 5.5B) and mean diffusivity (MD) (Fig. 5.5C), which reflect the directionality and magnitude of water diffusion, respectively. FA reflects the degree to which water diffusion is preferential to one direction, independent of the overall water diffusion coefficient. Values can range from 0, corresponding to isotropic diffusion that is equal in all directions, to 1, indicating anisotropic diffusion. FA values closer to 0 are found in regions where there is less myelination, relating to maturation, axonal loss in disease, or regions where there are many fibre crossings. FA values closer to 1 are found in highly myelinated, uniformly oriented and coherent fibre bundles

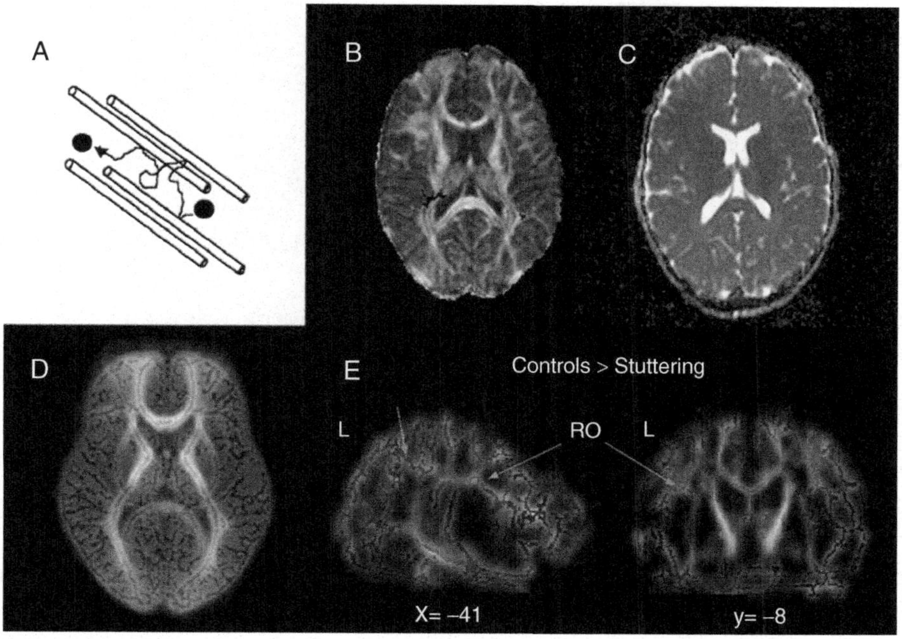

Fig. 5.5 A. Schematic view of water diffusion (water molecule is depicted as a solid sphere) restricted by highly aligned fibres (depicted as poles). B–C. Axial views of a 12-year-old brain scanned with a DTI sequence showing maps of the fractional anisotropy (FA) (B), and mean diffusivity (MD) (C). D. In tract-based spatial statistics (TBSS), individual FA maps are non-linearly aligned voxel-wise to an optimal target FA, typically one of the subjects whose FA map is normalized to a standard brain. An average of all of the aligned FA maps are created, and a 'skeleton' tract that is common to all subjects is created, shown here E. Only those voxels from each subject that are projected onto this skeleton is entered for across-subject statistics. Here, the result of the contrast between control and stuttering children are shown (Chang et al., 2008. Figure modified and reprinted here with permission). (See Plate section).

such as the corpus callosum. MD reflects the overall magnitude of water diffusion independent of anisotropy. In general, MD values are higher in the paediatric population compared to adults, owing to less myelination and higher water content in younger brains.

These measures are sensitive to changes in neural organization due to maturation as well as brain injury (Barnea-Goraly et al., 2005; Mukherjee and McKinstry 2006; Neil et al., 2002; Schmithorst et al., 2002; Snook et al., 2005b). The degree of anisotropy in certain white matter tracts has been shown to correlate positively with the development of reading skills, working memory, and other cognitive functions in normally developing school-age children (Beaulieu et al., 2005; Durston and Casey 2006; Klingberg 1999, 2000, 2006; Nagy et al. 2004). A comprehensive review on the application of DTI for studying white matter development in healthy children and clinical groups is available (Cascio et al., 2007).

Fractional anisotropy and MD are calculated for each voxel, and brain regions can be compared by contrasting these values extracted from ROIs. Conversely, FA and MD may be examined without pre-determined regions of interest, using a VBM-style analysis across the whole brain. Tract-based spatial statistics (TBSS) (Smith et al., 2006) provides a robust and sensitive method for such an analysis, which involves non-linear registration of each subject's FA map to a common target

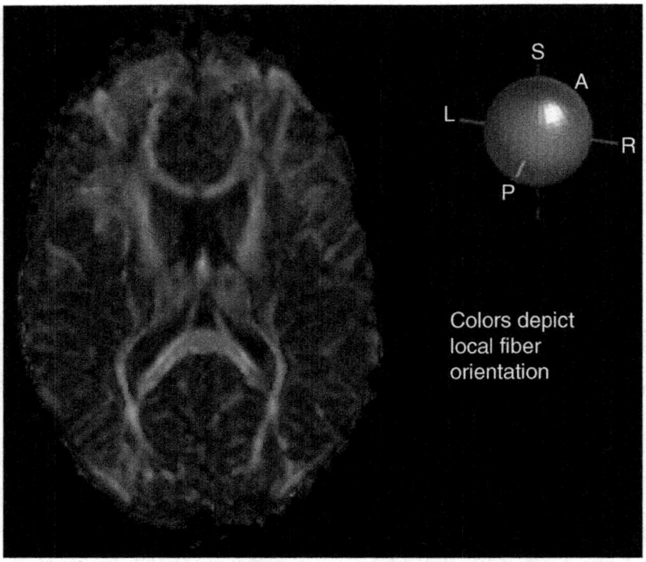

Fig. 5.6 Colour coded map illustrating the direction of fibres in three-dimensional space (See text for more detail). (See Plate section).

in standard space, and then calculating a 'skeletonized' white matter tract common to all subjects (Fig. 5.5D). Each subject's FA values that fall within this common tract are projected onto this tract, and between-subject statistics are computed to compare clinical groups on a voxel-to-voxel basis (Fig. 5.5E).

In addition to providing information on white matter microstructure, DTI allows visualization of white matter pathways by using colour coded maps of anisotropy, to illustrate the direction of fibres in three-dimensional space (Fig. 5.6). Tractography or fibre tracking is another method to examine white matter pathways by computing probable trajectories of fibre tracts between brain regions (Fig. 5.7). Typically, start and end points of a tract of interest are defined, and 'streamlines' that interconnect the two points are calculated by taking the primary direction of the water diffusion from each voxel (Croxson et al., 2005; Mori et al., 1999) (Fig. 5.7C). This method is not reliable in regions with fibre crossing or branching, or in grey matter regions, where there is increased uncertainty in path direction and reduced anisotropy, resulting in termination of tracking (Fig. 5.7D). For this reason, others have used probabilistic rather than deterministic tractography to enable tracking into deep grey matter (Behrens et al., 2003).

To analyse these fibre representations in a quantitative manner, anisotropy and other diffusion parameters can be extracted from the fibre tracts. Such an approach was used to quantify developmental changes in motor and somatosensory pathways in infants (Berman et al., 2005), and to examine pyramidal tracts in children with congenital hemiparesis compared to controls (Glenn et al., 2003).

As mentioned above on structural MRI, it is also important in DTI to ensure that children remain still during scanning. DTI is very susceptible to artefacts such as bright spots and spatial distortion from any metal implants (i.e., dental fillings) or air in the sinuses or the head, producing magnetic susceptibility artefacts (Basser and Jones 2002; Le Bihan et al., 2006). This may be circumvented by acquiring multiple copies of each image, eliminating images with too much artefact (Cascio et al., 2007), and correcting for distortions during pre-processing (Mangin et al., 2002; Rohde et al., 2004).

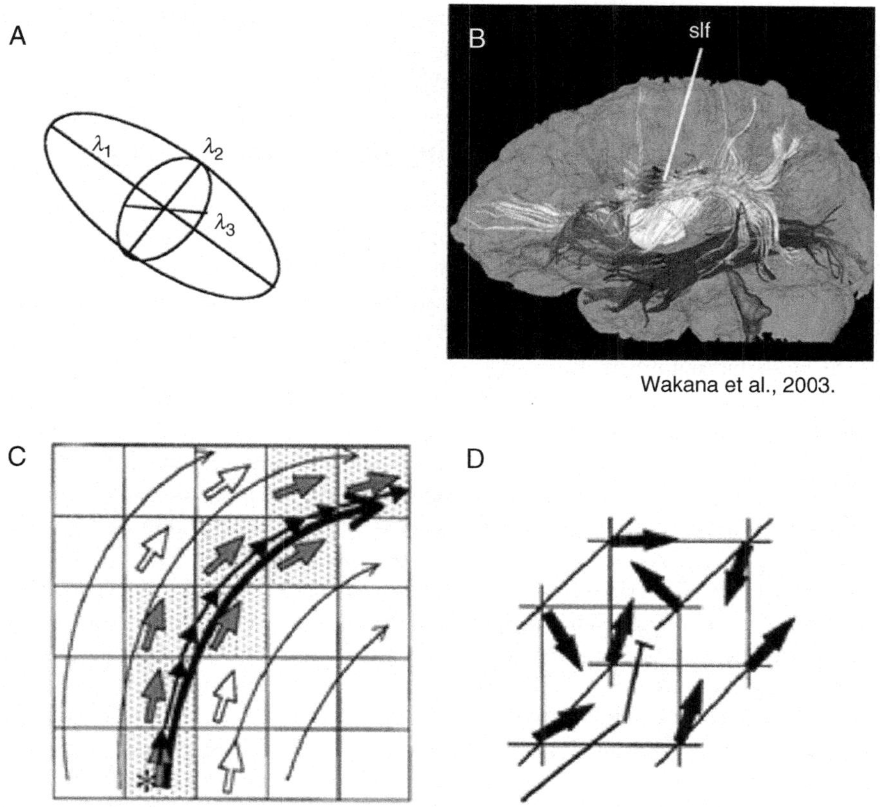

Fig. 5.7 A. Diffusion properties can be represented by an ellipsoid with three principal axes (λ_1, λ_2, λ_3), with the orientation of the main axis λ_1 ('first eigenvector') representing the average fibre direction. B. Three-dimensional depictions of association fibres including the superior longitudinal fasciculus (slf) using fibre tracking (after Wakana et al., 2003. Reprinted here with permission). C. Once the fibre direction is determined for each voxel, fibre tracking can proceed by taking the fibre direction at the centre of a voxel (asterisk) and change direction according to that of the neighbour. The actual fibres are represented as long curved arrows, and the average fibre directions in the voxels are represented as open arrows. The connected voxels resulting from tracking are shaded using small dots. D. When the fibre orientation becomes random, tracking is terminated (after Mori 1999. Reprinted here with permission).

In summary, structural MRI techniques have begun to provide unprecedented opportunities for *in vivo* examination of neuroanatomical changes accompanying normal and abnormal human brain development. The interpretation of grey matter changes measured through MRI including grey matter volume, density, cortical thickness, and sulcal/gyral patterns, is still not agreed upon. Although these measurements may reflect complex cellular mechanisms including dendritic remodelling, synaptic pruning, as well as the architecture of neurons, glia, and vasculature, this has yet to be determined. White matter structure changes measured through anisotropy, diffusivity, and DTI tractography are even more problematic; they may reflect changes in fibre tract organization, presence of crossing fibres, myelination, and pruning. One must keep in mind that, although MRI techniques provide detailed information, the biological bases for these changes and their underlying cellular mechanisms are still unclear and are topics of active investigation.

One may need to consider pairing the grey and white matter measurements derived through structural MRI, with behavioural measures (i.e., performance scores on a test), or measures of brain function during behaviour using fMRI, reviewed below.

5.3 **Examining brain activity during development using functional MRI (fMRI)**

In fMRI, the blood oxygen level dependent (BOLD) signal is an indirect measure of neural activity. When brain activity increases in a region, blood flow increases more than the actual oxygen consumption in that region, resulting in decreased de-oxygenated haemoglobin, which enhances the BOLD signal. An ideal experimental paradigm increases the BOLD signal in brain regions related to a task, but not others. By computing the percent change in the BOLD signal during a behaviour with another state such as rest, differences in neural activation between the states can be implied across the brain regions.

The original focus of functional brain imaging was to identify brain regions active for a particular function with the aim of identifying neural substrates involved in motor, sensory, or cognitive performance. Some have criticized this approach as overly simplistic and arbitrary where increases in the BOLD signal in certain brain regions were interpreted as being a 'center' in the brain for certain cognitive functions (Uttal 2003). More recently, functional neuroimaging paradigms have become focused more on neural networks as it has become evident that most functions involve inter-connected networks of neurons in the brain (Hubbard 2003). The designs are now more complex, and aimed at identifying brain networks active at different time points in the course of the task performance (Donaldson 2004).

Functional magnetic resonance imaging experiments can be run using 'block', 'event-related', or 'mixed' designs. Most studies examining speech and language have used either block- or event-related designs. In a block design, trials of each condition are grouped into blocks, which are either alternated or separated by rest blocks (Fig. 5.8A). For example, ten trials of a covert verb generation task can be performed in one block. Here the assumption is that the neural activation associated with verb generation is constant within that block. A rest block when no task is performed that is equal in length can be alternated with the task block. The neural activation associated with task performance can be measured by comparing the percent increase in the BOLD signal between the test block and the rest block. While simple and efficient, block designs have several limitations when used for speech research. Because any movement during fMRI data acquisition leads to severe movement artefacts, overt speech production will interfere with brain imaging results. In addition, speech produces changes in the air volume in the oral cavity causing artefacts. Speech-language research has typically used covert or imagined conditions when using block designs (Gaillard et al., 2003; Szaflarski et al., 2006). In addition, in experiments involving auditory stimuli presentation, scanner noise can mask the stimuli. Furthermore, when studying clinical groups such as people with stuttering, scanner noise likely will have an effect on fluency, which may be a confounding factor when examining the pattern of activation during speech production.

Event-related designs can circumvent some of these issues. Unlike in block designs, where trials are performed consecutively within a test block, in conventional event-related designs, discrete, short duration trials are presented randomly and are separated in time from previous events with various inter-trial intervals (ISI) (Huettel et al., 2004) (Fig. 5.8B). In sparse sampling designs, the time between successive scans is lengthened, so that brief silent periods occur between scans, which can be used for stimulus delivery and/or overt response (Eden et al., 1999; Hall et al., 1999) (Fig. 5.8C). Taking advantage of the hemodynamic response delay, which is typically 4–6 seconds

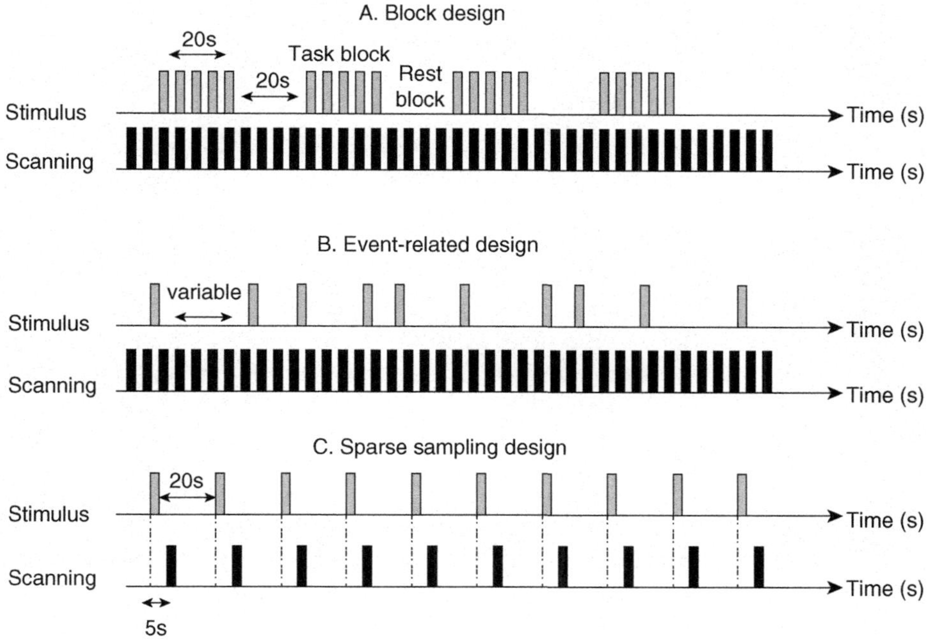

Fig. 5.8 Some fMRI experiment paradigms commonly used. Stimulus presentations are depicted as grey bars and scanning is depicted as black bars. A. Block design B. Event-related design C. Event-related design using sparse-sampling. In this example the scans are acquired 5 seconds following the onset of the stimuli to capture the peak of the hemodynamic response. Auditory stimuli can be presented in the absence of background scanner noise, and overt speech production can be performed without the concern of movement artefacts during the transient silent periods that occur in between the scans.

following a stimulus, the brain activation associated with a production or perception task (Fig. 5.9) are acquired 4–6 seconds after the onset of the task, effectively capturing the response peak without interference from noise and movement artefacts.

In paediatric fMRI, tasks need to be age appropriate, to compare similar performance levels across children. That is, a single task may require more effort and produce more errors in younger children. In addition, experimental runs may need to be kept shorter to maintain attention and cooperation throughout. Sufficient preparation and training in a calm, friendly environment, the use of procedures to minimize head movement using biofeedback, and creative ways to reinforce cooperation in task performance inside the scanner, have all been reported to be helpful in achieving successful fMRI sessions in children. For example, biofeedback techniques can help minimize head movement by using sensors around the head that pick up movement exceeding an acceptable range. When a child moves more than an acceptable range, they are notified through visual feedback delivered onto the screen. To increase cooperation in performing tasks inside the scanner, reward systems can be used, so that whenever a child successfully completes three or four trials, they are given a reward by a cartoon character that appears on screen, that can be coupled with a toy at the end of the session. A number of reviews discuss special considerations for acquisition, analysis, and interpretation for pediatric fMRI studies (Bookheimer 2000; Davidson et al., 2003; Gaillard et al., 2001; Poldrack et al., 2002). In the past decade, many studies have been conducted in school-age children, both healthy and with developmental disorders, using a variety of tasks to examine different cognitive modalities including speech/language, reading, memory,

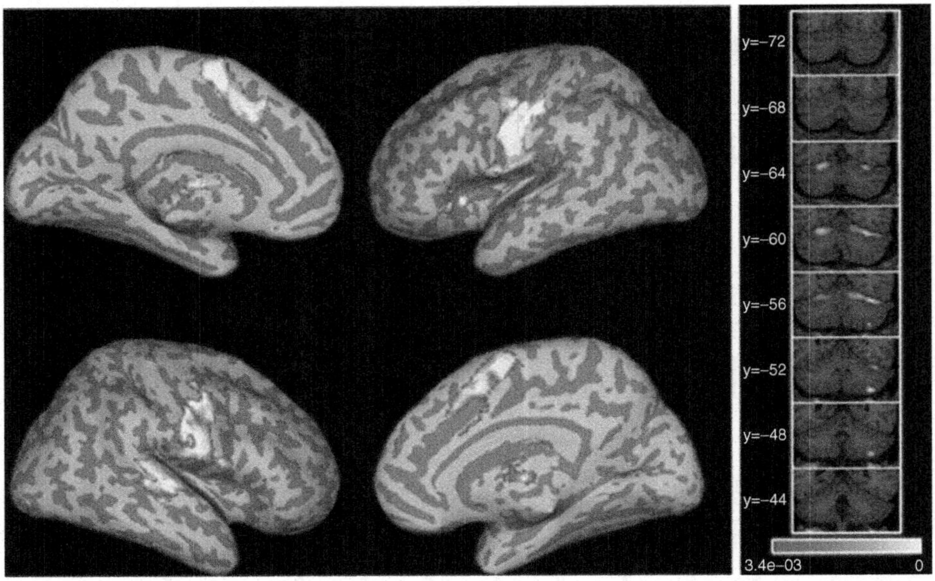

Fig. 5.9 Brain activation associated with overt speech production, captured with fMRI using a sparse sampling paradigm (Bohland and Guenther 2006) (figure reprinted here with permission). (See Plate section).

and self-regulation (Balsamo et al., 2002; Booth et al., 2001; Chiu et al., 2006; Gaillard et al., 2003; Holland et al., 2001; Luna et al., 2001; Marsh et al., 2006; Narain et al., 2003; Schmitz et al., 2006; Schweinsburg et al., 2005; Wilke et al., 2005; Wood et al., 2004). Notably, fMRI has also been successfully applied to sleeping infants by some investigators (Dehaene-Lambertz et al., 2002; Seghier et al., 2006).

A promising new area of research involves examining inter-regional functional connectivity (Friston et al., 1993; Horwitz 2003) during behavioural tasks (Bokde et al., 2001; Horwitz et al., 1998; Karunanayaka et al., 2007; Schmithorst et al., 2007). Correlations in BOLD fluctuations between regions can be examined to compare groups that differ in age, disorder status, or within subjects pre- and post-therapy, to investigate possible changes in functional connectivity associated with specific group standing. Here functional connectivity refers to correlation analyses of the similarity in BOLD signal changes over two regions, or between a seed region and the rest of the brain. No information is provided on causal relationships between brain regions. Effective connectivity, however, encompasses methods such as structural equation modelling (SEM) (McIntosh and Gonzalez-Lima 1994) and dynamic causal modelling (DCM) (Friston et al., 2003; Lee et al., 2006), which test hypotheses on causal relationships (directionality) between predetermined regions.

Recently, particular interest have been given to spontaneous BOLD fluctuations in the absence of stimulation or task performance that show correlations among functionally related regions in known anatomical systems (Fox and Raichle 2007). These fluctuations persist across different resting states, including sleep (Fukunaga et al., 2006) and anaesthesia (Peltier et al., 2005; Vincent et al., 2007), suggesting that they are an intrinsic property of the brain. As resting state connectivity analyses require no task performance and can be performed during sleep, they may be applied to younger children and infants.

5.4 Neural correlates of speech and language development during childhood

Apart from technical and practical challenges in conducting neuroimaging research in children, major challenges remain in interpreting structural and functional imaging results, in particular with respect to cognitive functions (Uttal 2003). Brain development is a highly interactive process, influenced by growth factors, gene expression, behaviour, environmental factors, and their complex interactions. The relationship between brain structure and function during development is poorly understood, although it is generally accepted that brain anatomy can constrain function, while function can in turn lead to neuroplastic changes in brain structure. Because dynamic changes occur throughout childhood and adolescence, adults and children cannot be compared on tasks (i.e., verb generation) even when they have similar performance levels. To achieve comparable levels of performance, children may employ different strategies than adults. For example, white matter tracts continue to grow throughout childhood and connectivity among regions may differ across the life span.

When considering developmental disorders, anomalous brain development in a particular region may in turn result in altered function in other brain regions due to compensatory or adaptive behaviours. Separating out cause and effect becomes impossible in such cases. Finding differences in brain structure and function in adults with a developmental disorder could thus reflect changes in the brain as a result of having a disorder as much as those differences that are the bases for the disorder. Large-scale longitudinal studies focusing on children with and without disorders may be helpful. Such studies on normally developing children are increasingly being reported, and are reviewed below. Similar longitudinal studies are needed to understand the neurological basis of developmental disorders such as stuttering.

5.4.1 Grey matter changes

Large-scale studies involving children from four years and beyond have found that the timing of grey matter growth differs for different regions of the brain. Consistently a more protracted growth pattern in the temporal lobe has been reported than in other cortical regions (Giedd 2004; Gogtay et al., 2004; Sowell et al., 2003, 2004a). In addition, cortical thickness increases in the left inferior frontal region are related to language development throughout childhood (Lu et al., 2006; Sowell et al., 2004a). Grey matter volume and thickness increase in most areas of the cortex in the preadolescent years, with the peak of the growth curve occurring later than most other regions for speech-language relevant regions, followed by a linear decrease later in life (Gogtay et al., 2004; Sowell et al., 2003).

In a longitudinal investigation of normally developing children scanned at two-year intervals between five and eleven years, cortical thickening in the left inferior frontal region was correlated with improving phonological processing scores but not hand motor skills (Lu et al., 2006). Grey matter thickening may reflect a proliferation of dendritic processes, synaptic connections or increases in soma size (Giedd 2004). Cortical maturation appears to involve both thickening and thinning of the cortex, the latter associated with dendritic pruning and myelination, supporting fine-tuning of already existing networks established earlier during development (Lu et al., 2006; Shaw et al., 2006). The temporal relationship between behavioural changes and the anatomical changes that support them are not clear. Changes in grey matter development and white matter development that improve signal transmission among different brain regions likely interact with behavioural changes occurring during development (Barnea-Goraly et al., 2005).

In one VBM study, proficiency in a second language and age at acquisition was related to grey matter density – the proportion of grey matter relative to white matter and CSF – in the left inferior parietal region (Mechelli et al., 2004). The more proficient subjects were on a second language, and the younger they were when they first acquired it, the higher the grey matter density was in this region. This suggests that differences in language experience during childhood results in subtle differences in cortical development. Conversely, one may speculate that the presence of a brain developmental difference due to genetic abnormalities could result in a speech disorder during early childhood that may have other more subtle effects on cortical development (Vargha-Khadem et al., 1998; Watkins et al., 2002).

These results suggest that function could drive structural changes, especially during the critical period of development, as even during adulthood structural changes can occur with extensive training or learning (Boyke et al., 2008; Draganski et al., 2006). As will be discussed in the following section, behaviour/function differences also affect white matter structure development; for instance, extensive piano practice leads to white matter plasticity especially when it occurs during younger age, when the fibre tracts are still undergoing maturation (Bengtsson et al., 2005). The authors suggested that increased neural activity associated with training can lead to increased myelination resulting in these white matter changes.

Perisylvian sulcal asymmetry in the sylvian fissure increases significantly from childhood to adulthood, and grey matter density in the latter group significantly correlates with increasing asymmetry in this region (Sowell et al., 2002). While evidence of perisylvian asymmetry exists in preverbal infants (Matsuzawa et al., 2001; Witelson and Pallie 1973), the increasing asymmetry with age suggests possible interactions between behaviour and brain plasticity. Differences in asymmetry patterns in the temporal regions, including the planum parietale and the planum temporale has been examined in several developmental disorders including dyslexia (Eckert and Leonard 2000; Heiervang et al., 2000; Leonard et al., 2001; Morgan and Hynd 1998), specific language impairment (Gauger et al., 1997), language and learning impaired children (Jernigan et al., 1991), and autism (Rojas et al., 2005). An excellent review on anatomical asymmetry using brain mapping can be found elsewhere (Toga and Thompson 2003).

Sex differences that are pronounced in adulthood (Allen et al., 2003; Gur et al., 1999; Luders et al., 2005; Szeszko et al., 2003) are also found in children; boys and girls differ in both global brain volume, local grey and white matter volume (Wilke et al., 2007), and degree of asymmetry (Blanton et al., 2004). On-going increases in white matter in the inferior frontal gyrus (IFG) are found in boys (age range 6–15) but not girls (age range 6–17), and boys show greater left IFG grey matter volume, possibly linked to gender differences in speech development (Blanton et al., 2004). Similarly, De Bellis et al. (2001) reported that males between the ages of 7 years and 17 years had more age-related grey matter decreases, indicating greater cerebral pruning, and more prominent increases in white matter volume and corpus callosal area compared to females (De Bellis et al., 2001). The authors suggested that such differences in patterns of brain development between boys and girls may explain the increased early onset of, and increased severity in neuropsychiatric disorders such as schizophrenia, which has been linked to excess elimination of synapses (Feinberg 1982). More specific to speech/language development, sex differences in cell packing density (Witelson et al., 1995) and anatomical asymmetry (Witelson 1991) have been reported in posterior temporal-parietal regions and in the left frontal lobe (Szeszko et al., 2003), regions known to support speech and language.

Age-related grey matter decreases may be based on neuronal pruning and the elimination of synapses; possible mechanisms to make neuronal transmission more focused and efficient. Similarly, increases in white matter possibly due to axonal growth and increased myelination may increase the speed of neurotransmission essential for information processing. Therefore, differences in grey matter volume and white matter increases between boys and girls may relate to differences in the incidence and vulnerability for developmental speech disorders between the two genders. In any case, it appears critical to take sex differences into account when conducting neuroimaging studies in children.

5.4.2 **White matter changes**

Unlike grey matter, white matter shows a linear developmental trajectory from early childhood continuing well onto adulthood, measured through increases in white matter volume/density, FA, and decreases in mean diffusivity with age (Barnea-Goraly et al., 2005; Paus et al., 2001; Schmithorst et al., 2002; Snook et al., 2005a). Like grey matter, white matter changes are associated with cognitive development (Mabbott et al., 2006; Nagy et al., 2004; Schmithorst and Holland 2007), effects of training (Bengtsson et al., 2005; Schmithorst and Wilke 2002), and reading ability (Beaulieu et al., 2005; Deutsch et al., 2005; Klingberg et al., 2000).

Faster and more efficient information transfer achieved through white matter growth and myelination may be critical in regions such as the left arcuate fasciculus, the major white matter bundle interconnecting the frontal-temporal regions. White matter density in the left arcuate fasiculus and age are positively correlated (Paus et al., 2001), and FA (Buchel et al., 2004; Parker et al., 2005) as well as fibre density (Nucifora et al., 2005; Vernooij et al., 2007) are highly asymmetric and greater on the left in adults. As mentioned in the previous section, gender differences in white matter asymmetry in adults have been reported in the left inferior frontal region; with higher FA in the left frontal lobe and greater leftward asymmetry in women compared to men, which correlated with better verbal comprehension and memory functioning (Szeszko et al., 2003). Decreases in white matter integrity when measured using FA in this tract, underlying the rolandic operculum on the left is associated with stuttering, both in adults (Sommer et al., 2002) and children (Chang et al., 2008). Similar white matter deficits were found underlying the bilateral temporoparietal regions in adults with reading difficulty, while diffusion anisotropy was significantly correlated with reading ability only on the left (Klingberg et al., 2000).

5.4.3 **Functional changes**

An fMRI study showed brain activity in response to speech stimuli had left-biased localization in infants as young as three months (Dehaene-Lambertz et al., 2002). This likely represents a strong genetic bias for speech processing favouring the left hemisphere, also consistent with structural MRI findings of greater asymmetry in the sylvian fissure and planum temporale early during foetal life (Chi et al., 1977; Witelson and Pallie 1973). These anatomical differences likely contribute to functional asymmetries for speech processing in the left hemisphere (Dehaene-Lambertz et al., 2006).

In one study, adults and children were found to exhibit comparable regions of left IFG and middle frontal gyrus activation during covert verbal fluency tasks, with a greater activation area and more right-sided activation in the children (Gaillard et al., 2000). Another study, involving larger groups of children and adults participating in verb generation and orthographic lexical retrieval tasks, showed no difference between the child and adult groups in localization of activation, or laterality of responses (Wood et al., 2004).

A large study of healthy children ($n = 332$) between ages 5 and 19, found BOLD increases with age in the left Broca's, middle frontal, Wernicke's, inferior parietal and anterior cingulate regions during a silent verb generation task (Schapiro et al., 2004). A longitudinal study of children between 5 years and 11 years on a silent verb generation task found age-related increases in activity in the language- and speech-related regions in the left and right hemispheres, and a decrease in activity in non-primary language regions such as the left posterior insula/extrastriate, superior frontal region, thalamus, and the right anterior cingulate (Szaflarski et al., 2006). Within this age range, there appears to be a strengthening in the activation of the language-related areas with a decrease in other areas, possibly representing more efficient language processing with age. Caution is needed in interpreting these findings, however, because differences in activity do not directly translate to either excitation or inhibition, and rapid temporal changes in neural activity are not well captured in fMRI. For example, excitatory neuronal firing cannot be differentiated from activity of inhibitory inter-neurons in functional neuroimaging.

A number of studies have started to examine functional networks involved in speech processing using functional and effective connectivity analyses of children while listening to stories (Karunanayaka et al., 2007; Schmithorst et al., 2007). Such studies can examine functional correlations and relationships between ROIs. These patterns are likely to change with development, and may differ between atypical and normally developing children. Combining functional connectivity analyses with methods probing structural connectivity such as diffusion tensor tractography may lead to better understanding of the functional and structural networks involved in speech and language development.

5.5 **Structural MRI study of children who stutter**

A number of structural MRI and functional neuroimaging (fMRI and PET) studies have been conducted on stuttering, but these studies have so far only focused on stuttering adults. Among these, PET involves measuring brain activity by injecting radioactive tracers into the bloodstream and examining its flow, metabolism, or receptor binding. PET is not further discussed here, as it involves exposure to ionizing radiation, and so its use in paediatric research is limited to cases with life-threatening disorders.

As was discussed in previous sections, due to significant structural and functional changes occurring between childhood and adulthood, there is a need to examine younger children to distinguish what changes might be a reaction to the disorder from what may be linked with the disorder itself. Recently we published a structural MRI study based on school-age (8–12 years) children (right-handed boys) who stutter (Chang et al., 2008). We found focal FA decreases on the left side in white matter tracts such as the arcuate fasciculus underlying the sensorimotor cortex (rolandic operculum). Decreased FA in this area was common for both persistent stuttering as well as those recovered from stuttering. Interestingly, the recovered group showed a non-significant trend of greater FA than both controls and the persistent group in a right hemisphere homologue region, a finding that warrants confirmation with larger groups to determine whether right-sided FA increase in this area correlates with recovery.

Our study replicates findings from an earlier study by Sommer et al. (2002), where left-sided FA decreases in the rolandic opercular region in adults who stutter were found compared to controls. The authors argued that stuttering is due to a left-sided white matter disruption that leads to disturbed timing in the speech-relevant brain areas, and that right hemisphere overactivation reported in earlier studies reflects a compensatory mechanism (Sommer et al., 2002). Whether the right hemisphere structure/function differences reflect compensatory effects of stuttering has been unclear. The left-sided decrease in white matter integrity found in both adults and now in children more clearly suggests, however, that this may be one of the important structural bases for the risk of stuttering. Although our school-age children who had persistent stuttering had been stuttering since two to four years of age, and are likely to have adopted some compensatory behaviours similar to adults, this cannot be said about the age-matched group of children who had recovered from stuttering, who had not been stuttering for at least two years prior to their study participation. The fact that both groups exhibited the same white matter differences compared to the control children however, suggests that this structural difference may be associated with the risk of developing stuttering, regardless of outcome. Future studies with larger samples are needed to confirm these findings.

Right hemisphere volumetric increases in the speech/language homologues that were reported previously based on adults (Foundas et al., 2001; Jancke et al., 2004) were not found in children who stutter when examining grey matter volume using optimized VBM (Chang et al., 2008). Children who stutter exhibited typical leftward asymmetry in volume, particularly in the planum temporale, a finding that also disagrees with decreased asymmetry found in adults by Foundas et al. (2001), although differences in methodology, group characteristics (i.e., right-handed males in our study versus mixed handedness males and females in Foundas et al., 2001) as well as age may account for the differences. A recent study examining sulcal morphology using asymmetry patterns in dextral adult males who stutter found comparable asymmetry patterns in adults who stutter, while increased sulcal connections were found only in the right perisylvian region (Cykowski et al., 2007). This suggests that right hemisphere enhancement may develop with continued stuttering into adulthood, although typical volumetric laterality may be maintained. Perhaps the STG increases found in children with persistent stuttering over those who recovered from stuttering are the result of continuing to stutter for 6–9 years after onset (Chang et al., 2008).

Another study examining adolescents and young adults (14–27 years) used both functional MRI and DTI to study functional and structural differences in stuttering participants (Watkins et al., 2007). This study replicated findings from earlier studies reporting over- and under-activated areas during speech production, but additionally found the bilateral ventral premotor cortex to be under-activated during articulation and speech production in stuttering participants. This area also showed less white matter integrity through FA analysis. The white matter tract underlying the ventral premotor region lies slightly more anterior to the unilateral left rolandic opercular region reported in Sommer et al. (2002) and Chang et al. (2008), but like the rolandic opercular region, also lies within the superior longitudinal fasciculus that likely serves as a critical tract for integrating motor and sensory information for efficient speech production. Unlike the unilateral deficit reported in previous studies, this study reports a bilateral deficit in their stuttering group (Watkins et al., 2007). Perhaps a more even sex ratio, as well as a wider age range used in this study (14–27 years) may have contributed to these differences: white matter development is actively taking place during childhood and adolescence (Paus 2005), possibly with a different pace in females versus males, particularly in the frontal region (Blanton et al., 2004). These issues need to be considered in future studies, and systematic comparisons between males and females who stutter may need to be conducted to clarify differences in findings.

In summary, our study based on children between 8 years and 12 years of age show that the greatest structural difference between stuttering children (persistent and recovered) and controls occurred in the GMV in the left inferior frontal region, and white matter tracts underlying the rolandic operculum, also on the left. These differences were similarly present in both persistent and recovered children, indicating that developmental deficits in this left-sided speech-language network may represent risk factors for developing childhood stuttering regardless of eventual recovery. These findings replicate studies based on adults reporting decreases in white matter integrity on the left hemisphere (Sommer et al., 2002), and comparable laterality in the perisylvian regions (Cykowski et al., 2007), but does not support the right-sided increases in volume in adults reported by others (Foundas et al., 2001; Jancke et al., 2004). Perhaps right-sided increases develop as people continue to stutter. Decreased white matter integrity in regions involved in the left superior longitudinal fasciculus and the arcuate fasciculus, which likely interconnect between frontal speech motor and posterior-temporal auditory regions, have now been found in adults (Sommer et al., 2002), adolescents (Watkins et al., 2007), and children (Chang et al., 2008), suggesting that this may be an important structural deficit that may contribute to the risk for stuttering.

5.6 Conclusion

Dynamic changes in brain structure and function occur throughout early childhood and adolescence, with critical cognitive skills and speech and language development actively taking place during this time. The neural correlates of normal development versus abnormal development due to a disorder are increasingly being studied, presenting opportunities to understand the neural basis for typical and atypical development better than ever before. Despite significant progress, many practical, technical, and interpretation challenges remain for the application of neuroimaging techniques in infants and younger children. In the future, multidisciplinary and multi-centre teams will be increasingly needed to solve some of the issues discussed in this chapter. Longitudinal as well as multimodality imaging using two or more different imaging techniques, may be needed to aid understanding of the processes involved in atypical development, and neuroplasticity related to speech and language disorders.

References

Allen, J. S., Damasio, H., Grabowski, T. J., Bruss, J., & Zhang, W. (2003). Sexual dimorphism and asymmetries in the gray-white composition of the human cerebrum. *Neuroimage*, 18(4), 880–894.

Ashburner, J. & Friston, K. J. (2000). Voxel-based morphometry – the methods. *Neuroimage*, 11(6 Pt 1), 805–821.

Balsamo, L. M., Xu, B., Grandin, C. B., Petrella, J. R., Braniecki, S. H., Elliott, T. K., et al. (2002). A functional magnetic resonance imaging study of left hemisphere language dominance in children. *Archives of Neurology*, 59(7), 1168–1174.

Barnea-Goraly, N., Menon, V., Eckert, M., Tamm, L., Bammer, R., Karchemskiy, A., et al. (2005). White matter development during childhood and adolescence: A cross-sectional diffusion tensor imaging study. *Cerebral Cortex*, 15(12), 1848–1854.

Beaulieu, C., Plewes, C., Paulson, L. A., Roy, D., Snook, L., Concha, L., et al. (2005). Imaging brain connectivity in children with diverse reading ability. *NeuroImage*, 25(4), 1266–1271.

Behrens, T. E. J., Johansen-Berg, H., Woolrich, M. W., Smith, S. M., Wheeler-Kingshott, C. A. M., Boulby, P. A., et al. (2003). Non-invasive mapping of connections between human thalamus and cortex using diffusion imaging. *Nature Neuroscience*, 6(7), 750–757.

Benasich, A. A., Choudhury, N., Friedman, J. T., Realpe-Bonilla, T., Chojnowska, C., & Gou, Z. (2006). The infant as a prelinguistic model for language learning impairments: Predicting from event-related potentials to behavior. *Neuropsychologia*, 44(3), 396–411.

Bengtsson, S. L., Nagy, Z., Skare, S., Forsman, L., Forssberg, H., & Ullen, F. (2005). Extensive piano practicing has regionally specific effects on white matter development. *Nature Neuroscience*, 8(9), 1148–1150.

Berman, J. I., Mukherjee, P., Partridge, S. C., Miller, S. P., Ferriero, D. M., Barkovich, A. J., et al. (2005). Quantitative diffusion tensor MRI fiber tractography of sensorimotor white matter development in premature infants. *Neuroimage*, 27(4), 862–871.

Bernal, J., Harmony, T., Rodriguez, M., Reyes, A., Yanez, G., Fernandez, T., et al. (2000). Auditory event-related potentials in poor readers. *International Journal of Psychophysiology*, 36(1), 11–23.

Blanton, R. E., Levitt, J. G., Peterson, J. R., Fadale, D., Sporty, M. L., Lee, M., et al. (2004). Gender differences in the left inferior frontal gyrus in normal children. *Neuroimage*, 22(2), 626–636.

Bohland, J. W. & Guenther, F. H. (2006). An fMRI investigation of syllable sequence production. *NeuroImage*, 32(2), 821–841.

Bokde, A. L. W., Tagamets, M. A., Friedman, R. B., & Horwitz, B. (2001). Functional interactions of the inferior frontal cortex during the processing of words and word-like stimuli. *Neuron*, 30(2), 609–617.

Bookheimer, S. Y. (2000). Methodological issues in pediatric neuroimaging. *Mental Retardation and Developmental Disabilities Research Reviews*, 6(3), 161–165.

Booth, J. R., Burman, D. D., Van Santen, F. W., Harasaki, Y., Gitelman, D. R., Parrish, T. B., et al. (2001). The development of specialized brain systems in reading and oral-language. *Child Neuropsychology*, 7(3), 119–141.

Boyke, J., Driemeyer, J., Gaser, C., Buchel, C., & May, A. (2008). Training-induced brain structure changes in the elderly. *Journal of Neuroscience*, 28(28), 7031–7035.

Buchel, C., Raedler, T., Sommer, M., Sach, M., Weiller, C., & Koch, M. A. (2004). White matter asymmetry in the human brain: A diffusion tensor MRI study. *Cerebral Cortex*, 14(9), 945–951.

Cascio, C. J., Gerig, G., & Piven, J. (2007). Diffusion tensor imaging: Application to the study of the developing brain. *Journal of the American Academy of Child and Adolescent Psychiatry*, 46(2), 213–223.

Chang, S. E., Erickson, K. I., Ambrose, N. G., Hasegawa-Johnson, M. A., & Ludlow, C. L. (2008). Brain anatomy differences in childhood stuttering. *NeuroImage*, 39(3), 1333–1344.

Chi, J. G., Dooling, E. C., & Gilles, F. H. (1977). Gyral development of human-brain. *Annals of Neurology*, 1(1), 86–93.

Chiu, C. Y. P., Schmithorst, V. J., Brown, R. D., Holland, S. K., & Dunn, S. (2006). Making memories: A cross-sectional investigation of episodic memory encoding in childhood using fMRI. *Developmental Neuropsychology*, 29(2), 321–340.

Croxson, P. L., Johansen-Berg, H., Behrens, T. E. J., Robson, M. D., Pinsk, M. A., Gross, C. G., et al. (2005). Quantitative investigation of connections of the prefrontal cortex in the human and macaque using probabilistic diffusion tractography. *Journal of Neuroscience*, 25(39), 8854–8866.

Cykowski, M. D., Kochunov, P. V., Ingham, R. J., Ingham, J. C., Mangin, J. F., Riviere, D., et al. (2007). Perisylvian Sulcal Morphology and Cerebral Asymmetry Patterns in Adults Who Stutter. *Cerebral Cortex*.

Davidson, M. C., Thomas, K. M., & Casey, B. J. (2003). Imaging the developing brain with fMRI. *Mental Retardation and Developmental Disabilities Research Reviews*, 9(3), 161–167.

Davies, P. L., Segalowitz, S. J., & Gavin, W. J. (2004). Development of response-monitoring ERPs in 7- to 25-year-olds. *Developmental Neuropsychology*, 25(3), 355–376.

De Bellis, M. D., Keshavan, M. S., Beers, S. R., Hall, J., Frustaci, K., Masalehdan, A., et al. (2001). Sex differences in brain maturation during childhood and adolescence. *Cerebral Cortex*, 11(6), 552–557.

Dehaene-Lambertz, G., Dehaene, S., & Hertz-Pannier, L. (2002). Functional neuroimaging of speech perception in infants. *Science*, 298(5600), 2013–2015.

Dehaene-Lambertz, G., Hertz-Pannier, L., & Dubois, J. (2006). Nature and nurture in language acquisition: Anatomical and functional brain-imaging studies in infants. *Trends in Neurosciences*, 29(7), 367–373.

Deutsch, G. K., Dougherty, R. F., Bammer, R., Siok, W. T., Gabrieli, J. D. E., & Wandell, B. (2005). Children's reading performance is correlated with white matter structure measured by diffusion tensor imaging. *Cortex*, 41(3), 354–363.

Donaldson, D. I. (2004). Parsing brain activity with fMRI and mixed designs: What kind of a state is neuroimaging in? *Trends in Neurosciences*, 27(8), 442–444.

Draganski, B., Gaser, C., Kempermann, G., Kuhn, H. G., Winkler, J., Buchel, C., et al. (2006). Temporal and spatial dynamics of brain structure changes during extensive learning. *Journal of Neuroscience*, 26(23), 6314–6317.

Durston, S. & Casey, B. J. (2006). What have we learned about cognitive development from neuroimaging? *Neuropsychologia*, 44(11), 2149–2157.

Eckert, M. A. & Leonard, C. M. (2000). Structural imaging in dyslexia: The planum temporale. *Mental Retardation and Developmental Disabilities Research Reviews*, 6(3), 198–206.

Eckert, M. A., Leonard, C. M., Wilke, M., Eckert, M., Richards, T., Richards, A., et al. (2005). Anatomical signatures of dyslexia in children: Unique information from manual and voxel based morphometry brain measures. *Cortex*, 41(3), 304–315.

Eden, G. F., Joseph, J. E., Brown, H. E., Brown, C. P., & Zeffiro, T. A. (1999). Utilizing hemodynamic delay and dispersion to detect fMRI signal change without auditory interference: The behavior interleaved gradients technique. *Magnetic Resonance in Medicine*, 41(1), 13–20.

Feinberg, I. (1982). Schizophrenia: Caused by a fault in programmed synaptic elimination during adolescence? *Journal of Psychiatric Research*, 17(4), 319–334.

Foundas, A. L., Bollich, A. M., Corey, D. M., Hurley, M., & Heilman, K. M. (2001). Anomalous anatomy of speech-language areas in adults with persistent developmental stuttering. *Neurology*, 57(2), 207–215.

Fox, M. D., & Raichle, M. E. (2007). Spontaneous fluctuations in brain activity observed with functional magnetic resonance imaging. *Nature Reviews Neuroscience*, 8(9), 700–711.

Friston, K. J., Frith, C. D., Liddle, P. F., & Frackowiak, R. S. (1993). Functional connectivity: The principal-component analysis of large (PET) data sets. *Journal of Cerebral Blood Flow and Metabolism*, 13(1), 5–14.

Friston, K. J., Harrison, L., & Penny, W. (2003). Dynamic causal modelling. *Neuroimage*, 19(4), 1273–1302.

Fukunaga, M., Horovitz, S. G., van Gelderen, P., de Zwart, J. A., Jansma, J. M., Ikonomidou, V. N., et al. (2006). Large-amplitude, spatially correlated fluctuations in BOLD fMRI signals during extended rest and early sleep stages. *Magnetic Resonance Imaging*, 24(8), 979–992.

Gaillard, W. D., Grandin, C. B., & Xu, B. (2001). Developmental aspects of pediatric fMRI: Considerations for image acquisition, analysis, and interpretation. *Neuroimage*, 13(2), 239–249.

Gaillard, W. D., Hertz-Pannier, L., Mott, S. H., Barnett, A. S., LeBihan, D., & Theodore, W. H. (2000). Functional anatomy of cognitive development – fMRI of verbal fluency in children and adults. *Neurology*, 54(1), 180–185.

Gaillard, W. D., Sachs, B. C., Whitnah, J. R., Ahmad, Z., Balsamo, L. M., Petrella, J. R., et al. (2003). Developmental aspects of language processing: fMRI of verbal fluency in children and adults. *Human Brain Mapping*, 18(3), 176–185.

Gauger, L. M., Lombardino, L. J., & Leonard, C. M. (1997). Brain morphology in children with specific language impairment. *Journal of Speech Language and Hearing Research*, 40(6), 1272–1284.

Giedd, J. N. (2004). Structural magnetic resonance imaging of the adolescent brain. *Annals of the New York Academy of Sciences*, 1021, 77–85.

Glenn, O. A., Henry, R. G., Berman, J. I., Chang, P. C., Miller, S. P., Vigneron, D. B., et al. (2003). DTI-based three-dimensional tractography detects differences in the pyramidal tracts of infants and children with congenital hemiparesis. *Journal of Magnetic Resonance Imaging*, 18(6), 641–648.

Gogtay, N., Giedd, J. N., Lusk, L., Hayashi, K. M., Greenstein, D., Vaituzis, A. C., et al. (2004). Dynamic mapping of human cortical development during childhood through early adulthood. *Proceedings of the National Academy of Sciences of the United States of America*, 101(21), 8174–8179.

Good, C. D., Johnsrude, I. S., Ashburner, J., Henson, R. N., Friston, K. J., & Frackowiak, R. S. (2001). A voxel-based morphometric study of ageing in 465 normal adult human brains. *Neuroimage*, 14(1 Pt 1), 21–36.

Gur, R. C., Turetsky, B. I., Matsui, M., Yan, M., Bilker, W., Hughett, P., et al. (1999). Sex differences in brain gray and white matter in healthy young adults: Correlations with cognitive performance. *Journal of Neuroscience*, 19(10), 4065–4072.

Hall, D. A., Haggard, M. P., Akeroyd, M. A., Palmer, A. R., Summerfield, A. Q., Elliott, M. R., et al. (1999). 'Sparse' temporal sampling in auditory fMRI. *Human Brain Mapping*, 7(3), 213–223.

Heiervang, E., Hugdahl, K., Steinmetz, H., Smievoll, A. I., Stevenson, J., Lund, A., et al. (2000). Planum temporale, planum parietale and dichotic listening in dyslexia. *Neuropsychologia*, 38(13), 1704–1713.

Holland, S. K., Plante, E., Byars, A. W., Strawsburg, R. H., Schmithorst, V. J., & Ball, W. S. (2001). Normal fMRI brain activation patterns in children performing a verb generation task. *Neuroimage*, 14(4), 837–843.

Horwitz, B. (2003). The elusive concept of brain connectivity. *Neuroimage*, 19(2), 466–470.

Horwitz, B., Rumsey, J. M., & Donohue, B. C. (1998). Functional connectivity of the angular gyrus in normal reading and dyslexia. *Proceedings of the National Academy of Sciences of the United States of America*, 95(15), 8939–8944.

Hubbard, E. M. (2003). A discussion and review of Uttal (2001) The New Phrenology. *Cognitive Science Online*, 1, 22–33.

Jancke, L., Hanggi, J., & Steinmetz, H. (2004). Morphological brain differences between adult stutterers and non-stutterers. *BMC Neurology*, 4(1), 23.

Jenkinson, M. & Smith, S. (2001). A global optimisation method for robust affine registration of brain images. *Medical Image Analysis*, 5(2), 143–156.

Jernigan, T. L., Hesselink, J. R., Sowell, E., & Tallal, P. A. (1991). Cerebral structure on magnetic-resonance-imaging in language-impaired and learning-impaired children. *Archives of Neurology*, 48(5), 539–545.

Karunanayaka, P. R., Holland, S. K., Schmithorst, V. J., Solodkin, A., Chen, E. E., Szaflarski, J. P., et al. (2007). Age-related connectivity changes in fMRI data from children listening to stories. *NeuroImage*, 34(1), 349–360.

Klingberg, T. (2006). Development of a superior frontal-intraparietal network for visuo-spatial working memory. *Neuropsychologia*, 44(11), 2171–2177.

Klingberg, T., Hedehus, M., Temple, E., Salz, T., Gabrieli, J. D. E., Moseley, M. E., et al. (2000). Microstructure of temporo-parietal white matter as a basis for reading ability: Evidence from diffusion tensor magnetic resonance imaging. *Neuron*, 25(2), 493–500.

Klingberg, T., Vaidya, C. J., Gabrieli, J. D. E., Moseley, M. E., & Hedehus, M. (1999). Myelination and organization of the frontal white matter in children: A diffusion tensor MRI study. *NeuroReport*, 10(13), 2817–2821.

Le Bihan, D. (2003). Looking into the functional architecture of the brain with diffusion MRI. *Nature Reviews Neuroscience*, 4(6), 469–480.

Lee, L., Friston, K., & Horwitz, B. (2006). Large-scale neural models and dynamic causal modelling. *NeuroImage*, 30(4), 1243–1254.

Leonard, C. M., Eckert, M. A., Lombardino, L. J., Oakland, T., Kranzler, J., Mohr, C. M., et al. (2001). Anatomical risk factors for phonological dyslexia. *Cerebral Cortex*, 11(2), 148–157.

Licht, R., Bakker, D. J., Kok, A., & Bouma, A. (1988). The development of lateral event-related potentials (ERPs) related to word naming: A four year longitudinal study. *Neuropsychologia*, 26(2), 327–340.

Lu, L. H., Leonard, C. M., Thompson, P. M., Kan, E., Jolley, J., Welcome, S. E., et al. (2006). Normal developmental changes in inferior frontal gray matter are associated with improvement in phonological processing: A longitudinal MRI analysis. *Cerebral Cortex*.

Luders, E., Narr, K. L., Thompson, P. M., Woods, R. P., Rex, D. E., Jancke, L., et al. (2005). Mapping cortical gray matter in the young adult brain: Effects of gender. *Neuroimage*, 26(2), 493–501.

Luna, B., Thulborn, K. R., Munoz, D. P., Merriam, E. P., Garver, K. E., Minshew, N. J., et al. (2001). Maturation of widely distributed brain function subserves cognitive development. *NeuroImage*, 13(5), 786–793.

Mabbott, D. J., Noseworthy, M., Bouffet, E., Laughlin, S., & Rockel, C. (2006). White matter growth as a mechanism of cognitive development in children. *NeuroImage*, 33(3), 936–946.

Maguire, E. A., Spiers, H. J., Good, C. D., Hartley, T., Frackowiak, R. S., & Burgess, N. (2003). Navigation expertise and the human hippocampus: A structural brain imaging analysis. *Hippocampus*, 13(2), 250–259.

Mangin, J. F., Poupon, C., Clark, C., Le Bihan, D., & Bloch, I. (2002). Distortion correction and robust tensor estimation for MR diffusion imaging. *Medical Image Analysis*, 6(3), 191–198.

Marsh, R., Zhu, H., Schultz, R. T., Quackenbush, G., Royal, J., Skudlarski, P., et al. (2006). A developmental fMRI study of self-regulatory control. *Human Brain Mapping*, 27(11), 848–863.

Matsuzawa, J., Matsui, M., Konishi, T., Noguchi, K., Gur, R. C., Bilker, W., et al. (2001). Age-related volumetric changes of brain gray and white matter in healthy infants and children. *Cerebral Cortex*, 11(4), 335–342.

McIntosh, A. R. & Gonzalez-Lima, F. (1994). Structural equation modeling and its application to network analysis in functional brain imaging. *Human Brain Mapping*, 2(1–2), 2–22.

Mechelli, A., Crinion, J. T., Noppeney, U., O'Doherty, J., Ashburner, J., Frackowiak, R. S., et al. (2004). Neurolinguistics: Structural plasticity in the bilingual brain. *Nature*, 431(7010), 757.

Mechelli, A., Price, C. J., Friston, K. J., & Ashburner, J. (2005). Voxel-based morphometry of the human brain: Methods and applications. *Current Medical Imaging Reviews*, 1, 105–113.

Morgan, A. E. & Hynd, G. W. (1998). Dyslexia, neurolinguistic ability, and anatomical variation of the planum temporale. *Neuropsychology Review*, 8(2), 79–93.

Mori, S., Crain, B. J., Chacko, V. P., & van Zijl, P. C. (1999). Three-dimensional tracking of axonal projections in the brain by magnetic resonance imaging. *Annals of Neurology*, 45(2), 265–269.

Mukherjee, P. & McKinstry, R. C. (2006). Diffusion tensor imaging and tractography of human brain development. *Neuroimaging Clinics of North America*, 16(1), 19–43, vii.

Nagy, Z., Westerberg, H., & Klingberg, T. (2004). Maturation of white matter is associated with the development of cognitive functions during childhood. *Journal of Cognitive Neuroscience*, 16(7), 1227–1233.

Narain, C., Scott, S. K., Wise, R. J. S., Rosen, S., Leff, A., Iversen, S. D., et al. (2003). Defining a left-lateralized response specific to intelligible speech using fMRI. *Cerebral Cortex*, 13(12), 1362–1368.

Neil, J., Miller, J., Mukherjee, P., & Huppi, P. S. (2002). Diffusion tensor imaging of normal and injured developing human brain – a technical review. *NMR Biomedicine*, 15(7–8), 543–552.

Nucifora, P. G. P., Verma, R., Melhem, E. R., Gur, R. E., & Gur, R. C. (2005). Leftward asymmetry in relative fiber density of the arcuate fasciculus. *Neuroreport*, 16(8), 791–794.

Parker, G. J., Luzzi, S., Alexander, D. C., Wheeler-Kingshott, C. A., Ciccarelli, O., & Lambon Ralph, M. A. (2005). Lateralization of ventral and dorsal auditory-language pathways in the human brain. *NeuroImage*, 24(3), 656–666.

Paterson, S. J., Heim, S., Friedman, J. T., Choudhury, N., & Benasich, A. A. (2006). Development of structure and function in the infant brain: Implications for cognition, language and social behaviour. *Neuroscience and Biobehavioral Reviews*, 30(8), 1087–1105.

Paus, T. (2005). Mapping brain maturation and cognitive development during adolescence. *Trends in Cognitive Sciences*, 9(2), 60–68.

Paus, T., Collins, D. L., Evans, A. C., Leonard, G., Pike, B., & Zijdenbos, A. (2001). Maturation of white matter in the human brain: A review of magnetic resonance studies. *Brain Research Bulletin*, 54(3), 255–266.

Peltier, S. J., Kerssens, C., Hamann, S. B., Sebel, P. S., Byas-Smith, M., & Hu, X. P. (2005). Functional connectivity changes with concentration of sevoflurane anesthesia. *Neuroreport*, 16(3), 285–288.

Poldrack, R. A., Pare-Blagoev, E. J., & Grant, P. E. (2002). Pediatric functional magnetic resonance imaging: Progress and challenges. *Topics in Magnetic Resonance Imaging*, 13(1), 61–70.

Rivera-Gaxiola, M., Silva-Pereyra, J., Klarman, L., Garcia-Sierra, A., Lara-Ayala, L., Cadena-Salazar, C., et al. (2007). Principal component analyses and scalp distribution of the auditory P150-250 and N250-550 to speech contrasts in Mexican and American infants. *Developmental Neuropsychology*, 31(3), 363–378.

Rohde, G. K., Barnett, A. S., Basser, P. J., Marenco, S., & Pierpaoli, C. (2004). Comprehensive approach for correction of motion and distortion in diffusion-weighted MRI. *Magnetic Resonance in Medicine*, 51(1), 103–114.

Rojas, D. C., Camou, S. L., Reite, M. L., & Rogers, S. J. (2005). Planum temporale volume in children and adolescents with autism. *Journal of Autism and Developmental Disorders*, 35(4), 479–486.

Sanders, L. D., Stevens, C., Coch, D., & Neville, H. J. (2006). Selective auditory attention in 3- to 5-year-old children: An event-related potential study. *Neuropsychologia*, 44(11), 2126–2138.

Schapiro, M. B., Schmithorst, V. J., Wilke, M., Byars, A. W., Strawsburg, R. H., & Holland, S. K. (2004). BOLD fMRI signal increases with age in selected brain regions in children. *Neuroreport*, 15(17), 2575–2578.

Schmithorst, V. J. & Holland, S. K. (2007). Sex differences in the development of neuroanatomical functional connectivity underlying intelligence found using Bayesian connectivity analysis. *NeuroImage*, 35(1), 406–419.

Schmithorst, V. J., Holland, S. K., & Plante, E. (2007). Development of effective connectivity for narrative comprehension in children. *NeuroReport*, 18(14), 1411–1415.

Schmithorst, V. J. & Wilke, M. (2002). Differences in white matter architecture between musicians and non-musicians: A diffusion tensor imaging study. *Neuroscience Letters*, 321(1–2), 57–60.

Schmithorst, V. J., Wilke, M., Dardzinski, B. J., & Holland, S. K. (2002). Correlation of white matter diffusivity and anisotropy with age during childhood and adolescence: A cross-sectional diffusion-tensor MR imaging study. *Radiology*, 222(1), 212–218.

Schmitz, N., Rubia, K., Daly, E., Smith, A., Williams, S., & Murphy, D. G. M. (2006). Neural correlates of executive function in autistic spectrum disorders. *Biological Psychiatry*, 59(1), 7–16.

Schweinsburg, A. D., Nagel, B. J., & Tapert, S. F. (2005). fMRI reveals alteration of spatial working memory networks across adolescence. *Journal of the International Neuropsychological Society*, 11(5), 631–644.

Seghier, M. L., Lazeyras, F., & Huppi, P. S. (2006). Functional MRI of the newborn. *Seminars in Fetal and Neonatal Medicine*, 11(6), 479–488.

Shafer, V. L., Shucard, D. W., Shucard, J. L., & Gerken, L. (1998). An electrophysiological study of infants' sensitivity to the sound patterns of English speech. *Journal of Speech, Language, and Hearing Research*, 41(4), 874–886.

Shaw, P., Greenstein, D., Lerch, J., Clasen, L., Lenroot, R., Gogtay, N., et al. (2006). Intellectual ability and cortical development in children and adolescents. *Nature*, 440(7084), 676–679.

Silva-Pereyra, J., Rivera-Gaxiola, M., & Kuhl, P. K. (2005). An event-related brain potential study of sentence comprehension in preschoolers: Semantic and morphosyntactic processing. *Cognitive Brain Research*, 23(2–3), 247–258.

Smith, S. M. (2002). Fast robust automated brain extraction. *Human Brain Mapping*, 17(3), 143–155.

Smith, S. M., Jenkinson, M., Johansen-Berg, H., Rueckert, D., Nichols, T. E., Mackay, C. E., et al. (2006). Tract-based spatial statistics: Voxelwise analysis of multi-subject diffusion data. *Neuroimage*, 31(4), 1487–1505.

Snook, L., Paulson, L. A., Roy, D., Phillips, L., & Beaulieu, C. (2005a). Diffusion tensor imaging of neurodevelopment in children and young adults. *NeuroImage*, 26(4), 1164–1173.

Snook, L., Paulson, L. A., Roy, D., Phillips, L., & Beaulieu, C. (2005b). Diffusion tensor imaging of neurodevelopment in children and young adults. *Neuroimage*, 26(4), 1164–1173.

Sommer, M., Koch, M. A., Paulus, W., Weiller, C., & Buchel, C. (2002). Disconnection of speech-relevant brain areas in persistent developmental stuttering. *Lancet*, 360(9330), 380–383.

Sowell, E. R., Peterson, B. S., Thompson, P. M., Welcome, S. E., Henkenius, A. L., & Toga, A. W. (2003). Mapping cortical change across the human life span. *Nature Neuroscience*, 6(3), 309–315.

Sowell, E. R., Thompson, P. M., Leonard, C. M., Welcome, S. E., Kan, E., & Toga, A. W. (2004a). Longitudinal mapping of cortical thickness and brain growth in normal children. *Journal of Neuroscience*, 24(38), 8223–8231.

Sowell, E. R., Thompson, P. M., Rex, D., Kornsand, D., Tessner, K. D., Jernigan, T. L., et al. (2002). Mapping sulcal pattern asymmetry and local cortical surface gray matter distribution in vivo: Maturation in perisylvian cortices. *Cerebral Cortex*, 12(1), 17–26.

Sowell, E. R., Thompson, P. M., & Toga, A. W. (2004b). Mapping changes in the human cortex throughout the span of life. *Neuroscientist*, 10(4), 372–392.

Stejskal, E. O. & Tanner, J. E. (1965). Spin diffusion measurements – spin echoes in presence of a time-dependent field gradient. *Journal of Chemical Physics*, 42(1), 288–&.

Szaflarski, J. P., Schmithorst, V. J., Altaye, M., Byars, A. W., Ret, J., Plante, E., et al. (2006). A longitudinal functional magnetic resonance imaging study of language development in children 5 to 11 years old. *Annals of Neurology*, 59(5), 796–807.

Szeszko, P. R., Vogel, J., Ashtari, M., Malhotra, A. K., Bates, J., Kane, J. M., et al. (2003). Sex differences in frontal lobe white matter microstructure: A DTI study. *NeuroReport*, 14(18), 2469–2473.

Thompson, P. M., Hayashi, K. M., Sowell, E. R., Gogtay, N., Giedd, J. N., Rapoport, J. L., et al. (2004). Mapping cortical change in Alzheimer's disease, brain development, and schizophrenia. *NeuroImage*, 23(SUPPL. 1).

Thompson, P. M., Lee, A. D., Dutton, R. A., Geaga, J. A., Hayashi, K. M., Eckert, M. A., et al. (2005). Abnormal cortical complexity and thickness profiles mapped in Williams syndrome. *Journal of Neuroscience*, 25(16), 4146–4158.

Thompson, P. M., Sowell, E. R., Gogtay, N., Giedd, J. N., Vidal, C. N., Hayashi, K. M., et al. (2005). Structural MRI and brain development. *Neuroimaging, Pt B*, 67, 285–+.

Tisserand, D. J., van Boxtel, M. P., Pruessner, J. C., Hofman, P., Evans, A. C., & Jolles, J. (2004). A voxel-based morphometric study to determine individual differences in gray matter density associated with age and cognitive change over time. *Cerebral Cortex*, 14(9), 966–973.

Toga, A. W. & Thompson, P. M. (2003). Mapping brain asymmetry. *Nature Reviews Neuroscience*, 4(1), 37–48.

Toga, A. W., Thompson, P. M., & Sowell, E. R. (2006). Mapping brain maturation. *Trends in Neurosciences*, 29(3), 148–159.

Uttal, W. R. (2003). *The New Phrenology: The Limits of Localizing Cognitive Processes in the Brain.* Cambridge, MA: MIT Press.

Vargha-Khadem, F., Watkins, K. E., Price, C. J., Ashburner, J., Alcock, K. J., Connelly, A., et al. (1998). Neural basis of an inherited speech and language disorder. *Proceedings of the National Academy of Sciences of the United States of America*, 95(21), 12695–12700.

Vernooij, M. W., Smits, M., Wielopolski, P. A., Houston, G. C., Krestin, G. P., & van der Lugt, A. (2007). Fiber density asymmetry of the arcuate fasciculus in relation to functional hemispheric language lateralization in both right- and left-handed healthy subjects: A combined fMRI and DTI study. *NeuroImage*, 35(3), 1064–1076.

Vincent, J. L., Patel, G. H., Fox, M. D., Snyder, A. Z., Baker, J. T., Van Essen, D. C., et al. (2007). Intrinsic functional architecture in the anaesthetized monkey brain. *Nature*, 447(7140), 83–U84.

Watkins, K. E., Smith, S. M., Davis, S., & Howell, P. (2007). Structural and functional abnormalities of the motor system in developmental stuttering. *Brain*, 131(Pt 1), 50–59.

Watkins, K. E., Vargha-Khadem, F., Ashburner, J., Passingham, R. E., Connelly, A., Friston, K. J., et al. (2002). MRI analysis of an inherited speech and language disorder: Structural brain abnormalities. *Brain*, 125, 465–478.

Wilke, M., Holland, S. K., Myseros, J. S., Schmithorst, V. J., & Ball, W. S. (2003). Functional magnetic resonance imaging in pediatrics. *Neuropediatrics*, 34(5), 225–233.

Wilke, M., Krageloh-Mann, I., & Holland, S. K. (2007). Global and local development of gray and white matter volume in normal children and adolescents. *Experimental Brain Research*, 178(3), 296–307.

Wilke, M., Lidzba, K., Staudt, M., Buchenau, K., Grodd, W., & Krageloh-Mann, I. (2005). Comprehensive language mapping in children, using functional magnetic resonance imaging: What's missing counts. *Neuroreport*, 16(9), 915–919.

Wilke, M., Schmithorst, V. J., & Holland, S. K. (2002). Assessment of spatial normalization of whole-brain magnetic resonance images in children. *Human Brain Mapping*, 17(1), 48–60.

Wilke, M., Schmithorst, V. J., & Holland, S. K. (2003). Normative pediatric brain data for spatial normalization and segmentation differs from standard adult data. *Magnetic Resonance in Medicine*, 50(4), 749–757.

Witelson, S. F. (1991). Neural sexual mosaicism: Sexual differentiation of the human temporo-parietal region for functional asymmetry. *Psychoneuroendocrinology*, 16(1–3), 131–153.

Witelson, S. F., Glezer, II, & Kigar, D. L. (1995). Women have greater density of neurons in posterior temporal cortex. *Journal of Neuroscience*, 15(5 Pt 1), 3418–3428.

Witelson, S. F. & Pallie, W. (1973). Left hemisphere specialization for language in newborn – neuroanatomical evidence of asymmetry. *Brain*, 96(Sep), 641–&.

Wood, A. G., Harvey, A. S., Wellard, R. M., Abbott, D. F., Anderson, V., Kean, M., et al. (2004). Language cortex activation in normal children. *Neurology*, 63(6), 1035–1044.

Chapter 6

Motor speech profile in relation to site of brain pathology: a developmental perspective

Angela Morgan, Frédérique Liégeois, and Faraneh Vargha-Khadem

Abstract

Few reports exist on motor speech profiles of children with congenital or acquired brain damage, relating the speech disorder to its compromised neural substrate. Here, we examine motor speech characteristics in representative cases with: a) speech and orofacial dyspraxia resulting from mutation of the *FOXP2* gene; b) dysarthria resulting from the resection of posterior fossa tumour, and c) dysarthria associated with hemispherectomy for treatment of intractable epilepsy. The neuropathology that is implicated in each type of motor speech disorder is considered with the aim of identifying those aspects of the motor circuitry that may have become disrupted as a result of the brain damage. The role of bilateral versus unilateral neuropathology, and the involvement of the fronto-striatal and fronto-cerebellar loops in dyspraxia and dysarthria are discussed.

6.1 **Introduction**

By the end of the first decade of life, children have acquired all of the speech sounds of their mother tongue, and are able to comprehend and produce grammatically complex sentences. In parallel, they have mastered the motor skill of fluent speech execution and the ability to rapidly produce perfectly intelligible yet phonetically complex utterances. These linguistic and motor speech skills are mastered with little apparent effort in typically developing children.

While much is known about the relationship between motor speech dysfunction and the underlying brain pathology in adults, the paediatric literature on congenital or acquired persistent motor speech disorders is relatively sparse. Existing reports focus primarily on motor speech performance with limited information about the brain abnormality responsible for the disorder. A possible reason for the dearth of reported cases of chronic motor speech disorders in children is that the increased propensity for recovery and/or reorganization of speech resulting from neuronal plasticity reduces the severity of the disorder in the long term.

In the light of the above, this chapter provides an overview of three different types of motor speech problems associated with neurodevelopmental disorders: (a) Congenital orofacial and speech dyspraxia resulting from the mutation of the *FOXP2* gene; (b) ataxic-flaccid dysarthria after surgical treatment of posterior fossa tumour acquired late in childhood; and (c) unilateral upper motor neuron dysarthria (flaccid-ataxic variant) after hemispherectomy performed in childhood for control of intractable epilepsy. By systematically contrasting the motor speech profiles of cases from each of these aetiological categories, the neural substrates implicated in the motor speech circuitry will be examined.

6.2 **Orofacial and speech dyspraxia resulting from the mutation of the *FOXP2* gene**

6.2.1 **Adult-onset versus developmental apraxia of speech**

In adulthood, *acquired* apraxia of speech (AOS) is typically associated with unilateral left-sided lesions in the inferior frontal gyrus (Hillis et al., 2004). To date, studies of children with pre- or perinatally acquired left-sided cortical lesions affecting the anterior speech and language territory have systematically reported on language outcome only (Bates et al., 2001; Mosch et al., 2005), with infrequent and anecdotal reporting of any co-morbid motor speech deficits. Where case studies of motor speech problems resulting from subcortical infarcts are reported, the pathology affecting different components of the orofacial and orovocal systems is not specified (e.g., Tallal et al., 1994). It is therefore not clear whether the absence of systematic reporting on motor speech status has resulted in AOS deficits in children being overlooked, or whether such conditions simply do not occur in childhood.

In contrast to *acquired* AOS in children, idiopathic congenital or developmental childhood apraxia of speech (CAS) has been thoroughly characterized (see American Speech and Hearing

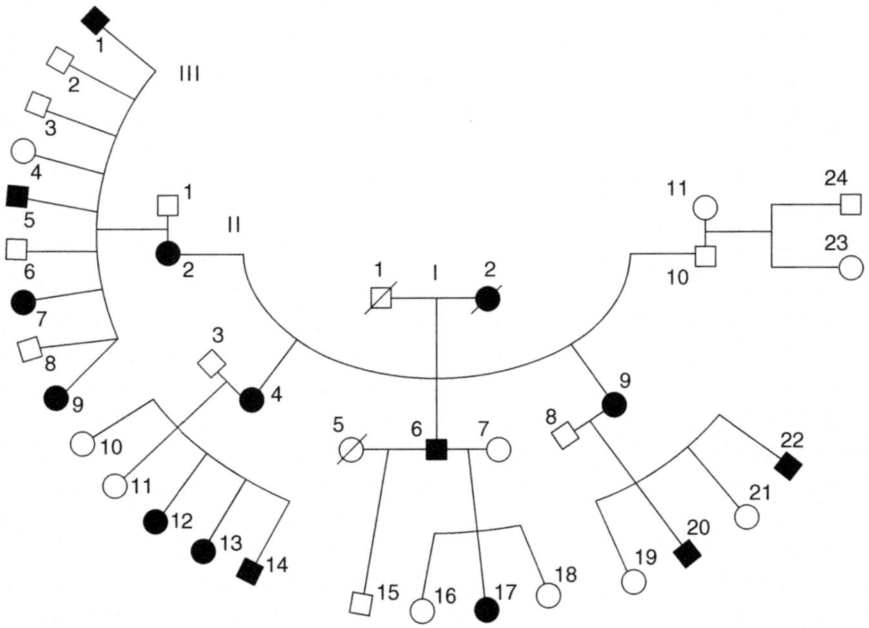

Fig. 6.1 Pedigree of the KE family. I, II, and III mark the generations. Shaded symbols designate affected status; circles, females; squares, males. Cases 1 and 2 are III-7 and III-20, respectively. Copyright (1998) National Academy of Sciences, USA.

Association Position Statement and Technical Report on CAS, 2007 for review). Furthermore, the neural substrate for one subtype of CAS, caused by the disruption of the *FOXP2* gene, has been identified through a series of structural and functional magnetic resonance imaging (MRI) studies of the three-generational KE family (see Fig. 6.1, Family Pedigree), where 15 of the 30 members are affected with an inherited form of orofacial and speech dyspraxia.

6.2.2 **Speech profile of the affected KE family members**

Despite attending speech and language units, and receiving intensive speech therapy throughout childhood and adolescence, affected members of the KE family present with a severe and persistent speech disorder. The speech dyspraxia in this group varies in severity, but is relatively homogeneous with regard to the pattern of diagnostic features and the underlying core deficits. The affected family members (including the two cases detailed here) present with a moderate to severe speech disorder that markedly affects intelligibility. Interestingly, despite varying levels of severity of functional speech outcome during adult life, the affected family members demonstrate underlying weakness in their speech motor system when challenged by demanding articulatory tasks. For example, in comparison to control participants, severe breakdown is noted in timing and accuracy of performance on a diadochokinetic task that involves production of alternating syllables and consonant clusters (e.g., pla-kra-ta). Altogether, the speech dyspraxia in the KE family is reported to be similar to both adult AOS (Watkins et al., 2002a) and CAS (Liégeois et al., 2007).

6.2.3 **Neuropathology associated with the speech and language disorder in the affected KE members**

Despite the normal appearance of the MRI scans on radiological examination, quantitative analyses of these same scans, relative to those obtained from the unaffected family members and controls, revealed subtle but significant differences. Thus, voxel-based morphomerty (VBM) revealed less grey matter density, subsequently referred to as 'morphological' brain abnormalities, in certain regions while functional MRI studies showed anomalous patterns of brain activity during language tasks.

In line with gene expression studies of *FOXP2/Foxp2*[1] in the brain of human and mouse embryo (Lai et al., 2003), VBM analyses revealed bilateral abnormalities in a number of motor-related cortical and subcortical areas including abnormally low levels of grey matter in the head of the caudate nucleus, inferior frontal gyrus (Broca's area), the precentral gyrus, the temporal pole, and the ventral cerebellum (lobules VIIB and VIIIB) (Belton et al., 2003; Fig. 6.2). Abnormal increases in grey matter were noted in the posterior part of the superior temporal gyrus (Wernicke's area), the angular gyrus and the putamen (Belton et al., 2003).

In relation to the neural substrate underlying speech, three functional MRI (fMRI) studies were conducted comparing activation patterns in the affected and unaffected KE members (Liégeois et al., 2003). The fMRI paradigms included silent verb generation (i.e., generating verbs using 'internal speech'), spoken verbs in response to nouns heard over headphones, and word repetition. Consistent with the structural imaging findings, fMRI tasks revealed under-activation in affected relative to unaffected KE members in the putamen, Broca's area, and the right hemisphere homologue of Broca's region (Liégeois et al., 2003).

[1] Standard gene nomenclature denotes that human gene symbols are italicized and in uppercase (e.g., *FOXP2*) and mice gene symbols are italicized with the first letter in uppercase and the remaining letters in lowercase (*Foxp2*).

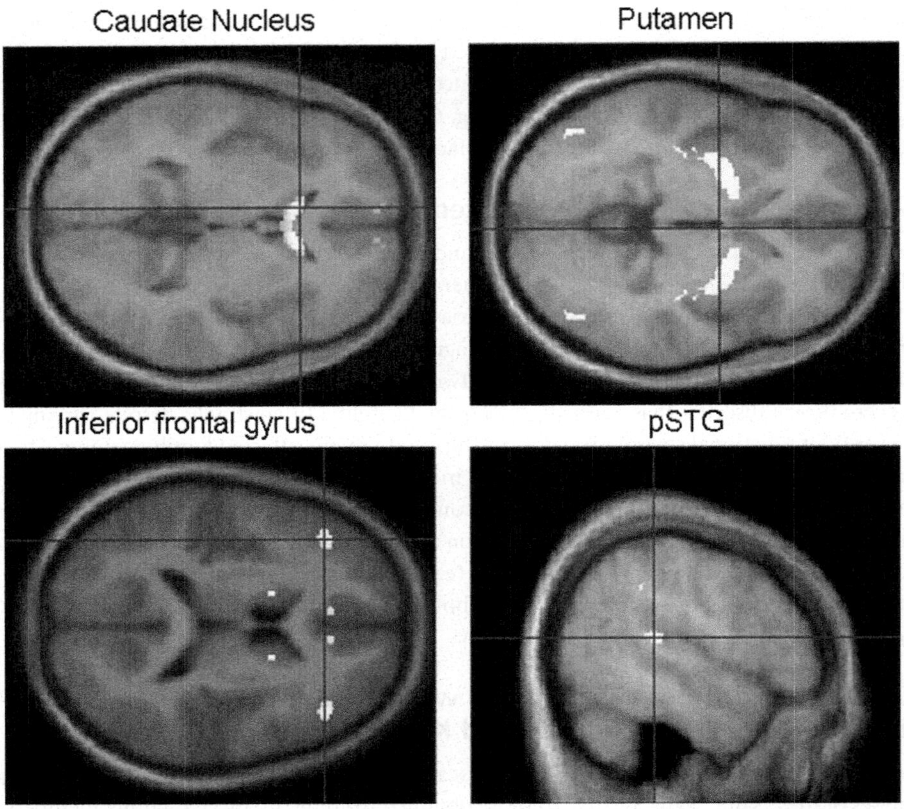

Fig. 6.2 Morphological abnormalities demonstrating regions of reduced (left column) and increased (right column) grey matter density in affected KE family members compared to unaffected members, using VBM. For details see Belton et al., 2003. (See Plate section).

6.2.4 **Case presentation**

Table 6.1 provides details of speech dyspraxic and dysarthric features in two affected KE members from the third generation, Cases 1 and 2 (III-7 and III-20, respectively, Fig. 6.1). At the time of testing, Cases 1 and 2 were young adults, and presented with a range of features consistent with the developmental form of speech dyspraxia, including phonemic level errors of substitution, omission, addition, transposition, and distortion of both consonants and vowels, and more frequent errors with increases in the length or complexity of phonemic sequences (see Table 6.1, 'key features of speech dyspraxia'). Features of spastic dysarthria included a low and monotonous pitch, a strained-strangled (Case 1) or hoarse-breathy voice (Case 2), and hypernasality. In addition, a limited number of other speech features not traditionally associated with spastic dysarthria were noted (i.e., alternating loudness, prolonged phonemes) (see Table 6.1, 'key features of dysarthria').

One of the striking dysarthric features is a disturbance of oral-nasal resonance. Nasality has a profound impact on 'naturalness ratings' of speech production. The impact of disturbed nasal resonance is highlighted by self-reports of some of the affected members stating that the general public frequently ask them whether they are deaf because they sound as though they have 'deaf speech'. Overall, the dysarthric features can be classified as mixed, but predominantly spastic with characteristic low pitch, reduced stress, and a breathy voice (Morgan et al., 2005).

Table 6.1 Neural and speech profiles of cases across three different neurodevelopmental aetiologies

	Case 1	Case 2	Case 3	Case 4	Case 5	Case 6
Aetiology	Genetic disruption: FOXP2 mutation	Genetic disruption: FOXP2 mutation	Posterior fossa tumour (astrocytoma)	Posterior fossa tumour (astrocytoma)	Hemispherectomy (LC1) (intractable epilepsy associated with congential dysplasia)	Hemispherectomy (RC4) (intractable epilepsy associated with hemimegan-cephaly)
Neural pathology	Bilateral involvement: head of caudate nucleus, pars opercularis (Broca's and R homologue), precentral gyrus, ventral cerebellar lobules: VIIB, VIIIB, temporal pole; posterior superior temporal gyrus, angular gyrus	Bilateral involvement: head of caudate nucle-us, pars opercularis (Broca's and R homo-logue), precentral gyrus, ventral cerebellar lobules: VIIB, VIIIB, temporal pole; posterior superior temporal gyrus, angular gyrus	Vermis + RH cerebellum: Ventral lobules: V, VI; Medial lobules: VI, CrusI, CrusII; Lateral lobules: CrusI, CrusII, VII, VIII	LH cerebellum: Lateral lobules: CrusII, VII, VIII	LH cerebrum surgically removed	RH cerebrum surgically removed
Age at onset of neuropathology	Congenital	Congenital	6 years	7 years 6 months	Onset of seizures at 2;0 years; hemi-spherectomy at 13 years 10 months	Onset of seizures at 7 months; hemispherectomy at 4 years 2 months
Age at assessment	23 years	31 years	10 years 5 months	11 years 9 months	21 years 2 month	13 years 10 months
Elapsed time post-surgery	NA	NA	4 years 5 months	4 years 3 months	7 years 4 months	9 years 8 months
Gender	Female	Male	Female	Male	Male	Male
Motor speech diagnosis	Moderate verbal dyspraxia, moderate oral apraxia, and concomitant moderate spastic dysarthria	Severe verbal dyspraxia, moderate oral apraxia, and concomitant moder-ate spastic dysarthria	Mild flaccid-ataxic dysarthria	Mild flaccid-ataxic dysarthria	Mild unilateral upper motor neuron dysar-thria (flaccid-ataxic variant)	Mild unilateral upper motor neuron dysar-thria (flaccid-ataxic variant)

(Continued)

Table 6.1 (Cont.) Neural and speech profiles of cases across three different neurodevelopmental aetiologies

	Case 1	Case 2	Case 3	Case 4	Case 5	Case 6
Key features of verbal dyspraxia	Phonemic-level errors: substitution, omission, addition, transposition, distortion, voicing Vowel errors Visible searching Abnormal prosody ↑errors with ↑in phonemic sequence/complexity ↓errors in automatic than volitional speech	Phonemic-level errors: substitution, omission, addition, transposition, distortion, voicing Vowel errors Visible searching Abnormal prosody ↑errors with ↑in phonemic sequence/complexity ↓errors in automatic than volitional speech	Nil dyspraxia	Nil dyspraxia	Nil dyspraxia with exception of syllable sequencing difficulties on DDK (i.e., omissions, substitutions or additions of phonemes during DDK task)	Nil dyspraxia with exception of syllable sequencing difficulties on DDK (i.e., omissions, substitutions or additions of phonemes during DDK task)
Key features of dysarthria	Monopitch Reduced pitch Vocal tremor Alternating loudness, Strained-strangled harsh voice Reduced rate Imprecise consonants Hyponasality Distorted vowels Irregular articulatory breakdowns	Monopitch Reduced pitch Monoloudness Alternating loudness Hoarse-breathy voice (continuous) Hyponasality Reduced rate Short phrases Increased rate in segments Distorted vowels	Monopitch Vocal tremor Monoloudness Reduced overall loudness Breathy voice (transient) Reduced rate Imprecise consonants Hypernasality	Monopitch Hoarse voice Forced respiration Reduced stress Reduced rate Imprecise consonants	Increased pitch Monopitch Vocal tremor Hoarse, breathy voice (transient) Reduced rate Short phrases Increased rate in segments Reduced stress Prolonged intervals Inappropriate silences	Increased pitch Monopitch Vocal tremor Monoloudness Loudness decay Harsh, hoarse, breathy (transient) voice Reduced rate Short phrases Increased rate in segments Reduced stress

	Prolonged phonemes Excess and equal stress	Irregular articulatory breakdowns Prolonged phonemes Excess and equal stress			Imprecise consonants Prolonged phonemes Hypernasality Audible inspiration	Prolonged intervals Inappropriate silences Imprecise consonants Prolonged phonemes Imprecise vowels Hypernasality Audible inspiration Weak pressure consonants
Articulation errors	/r/, /th/, /ts/, /sh/*v	/r/, /th/, /ts/, /sh/	Nil	Nil	Nil	Nil
Phonological errors	^Cluster reduction, weak syllable deletion, deaffrication, final consonant de-voicing, fronting fricatives, gliding, stopping fricatives, post-vocalic voicing	^Cluster reduction, weak syllable deletion, deaffrication, final consonant de-voicing, fronting fricatives, gliding, stopping fricatives	Nil	Nil	Nil	Nil
Single-word intelligibility (%)	70	44	98	94	100	85

^Rated using Goldman-Fristoe and phonological errors determined based on Dodd and Iacono (1989), Dodd (1995).

Spastic dysarthria is most commonly associated with bilateral damage to the upper motor neurons of the pyramidal or extra-pyramidal tracts (Urban et al., 2006; Ziegler and von Cramon 1986). It is therefore possible that the spastic features reported in Cases 1 and 2 result from abnormality in the motor and premotor regions and associated pathways.

Numerous instances of spastic dysarthria have been reported in adults in association with bilateral cortical involvement (or upper motor neuron lesions), including progressive motor neuron disease (Duffy et al., 2007), acquired cerebrovascular accidents (Thompson et al., 1995), and traumatic brain injury (Ziegler and von Cramon 1986). Similarly, acquired spastic dysarthria in children is sometimes reported after bilateral damage to the frontal cortex, resulting for example, from diffuse axonal injury associated with traumatic brain injury (Cahill et al., 2005; Morgan et al., 2007). Persistent dysarthria resulting from congenital aetiologies is also typically reported as spastic, and may co-occur with non-speech orofacial and speech apraxia, particularly in children with bilateral perisylvian syndromes, such as suprabulbar palsy, or Worster-Drought syndrome (Suresh and Deepa 2004; Clark et al., 2000; Worster-Drought 1974, 1956).

The co-morbidity of speech dyspraxia and dysarthria was recently reported in a mother and daughter with a 7;13 translocation affecting *FOXP2* (Shriberg et al., 2006). Although it is difficult to directly compare the phenotype of cases with translocations disrupting two chromosomes to those with a mutation on one chromosome, it is noteworthy that Shriberg and colleagues report both speech dyspraxia and dysarthria as the core phenotype of their patients.

Despite the presence of abnormalities in the basal ganglia (specifically in the caudate and the putamen) in the affected KE members, the dysarthric features of the two cases presented here cannot be classified as either hyperkinetic or hypokinetic as documented in adult patient groups with neostriatal pathology. Specifically, Cases 1 and 2 do not present with any form of abnormal, involuntary movement disorder, nor do they present with the distinctive pattern of speech production associated with either hyper or hypokinesia (Darley et al., 1969).

6.2.5 Fronto-striatal pathology and dyspraxia

As indicated above, speech dyspraxia is the most prominent diagnostic feature in the affected KE members. In adults, acquired AOS has been frequently associated with the disruption of the posterior part of the inferior frontal gyrus, or Broca's area, with this having been recently reported in a comprehensive study of 80 cases of adult-acquired left hemisphere stroke (Hillis et al., 2004). Other authors have linked AOS to damage to the left insular cortex in stroke patients (Dronkers 1996; Ogar et al., 2006). In relation to children, there are two reported cases in the literature of AOS associated with damage to Broca's area and its homologue on the right side, and direct and/or indirect bilateral damage to the basal ganglia (Vargha-Khadem et al., 1985; Tallal et al., 1994).

The link between *unilateral* basal ganglia damage and dyspraxia in childhood is less clear. An early study by Aram and colleagues (Aram et al., 1983) reported the case of a seven-year-old girl with an infarct to the left putamen, the anterior limb of the internal capsule, and the lateral aspect of the head of the caudate nucleus. The patient showed transient mutism and oral apraxia, but not speech dyspraxia. Similarly, the study of a group of patients with childhood-acquired unilateral infarcts confined to the basal ganglia failed to show any evidence of speech dyspraxia (Rowan 2003; Rowan et al., 2007).

The findings in the KE family along with the few paediatric reports in the literature, highlight the role of the fronto-striatal network in the early acquisition of speech motor sequences that are critical for the typical development of intelligible speech (see Fig. 6.3). In addition, the findings support the hypothesis that in the absence of intellectual or sensory restrictions, chronic speech deficits in children are the consequence of bilateral damage to the thalamocortical speech and language networks (Vargha-Khadem et al., 1985, Tallal et al., 1994; Landau and Kleffner 1957).

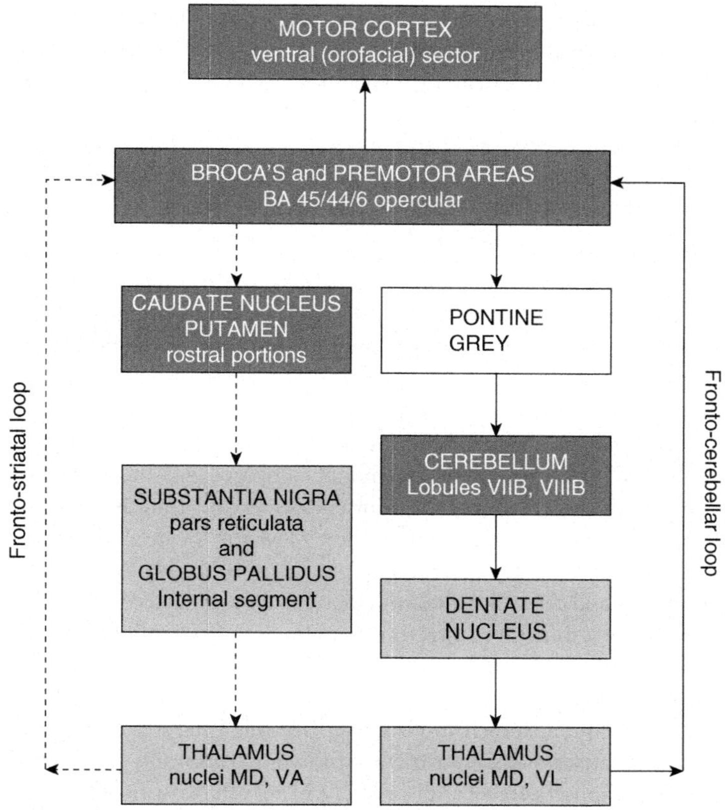

Fig. 6.3 Proposed model for *FOXP2*-dependent speech and language circuit, derived from both gene expression (light and dark grey boxes) studies and KE family morphological and functional brain abnormalities (dark grey boxes). BA, Brodmann's area. (Adapted from Figure 4, Vargha-Khadem et al., 2005; see Figure 3 in same article for a full description of other brain regions where *FOXP2/Foxp2* is expressed).

Thus, in the KE family bilateral cortico-striatal abnormality may be the main cause of persistent speech and orofacial dyspraxia. Interestingly, this dyspraxia is not associated with gross limb apraxia (Watkins et al., 2002a), suggesting that the latter may be subserved by a different neural subsystem. Whether highly skilled movements of the fingers and the hands, such as those required for expert typing or for playing musical instruments require the same coarticulation abilities as speech, and therefore rely on the same cortico-striatal pathway, remains to be determined (Vargha-Khadem et al., 2005).

6.2.6 **Fronto-striatal pathology and dysarthria**

As noted above (see 6.2.4, Case Presentation), the features of spastic dysarthria described in KE Cases 1 and 2 are not consistent with those reported for adults with degenerative disorders resulting in hyperkinetic or hypokinetic dysarthria associated with basal ganglia pathology. The lack of consistency may be due to a number of underlying pathological processes that characterize the features of each aetiological condition. It is clear, however, that in adult-onset conditions such as Parkinson's Disease or Huntington's Disease, the motor circuitry, including the components regulating motor speech production, had developed, and was functioning normally prior to the onset of the degenerative process. Such is not the case with the heritable *FOXP2* abnormality, where the motor circuitry is abnormal from the start, and fails to develop to the requisite standard to subserve fine oromotor control (Vargha-Khadem et al., 2005). It is therefore difficult to determine which aspects of frontostriatal function/dysfunction result in the spastic dysarthria that is reported in the KE members presented here.

6.2.7 Cerebellar pathology and speech dyspraxia

The neuroimaging studies of the KE family (Belton et al., 2003; Liégeois et al., 2003; Watkins et al., 2002b), and gene expression studies of FOXP2/Foxp2 highlight the importance of the inferior-frontal cerebellar loop in setting up the motor circuitry during development. Gene expression studies in both human and mouse embryo implicate the cerebellum as an early site of *Foxp2* expression (Lai et al., 2003), and possibly a critical site for the development of motor skill given the abundance of evidence linking this structure with motor skill learning (Jackson et al., 2003). A recent study on mice with a point mutation identical to the one in the KE family suggested reduced rates of motor learning in the mutant compared with the wild type (Groszer et al., 2008). In addition, although the average running speed was similar in the two groups of mice on day 1, the subsequent rate of increase was significantly lower in the heterozygous mice, as was the final running speed. Another study of mice with one disrupted copy of *Foxp2* reported impaired ultrasonic vocalization and cerebellar abnormalities, most pronounced in the Purkinje cells (Shu et al., 2005). Although it is difficult to directly extend findings from rodents to humans, the cross-species evidence suggests that *Foxp2*/ *FOXP2* plays a role in cerebellar structure and function, with the ultimate goal of achieving finely tuned, and timed, motor control.

A role for the cerebellum in speech and language has long been suggested (Ackermann, et al., 2007 for a review). Mutism and dysarthria are the most commonly reported speech-related manifestations of acute-onset cerebellar disorders, and are often associated with limb and orofacial dyspraxia, dysphagia, emotional regression, and/or language deficits (e.g., after removal of astrocytoma or medulloblastoma in children, Aarsen et al., 2004; see Schmahmann and Pandya 2008, for a summary).

Within the context of the core deficits of speech and orofacial dyspraxia in the affected KE members, it is difficult to identify the contributions of the inferior frontal cerebellar loop as distinct from those of the inferior frontal basal ganglia loop, given that sectors within both loops show abnormal structure and/or function in the neuroimaging studies (see Fig. 6.3; Vargha-Khadem et al., 2005). A parsimonious conclusion based on the available data is that the *FOXP2* gene may be critical for the development of the motor circuitry, in particular the putative fronto-striatal and fronto-cerebellar networks associated with the selection, planning, and execution of speech, and non-speech oromotor sequences.

6.3 Speech profile following surgery for posterior fossa tumour

The posterior fossa region encompasses the area below the tentorium, incorporating the cerebellum and the fourth ventricle. Tumours occurring in this region are typically treated via surgical removal of the tumour mass, and in malignant cases radiotherapy and chemotherapy follows surgical treatment (Ibrahim and Appleton 2004).

Dysarthria frequently occurs during the acute recovery period from surgical removal of a posterior fossa tumour (PFT) in children, though less commonly in adults (Catsman-Berrevoets et al., 1999; Ildan et al., 2002; Murdoch and Hudson-Tennent 1994; Pollack et al., 1995). In some cases, the dysarthria is chronic and may persist for more than five years post-surgery (Cornwell et al., 2003a; Huber et al., 2006). A subgroup of children undergoing surgical treatment for PFT may also develop mutism and subsequent dysarthria (MSD) post-surgery (see de Smet 2007, for review). It has been proposed that post-operative mutism may in fact be a very severe form of dysarthria, or anarthria, and, as such, mutism and dysarthria may share a similar neural substrate (Ackermann and Ziegler 1994; van Mourik et al., 1998; van Calenbergh 1995). The dysarthria that emerges following surgical removal of PFT is characterized as ataxic and/or flaccid in nature (Cornwell et al., 2003a, 2004; Murdoch and Hudson-Tennent 1994).

6.3.1 The neuropathology associated with posterior fossa tumours and their treatment

The neuropathology giving rise to disturbances of speech and language following PFT resection is often limited with respect to definition of the site of involvement, i.e., left or right cerebellar hemispheres, or midline cerebellar vermal regions (but see Ozimek et al., 2004; Richter et al., 2005, for exceptions). In studies that relate the neuropathology specifically to disturbances of speech and language, the emphasis is on the pathophysiology of mutism, with or without dysarthria (Ozgur et al., 2006; van Dongen et al., 1994; Steinbok et al., 2003; Ersahin et al., 1996), rather than on dysarthria per se. In recent years, quantitative structural and functional MRI techniques, and access to atlas of the cerebellum (e.g., Schmahmann et al., 2000) have allowed the regions and lobules involved in task performance to be identified with increased precision. For the two patients (Cases 3 and 4) presented here, the cerebellar territories invaded by the tumour and the surgery were identified using the anatomical distinctions between the cerebellar lobules adopted by Schmahmann and colleagues (Schmahmann et al., 2000) in their MRI atlas of the cerebellum (Whiting, 2005 see Table 6.1). In Case 3, the tumour encroached the midline vermal regions, and the right cerebellar hemisphere with involvement of the ventral, medial, and lateral lobules. The tumour in Case 4 was in the left cerebellar hemisphere and involved the lateral lobules only.

6.3.2 Case presentation

The two patients reported here had onset of cerebellar astrocytoma after the age of five years. Treatment consisted of surgical resection of the benign tumour, with no post-surgical radiotherapy or chemotherapy. Despite the absence of post-surgical mutism, both patients continued to suffer from a mild, but chronic flaccid-ataxic dysarthria when assessed more than four years after the resection of the tumour (see Table 6.1). The ataxic component of the dysarthria was characterized primarily by phonatory-prosodic insufficiency, including monotonous pitch and loudness, and a hoarse or breathy voice. Articulatory breakdown was also present, signalled by imprecise consonant production as a result of subtle unilateral weakness of cranial nerves VII (slow speech rate, vowel distortions) and XII (consonant imprecision). This profile is consistent with previous perceptual (Cornwell et al., 2003a, b; Murdoch and Hudson-Tennent 1994) and acoustic (Cornwell et al., 2004) reports of flaccid-ataxic dysarthia in children with PFT. Differential diagnosis confirmed the absence of spastic, hyperkinetic, and hypokinetic dysarthria given that the children did not demonstrate tonal spasticity, or abnormal involuntary movements affecting their speech (Darley et al., 1969a). Furthermore, there was no evidence of speech or orofacial dyspraxia, nor any features of developmental articulation or phonological deficits.

6.3.3 Cerebellar pathology and dysarthria

A number of risk factors have been used to predict dysarthria after surgical resection for PFT. These include the presence of post-surgical mutism, the type and size of tumour, the presence of hydrocephalus, the need for further treatment with radiotherapy and/or chemotherapy, and the site of neuropathology associated with the tumour and its resection (see Huber et al., 2006; de Smet et al., 2007, for further discussion). None of these factors in isolation predict dysarthria, but the site of neuropathology is an important variable inasmuch as its consequences can be evaluated in relation to disruptions in function, and to interference with neuroanatomical pathways.

In patients who have developed dysarthria following PFT treatment, the site of cerebellar pathology can be used to address several questions: first, does dysarthria emerge after unilateral (left or right), or bilateral cerebellar damage? A related issue is whether the cerebellar hemispheres show specialization for speech and language, mirroring the well-documented cortical specialization for this function. Second, is the dysarthria directly related to disruption of specific cerebellar lobules? Third, does dysarthria emerge because of disruption of white matter pathways subserving speech, specifically, the dentate-thalamic-cerebellar pathway? Each of these questions will be addressed here in relation to the two case presentations.

There is lack of consensus about the role of unilateral versus bilateral cerebellar pathology resulting in dysarthric speech. A number of studies involving adult patients conclude that only left cerebellar hemisphere damage disrupts speech (Amarenco et al., 1991; Lechtenberg and Gilman 1978). In contrast, reports based on adult patients with ischaemic infarcts indicate that dysarthria may result from unilateral lesions of either the left or the right cerebellar hemisphere (Ackermann et al., 1992), suggesting an absence of asymmetry of function at the cerebellar level.

The two patients presented here had the diagnosis of cerebellar astrocytoma, and showed similar ratings of severity of dysarthria. Nevertheless, the site of neuropathology in each case was markedly different, with Case 3 showing involvement of the vermis and three medial lobules extending to the right cerebellar hemisphere, and Case 4 showing only left cerebellar hemisphere pathology (see Table 6.1). The present findings are therefore in line with those reported for adults with ischaemic infarcts (Ackermann et al., 1992), suggesting that bilateral cerebellar damage is not a prerequisite for the emergence of mild, yet chronic dysarthria. Furthermore, the finding that damage to either cerebellar hemisphere can lead to dysarthria suggests an absence of specialization at the level of the cerebellum for the motor control of speech.

Regarding the role of specific cerebellar lobules in dysarthric speech, studies of adult patients with ischaemic lesions implicate the paravermal region of the superior cerebellum, corresponding to paravermal lobules VI and VII, or Crus I, (Ackermann et al., 1992; Amarenco et al., 1991; Lechtenberg and Gilman 1978). The dysarthria in these adult patients is characterized as ataxic (Ozimek et al., 2004). There is evidence to suggest, however, that children may have ataxic dysarthria resulting from neuropathology that is different from that documented in adults (see Ackermann et al., 1992; Ozimek et al., 2004). Of the two paediatric cases presented here, only Case 3 had a cerebellar lesion that extended into lobules VI and VII. Interestingly, however, previous case studies of dysarthria (Ozimek et al., 2004; Richter et al., 2005) and the two cases presented here had involvement of lobules VII and VIII, consistent with cerebellar pathology in the KE family. Advances in MR imaging and development of quantitative techniques to assess the integrity of white matter tracts (Habas and Cabanis 2007; Salamon et al., 2007) provide the opportunity to test the commonly supported hypothesis that dysarthria, or specifically MSD, may emerge because of the disruption of the white matter pathway connecting the dentate nuclei to the supplementary motor area via the thalamus (Crutchfield et al., 1994; van Calenbergh et al., 1995; Dietze and Mickle 1990; Kusano et al., 2006; van Dongen et al., 1994; Pollack et al., 1995; Rekate et al., 1985). Disruption of this pathway in adult patients has been associated with ataxic dysarthria. However, in line with previous paediatric case reports, both cases documented in this chapter demonstrated a mixed flaccid-ataxic dysarthria (Cornwell et al., 2003a, b; Murdoch and Hudson-Tennent 1994; van Dongen et al., 1994; van Mourik et al., 1998).

Flaccid dysarthria is most commonly associated with disruption of the lower motor neurons of the corticobulbar pathway (i.e., cranial nerve nuclei, or the axons between the brainstem nuclei and the spinal cord to the speech musculature). Given the behavioural features of ataxic-flaccid dysarthria, and the close association of the posterior fossa region to the brainstem via the floor of the fourth ventricle, it is plausible that dysarthria in children with PFT may be a reflection of disruption of both corticocerebellar and corticobulbar white matter pathways.

6.4 Dysarthria associated with hemispherectomy

Hemispherectomy is the surgical removal of a cerebral hemisphere for the treatment of intractable epilepsy (Nogueira et al., 2006). The procedure is well-tolerated in children and results in significantly improved seizure control and good neurological outcome, except for the presence of hemiplegia which in most cases is established before surgery (van Empelen et al., 2004). Motor skills on the contralesional side may remain impaired post-surgery, or may become exacerbated if only a mild degree of hemiplegia was present prior to surgery (van Empelen et al., 2004; Devlin et al., 2003; Leonhardt et al., 2001; Maehara et al., 2002). While the majority of patients are reported to have relatively preserved gross motor function, with preserved ability for walking and moving their upper limbs without assistance, fine motor movements are severely restricted. In particular, hand and finger movements are limited because of increased spasticity and poor sensory feedback. In addition, there is almost complete absence of pincer grip and individual finger movements (Dijkerman et al., 2008; Holloway et al., 2000, Kossoff et al., 2003; Leonhardt et al., 2001; van Empelen et al., 2004). These motor deficits persist irrespective of the hemispheric side of removal, and regardless of the aetiology and/or age at acquisition of the seizure-inducing lesion, suggesting only limited capacity for reorganization of contralesional sensorimotor control of the hand and fingers.

In contrast, there is an impressive rescue and/or reorganization of language and basic communication skills after sufficiently early unilateral lesions leading to hemispherectomy (Liégeois et al., 2008; Pulsifer et al., 2004; Vargha-Khadem et al., 1997). Speech and language status after hemispherectomy is related to a number of factors, with older at age at onset of pathology affecting the left hemisphere predicting poor outcome (Patterson et al., 1989; Vargha-Khadem, et al., 1991; Rankin and Vargha-Khadem 2007). Of note, near normal every day language and fluent speech after left hemispherectomy is reported in children with congenital damage (Liégeois et al., 2008; Mariotti et al., 1998; Vargha-Khadem et al., 1991), whereas in patients with damage acquired after the age of five years, dysphasic symptoms emerge (Boatman et al., 1999; Patterson et al., 1989; Vargha-Khadem et al., 1991).

Despite the distinction between fine motor control of the upper limb, and language status post-hemispherectomy, speech characteristics (AOS or dysarthria) have not been systematically investigated. In this context, paediatric cases presenting with dysarthria after unilateral cortical lesions are extremely rare, and detailed investigation of their speech deficits informs about the potential for compensatory processes involved in motor speech function in the isolated hemisphere.

6.4.1 Neuropathology caused by the surgical procedure of hemispherectomy

The standard anatomical hemispherectomy involves the removal of most of one cerebral hemisphere, including the insular cortex and variable portions of the basal ganglia (see Fig. 6.4A). Although the effectiveness of the standard procedure for control of seizures is well established, there have been late complications in the form of haemosiderosis and hydrocephaly (Smith et al., 2005; Tinuper et al., 1988). To avoid late complications, several modifications to the standard

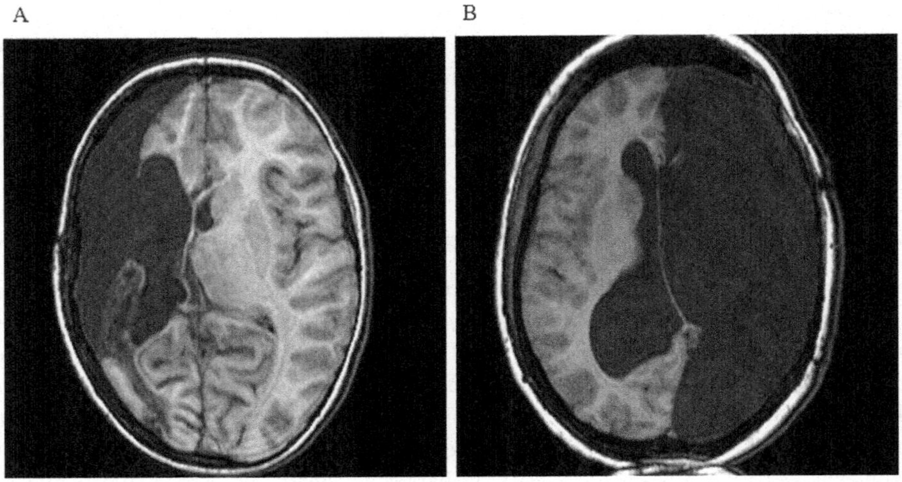

Fig. 6.4 Axial views of T1-weighted MRI scans of patients with hemispherectomy. A: Left functional hemispherectomy; B: Right anatomical hemispherectomy.

procedure have been introduced (e.g., Adam's Modification, Adams 1983; functional hemispherectomy, Tinuper et al., 1988; Rasmussen and Villemure 1989), with the currently preferred method placing the emphasis on disconnecting procedures rather than extensive resective surgery (Smith et al., 2005). In functional hemispherectomy, the central cortical region is removed, including the parasagittal tissue and the cingulate gyrus. This is then followed by a temporal lobectomy, including the amygdala and the hippocampus, and undercutting the white matter connections of the remaining portions of the frontal lobe and the parietal lobes from the brain stem and the opposite hemisphere. This procedure isolates the frontal and parieto-occipital poles from the rest of the brain while preserving the blood supply to these regions, and enables the complete disconnection of neural pathways that allow interhemispheric communication [Fig. 6.4B; (Schramm 2002; see Nogueria et al., 2006, for a review of the surgical procedures)]. Of particular relevance to this chapter, all hemispherectomy procedures involve removal of the sensorimotor, primary motor, and premotor cortices. Thus, both pyramidal and extrapyramidal tracts are unilaterally severed. At the brain stem level, all cranial nerves in a hemispherectomized patient still receive either ipsilateral or contralateral input from the remaining hemisphere, except one set of cranial nerves (VII and XII) which lose only their contralateral input from the pyramidal tract. The functional correlate of this disconnection is consistent with the profile of unilateral upper motor neuron dysarthria (ataxic-flaccid variant), as documented in the two hemispherectomy cases reported here.

6.4.2 **Case presentation**

Table 6.1 presents the speech profiles of two children who have undergone hemispherectomy for relief from intractable epilepsy. An anatomical hemispherectomy on the right side, and a functional hemispherectomy on the left side are included to contrast the effects of side of surgical removal on motor speech outcome. In both cases the epileptic seizures were induced by a developmental malformation that had developed in the pre- or perinatal period (i.e., cortical dysplasia, Case 1; hemimegalencephaly, Case 2), and the hemiplegia had been diagnosed within the first six months of life. Because speech assessment was not carried out pre-operatively, it cannot be concluded that the observed deficits post-surgery are a consequence of hemispherectomy per se. As with hemiplegia which commonly occurs prior to hemispherectomy, motor speech deficits may also have been present due to the pre-existing congenital brain pathology, or may have emerged or been exacerbated due to the later developing epileptic disorder. At the time of assessment more than seven years post-surgery, both cases were seizure-free, and were more than seven years of age (i.e., when articulation, phonological, and oromotor skills are expected to have matured to ensure that any speech difficulties were less likely to be caused by a developmental lag).

Despite the differences in hemispheric side of removal, the speech profile of the two patients post-hemispherectomy was relatively consistent. Thus, both cases presented with a very mild form of unilateral upper motor neuron dysarthria (flaccid-ataxic variant). Multiple dimensions of speech were affected either because of neuromuscular weakness (i.e., flaccid dysarthria) or lack of coordination and reduced muscle tone impacting on the force, range, timing, and direction of speech movements (ataxic dysarthria, Darley et al., 1969a, b). The ataxic-related speech deficits impacted upon articulation and prosody (e.g., increased rate in segments, inappropriate silences), and phonation (i.e., monopitch, monoloudness, hoarse breathy voice, increased pitch). The flaccid dysarthria was also denoted by articulatory breakdown (with features of consonant imprecision and slow rate), associated with VIIth and XIIth cranial nerve deficits. It is noteworthy that the neuropathology affecting the cranial nerves following hemispherectomy is typically bilateral. The pervasive compromise suffered by these nerves may contribute to the child's inability to compensate for articulatory imprecision. Further, hypernasality was present, more likely because of the involvement of the 9th cranial nerve. Differential diagnosis confirmed the absence of spastic, hyperkinetic, or hypokinetic dysarthria as neither case showed the distinctive features of spasticity or abnormal involuntary movement (Darley et al., 1969a, b).

6.4.3 Speech outcome and extensive unilateral cerebral resection

As previously reported for contralesional distal movements of the hand and fingers (van Empelen et al., 2004), both cases had deficits in the execution of speech movements (i.e., dysarthria), irrespective of side of surgery. Despite high intelligibility, both cases demonstrated mild but chronic dysarthria that disrupted the naturalness of their speech. Multiple aspects of utterances, including phonation, orofacial coordination, and articulation, were impaired, and the profile did not correspond directly to any dysarthric profile previously reported in the paediatric literature (van Mourik et al.,1997). Rather, the profile documented in these paediatric patients was consistent with that from an adult patient who had undergone left hemispherectomy at the age of five (Vanlancker-Sidtis 2004). This patient had appropriate pragmatic skills, but showed asymmetrical mouth movements, effort on velar consonant repetition, and difficulty with repeating phonetically complex items. On the basis of the two cases reported here, we suggest that extensive unilateral brain damage leading to hemispherectomy may be sufficient to result in a mild but persistent dysarthria.

Specifically, the deviant speech features demonstrated by cases 5 and 6 are consistent with the characteristics of unilateral upper motor neuron (UUMN) dysarthria- flaccid and ataxic variant- described in adults. UUMN dysarthria is also concomitant with hemiplegia, but it typically occurs due to stroke, and is usually transient (Duffy 2005). In adulthood, UUMN frequently affects both the direct pyramidal speech pathway responsible for the fine coordination of skilled movements, and the indirect extrapyramidal pathway involved in the regulation of reflexes and control of posture and tone (Duffy 2005). It is therefore not surprising that after hemispherectomy features concomitant with UUMN such as hemiplegia, impairment of fine-skilled movements, and central facial and tongue weakness are observed as a consequence of damage to these pathways.

Adults with UUMN frequently experience co-morbid AOS when the left hemisphere is affected (Duffy 2005). Neither the left-, nor the right-hemispherectomy cases presented here experienced non-speech oral or speech dyspraxia. Both cases presented with congenital neurological abnormality, and it is possible that planning and sequencing deficits may be a feature of late childhood-onset left hemisphere pathology. Stark and colleagues (1995) briefly described the speech of two hemispherectomy patients (one left, one right, assessed at the age of nine to ten years), in whom epilepsy had started after a short period of normal development (one to two years). When examined more than two years post-surgery, speech production was found to be unimpaired and at a normal rate for monosyllabic and bisyllabic words, but both patients were unable to repeat three syllable nonwords accurately at a rapid rate (i.e., /pataka/). The absence of consistent dyspraxic deficits after left or right hemispherectomy in the patients described here suggests that the contralesional hemisphere has good potential for rescuing of speech planning and sequencing. Furthermore, despite speech being subserved by a single hemisphere, both children were highly intelligible, indicating relatively favourable long-term speech outcome after hemispherectomy.

6.5 **Summary**

The aim of this chapter was to characterize the profiles of three different developmental forms of motor speech disorder in relation to brain circuits involved in the coordination of orofacial musculature. Representative cases with (a) verbal and orofacial dyspraxia and spastic dysarthria resulting from the mutation of the FOXP2 gene, (b) flaccid-ataxic dysarthria post-surgical treatment of posterior fossa tumour, and (c) unilateral upper motor neuron dysarthria (flaccid-ataxic variant) associated with hemispherectomy for treatment of intractable epilepsy, were presented. Characteristic features of each disorder were discussed in terms of the neural substrate/s implicated in planning/programming, and execution of motor speech. Neuroanatomical and functional neuroimaging findings suggest that these aspects of motor speech performance rely on parallel and partly overlapping neural networks subserved by the basal ganglia and the cerebellum.

All six case studies representing the three aetiological conditions exhibited dysarthria, albeit different variants (i.e., spastic, flaccid ataxic), implicating the compromise of the speech execution network in each case. This suggests that after focal excisions of the cerebellum, or after the removal of an entire cerebral hemisphere, the remaining brain regions do not fully rescue speech execution capability, implying that the neural substrates subserving this ability must be intact bilaterally to permit normal execution of speech. Bilateral disruption of the neostriatal and/or cerebellar networks, (exemplified by the affected KE cases) may additionally contribute to the severity of the dysarthria (moderate in the two affected KE cases, and mild in the four cases post tumour or hemispheric resection).

Of the six developmental cases, only two (affected KE members) exhibited verbal and orofacial dyspraxia. While *unilateral* lesions of the left hemisphere in adults can lead to chronic speech dyspraxia as a result of disruption of the planning/programming system, such an outcome is seen in children only after *bilateral* pathology of the critical networks. The chronic speech dyspraxia documented in the affected members of the KE family is therefore likely to be the result of *bilateral* pathology in the basal ganglia and the cerebellar loops. The absence of speech dyspraxia post-surgical treatment of posterior fossa tumour, or hemispherectomy suggests that the planning/programming system in children can be rescued either by a single cerebral hemisphere, or subserved by the intact regions of the cerebellum.

Altogether these findings indicate that during development motor speech outcome differs depending on whether neuropathology is bilateral or unilateral, and whether it affects the planning/programming neural system, and/or the execution system and its control loops. For clinical practice, we suggest that the comparison with adult outcome studies is of limited relevance. Diagnostic and prognostic indicators of motor speech outcome in children will benefit from the development of a functional classification of speech disorders in relation to their underlying neuropathology.

References

Aarsen, F.K., Van Dongen, H.R., Paquier, P.F., Van Mourik, M. & Catsman-Berrevoets, C.E. (2004). Long-term sequelae in children after cerebellar astrocytoma surgery. *Neurology*, 27, 62(8):1311–6.

American Speech-Language-Hearing Association. (2007). *Childhood Apraxia of Speech* [Position Statement]. Available at: www.asha.org/policy.

Ackermann, H., Vogel, M., Petersen, D. & Poremba, M. (1992). Speech deficits in ischaemic cerebellar lesions. *Journal of Neurology*, 2394: 223–7.

Ackermann, H. & Ziegler, W. (1994). Mutism in central motor disorders: a review of the literature. *Fortschritteder Neurologie Psychiatrie*, 62,9:337–44.

Ackermann, H., Mathiak, K. & Riecker, A. (2007). The contribution of the cerebellum to speech production and speech perception: clinical and functional imaging data. *Cerebellum*, 6(3):202–13.

Adams, C.B. (1983). Hemispherectomy: a modification. *Journal of Neurology Neurosurgery & Psychiatry*, 46(7):617–19.

Amarenco, P., Chevrie-Muller, C., Roullet, E. & Bousser, M.G. (1991). Paravermal infarct and isolated cerebellar dysarthria. *Annals of Neurology*, 30: 211–13.

Aram, D.M., Rose, D.F., Rekate, H.L. & Whitaker, H.A. (1983). Acquired capsular/striatal aphasia in childhood. *Archives of Neurology & Psychiatry*, 40(10):614–7.

Bates, E., Reilly, J., Wulfeck, B. et al. (2001). Differential effects of unilateral lesions on language production in children and adults. *Brain andLanguage*, 79:223–65.

Belton, E., Salmond, C.H., Watkins, K.E., Vargha-Khadem, F. & Gadian, D.G. (2003). Bilateral brain abnormalities associated with dominantly inherited verbal and orofacial dyspraxia. *Human Brain Mapping*, 18:194 –200.

Boatman, D., Freeman, J., Vining, E. et al. (1999). Language recovery after left hemispherectomy in children with late-onset seizures. *Annals of Neurology*, 46:579–86.

Cahill, L.M., Murdoch, B.E. & Theodoros, D.G. (2005). Articulatory function following traumatic brain injury in childhood: a perceptual and instrumental analysis. *Brain Injury*, 19:41–58.

Catsman-Berrevoets, C.E., van Donegen, H.R., Mulder, P.G.H., Geuze, D.P., Paquier, P.F. & Lequin, M.H. (1999). Tumour type and size are high risk factors for the syndrome of cerebellar mutism and subsequent dysarthria. *Journal of Neurology Neurosurgery & Psychiatry*, 67:755–7.

Cornwell., P.L., Murdoch, B.E., Ward, E.C. & Morgan, A.T. (2003a). Dysarthria and dysphagia as long-term sequelae in a child treated for posterior fossa tumour. *Pediatric Rehabilitation*, 6(2): 67–75.

Cornwell, P.L., Murdoch, B.E., Ward, E.C. & Morgan, A.T. (2003b). Dysarthria and dysphagia following treatment for a fourth ventricle choroid plexus papilloma. *Journal of Clinical Neuroscience*, 10(4): 506–12.

Cornwell, P.L., Murdoch, B.E., Ward, E.C. & Kellie, S. (2004). Acoustic investigation of vocal quality following treatment for childhood cerebellar tumour. *Folia Phoniatrica et Logopaedica*, 56: 93–107.

Clark, M., Carr, L., Reilly, S. & Neville, B.G. (2000). Worster-Drought syndrome, a mild tetraplegic perisylvian cerebral palsy. Review of 47 cases. *Brain*, 123(10): 2160–70.

Crutchfield, J.S., Sawaya, R., Meyers, C.A. & Moore III, B.D. (1994). Transient mutism after posterior fossa surgery. *Childs Nervous System*, 10:275–8.

de Smet, H.J., Baillieuxa, H., Catsman-Berrevoets, C., De Deyn, P.P., Marie, P. & Paquiera, P.F. (2007). Postoperative motor speech production in children with the syndrome of 'cerebellar' mutism and subsequent dysarthria: a critical review of the literature. *European Journal Paediatric Neurology*, 11(4):193–207.

Darley, F.L., Aronson, A.E. & Brown, J.R. (1969a). Differential diagnostic patterns of dysarthria. *Journal of Speech, Language, and Hearing Research*, 12:246–69.

—— (1969b). Clusters of deviant speech dimensions in the dysarthrias. *Journal of Speech, Language, and Hearing Research*, 12:462–96.

Devlin, A.M., Cross, J.H. & Harkness, W. et al. (2003). Clinical outcomes of hemispherectomy for epilepsy in childhood and adolescence. *Brain*, 126:556–66.

Dietze, D.D.J. & Mickle, J.P. (1990) Cerebellar mutism after posterior fossa surgery. *Pediatric Neurosurgery*, 16:25–31.

Dijkerman, H.C., Vargha-Khadem, F., Polkey, C.E. et al. (2008). Contralateral and ipsilateral sensorimotor function after hemispherectomy:differences between distal and proximal function. Neuropsychologia, 12, 46(3):886–901.

Dronkers, N.F. (1996). A new brain region for coordinating speech articulation. *Nature*, 14, 384(6605):159–61.

Duffy, J.R. (2005). *Motor Speech Disorders. Substrates, Differential Diagnosis and Management (2nd edn).* St Louis: Elsevier Mosby.

Duffy, J.R., Peach, R.K. & Strand, E.A. (2007). Progressive apraxia of speech as a sign of motor neuron disease. *American Journal of Speech-Language Pathology*, 16(3): 198–208.

Ersahin, Y., Mutluer, S., Cagli, S. & Duman, Y. (1996). Cerebellar mutism: report of seven cases and review of the literature. *Neurosurgery*, 381: 60–6.

Groszer, M., Keays, D.A., Deacon, et al. (2008). Impaired synaptic plasticity and motor learning in mice with a point mutation implicated in human speech deficits. *Current Biology*, 11, 18(5):354–62.

Habas, C. & Cabanis, E.A. (2007). Anatomical parcellation of the brainstem and cerebellar white matter: a preliminary probabilistic tractography study at 3 T. *Neuroradiology*, 49: 849–63.

Hillis, A.E., Work, M., Barker, P.B. et al. (2004). Re-examining the brain regions crucial for orchestrating speech articulation. *Brain*, 127:1479–87.

Holloway, V., Gadian, D.G., Vargha-Khadem, F. et al. (2000).The reorganization of sensorimotor function in children after hemispherectomy. A functional MRI and somatosensory evoked potential study. *Brain*, 123:2432–44.

Huber, J.F., Bradley, K., Spiegler, B.J. & Dennis, M. (2006). Long-term effects of transient cerebellar mutism after cerebellar astrocytoma or medulloblastoma tumor resection in childhood. Childs Nervous System, 22(2):132–8.

Ibrahim, K. & Appleton, R. (2004). Seizures as the presenting symptom of brain tumours in children. *Seizure*, 13(2):108–12.

Ildan, F., Tuna, M., Erman, T., Gocer, A.I., Zeren, M. & Cetinalp, E. (2002). The evaluation and comparison of cerebellar mutism in children and adults after posterior fossa surgery: report of two adult cases and review of the literature. *Acta Neurochirurgica*, 144, 463–73.

Jackson, P.L., Lafleur, M.F., Malouin, F., Richards, C.L., & Doyon, J. (2003). Functional cerebral reorganization following motor sequence learning through mental practice with motor imagery. *Neuroimage*, 20:1171–80.

Kossoff, E.H., Vining, E.P., Pillas, D.J., Pyzik, P.L., Avenillo, A.M., Carson, B.S. & Freeman, J.M. (2003). Hemispherectomy for intractable unihemispheric epilepsy etiology vs outcome. *Neurology*, 61:887–90.

Kusano, Y., Tanaka, Y., Takasuna et al. (2006). Transient cerebellar mutism caused by bilateral damage to the dentate nuclei. *Journal of Neurosurgery*, 104:329–31.

Lai, C.S., Gerrelli, D., Monaco, A.P., Fisher, S.E. & Copp, A.J. (2003). FOXP2 expression during brain development coincides with adult sites of pathology in a severe speech and language disorder. Brain, 126:2455–62.

Lechtenberg, R. & Gilman, S. (1978). Speech disorders in cerebellar disease. *Annals of Neurology*, 34, 285–90.

Leonhardt, G., Bingel, U., Spiekermann, G. et al. (2001). Cortical activation in patients with functional hemispherectomy. *Journal of Neurology*, 248:881–8.

Liégeois, F., Baldeweg, T., Connelly, A., Gadian, D.G., Mishkin, M., & Vargha-Khadem, F. (2003). Language fMRI abnormalities associated with FOXP2 gene mutation. Nature Neuroscience, 6(11):1230–7.

Liégeois, F., Morgan, A.T. & Vargha-Khadem, F. (2007). Neurogenetic bases of speech and language disorders. In: D Coch, G Dawson, & KW Fischer, (2nd edn). *Human Behaviour and the Developing Brain: Atypical Development.* New York: Guilford Press.

Liégeois, F., Cross, J.H., Polkey, C., Harkness, W. & Vargha-Khadem, F. (2008). Language after hemispherectomy in childhood: contributions from memory and intelligence. *Neuropsychologia*, 46(13):3101–7.

Landau, W.M. & Kleffner, F.R. (1957). Syndrome of acquired aphasia with convulsive disorder in children. *Neurology*, 7, 8:523–30.

Maehara, T., Shimizu, H., Kawai, K. et al. (2002). Postoperative development of children after hemispherotomy. *Brain Development*, 24:155–60.

Mariotti, P., Iuvone, L., Torrioli, M.G. et al. (1998). Linguistic and non-linguistic abilities in a patient with early left hemispherectomy. *Neuropsychologia*, 36:1303–12.

Morgan, A., Liégeois, F., Vogel, A., Connelly, A. & Vargha-Khadem, F. (2005). Electropalatography findings and functional brain abnormalities associated with an inherited speech disorder. *4th International EPG Symposium*, Edinburgh, UK, 29–30 Sept.

Morgan, A.T., Liégeois, F. & Occomore, L. (2007). Electropalatography treatment for persistent dysarthria subsequent to paediatric acquired brain injury. *Brain Injury*, 1–11.

Mosch, S.C., Max, J.E. & Tranel, D. (2005). A matched lesion analysis of childhood versus adult-onset brain injury due to unilateral stroke: another perspective on neural plasticity and recovery of social functioning. *Cognitive and Behavioral Neurology*, 18:5–17.

Murdoch, B.E. & Hudson-Tennent, L.J. (1994). Speech disorders in children treated for posterior fossa tumours: ataxic and developmental features. *European Journal Disorders in Communication*, 29:379–97.

Nogueira, D.A., Marino, R., Jr., Aguiar, P.H. et al. (2006). Hemispherectomy: a schematic review of the current techniques. *Neurosurgical Review*, 29:97–102.

Ogar, J., Willock, S., Baldo, J., Wilkins, D., Ludy, C. & Dronkers N. (2006).Clinical and anatomical correlates of apraxia of speech. *Brain and Language*, 97(3):343–50.

Ozgur, B.M., Berberian, J., Aryan, H.E., Meltzer, H.S. & Levy, M.L. (2006). The pathophysiologic mechanism of cerebellar mutism. *Surgical Neurology*, 66(1):18–25.

Ozimek, A., Richter, S., Hein-Kropp, C. et al. (2004). Cerebellar mutism. report of four cases. *Journal of Neurology*, 251:963–72.

Patterson, K., Vargha-Khadem, F. & Polkey, C.E. (1989). Reading with one hemisphere. *Brain*, 112(pt1):39–63.

Pollack, I.F., Polinko, P., Albright, A.L., Towbin, R. & Fitz, C. (1995). Mutism and pseudobulbar symptoms after resection of posterior fossa tumors in children: incidence and pathophysiology. *Neurosurgery*, 37:885–93.

Pulsifer, M.B., Brandt, J., Salorio, C.F., Vining, E.P., Carson, B.S. & Freeman, J.M. (2004). The cognitive outcome of hemipherectomy in 71 children. *Epilepsia*, 45:243–54.

Rankin, P. & Vargha-Khadem, F. (2007). Neuropsychological evaluation – children. In: *Epilepsy: A Comprehensive Textbook*, Engel, J. & Pedley, T.A. (eds) Philadelphia: Lippincott Williams & Wilkins.

Rasmussen, T. & Villemure, J.G. (1989). Cerebral hemispherectomy for seizures with hemiplegia. *Cleveland Clinic Journal of Medicine*, 56 Suppl (Pt1): S62–68; S79–83.

Rekate, H.L., Grubb, R.L., Aram, D.M., Hahn, J.F. & Ratcheson, R.A. (1985) Muteness of cerebellar origin. *Archives of Neurology and Psychiatry*, 42: 697–8.

Richter, S., Schoch, B., Ozimek, A. et al. (2005). Incidence of dysarthria in children with cerebellar tumors: a prospective study. *Brain and Language*, 92: 153–67.

Rowan, A.F. (2003). Speech and language outcome after unilateral basal ganglia infarction acquired during childhood: a combined neuropsychological and neuroimagine study. PhD thesis, 2003. University College London.

Rowan, A., Vargha-Khadem, F., Calamante, F. et al. (2007). Cortical abnormalities and language function in young patients with basal ganglia stroke. *Neuroimage*, 36(2):431–40.

Salamon, N., Sicotte, N., Drain et al. (2007). White matter fiber tractography and color mapping of the normal human cerebellum with diffusion tensor imaging. *Journal of Neuroradiology*, 34:115–28.

Schramm, J. (2002). Hemispherectomy techniques. *Neurosurgical Clinics of North America*, 13, 1:113–34.

Schmahmann, J.D., Dojon, J., Toga, A.W., Petrides, M. & Evans, C.A. (2000). *MRI Atlas of the Human Cerebellum*. San Diego: Academic Press.

Schmahmann, J.D. & Pandya, D.N. (2008) Disconnection syndromes of basal ganglia, thalamus, and cerebrocerebellar systems. *Cortex*, 44(8):1037–66.

Shriberg, L.D., Ballard, K.J., Tomblin, J.B., Duffy, J.R., Odell, K.H. & Williams, C.A. (2006). Speech, prosody, and voice characteristics of a mother and daughter with a 7;13 translocation affecting FOXP2. *Journal of Speech, Language and Hearing Research*, 49(3):500–25.

Shu, W., Cho, J.Y., Jiang, Y. et al. (2005). Altered ultrasonic vocalization in mice with a disruption in the Foxp2 gene. *Proceedings of the National Academy of Sciences of the United States of America*, 102(27):9643–8.

Smith, J.R., Rountas, K.N. & Lee, M.R. (2005). Hemispherectomy: description of surgical technique. *Childs Nervous System*, 21(6): 466–72.

Stark, R.E., Bleile, K., Brandt, J. et al. (1995). Speech-language outcomes of hemispherectomy in children and young adults. *Brain and Language*, 51:406–21.

Steinbok, P., Cochrane, D.D., Perrin, R. & Price, A. (2003). Mutism after posterior fossa tumour resection in children: incomplete recovery on long-term follow-up. *Pediatric Neurosurgery*, 39(4):179–83.

Suresh, P.A. & Deepa, C. (2004). Congenital suprabulbar palsy: a distinct clinical syndrome of heterogeneous aetiology. *Developmental Medicine and Child Neurology*, 46(9):617–25.

Tallal, P., Jernigan, T.L. & Trauner, D. (1994). Developmental bilateral damage to the head of the caudate nuclei: implications for speech-language. *Pathology Journal of Medical Speech – Language Pathology*, 2: 23–8.

Thompson, E.C., Murdoch, B.E. & Stokes, P.D. (1995). Lip function in subjects with upper motor neuron type dysarthria following cerebrovascular accidents. *European Journal Disorders in Communication*, 30(4):451–66.

Tinuper, P., Andermann, F., Villemure, J.G., Rasmussen, T.B. & Quesney, L.F. (1988). Functional hemispherectomy for treatment of epilepsy associated with hemiplegia: rationale, indications, and comparisons with callosotomy. *Annals of Neurology*, 24(1):27–34.

Urban, P.P., Rolke, R., Wicht, S. et al. (2006). Left-hemispheric dominance for articulation: a prospective study on acute ischaemic dysarthria at different localizations. *Brain*, 129, 767–77.

van Calenbergh, F., Van De Laar, A., Plets, C., Goffin, J. & Casear, P. (1995). Transient cerebellar mutism after posterior fossa surgery in children. *Neurosurgery*, 37:894–8.

van Dongen, H.R., Catsman-Berrevoets, C.E. & van Mourik, M. (1994). The syndrome of 'cerebellar' mutism and subsequent dysarthria. *Neurology*, 44:2040–6.

van Empelen, R., Jennekens-Schinkel, A., Buskens, E. et al. (2004). Functional consequences of hemispherectomy. *Brain*, 127:2071–9.

van Mourik, M., Catsman-Berrevoets, C.E., Paquier, P.F. et al. (1997). Acquired childhood dysarthria: review of its clinical presentation. *Pediatric Neurology*, 17:299–307.

van Mourik, M., Catsman-Berrevoets, C.E., Yousef-Bak, E., Paquier, P.F. & van Dongen, H.R. (1998). Dysarthria in children with cerebellar or brainstem tumors. *Pediatric Neurology*, 18(5):411–4.

Vanlancker-Sidtis D. (2004). When only the right hemisphere is left: studies in language and communication. *Brain and Language*, 91:199–211.

Vargha-Khadem, F., Watters, G.V. & O'Gorman, A.M. (1985). Development of speech and language following bilateral frontal lesions. *Brain and Language*, 25(1):167–83.

Vargha-Khadem, F., Isaacs, E.B., Papaleoudi, H. et al. (1991). Development of language in six hemispherectomized patients. *Brain*, 114:473–95.

Vargha-Khadem, F., Carr, L.J., Isaacs, E., Brett, E., Adams, C. & Mishkin, M. (1997) Onset of speech after left hemispherectomy in a nine-year-old boy. *Brain*, 120: 159–82.

Vargha-Khadem, F., Gadian, D.G., Copp, A. & Mishkin, M. (2005). FOXP2 and the neuroanatomy of speech and language. *Nature Reviews Neuroscience*, 6(2):131–8.

Watkins, K.E., Dronkers, N.F. &Vargha-Khadem, F. (2002a). Behavioural analysis of an inherited speech and language disorder: comparison with acquired aphasia. Brain, 125:452–64.

Watkins, K.E., Vargha-Khadem, F., Ashburner, J. et al. (2002b). MRI analysis of an inherited speech and language disorder: structural brain abnormalities. Brain, 125:465–78.

Whiting, B.A. (2005). Motor and cognitive function in children with neurodevelopmental versus acquired pathology of the cerebellum. PhD thesis, 2005. University College London.

Worster-Drought, C. (1974). Suprabulbar paresis. congenital suprabulbar paresis and its differential diagnosis, with special reference to acquired suprabulbar paresis. Developmental Medicine and Child Neurology, Supplement, 30:1–33.

Worster-Drought, C. (1956). Congenital suprabulbar paresis. *Journal of Laryngology & Otology*, 70, 8:453–63.

Ziegler, W. & von Cramon, D. (1986). Spastic dysarthria after acquired brain injury: an acoustic study. *British Journal of Disorders of Communication*, 21(2):173–87.

Chapter 7

Cerebral control of motor aspects of speech production: neurophysiological and functional imaging data

Hermann Ackermann and Axel Riecker

Abstract

So far, studies of the brain mechanisms of speech motor control predominantly had to rely upon the analysis of dysarthric deficits in patients with focal cerebral lesions or neurodegenerative diseases, restricted to defined central-motor subsystems. Depending upon 'natural' events, these data, however, are often confounded by individual variation in the severity and/or localization of the respective disorders and, thus, do not always allow for unambiguous conclusions. As an alternative, functional imaging techniques such as positron emission tomography (PET) or functional magnetic resonance imaging (fMRI) have been exploited during the past years for the investigation of the cerebral networks underlying speech production. Functional imaging studies, based upon the production/repetition of lexical and non-lexical mono- or polysyllabic items, point at a 'minimal brain network' of motor aspects of speech production, encompassing the supplementary motor area (SMA) within the medial wall of the frontal lobe, opercular parts of the precentral gyrus and posterior components of the inferior frontal gyrus (Broca's area), the anterior insula at the floor of the lateral sulcus, the 'mouth region' of primary sensorimotor cortex, the basal ganglia, thalamus, and the cerebellar hemispheres. Depending upon task demands and the selected activation contrasts, hemodynamic responses of other cerebral structures such as the superior temporal gyrus and lower parietal areas may emerge as well. Most noteworthy, functional imaging techniques now begin to provide new insights into the pathomechanisms of dysarthric deficits such as abnormalities of speaking rate in Parkinson's disease or in cerebellar ataxia.

7.1 **Introduction**

Clinical investigations, based upon patients with brain lesions or neurodegenerative diseases, indicate the motor level of speech production to encompass at least three distinct processing stages (for references see Ackermann and Ziegler 2010):

(i) Damage to SMA of the language-dominant hemisphere spares articulatory and phonatory functions but may result in a significant decrease of speech production, giving rise to a variant of transcortical motor aphasia. Therefore, starting mechanisms of speech production – initiating and maintaining an ongoing and fluent verbal stream – are assumed to depend upon this mesiofrontal structure.

(ii) Lesions of left-hemisphere rostral perisylvian cortex (posterior parts of the inferior frontal gyrus [IFG] = Broca's region, opercular [premotor] areas of the ventral, i.e., lower precentral gyrus) and / or ipsilateral anterior insula may cause apraxia of speech (AOS), a syndrome characterized by articulatory breakdown in the absence of elementary motor deficits such as paresis or increased tone of vocal tract muscles. As a consequence, these areas are assumed to participate in the construction of the phonetic make-up of an utterance (motor planning / programming) prior to the innervation of vocal tract musculature.

(iii) The generation of the neural signals 'steering' the respiratory, laryngeal, and supralaryngeal muscles during speech production (motor execution) must be bound to the corticobulbar system as well as cortico-subcortical motor loops, traversing the basal ganglia and the cerebellar hemispheres, since disorders of these networks give rise to distinct types of dysarthria.

In order to further elaborate these clinical data, functional imaging and electrophysiological studies addressing the cerebral organization of speech motor control are reviewed.

7.2 **Cortical representation of vocal tract muscles: direct and transcranial brain stimulation**

Electrical stimulation mapping during brain surgery revealed a comprehensive representation of the human body, extending across the precentral gyrus and adjacent parts of the medial wall of the frontal lobe (see Woolsey et al., 1979 for a review; Fig. 7.1).

More recent studies, based upon non-invasive techniques (transcranial electrical or magnetic brain stimulation), were able to corroborate these findings (e.g., Khedr and Aref 2002; Rödel et al., 2003). At the level of cytoarchitectural organization, this now well-established 'motor homunculus' is assumed to involve primary motor (Brodmann area (BA) 4) and adjacent parts of premotor cortex (BA 6). Among the various vocal tract structures, the tongue has been analysed in more detail: using chronically implanted subdural electrode grids in patients with drug-resistant seizures, a rather broad cortical representation of lingual muscle groups could be documented (range in rostro-caudal direction = 7.5 cm across subjects, 4.5 cm anterior, and 3.0 cm posterior to the central sulcus), encroaching, most presumably, upon posterior parts (BA 44 and 45) of IFG (Urasaki et al., 1994). Both arrest of alternating movements as well as involuntary excursions (pulling back or lateral deviation) were observed during electrical stimulation. It remains to be established in how far technical constraints such as current spread account for the considerably large 'tongue area' or whether this vocal tract structure is associated with multiple motor representation fields (Huang et al., 1988, 1989a, 1989b).

Several reports, published in the 1930s, noted instances of 'grunts and groans' as well as 'clear, sustained vowel cries' during intraoperative electrical surface stimulation of the lower motor strip in awake subjects (review in Penfield and Roberts 1959). Subsequent systematic 'speech-area mapping' studies at the Montreal Neurological Institute within a programme of surgical treatment for medically refractory focal epilepsy found electrical excitation of precentral and – less frequently – postcentral orofacial areas at either side to elicit vocalizations in terms of a 'sustained or interrupted vowel cry, which at times may have a consonant component'. Besides the lateral surface of the hemispheres, electrical stimulation of the supplementary motor area (SMA) within the medial wall of the frontal lobes may elicit involuntary vocal emissions (Penfield and Roberts 1959, see also Paus et al., 1993, p. 466). In parentheses, the designation 'supplementary

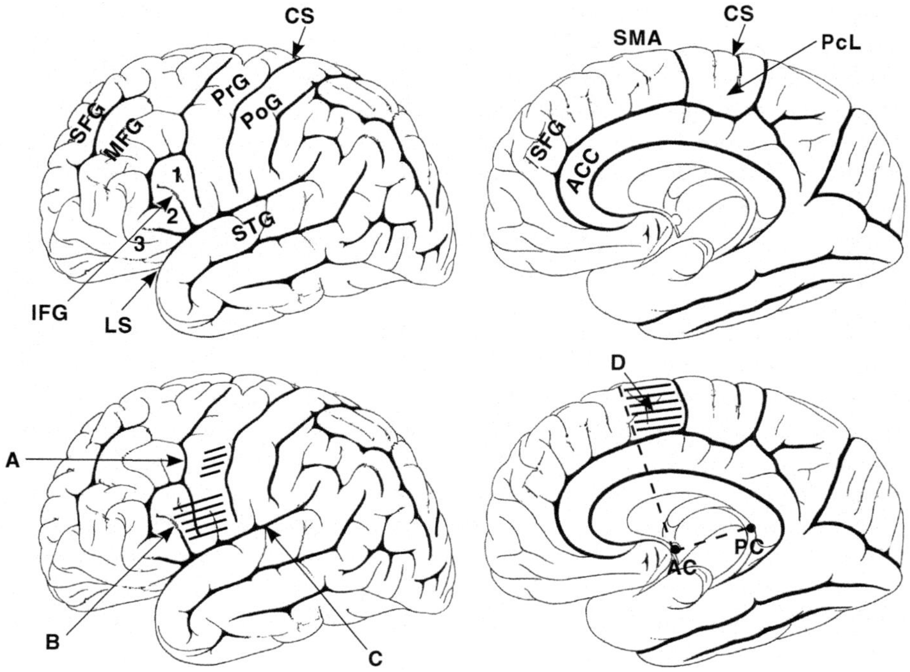

Fig. 7.1 Upper row, left. Several major gyri and sulci of the lateral aspect of the left hemisphere: IFG = inferior frontal gyrus, segregating into an opercular (1), triangular (2), and an orbital part (3), MFG = middle frontal gyrus, SFG = superior frontal gyrus, PrG = precentral gyrus, PoG = postcentral gyrus, STG = superior temporal gyrus, LS = lateral sulcus (Sylvian fissure), CS = central sulcus (Rolandic sulcus). Upper row, right. Medial wall of the left hemisphere: the posterior part of SFG houses the so-called supplementary motor area (SMA 6), i.e., the medial extension of Brodmann area (BA) 6, the dashed line perpendicular to a plane through anterior (AC) and posterior commissure (PC) roughly corresponds to the anterior limit of SMA 6 (= SMA proper), PcL = paracentral lobule, i.e., the medial extension of PrG and PoG, ACC = anterior cingulate cortex.

Lower row. The shaded areas (horizontal lines) refer to the cortical regions engaged in speech motor control: bilateral primar motor cortex (A), opercular part of left IFG and lower left PrG (B), left SMA proper (D). In addition, the rostral part of intrasylvian cortex (anterior insula) in the depth of the lateral sulcus (LS) is assumed to contribute to speech motor control (C). The location of the first two regions (A,B) has been derived from the respective areas of maximum hemodynamic activation as reported by a recent meta-analysis (Fox et al., 2001)

motor area' traces back to these observations (Fig. 7.1). These effects may emerge at either side of the brain, but more often in association with the language-dominant hemisphere. Furthermore, involuntary repetitions of syllables and words, e.g., during counting, could be observed. Electrical stimulation of further rostral regions such as the anterior cingulate cortex (ACC), by contrast, fails to evoke involuntary vocal behaviour in humans. As compared to precentral areas, SMA responses may show a more complex acoustic pattern, e.g., in terms of loudness and pitch fluctuations. Penfield and Welch (1951), therefore, suggested mesiofrontal areas to contribute to the prosodic modulation of verbal utterances (as alternative models, right-hemisphere dorsolateral frontal cortex [Ross 1981] or the basal ganglia [van Lancker Sidtis et al., 2006] have been assumed to control speech prosody). Production of 'intelligible words', however, was never observed under these conditions. Since, furthermore, the observed involuntary 'cries', by and large, do not display the perceptual qualities of (well-articulated) speech sounds, a direct impact upon the motor execution apparatus rather than higher order phonological operations must be assumed.

Apart from vocalizations, exclusively bound to the motor strip and SMA, electrical surface stimulation may result in 'an inability to vocalize spontaneously' ('speech arrest', Penfield and Roberts 1959; for a more recent approach to the study of speech arrest, based upon transcranial magnetic stimulation, see Pascual-Leone et al., 1991). At the level of the right hemisphere, speech arrest can only be elicited at vocalization-related areas. By contrast, the respective susceptible zone of the language-dominant side extends both to IFG and temporoparietal regions (Ojemann 1994). Principally, speech arrest could reflect disruption of either speech motor control mechanisms ('motor speech arrest') or preceding higher order processes of language formulation such as the generation of the sound structure of verbal utterances. Apart from pre- and postcentral areas, systematic exploration of perisylvian cortex found motor speech arrest to be limited to a small segment of posterior IFG, a zone where also orofacial motor responses could be elicited. At that location, electrical stimuli were able to interrupt all verbal utterances, irrespective of task condition, and to compromise even the ability to mimic single orofacial gestures. Using chronically indwelling subdural electrode grids, subsequent investigations were able to corroborate the suggestion that this area represents a 'final motor pathway' of the cerebral circuitry engaged in speech production (Lesser et al., 1984).

Verbal hesitations or slurred articulation could be observed – though rather infrequently – at about the same locations (lower half of the precentral convolution and posterior IFG) as where speech arrest was elicited (Penfield and Roberts 1959). Subsequent stimulation mapping studies reported sporadic instances of dysarthric deficits following stimulation of the lower motor strip (1/5 patients tested; Ojemann 1979).

7.3 Time course of brain activity related to speech motor control: electro- and magnetoencephalographic measurements

Electro- (EEG) and magnetoencephalographic (MEG) techniques represent the most direct approach available in healthy humans to the investigation of the neural correlates of distinct sensorimotor or cognitive tasks. Given a multitude of adequately spaced EEG electrodes or MEG sensors, functional brain maps can be computed on the basis of these data. Measurements of evoked electrical potentials or magnetic field strengths at the scalp are a widely used approach to the study of speech sound perception (for a review see Ackermann et al., 2006). By contrast, only few EEG and MEG analyses addressing cerebral speech motor control have been conducted so far. For example, recordings of the readiness potential preceding word utterances revealed a bilateral distribution of slow brain negativity starting at about 1.5 s prior to the onset of speech, significant left-lateralization effects being restricted to a very late time interval of this foreperiod (Deecke et al., 1986). Furthermore, using chronically implanted subdural electrodes, neurophysiological investigations in epileptic patients were able to obtain movement-related potentials over left SMA, associated with self-paced tongue protrusions and vocalizations (Ikeda et al., 1992; only left side explored). Similar to the upper limbs, thus, mesiofrontal areas encompassing SMA appear to participate in the control of internally triggered human orofacial movements and vocal behaviour ('starting mechanism of speech'; Botez and Barbeau 1971). The comparison of magnetic field changes bound to the production of visually triggered lexical items and vowel-like sounds, respectively, suggests the subsequent generation of verbal utterances to evolve across two processing stages that, tentatively, can be assigned to ventrolateral frontal cortex (Broca's area and its right-hemisphere analogue) and to sensorimotor representation areas. Clear-cut lateralization effects could not be observed (Sasaki et al., 1996).

7.4 Hemodynamic functional imaging of the phonetic/articulatory stage of speech production

7.4.1 Physiological and technical background of functional imaging

On the basis of animal experimentation, an 'automatic' increase of regional cerebral blood flow (rCBF) in response to local variations of neural activity was first suggested in the late nineteenth century ('neurovascular coupling'; for references see Ackermann et al., 2004a). Thus, hemodynamic measurements should provide – with some reservations – a means for the identification of cerebral structures engaged in distinct sensorimotor or cognitive tasks. At this time, hemodynamic positron emission tomography (PET) and functional magnetic resonance imaging (fMRI) represent the two most important brain imaging techniques, applied to the investigation of the brain mechanisms of speech motor control. Alternatives such as functional near-infrared spectroscopy (fNIRS) have not yet been applied to this research area. During PET scanning, the subject's head is placed within a corona of radiation detectors, electronically coupled by so-called coincidence circuits. Following the injection of a small amount of ^{15}O-labeled water, the radioactive substance accumulates at the level of the cerebral cortex in direct proportion to local blood flow and, thus, local neural activity. Besides rCBF, metabolic processes such as glucose consumption show a strong correlation with the degree of neural activity. Using a feasible biological probe, PET also allows for the calculation of local cerebral metabolic rates for glucose (lCMRGlc) within distinct brain structures. Because of a rather long delay between administration of the tracer and subsequent measurements, extending across tens of minutes, this method is of limited relevance for the study of speech motor control in normal subjects, but has been used, e.g., to compare the distribution of hypometabolic areas with speech motor deficits in patients suffering from olivo-ponto-cerbellar atrophy (Kluin et al., 1988).

In contrast to PET, the more recent technique of fMRI represents a completely non-invasive procedure, based on the detection of endogenous tissue contrasts. Furthermore, this technique offers superior spatial resolution approximating that of anatomical MR imaging. However, articulatory gestures during spoken language production may give rise to motion-induced BOLD (=blood oxygenation level dependent) signal changes that, eventually, confound the effects of experimental tasks. Some early studies considered silent speech as a surrogate of overt verbal utterances, assuming that these two conditions recruit overlapping networks of cerebral structures (e.g., Wildgruber et al., 1996). As an alternative, several procedures have been introduced that may disentangle speech-related movement artefacts and task-induced hemodynamic responses. For example, verbal utterances can be restricted to pauses of image acquisition, taking advantage of the physiological delay of the hemodynamic response to a given task (Birn et al., 1999; Gracco et al., 2005; see also chapter 5 this volume by Chang and Ludlow).

7.4.2 Cerebral correlates of speech motor control: meta-analyses of functional imaging studies

The first systematic account of the brain circuitry underlying motor aspects of speech production emerged as a by-product of a PET investigation of lexical aspects of single-word processing (Petersen et al., 1989). Subjects were confronted with a set of tasks of increasing complexity: (a) fixation of a sign appearing on a screen, (b) passive exposure to written or spoken English nouns, (c) spoken repetition of auditorily or visually applied items, and (d) generation of a verb semantically related to the presented noun (hierarchical design). It was assumed that subtraction of the hemodynamic responses to the second stage of performance, i.e., passive viewing of or listening to words, from the rCBF effects bound to the third level, i.e., loud repetition of the nouns, should isolate the brain areas related to speech motor control. Besides activation of SMA, bilateral responses of sensorimotor cortex and anterior–superior portions of the cerebellum could be noted. Furthermore, and quite unexpected, an activation spot 'buried' in the depth of the lateral sulcus emerged whereas, by contrast, both Broca`s area and basal ganglia did not show any significant hemodynamic effects. In line with several sporadic observations (for references see Ackermann et al., 2004a), a subsequent PET study based upon the repetition of auditorily applied nouns (versus stimulus anticipation) was able to assign the intrasylvian response to the anterior insula (Wise et al., 1999; significant effects restricted to the left side).

More than 80 functional imaging studies addressing single-word processing (picture naming, verb/noun generation, word/pseudoword reading and listening) have been published so far. Using these data, a comprehensive meta-analysis tried to delineate the cerebral correlates of several distinct stages of speech production: lexical selection, phonological code retrieval, syllabification, phonetic/articulatory processes, and self-monitoring (Indefrey and Levelt 2004). As a basic assumption, this review suggested overt tasks to engage both syllabification and phonetic/articulatory operations whereas silent verbal performance should, more or less, spare the latter stage. The contrast of overt (aloud) and covert (silent) conditions, thus, might allow for the delineation of motor aspects of speech production, 'downstream' to language formulation. A comparison of the two modes of single-word production resulted in the identification of altogether 17 cerebral structures associated with phonetic/articulatory operations, 12 of them pertaining to the central-motor system, e.g., ventral parts of sensorimotor cortex, dorsolateral premotor areas, SMA, thalamus, cerebellum, and the midbrain. The remaining five brain regions, among others, right-hemisphere posterior IFG and occipital areas, lack a direct relationship to movement control. Rather than phonetic/articulatory processing, most noteworthy, intrasylvian cortex was found to be associated with phonological code retrieval and Broca's area was found to mediate syllabification processes. At the lateral surface of the left hemisphere, the cortical area linked to motor aspects of speech production roughly encompasses the lateral third of sensorimotor cortex, bounded by the pre- and postcentral sulci as well as the Sylvian fissure, but excluding posterior IFG. As a consequence, this review failed to differentiate between primary motor and opercular premotor components of speech motor control, a functional compartmentalization indicated, e.g., by direct electrical cortex stimulation (see above). Furthermore, these data are at some variance with a probabilistic topographic description of the 'mouth region' – to be more specific, the primary sensorimotor representation of all muscles engaged in speech production – based upon a series of functional imaging studies (overt speech tasks such as reading/repetition of single words, counting etc.; Fox et al., 2001). The observed clusters of activated voxels, extending within both hemispheres across a distance of about 2 cm along the three Talairach coordinates, were strictly separated from hemodynamic responses arising within Broca's area (BA 44) and the opercular portion of precentral gyrus (BA 6; see figure 7.1 above).

In order to obtain a more refined model of the compartmentalization of posterior IFG and the ventral (lower) precentral convolution, a more recent meta-analysis compiled 43 functional imaging studies with a focus on the phonological level of speech production (Vigneau et al., 2006). On the basis of these data, it was assumed that the lower frontal convexity encompasses three distinct levels of phonetic /articulatory processing, i.e., 'an upper motor area for mouth motion control, a lower premotor area in the precentral gyrus that is dedicated to pharynx and tongue fine-movement coordination, and a sensory-motor integration region in the Rolandic operculum' (p. 1419). However, visual inspection of the displayed maps reveals a rather continuous area of hemodynamic activation, and the observed responses within the lateral convexity of the frontal lobe do not easily segregate into three distinct clusters. Whereas precentral activation, indeed, encroaches upon the primary motor area of vocal tract musculature (see for comparison the probabilistic description of the 'mouth area' in Fox et al., 2001), the separation of a 'lower premotor pharynx and tongue region' subserving 'fine-movement coordination' from a 'sensory-motor integration region in the Rolandic operculum' is not unambiguously supported by the obtained data. Furthermore, it remains unclear, in how far 'fine-movement coordination' and 'sensory-motor integration' differ from each other in terms of motor control processes.

7.4.3 Contribution of the basal ganglia and the cerebellum to syllable rate control

7.4.3.1 Hemodynamic rate/response functions

The meta-analyses referred to are based upon studies not specifically designed for the investigation of the cerebral correlates of the articulatory/phonetic stage of spoken language. As an alternative, more focused functional imaging studies can be expected to provide a more fine-grained display of the cerebral organization of speech motor control. As compared to the production of lexical items or pseudo-words, syllable repetitions represent a more direct probe of articulatory performance, lacking any significant impact of perceptual processes, grapheme-phoneme transformation, lexical or syntactic operations. Furthermore, this task performed as fast as possible (oral diadochokinesis) has been claimed to represent a sensitive and – within some limits – specific overall measure of dysarthric deficits (Kent et al., 1987; but see Weismer in his recent papers on this topic). For example, a reduced maximum speech tempo has been observed in patients with spastic or ataxic dysarthria. By contrast, subgroups of patients with Wilson`s or Parkinson`s disease even may exhibit 'speech hastening', i.e., involuntary acceleration of speaking rate, while speech tempo, otherwise, is found largely unimpaired in these disorders (Duffy 2005). In order to futher elucidate the differential contribution of the various components of the cerebral speech motor network to rate control, a fMRI study of our group measured hemodynamic brain activation during syllable repetitions at different rates (2.0, 2.5, 3.0, 4.0, 5.0, 6.0 Hz), synchronized either to an auditory pacing signal or produced in an self-paced manner (Riecker et al., 2005; 2006). Significant hemodynamic main effects, calculated across all repetition rates (versus passive listening to the acoustic pacing signals), emerged within SMA, primary sensorimotor areas, opercular premotor cortex, encroaching upon Broca's region, anterior insula, thalamus, basal ganglia, and cerebellum (two separate clusters of activated voxels at either side). Ventrolateral frontal and intrasylvian cortex as well as the caudate nucleus showed left-lateralized responses whereas the other components displayed a rather bilateral activation pattern.

Since damage to these cerebral structures compromises verbal behaviour, giving rise to dysarhria, AOS or transcortical motor aphasia (see above), these findings are in good accord with clinical data. As a second step of signal analysis, hemodynamic rate /response functions were calculated. SMA, opercular premotor as well as sensorimotor cortex, anterior insula, and the thalamus showed a positive linear rate /response relationship, i.e., an increase of the BOLD signal in parallel with syllable repetition rate ('hemodynamic mass effect'). Most noteworthy, the cerebellar activation clusters at either side were characterized by a step-wise increase of the BOLD signal between 3 Hz and 4 Hz. Furthermore, silent (covert) syllable repetitions yielded similar results (Wildgruber et al., 2001). A series of acoustic studies of our group has revealed syllable rate not to fall below a value of 3 Hz in patients with ataxic dysarthria during oral diadochokinesis and sentence production tasks (Hertrich and Ackermann 1997). These clinical and

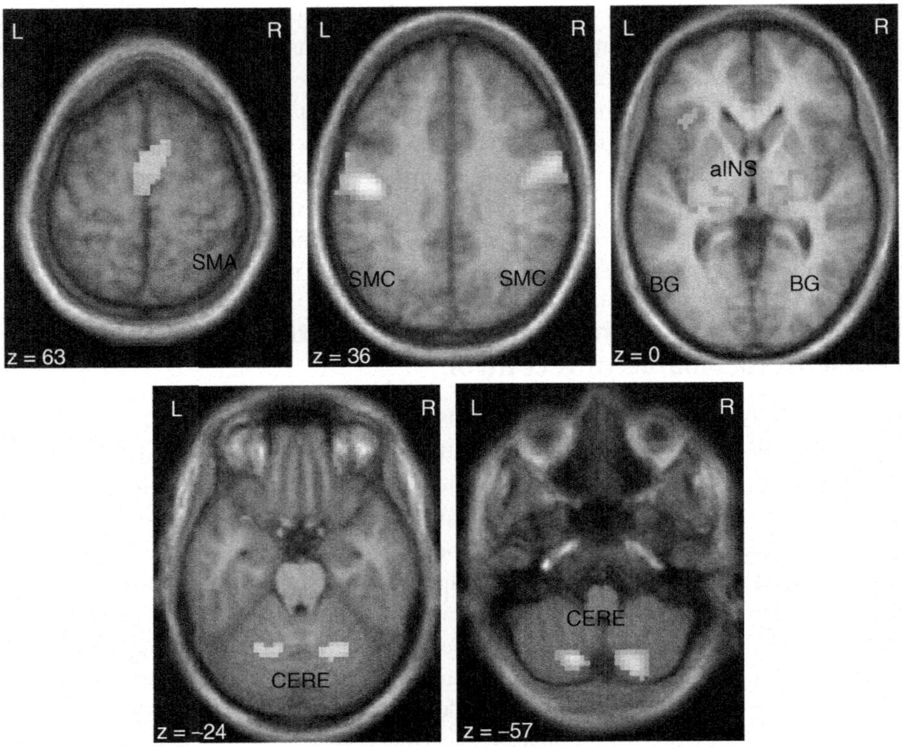

Fig. 7.2 Hemodynamic main effects during syllable repetitions computed across all six frequency conditions and subjects (gray areas), displayed on transverse sections of the averaged anatomic reference images (z = distance to the intercommissural plane; L = left hemisphere, R = right hemisphere): Significant responses emerged within SMA, bilateral sensorimotor cortex (SMC), bilateral basal ganglia (BG), left anterior insula (aINS), left inferior frontal gyrus (not shown), and both cerebellar hemispheres (CERE; from left to right). Analysis of the relationship between syllable frequency and hemodynamic activation revealed linear rate/response functions in all components of the cerebral network of speech motor control, apart from the basal ganglia: Bilateral putamen/ pallidum and left caudate nucleus showed, unexpectedly, a negative rate/response function. Group averages of hemodynamic activation within the various components of the cerebral network of speech motor control, calculated separately for the six stimulus frequencies considered, indicate the linear rate/response function of both the superior and inferior cerebellar 'spots' at either side to be characterized by a step-wise increase of the BOLD (= blood oxygenation level dependent) signal at about 3 Hz. (See Plate section).

functional imaging data, taken together, could indicate that the cerebellum supports the sequencing of the successive syllables of verbal utterances and, on these grounds, 'pushes' speaking rate beyond a level of about 3 Hz (see Ackermann et al., 2004b for a further discussion). However, syllable repetitions and connected speech may differ – at least to some extent – in their underlying motor control mechanisms (Ziegler 2002). Any inferences from brain activation data based upon syllable repetition paradigms to sentence production, hence, must still be considered with some precautions.

As a novel finding, parametric signal analysis revealed a negative linear relationship between syllable rate and hemodynamic responses within the basal ganglia (bilateral putamen / pallidum, left caudate nucleus). In accordance with these data, recent PET studies reported an inverse relationship between a volume-mean normalized measure of regional cerebral blood flow and syllable frequency at the level of right caudate nucleus both in normal speakers and ataxic subjects (Sidtis et al., 2003, 2006). On a global scale, thus, the basal ganglia seem to be characterized by a decline of hemodynamic activation in parallel with an increase of motor demands, at least during repetitive movements. Conceivably, this negative rate / response profile reflects a more efficient organization of faster movements. In contrast to other central-motor disorders, patients suffering from an idiopathic Parkinsonian syndrome, as a rule, do not show a lowered maximum repetition rate during oral diadochokinesis tasks (see, e.g., Ackermann et al., 1993; 1997). Given a reverse relationship between speech tempo and neural activity, dysfunctions of the relevant components of the basal ganglia can be expected to spare this aspect of verbal behaviour – at least during less advanced stages of the disease.

7.4.3.2 Motor preparation/initiation and movement execution during syllable repetitions

Besides the calculation of rate/response relationships, the time series of the BOLD signal across syllable repetitions derived from the various components of the cerebral network of speech motor control were compared to each other (functional connectivity analysis; for further details see Riecker et al., 2005). Most noteworthy, these areas segregated into two clusters: (a) SMA, Broca's area, anterior insula, superior cerebellum, on the one hand, and (b) sensorimotor cortex, thalamus, basal ganglia, inferior cerebellum, on the other hand, were found to be interconnected each by high (0.75–0.9) and very high (> 0.9) correlation coefficients.

In order to further characterize the temporal behaviour of the BOLD signal within these functionally associated brain areas, a voxel-wise comparison of the measured BOLD signal changes with the canonical hemodynamic response function was conducted. As a rule, the onset of cerebral hemodynamic responses to a perceptual, motor or cognitive task is delayed by about two seconds, and the decline of the elevated BOLD signal towards rest level starts at a similar interval after offset of stimulation or behavioural performance. This temporal profile of hemodynamic activation could be observed at the level of sensorimotor cortex, and visual analysis revealed a similar pattern within the basal ganglia (left putamen/pallidum and left caudatum), the thalamus as well as inferior aspects of the cerebellar hemispheres. In consideration of the time course of the BOLD signal, this network seems to subserve motor execution processes in terms of either the generation of motor control signals steering the 'speech apparatus' or in the transmission and processing of reafferent input. By contrast, the hemodynamic responses of the second cluster of cerebral structures were characterized by a markedly earlier onset and a shorter duration. Taking into account the available clinical data (see above), this second network might be linked to preparatory activities or movement initiation mechanisms. Most noteworthy, the two separate cerebellar clusters of activated voxels appear to participate in different aspects of speech motor control, and the superior responses, obviously, operate in concert with cerebral structures engaged in prearticulatory processes.

7.4.4 The impact of syllable sequencing, syllable complexity, and syllable frequency upon hemodynamic activation patterns during verbal tasks

A widespread and mostly bilateral pattern of hemodynamic activation was found to be associated with the production of the isolated vowel 'ah', including precentral gyrus, mesiofrontal areas, posterior insula, superior temporal lobe, thalamus, basal ganglia, red nucleus, and the cerebellum (Sörös et al., 2006; see Riecker et al., 2000b for a fMRI study of a similar design). Since this task had been contrasted with a rest condition, a variety of speech-unspecific responses must be

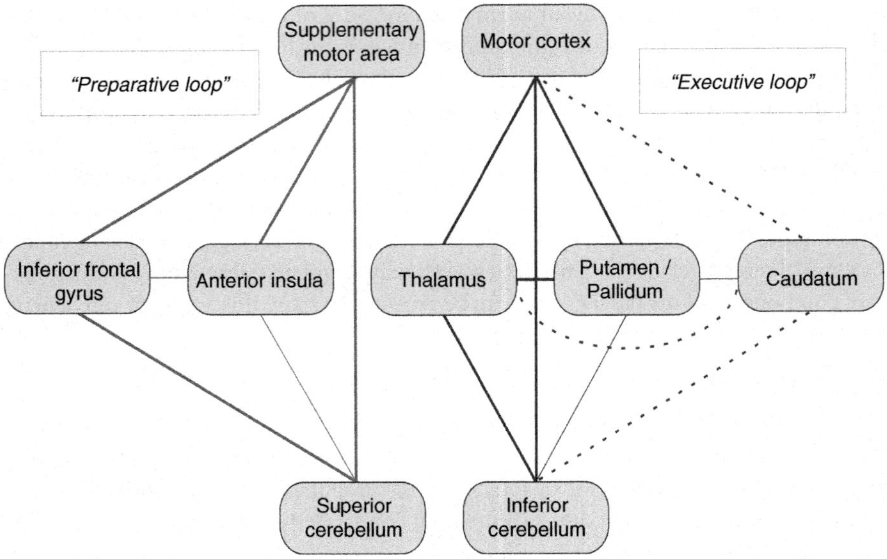

Fig. 7.3 Quantitative functional connectivity analyses: computed correlation coefficients across the time series of the BOLD (= blood oxygenation level dependent) signal within the volumes of interest considered, i.e., the areas of a significant hemodynamic main effect (bold lines = correlation coefficient >0.9, thin lines = 0.75 – 0.9, low and intermediate correlations not depicted; see Riecker et al., 2005, for further details). (See Plate section).

expected, besides the cerebral correlates of articulatory/phonatory functions. For example, the authors refer to 'self-awareness of movement' as an explanation of the observed bilateral recruitment of the posterior insula. Furthermore, there is some evidence that rest conditions represent a specific activation state, confounding, eventually, the effects of any experimental tasks (e.g., Raichle et al., 2001). Comparison of CV utterances ('pa', 'ta', or 'ka') and the polysyllabic item 'pataka' with the vowel task revealed hemodynamic responses at the level of the temporal lobes (CV and 'pataka') as well as the basal ganglia and the cerebellum ('pataka'). Most presumably, the additional subcortical BOLD signal changes reflect the enhanced motor control demands in association with syllable sequencing, whereas the rather extensive responses of the temporal gyri were explained in terms of central-auditory and phonological processing. Unexpectedly, production of the polysyllabic item elicited neither activation of opercular premotor nor of the anterior insular cortex of the left hemisphere, though damage to these regions may give rise to severe disruption specifically of the polysyllabic variant of syllable repetition tasks (see below).

The prearticulatory phase of spoken language production is assumed to encompass, among others, the generation of a motor programme or a phonetic plan, respectively, providing the input to the execution apparatus (e.g., Levelt et al., 1999). Dysfunctions of this stage of speech motor control may give rise to AOS. As a salient neuroanatomical characteristic, this syndrome is bound to lesions of the language-dominant hemisphere, almost exclusively left-sided infarctions within the area of blood supply of the middle cerebral artery (see Ziegler 2008 for a recent review). By contrast, unilateral supratentorial lesions rarely – if at all – give rise to severe and persisting dysarthria. Hence, unlike more basic motor execution processes, assumed to be organized in a bilateral fashion, the higher-order planning aspects of speech motor control show the same cerebral lateralization effects as the 'core psycholinguistic language functions' (Caplan 1987). The intra-hemispheric lesion site of AOS, however, is still a matter of dispute (Ziegler 2008). Based upon clinico-neuroanatomical correlation studies, the major hypotheses either focus upon posterior parts of the left IFG (Hillis et al., 2004), ipsilateral anterior insular cortex (Dronkers 1996), or the 'face/mouth area' of the motor strip of the language-dominant hemisphere, including adjacent white matter structures as well as the anterior limb of the internal capsule (e.g., Schiff et al., 1983).

Since AOS is assumed to reflect a deficit in the 'programming' of vocal tract movements and since the demands on 'motor planning' must be expected to increase with utterance length, a recent fMRI study suggested hemodynamic activation of the insula to covary with this parameter of spoken language (Shuster and Lemieux 2005). Indeed, overt (versus silent) repetition of mono- and multisyllabic nouns was found to be associated with hemodynamic responses arising at the floor of the Sylvian fissure. Whereas, however, the longer items yielded significantly enhanced activation of the inferior parietal lobule, the precentral convolution (BA 6), and posterior parts of IFG (BA 44) of the left hemisphere each, a comparable effect of intrasylvian structures did not emerge. Thus, although both the ventrolateral convexity of the frontal lobe and the insular cortex in the depth of the lateral sulcus seem to pertain to the articulatory/phonetic network of speech production, these structures might subserve different control mechanisms.

Phonotactic rules, e.g., of the German or English language, allow for a variety of syllable onset structures (V, CV, CCV). Besides utterances length, in terms of the number of enclosed syllables, consonant clusters might pose higher demands on articulatory/phonetic control mechanisms as compared to CV units (Aichert and Ziegler 2004). A recent elaborate fMRI study used four tri-syllabic items ('ta-ta-ta'/'ka-ru-ti'/'stra-stra-stra'/'kla-stri-splu'), systematically varied in sequence complexity (the same three versus three different items in a row) and syllabic onset complexity (CV versus CCCV onset), as test materials (Bohland and Guenther 2006, see Guenther et al., 2006a, b for an attempt to integrate fMRI results with a computation model of speech production). Since the experimental design included both GO and NOGO trials, overt task performance could be contrasted with a state of being prepared to produce the same items. The 'minimal cerebral network of overt speech production', in terms of the conjunction of hemodynamic activation across the four test materials considered (versus baseline), was found to encompass, among others, post- and precentral gyrus, encroaching upon posterior IFG, anterior insula, superior temporal cortex, SMA, basal ganglia, thalamic areas, and superior components of the cerebellar hemispheres. Significant left-lateralization effects emerged at the level of intrasylvian cortex. In contrast, posterior IFG and sensorimotor cortex failed to display comparable side-differences of hemodynamic activation. The contrast of GO and NOGO trials revealed, by and large, the same response pattern. An increase of stimulus complexity in either dimension yielded, as expected, enhanced activation of at least some components of the 'basic speech network'. It remains, however, unsettled in how far additional demands upon motor execution mechanisms or motor planning processes contribute to these observed effects.

The still most elaborated contemporary model of language production (e.g., Levelt et al., 1999) assumes phonetic planning to be centered around the retrieval and assembly of syllable-sized motor programmes. Within this conceptual framework, the computational load of higher-order aspects of speech motor control must be expected to vary, in the first instance, with syllable frequency rather than articulatory complexity: the encoding of high-frequency items simply requires access to a 'mental syllabary', i.e., a store of highly automatized, precompiled, holistic motor routines representing entire syllable structures, whereas syllables of a low frequency of occurrence must be assembled from smaller bits, e.g., from phonemes, a route requiring enhanced effort and, thus, posing higher demands upon phonetic planning (Cholin et al., 2006). In line with these suggestions, AOS subjects produce more errors in association with low- as compared to high-frequency syllables (Aichert and Ziegler 2004; Staiger and Ziegler 2008). On the basis of the Levelt-model of language production, experimental variation of syllable frequency, thus, should represent the most adequate probe of phonetic encoding operations. However, apart from a small number of studies of visual word processing (Carreiras et al., 2006), the available functional imaging studies of speech motor control have not strictly controlled for this parameter. For example, the test materials considered by Shuster and Lemieux (2005) were controlled for *word*, but not for *syllable* frequency. It cannot be ruled out, therefore, that the monosyllabic items predominantly consisted of low-frequency syllables while their longer cognates were composed of high-frequency syllables. As a consequence, the expected impact of word length upon phonetic encoding processes might have been masked, and the observed distributional pattern of hemodynamic responses could reflect unspecific effects of the longer test materials, e.g., increased articulatory effort. With respect to the dimension *within-syllable complexity* of the investigation by Bohland and Guenther (2006), items with an initial consonant cluster are often less frequent than simple CV units. Variation of this factor, thus, also might be confounded by syllable frequency. In order to accomplish a more precise differentiation of the stage of phonetic planning from motor execution processes, as conceptualized in current psycholinguistic models, the test materials of a recent fMRI study of our group were systematically controlled for syllable frequency (Riecker et al., 2008). As a second factor, complexity of syllable onset was varied in an orthogonal fashion to the former dimension. The Levelt-model predicts that the neural network engaged in speech motor planning is predominantly sensitive to changes in syllable frequency and only within the domain of low-frequency items to variation in onset structure. A cognitive subtraction approach revealed a significant main effect of syllable onset complexity (CCV versus CV) – but not the expected impact of syllable frequency (low- versus high-frequency items) – at the level of left posterior IFG, left anterior insula and both cerebellar hemispheres. Assuming left fronto-opercular and intrasylvian cortex to participate in speech motor planning, this process appears to be sensitive to the phonetic/phonological complexity of syllable structure rather than syllable frequency. Since the brain lesions of AOS patients commonly involve the above structures, these results help to explain why complex syllables are particularly challenging to patients with AOS (Staiger and Ziegler 2008). However, the obtained data are at variance with the Levelt-model of speech production which would predict that the variation of the onset complexity should have no impact on the production of high-frequency syllables since all of them are stored as precompiled as 'motor plans'. Nevertheless, there seems to be a more subtle influence of syllable frequency on phonetic planning processes which deserves further elucidation: calculation of the time series of hemodynamic activation within the various cerebral structures engaged in speech motor control revealed this factor to enhance functional connectivity between Broca's area and ipsilateral anterior insula (see Riecker et al., 2005, for further details of this approach).

Notwithstanding some discrepancies, a variety of PET and fMRI studies point, taken together, at a 'minimal brain network' (Bohland and Guenther 2006) of motor aspects of speech production, encompassing SMA within the medial wall of the frontal lobe, opercular parts of the precentral gyrus and/or posterior IFG (Broca's area), the anterior insula at the floor of the lateral sulcus, the 'mouth region' of primary sensorimotor cortex, the basal ganglia, and the cerebellar hemispheres. Early and late bilinguals seem to recruit essentially the same brain circuitry during production of verbal utterances (Frenck-Mestre et al., 2005). Depending upon task demands and the selected activation contrasts, hemodynamic responses in other areas, e.g., the superior temporal gyrus and lower parietal areas, may emerge as well.

So far, only sparse data on the modifications of the 'minimal brain network' of speech production in patients suffering from AOS or dysarthria are available. In Parkinson's disease, e.g., reduced hemodynamic activation of the primary motor 'orofacial area' (right hemisphere) and the cerebellum concomitant with enhanced responses of SMA during sentence productions could be noted (Pinto et al., 2004). Especially, the susceptibility to movement artifacts, e.g., in patients with tremor, constrains the application of fMRI to clinical populations. As a further problem, brain pathology may have an impact upon the temporal dynamics of the BOLD signals (e.g., Bonakdarpour et al., 2007).

7.4.5 Covert generation of verbal utterances ('inner speech')

Internal speech has been considered a 'prearticulatory, but otherwise fully parsed speech code' (Levelt 1989). As a consequence, the investigation of covert verbal utterances might provide a 'window' into preparatory activities preceding actual performance of movement sequences and allow for the delineation of the cerebral correlates of motor programming or planning processes (Jeannerod 1994). In order to delineate the cerebral network mediating covert or imagined verbal utterances, a fMRI study of our group asked subjects to produce 'automatic speech' such as the ongoing recitation of the months of the year. By contrast to the production of single nouns, this task provides an opportunity to address fluent or connected verbal output, in the absence of any relevant demands on lexical retrieval or syntactic processing. Since 'automatic speech' can be expected to elicit a rather monotonous mode of speech production, no significant confounding impact of intonational suprasegmental patterns must be expected. As a control condition, participants reproduced a nonlyrical tune drawn from a serenade in order to avoid any retrieval of propositional materials. Whereas covert speech was found to elicit exclusive activation of the left precentral gyrus as well as the right cerebellar hemisphere, silent singing resulted in an opposite response pattern encompassing right premotor cortex and superior aspects of the left cerebellar hemisphere (Ackermann et al., 1998; Riecker et al., 2000a). These findings corroborate the suggestion that superior parts of the cerebellum are engaged in prearticulatory operations of speech motor control (see above). As a precaution, it must, however, be taken into account that inner speech might be associated with subliminal activity of the tongue musculature (Sokolov 1972).

At some variance with our data, a recent fMRI study found silent single-word repetition to be associated with a more wide-spread network of cerebral structures, including right-hemisphere areas, even in contrast to overt production of the same items (Shuster and Lemieux 2005). Most presumably, the much more restricted activation pattern during 'automatic speech' reflects the simplicity of this task, lacking, e.g., significant demands upon lexical retrieval or prosodic modulation.

7.4.6 Comparison of verbal and nonverbal orofacial movements

Similar to transcranial or direct brain stimulation studies, fMRI measurements of the hemodynamic responses to a variety of upper and lower limb movements (single-joint excursions, motor sequences) as well as nonspeech orofacial activities (lip pursing) also revealed human motor cortex to be organized as a topographic body map (Lotze et al., 2000). Furthermore, as expected, lip pursing yielded a highly symmetrical response pattern extending across the pre- and postcentral gyrus. By contrast, verbal utterances often – but not unanimously – were found to yield lateralization effects towards the left hemisphere at the level of sensorimotor cortex (Wildgruber et al., 1996; Riecker et al., 2000a; Loucks et al., 2007).

Early functional imaging studies of word processing had used a compound subtraction procedure in order to separate cognitive (lexical retrieval) and motor aspects (articulation/phonation) of language processing (e.g., Petersen et al., 1989). As a probe of the validity of this approach, Sidtis and coworkers (1999) applied the principles of 'decomposition logic' on speech motor control itself. On these grounds, syllable repetitions might be conceived of as the 'sum' of lip closure movements and laryngeal activity. Thus, the activation pattern bound to phonation tasks (minus baseline) must be expected to equal the difference in hemodynamic responses to lip gestures and syllable repetitions. Besides a baseline condition, i.e., subjects being quiet and awake, three activation tasks were considered for analysis: (a) iteration of the syllables 'pa', 'ta', and 'ka' as fast as possible, (b) sustained production of the vowel 'a', and (c) repetitive lip closures. The PET measurements failed to document any task additivity under these conditions. Most noteworthy, the 'simpler' tasks of sustained phonation and lip closure movements yielded more spacious clusters of 'active voxels' within several regions than the ostensibly higher motor control demands linked to syllable repetitions. Two fMRI studies also found nonspeech orofacial movements to yield more extensive hemodynamic responses than linguistic test materials (Wildgruber et al., 1996: vertical nonspeech tongue movements, the lips being closed, versus highly overlearned word strings; Riecker et al., 2000b: horizontal tongue movements, the mouth open, versus reiteration of nonsense test materials differing in articulatory/phonetic complexity). Presumably, nonspeech orofacial tasks are associated with increased effort as compared to coarticulated mono- and polysyllabic items ('movement fractionation' versus 'nonindividualized' motor control; see Riecker et al., 2000b).

As a rule, the various speech sounds of human languages are generated by means of distinct glottal and/or supralaryngeal modulations of the expiratory air stream. Most noteworthy, a recent fMRI study found a by and large similar cerebral network to be associated with speech phonation (syllable repetitions, sustained vowel productions) and voluntary prolonged oral exhalation (Loucks et al., 2006). However, hemodynamic responses of SMA were restricted to the verbal utterances. These findings are in line with the notion of a mesiofrontal speech initiation mechanism, although other differences between the two conditions might also contribute to the differential involvement of SMA.

7.5 Conclusions

(i) A variety of PET and fMRI studies, based upon the production / repetition of lexical and non-lexical mono- or polysyllabic items, point at a 'minimal brain network' of motor aspects of speech production, encompassing SMA within the medial wall of the frontal lobe, opercular parts of the precentral gyrus and posterior IFG (Broca's area), the anterior insula at the floor of the lateral sulcus, the 'mouth region' of primary sensorimotor cortex, the basal ganglia, thalamus, and the cerebellar hemispheres. Most presumably, hemodynamic activation is lateralized towards the left side within SMA, opercular premotor cortex and anterior insula. Depending upon task demands and the selected activation contrasts, hemodynamic responses of other cerebral structures such as the superior temporal gyrus and lower parietal areas may emerge as well.

(ii) The available – still very limited – neurophysiological data provide first insights into the time course of brain activity across the cortical components of speech motor control: whereas mesiofrontal cortex (SMA) is found to participate in the internal triggering of orofacial movements and vocal behaviour, the subsequent generation of verbal utterances appears to engage in a serial fashion Broca's area and primary motor cortex. Conceivably, the anterior insula operates – depending upon task demands – in concert with the dorsolateral components of the frontal lobe.

(iii) As expected, calculation of rate/response functions based upon functional imaging studies of syllable repetitions revealed a parallel increase of hemodynamic responses and motor demands ('mass activation effect') within SMA, premotor and primary sensorimotor cortex, anterior insula, and thalamus. By contrast, negative linear relationship between syllable rate and hemodynamic response emerged at the level of the basal ganglia (putamen/pallidum and caudate nucleus). Conceivably, these data – reflecting a more efficient organization of faster movements – provide a basis for the explanation of a mostly normal or even accelerated syllable rate during oral diadochokinesis tasks and sentence productions in patients with Parkinson's disease. The cerebellar activation clusters included at either side voxels with a step-wise increase of the BOLD signal between 3 Hz and 4 Hz both during overt and covert syllable repetitions. In line with these findings, a series of acoustic studies indicate that syllable rate does not fall below a value of 3 Hz in patients with ataxic dysarthria. Thus, the cerebellum might be instrumental in 'pushing' speech rate beyond a level of about 3 Hz.

(iv) Opercular premotor areas of the left hemisphere (ventral, i.e., lower precentral convolution and posterior IFG) as well as the ipsilateral anterior insula have been assumed to participate in the construction of the phonetic make-up of an utterance prior to innervation of vocal tract musculature. In order to further specify the functional characteristics of these areas, a series of studies used test materials systematically varied in phonetic /phonological or psycholinguistic parameters such as syllable /word frequency and onset complexity. Both the opercular and the intrasylvian components of the cerebral speech motor control circuit turned out to be more sensitive to 'articulatory load' than syllable frequency. Unfortunately, however, the available data do not yet provide unambiguous evidence for a differential contribution of opercular premotor cortex and anterior insula to acoustic communication in our species.

(v) Two distinct hemodynamic responses within either cerebellar hemisphere emerged during syllable repetitions. Functional connectivity analyses found the inferior 'activation spot' to operate in concert with sensorimotor cortex, basal ganglia, and thalamus. By contrast, the time course of the other cerebellar response, at a more superior location, was correlated with the temporal dynamics of the BOLD signal obtained from SMA, Broca's area, and anterior insula, i.e., cerebral areas engaged in speech motor initiation, preparation, and planning. Furthermore, 'internal speech' yielded activation of the superior, but not of the inferior cerebellar activation spot. At least the superior parts of the cerebellum, thus, appear to cooperate with structures primarily engaged in prearticulatory processes of speech motor control.

References

Ackermann H, Gröne BF, Hoch G and Schönle PW (1993). Speech freezing in Parkinson's disease: A kinematic analysis of orofacial movements by means of electromagnetic articulography. *Folia Phoniatrica*, **45**, 84–9.

Ackermann H, Konczak J and Hertrich I (1997). The temporal control of repetitive articulatory movements in Parkinson's disease. *Brain and Language*, **56**, 312–9.

Ackermann H, Wildgruber D, Daum I and Grodd W (1998). Does the cerebellum contribute to cognitive aspects of speech production? A functional magnetic resonance imaging (fMRI) study in humans. *Neuroscience Letters*, **247**, 187–90.

Ackermann H, Riecker A and Wildgruber D (2004a). Functional brain imaging of motor aspects of speech production. In B Maassen, RD Kent, HFM Peters, PHHM van Lieshout and W Hulstijn, eds. *Speech Motor Control in Normal and Disordered Speech*, pp. 85–111. Oxford University Press, Oxford.

Ackermann H, Mathiak K and Ivry RB (2004b). Temporal organization of 'internal speech' as a basis for cerebellar modulation of cognitive functions. *Behavioral and Cognitive Neuroscience Reviews*, **3**, 14–22.

Ackermann H, Hertrich I, Lutzenberger W and Mathiak K (2006). Functional neuroanatomy of speech sound perception: Clinical and imaging data. *Aktuelle Neurologie*, **33**, 218–31 (German).

Ackermann H and Ziegler W (2010). Brain mechanisms underlying speech motor control. In WJ Hardcastle and J Laver, eds. *The Handbook of Phonetic Sciences*, 2nd edn, in press. Blackwell, Malden, MA.

Aichert I and Ziegler W (2004). Syllable frequency and syllable structure in apraxia of speech. *Brain and Language*, **88**, 148–59.

Birn RM, Bandettini PA, Cox RW and Shaker R (1999). Event-related fMRI of tasks involving brief motion. *Human Brain Mapping*, **7**, 106–14.

Bohland JW and Guenther FH (2006). An fMRI investigation of syllable sequence production. *NeuroImage*, **32**, 821–41.

Bonakdarpour B, Parrish TB and Thompson CK (2007). Hemodynamic response function in patients with stroke-induced aphasia: Implications for fMRI data analysis. *NeuroImage*, 36, 322–31.

Botez MI and Barbeau A (1971). Role of subcortical structures, and particularly of the thalamus, in the mechanisms of speech and language: A review. *International Journal of Neurology*, **8**, 300–20.

Caplan D (1987). *Neurolinguistics and linguistic aphasiology: An introduction.* Cambridge University Press, Cambridge.

Carreiras M, Mechelli A and Price CJ (2006). Effect of word and syllable frequency on activation during lexical decision and reading aloud. *Human Brain Mapping*, **27**, 963–72.

Cholin J, Levelt WJM and Schiller N (2006). Effects of syllable frequency in speech production. *Cognition*, **99**, 205–35.

Deecke L, Engel M, Lang W and Kornhuber HH (1986). Bereitschaftspotential preceding speech after holding breath. *Experimental Brain Research*, **65**, 219–23.

Dronkers NF (1996). A new brain region for coordinating speech articulation. *Nature*, **384**, 159–61.

Duffy JR (2005). *Motor Speech Disorders: Substrates, Differential Diagnosis, and Management, 2nd edn.* Elsevier Mosby, St. Louis, MO.

Fox PT, Huang A, Parsons LM, Xiong JH, Zamarippa F, Rainey L and Lancaster JL (2001). Location-probability profiles for the mouth region of human primary motor-sensory cortex: Model and validation. *NeuroImage*, **13**, 196–209.

Frenck-Mestre C, Anton JL, Roth M, Vaid J and Viallet F (2005). Articulation in early and late bilinguals' two languages: Evidence from functional magnetic resonance imaging. *Neuroreport*, **16**, 761–5.

Gracco VL, Tremblay P and Pike B (2005). Imaging speech production using fMRI. *NeuroImage*, **26**, 294–301.

Guenther FH, Ghosh SS and Tourville JA (2006a). Neural modelling and imaging of the cortical interactions underlying syllable production. *Brain and Language*, **96**, 280–301.

Guenther FH, Ghosh SS, Nieto-Castanon A and Tourville JA (2006b). A neural model of speech production. In J Harrington and M Tabain, eds. *Speech Production: Models, Phonetic Processes, and Techniques*, pp. 27–39. Psychology Press, New York, NY.

Hertrich I and Ackermann H (1997). Acoustic analysis of durational speech parameters in neurological dysarthrias. In Y Lebrun, ed. *From the Brain to the Mouth: Acquired Dysarthria and Dysfluency in Adults*, pp. 11–47. Kluwer, Dordrecht.

Hillis AE, Work M, Barker PB, Jacobs MA, Breese EL and Maurer K (2004). Re-examining the brain regions crucial for orchestrating speech articulation. *Brain*, **127**, 1479–87.

Huang CS, Sirisko MA, Hiraba H, Murray GM and Sessle BJ (1988). Organization of the primate face motor cortex as revealed by intracortical microstimulation and electrophysiological identification of afferent inputs and corticobulbar projections. *Journal of Neurophysiology*, **59**, 796–818.

Huang CS, Hiraba H and Sessle BJ (1989a). Input–output relationships of the primary face motor cortex in the monkey (Macaca fascicularis). *Journal of Neurophysiology*, **61**, 350–62.

Huang CS, Hiraba H, Murray GM and Sessle BJ (1989b). Topographical distribution and functional properties of cortically induced rhythmical jaw movements in the monkey (Macaca fascicularis). *Journal of Neurophysiology*, **61**, 635–50.

Ikeda A, Lüders HO, Burgess RC and Shibasaki H (1992). Movement-related potentials recorded from supplementary motor area and primary motor area. *Brain*, **115**, 1017–43.

Indefrey P and Levelt WJM (2004). The spatial and temporal signatures of word production components. *Cognition*, **92**, 101–44.

Jeannerod M (1994). The representing brain: Neural correlates of motor intention and imagery. *Behavioral and Brain Sciences*, **17**, 187–202.

Kent RD, Kent JF and Rosenbek JC (1987). Maximum performance tests of speech production. *Journal of Speech and Hearing Disorders*, **52**, 367–87.

Kent RD (1997). *The Speech Sciences*. Singular, San Diego, CA.

Khedr EM and Aref EE (2002). Electrophysiological study of vocal-fold mobility disorders using a magnetic stimulator. *European Journal of Neurology*, **9**, 259–67.

Kluin KJ, Gilman S, Markel DS, Koeppe RA, Rosenthal G and Junck L (1988). Speech disorders in olivopontocerebellar atrophy correlate with positron emission tomography findings. *Annals of Neurology*, **23**, 547–54.

Lesser RP, Lueders H, Dinner DS, Hahn J and Cohen L (1984). The location of speech and writing functions in the frontal languge area: Results of extraoperative cortical stimulation. *Brain*, **107**, 275–91.

Levelt WJM (1989). *Speaking: From Intention to Articulation*. MIT Press, Cambridge, MA.

Levelt WJM, Roelofs A and Meyer AS (1999). A theory of lexical access in speech production. *Behavioral and Brain Sciences*, **22**, 1–75.

Lotze M, Erb M, Flor H, Huelsmann E, Godde B and Grodd W (2000). fMRI evaluation of somatotopic representation in human primary motor cortex. *NeuroImage*, **11**, 473–81.

Loucks TMJ, Poletto CJ, Simonyan K, Reynolds CL and Ludlow CL (2007). Human brain activation during phonation and exhalation: Common volitional control for two upper airway functions. *NeuroImage*, **36**, 131–43.

Ojemann GA (1979). Individual variability in cortical localization of language. *Journal of Neurosurgery*, **50**, 164–9.

Ojemann GA (1994). Cortical stimulation and recording in language. In A Kertesz, ed. *Localization and Neuroimaging in Neuropsychology*, pp. 35–55. Academic Press, San Diego, CA.

Pascual-Leone A, Gates JR and Dhuna A (1991). Induction of speech arrest and counting errors with rapid-rate transcranial magnetic stimulation. *Neurology*, **41**, 697–702.

Paus T, Petrides M, Evans AC and Meyer E (1993). Role of the human anterior cingulate cortex in the control of oculomotor, manual, and speech responses: A positron emission tomography study. *Journal of Neurophysiology*, **70**, 453–69.

Penfield W and Roberts L (1959). *Speech and Brain Mechanisms*. Princeton University Press, Princeton, NJ.

Penfield W and Welch K (1951). The supplementary motor area of the cerebral cortex: A clinical and experimental study. *Archives of Neurology and Psychiatry*, **63**, 289–317.

Petersen SE, Fox PT, Posner MI, Mintun M and Raichle ME (1989). Positron emission tomographic studies of the processing of single words. *Journal of Cognitive Neuroscience*, **1**, 153–70.

Pinto S, Thobois S, Costes N et al. (2004). Subthalamic nucleus stimulation and dysarthria in Parkinson's disease: A PET study. *Brain*, **127**, 602–15.

Raichle ME, MacLeod AM, Snyder AZ, Powers WJ, Gusnard DA and Shulman GL (2001). A default mode of brain function. *Proceedings of the National Academy of Sciences*, **98**, 676–82.

Riecker A, Ackermann H, Wildgruber D, Dogil G and Grodd W (2000a). Opposite hemispheric lateralization effects during speaking and singing at motor cortex, insula and cerebellum. *NeuroReport*, **11**, 1997–2000.

Riecker A, Ackermann H, Wildgruber D, Meyer J, Dogil G, Haider H and Grodd W (2000b). Articulatory/phonetic sequencing at the level of the anterior perisylvian cortex: A functional magnetic resonance imaging (fMRI) study. *Brain and Language*, **75**, 259–76.

Riecker A, Mathiak K, Wildgruber D, Erb M, Hertrich I, Grodd W and Ackermann H (2005). fMRI reveals two distinct cerebral networks subserving speech motor control. Neurology, **64**, 700–6.

Riecker A, Kassubek J, Gröschel K, Grodd W and Ackermann H (2006). The cerebral control of speech tempo: Opposite relationship between speaking rate and BOLD signal changes at striatal and cerebellar structures. *NeuroImage*, **29**, 46–53.

Riecker A, Brendel B, Ziegler W, Erb M, and Ackermann H (2008). The influence of syllable onset complexity and syllable frequency on speech motor control. *Brain and Language*, **107**, 102–13.

Rödel RMW, Laskawi R and Markus H (2003). Tongue representation in the lateral cortical motor region of the human brain as assessed by transcranial magnetic stimulation. *Annals of Otology, Rhinology & Laryngology*, **112**, 71–6.

Ross ED (1981). The aprosodias: Functional-anatomic organization of the affective components of language in the right hemisphere. *Archives of Neurology*, **38**, 561–9.

Sasaki K, Nambu A, Tsujimoto T, Matsuzaki R, Kyuhou S and Gemba H (1996). Studies on integrative functions of the human frontal association cortex with MEG. *Brain Research Cognitive Brain Research*, **5**, 165–74.

Schiff HB, Alexander MP, Naeser MA and Galaburda AM (1983). Aphemia: Clinical-anatomic correlations. *Archives of Neurology*, **40**, 720–7.

Shuster LI and Lemieux SK (2005). An fMRI investigation of covertly and overtly produced mono- and multisyllabic words. *Brain and Language*, **93**, 20–31.

Sidtis JJ, Strother SC, Anderson JR and Rottenberg DA (1999). Are brain functions really additive? *NeuroImage*, **9**, 490–6.

Sidtis JJ, Strother SC and Rottenberg DA (2003). Predicting performance from functional imaging data: Methods matter. *NeuroImage*, **20**, 615–24.

Sidtis JJ, Gomez C, Groshong A, Strother SC and Rottenberg DA (2006). Mapping cerebral blood flow during speech production in hereditary ataxia. *NeuroImage*, **31**, 246–54.

Sörös P, Sokoloff LG, Bose A, McIntosh AR, Graham SJ and Stuss DT (2006). Clustered functional MRI of overt speech production. *NeuroImage*, **32**, 376–87.

Sokolov AN (1972). *Inner Speech and Thought.* Plenum, New York, NY.

Staiger A and Ziegler W (2008). Syllable frequency and syllable structure in the spontaneous speech production of patients with apraxia of speech. Aphasiology, **22**(11), 1201–15.

Urasaki E, Uematsu S, Gordon B and Lesser RP (1994). Cortical tongue area studied by chronically implanted subdural electrodes – with special reference to parietal motor and frontal sensory responses. *Brain*, **117**, 117–32.

Van Lancker Sidtis D, Pachana N, Cummings JL and Sidtis JJ (2006). Dysprosodic speech following basal ganglia insult: Toward a conceptual framework for the study of the cerebral representation of prosody. *Brain and Language*, **97**, 135–53.

Vigneau M, Beaucousin V, Hervé PY, Duffau H, Crivello F, Houdé O, Mazoyer B and Tzourio-Mazoyer N (2006). Meta-analyzing left hemisphere language areas: Phonology, semantics, and sentence processing. *NeuroImage*, **30**, 1414–32.

Wildgruber D, Ackermann H, Klose U, Kardatzki B and Grodd W (1996). Functional lateralization of speech production at primary motor cortex: A fMRI study. *NeuroReport*, **7**, 2791–5.

Wildgruber D, Ackermann H and Grodd W (2001). Differential contributions of motor cortex, basal ganglia, and cerebellum to speech motor control: Effects of syllable repetition rate evaluated by fMRI. *NeuroImage*, **13**, 101–9.

Wise RJS, Greene J, Büchel C and Scott SK (1999). Brain regions involved in articulation. *Lancet*, **353**, 1057–61.

Woolsey CN, Erickson TC and Gilson WE (1979). Localization in somatic sensory and motor areas of human cerebral cortex as determined by direct recording of evoked potentials and electrical stimulation. *Journal of Neurosurgery*, **51**, 476–506.

Ziegler W (2002). Task-related factors in oral motor control: Speech and oral diadochokinesis in dysarthria and apraxia of speech. *Brain and Language*, **80**, 556–75.

Ziegler W (2008). Apraxia of speech. In G Goldenberg and B Miller, eds. *Handbook of Clinical Neurology*, vol. 88 (3rd series), *Neuropsychology and Behavioral Neurology*, pp. 269–85. Elsevier, London.

Section 3

Speech motor development

Chapter 8

Dynamic interaction of motor and language factors in normal and disordered development

Lisa Goffman

Abstract

Language and motor skills co-develop in normal and language disordered children. The aim of this chapter is to report on empirical findings detailing interactions between language and motor domains in normally developing and language disordered learners. It is shown that speech motor variability may serve as an index of learning, one that changes as a function of both perceptual and production input. Further, articulatory and linguistic production units interact in complex ways, with changes in segmental, lexical, and prosodic variables showing broadly distributed effects on speech motor output. Finally, as demonstrated in previous studies, language and generalized motor impairments co-occur. However, the specific nature of these interactions is complex, with speech motor skills implicated, but no evidence of a generalized timing deficit. Empirical data of this sort will ultimately contribute to a more comprehensive model of language production that incorporates perceptual, language, and speech motor components.

8.1 Introduction

The neural organization for language and movement are highly interactive (e.g., Arbib 2006; Kent 2004). Consistent with common neural organization, behavioural evidence from developmental disorders reveals a high degree of co-occurrence of cognitive-linguistic and motor deficits (e.g., Diamond 2000; Hill 2001). Such clear interactions between language and action have only minimally found their way into models of language production in children. Theoretical accounts of children's language production emphasize the acquisition of phonology, the lexicon, and grammar, with little attention to associated speech motor processes. The broad aim of this chapter is to report on recent findings that assess how language and motor skills co-develop in normal and disordered language learners. The basic premise of these studies is that the trajectory of acquisition of children's language production is influenced by both language and motor domains. Language acquisition is particularly difficult for some children, such as those with language disorders, though it remains unclear when and how language or motor aspects serve as a primary constraining factor. Ultimately, an empirical data base is critical in informing models of normal and disordered language acquisition.

In the present chapter, I will develop three themes related to language and motor interactions. One critical developmental construct involves learning. Children must acquire new language structures while their speech motor systems are also in a period of developmental change. Much of my current work is concerned with speech motor variability as an index of plasticity and of learning. A second theme involves the size and nature of language and articulatory speech production units. The syllable has often been seen as the predominant unit of speech motor control (MacNeilage and Davis 2000; Cholin et al., 2006; Levelt and Wheeldon 1994). I suggest that, even for young children, units larger than the syllable directly influence motor commands to the muscles involved in articulation. Finally, as a third theme, I will turn to the co-occurrence of language and speech motor, as well as general motor, deficits in children with specific language impairment (SLI). Children with language disorders serve as an important test case for assessing how language and motor systems interact, and understanding how language or motor aspects constrain output has critical implications for theoretical accounts as well as for the development of optimal interventions for these children.

8.2 Theme 1: speech motor variability as an index of learning and plasticity

8.2.1 Production variability

A primary analytic approach we have employed focuses on articulatory variability in the movement signal on repeated trials (Smith et al., 1995, 2000). The interpretation of variability has been debated (e.g., Van Lieshout and Namasivayam, Chapter 11 this volume; Stathopoulos 1995). In studies of speakers with disorders, increased articulatory variability is viewed as a sign of reduced coordinative ability. Similarly, older adults also often show increased movement variability, again interpreted as an indicator of a degraded speech motor control system (Kleinow et al., 2001; Wohlert 1996). However, variability also may be a positive attribute of a biological system. Thelen and her colleagues beautifully articulate how young children demonstrate increased variability in the context of a developmental task, such as learning to reach (Thelen and Smith 1994; Thelen et al., 1994). As Thelen and Smith (1994) point out, variability is 'an important concomitant of transitions to new forms (p. 87)'.

Changes in movement variability may provide an index of learning, even when more overt production measures, such as perceived segmental accuracy, remain stable. It has become obvious that perceptually based transcription does not always provide an accurate measure of language representations. For example, acoustic and kinematic measures have been used to determine covert contrasts, such as segmental or morphological contrasts that are present in the physical signal, but not realized perceptually (Owen and Goffman 2007; Scobbie et al., 2000). As an example, some children with articulation disorders have been shown to produce more posterior movements for the production of a /k/ than a /t/ target, even though both are realized perceptually as /t/ (Gibbon 1999). These children's articulatory movement patterns reveal that /t/ and /k/ are distinct categories, even though both productions are transcribed as [t] (Gibbon 1999). In this case, discrete segmental categories have emerged, but are not overtly produced. Motor-based analyses have the potential to provide a sensitive index of developmental change that is not apparent in perceptually based transcription approaches.

Indeed, the time course of speech motor development is protracted (Smith and Goffman 1998; Smith and Zelaznik 2004; Walsh and Smith 2002). Children who are developing normally show significantly more variable oral movement trajectories than adults, even into adolescence (Smith and Zelaznik 2004; Walsh and Smith 2002). Thus, children are variable oral movement generators well beyond the age at which they have overtly mastered the segmental units of their language.

Such flexibility in motor performance may also relate to flexibility in language performance. In studies of language perception, some aspects of language, such as syntax and phonology, are known to be more learnable prior to adolescence, as demonstrated, for example, in second language learning. Weber-Fox and Neville (1996) tested English–Chinese bilingual adult speakers who had been exposed to English at different ages, ranging from one year to after sixteen years of age. Analyses of accuracy and of event-related potentials (ERPs) showed that even the speakers exposed to English at one year to three years were different from their monolingual peers in their syntactic processing. The accuracy of responses as well as the distribution and time course of ERP responses differed between these highly proficient second language speakers and those exposed to English from birth. However, processing of sentences that contained semantic anomalies only differed in Chinese–English bilingual speakers who were not exposed to English until adolescence. These results reveal that neural subsystems underlying syntactic and semantic processing have different sensitive periods.

Returning to speech production, in a study of nine- and ten-year-old children and adults, Walsh et al. (2006) asked whether changes in short-term variability may index the acquisition of a novel phonetic sequence. Two sources of variability were assessed. One source, neuromotor or background noise (Newell et al., 2006) was not expected to change over the course of a short-term (20 min) speech motor learning task. Children are, on average, more variable movement generators than adults due to higher inherent neuromotor noise. However, a second type of variability was thought to be related to practice and task demands, or to short-term learning (Deutsch and Newell 2004). This source of variability was predicted to change with alterations in task demands, perhaps even over a very short time period.

In this experiment, children and adults imitated novel nonwords of varying lengths, ranging from one (e.g., [maeb]) to four (e.g., [maebsheltaldoyb]) syllables. These recorded stimuli were produced naturally and were not controlled for stress pattern. As expected, nine- to ten-year-olds were more variable overall than were adults. The more interesting finding was related to short-term learning. When the first five productions of a nonword were compared with the last five productions, the adults showed no differences in articulatory variability. However, the children showed reduced variability in the last five productions, but only on the more complex 3 and 4 syllable nonwords; it is only in producing nonword forms that are at the edge of their capacities that such learning effects emerged. This short-term production experience influenced speech motor coordination in the children. The adults did not show such flexibility, but it was unclear whether this was because of a reduced capacity to learn or because the task was relatively easy for adults and was not in a range that required learning. A follow-up study supported the latter interpretation, as young adults did show a short-term learning effect when the nonwords were made more difficult (Sasisekaran, Smith, Sadagopan, and Weber-Fox, in progress).

The short-term transitions in variability observed in these studies of the acquisition of novel words may help to explain why second language learning is considerably more difficult for adults than children (Flege et al., 1999). In a study of adult second language learners, Chakraborty et al. (2008) observed no differences in articulatory variability in sentences produced in the first versus the second language, the assumption being that increased articulatory variability is an indicator of a more flexible system. Children show short-term changes in articulatory variability (Walsh et al., 2006) and are also more facile at learning a second language compared with adults. Adult learners demonstrate reduced flexibility along with a reduced capacity to learn.

The Chakraborty et al. (2008) study included adult speakers whose first language was Bengali and second language English. The initial age of exposure to English ranged from 8 months to 10 years, though all lived in India for 22–32 years before moving to the United States. These speakers varied in English proficiency, but all learned Bengali as young children and used English in school. Speakers who were judged as highly proficient in English were exposed to

English relatively early. These speakers also performed at relatively high levels on the Speaking Grammar subtest of the *Test of Adolescent and Adult Language* (TOAL-3; Hammill et al., 1994). All participants were residing in an English speaking country at the time the data were obtained.

Speakers produced three English sentences and three Bengali sentences that were closely matched for stress and segmental content (e.g., 'Buy Bobby a puppy' in English paired with 'baba pepe khabe' ([baba pepe k^habe]; 'daddy will eat papaya', in Bengali). For these adult speakers, both first and second language sentences were produced with highly stable articulatory movement trajectories; there were no differences between monolingual English speakers and Bengali–English bilingual speakers in the production of English sentences. First and second language and articulatory movement trajectories were similar to those observed in adult monolingual speakers of English. In their production of these syntactically and semantically simple sentences, adult late learners did not demonstrate increased variability in their articulatory systems for their second language. This was even the case for less proficient, highly accented, speakers. These data show the expected lack of plasticity in later learners and provide indirect evidence that lower articulatory variability may also imply decreased flexibility, since these heavily accented late learners were relatively fixed in their articulatory patterning. It is critical to assess structures in the second language that are more complex than those studied here or that are not consistent with the characteristics of the speakers first language to fully understand how speech motor plasticity relates to second language acquisition.

As suggested in the above paragraphs, measures of articulatory variability provide an index of global developmental change that is reduced over the time course of many years into young adulthood. In addition, changes in articulatory variability were observed in short-term production-based learning of novel words in children (Walsh et al., 2006). However, variability did not increase in adult language learners producing a second language in which they demonstrated rather poor proficiency (Chakraborty et al., 2008). Thus, variability may be viewed as an index of flexibility and is increased in a system that is still in a period of learning.

An additional sort of learning involves the influence of changes in perceptual input on speech motor variability. One approach to investigating the influence of perception on production is to study changes in speech motor variability in children who have received a cochlear implant. These children are likely to have normal language processing capacities, but have been deprived of auditory input. In a preliminary investigation of a seven-year-old boy, we assessed changes in speech motor variability pre- and post-cochlear implant (Goffman et al., 2002). We asked whether new auditory input would result in changes in speech motor variability. This child experienced meningitis at three years and lost his hearing. He received a multichannel cochlear implant at age seven years.

In the experimental task, the child produced multiple renditions of the words 'man', 'pan', and 'fan' embedded in the phrase 'I see a... again'. Articulatory variability was assessed pre-implant and at two-month intervals post-implant for one year. Pre-implant, the child produced spatiotemporal variability that was slightly higher than expected, similar to that of younger normally developing peers (i.e., four-year-olds). At two to four months post-implant, his ability to produce consistent articulatory movements on multiple trials became quite disrupted. His movement variability increased significantly for all three words produced. By six months post-implant, the variability of his articulatory movements decreased markedly, now to values similar to his age-matched peers (i.e., seven-year-olds). His productions remained stable for the remaining six months of the study. Importantly, transcription analysis showed that he produced the target words correctly throughout. The new auditory input initially destabilized his articulatory system during the early period of learning, suggesting that changes in auditory input lead to modification of a flexible system. It would be important to see if such effects appear in adult implant recipients.

8.2.2 Influences of perceptual learning on production variability

Another potentially valuable way to assess the role of perceptual input on speech motor learning draws on paradigms used in infant studies. In these studies, infants are presented with different kinds of input and engage in short-term learning. Often the goal is to determine whether infants show processing capacities that may be relevant for language learning. For example, infants may be presented with syllable sequences that show different segmental co-dependencies or stress patterns to assess their use of cues for parsing words and phrases from the input (Saffran et al., 1996; Seidl 2007). Word learning may be evaluated by presenting novel pictures paired with novel phonetic forms and determining how infants acquire these new words (Hollich et al., 2007; Werker et al., 2002). Infants demonstrate remarkable capacities to parse words and sentences and learn new words based on rather sparse perceptual input. These early capacities must relate to the emergence of words and sentences in production, though little work has directly investigated how early perceptual skills relate to production. In a retrospective study, it was shown that early performance on speech segmentation tasks predicts vocabulary size at 24 months, and language, but not cognitive, status at 4 years (Newman et al., 2006). Thus, it appears that some aspects of speech processing, that is the ability to segment the speech stream, are important for later language production.

Infants' perceptual systems develop early and are sensitive to many stimuli that may be relevant for language learning. Gomez and Gerken (1999) demonstrated that, by 12 months, infants are able to extract rules for a simple artificial grammar. After only a few minutes of familiarization with the grammar, infants are able to distinguish well-formed novel strings from those that violate the word order of the input grammar. Infants learned non-adjacent dependencies similar to those required in grammatical learning. Adults with a history of language disorders showed difficulty with this type of 'grammatical' learning (Plante et al., 2002).

Paralleling morphosyntactic learning, non-linguistic prerequisites also seem to exist in the acquisition of prosodic structure. By seven months, infants are sensitive to probabilities of co-occurrence across syllables which they may use to subsequently formulate constraints on their language's foot structure (Thiessen and Saffran 2003). This perceptual capacity may influence their sensitivity to lexical stress at eight months (Johnson and Jusczyk 2001; Jusczyk et al., 1999; Thiessen and Saffran 2003). Both statistical and stress cues are thought to allow infants to parse the speech stream into individual words and thus these cues play an important role in later word learning. However, we don't know how perceptual learning of this kind relates to language production later in development. The interaction between perceptual capacities and language representations is complex. For example, although newborn infants are sensitive to voicing contrasts, 14-month-olds cannot use these perceptual capacities to differentiate similar sounding words (Werker et al., 2002). Vocabulary size influences how perceptual capacities are invoked in word learning, with 14-month-olds showing diminished abilities compared with far younger infants (Werker et al., 2002). Thus, there are likely reciprocal interactions between vocabulary size and perceptual capacities. In general, perceptual processing capacities, even those that emerge very early, have not been explicitly linked to language or motor aspects of production.

What is notable here is that production learning significantly lags perceptual learning and, further, that there has been very little investigation of how perceptual input influences language learning, especially in the production domain. In some current studies, we are attempting to integrate some of the approaches in studying perceptual learning and assessing influences on production processes.

Borrowing from studies of infant perceptual learning, we investigated how word learning interacts with speech motor implementation. In many models of language production, most notably

Levelt's, lexical processing does not interact directly with articulation (e.g., Levelt et al., 1999). However, in this study, we asked whether manipulation of an object referent associated with a nonsense lexical form has direct effects on the output of the speech motor system (Heisler et al., in press; Heisler 2004). That is, does assigning a nonsense word a visual referent (i.e., semantic meaning) influence speech motor variability? In order to obtain a baseline of speech motor performance without any semantic content, children were initially asked to repeat four two-syllable nonsense words that were controlled for phonotactic frequency (e.g., 'pafkub'). They looked at a computer screen with a checkerboard pattern during production of all four nonwords. In a perceptual input phase that immediately followed, two of these four words were assigned a visual referent, while two continued to be presented without meaning (i.e., while the children looked at a checkerboard). The children then produced the words again, just as they did initially, while looking at a checkerboard pattern. Children's articulatory movement variability was lower in the post-test than the pre-test when a referent was assigned but remained constant when no semantic meaning was applied. Lexical status influenced articulatory variability.

The finding that a change in lexical status has a direct effect on speech motor output is not predicted by existing models (Levelt et al., 1999; but see Rapp and Goldrich 2006). However, the present results suggest a direct link between semantic processing and speech motor output. Further, short-term learning occurs not only as a function of motor practice (Walsh et al., 2006), but also of changes in semantic status acquired through perceptually based learning. It seems a very promising domain of enquiry to assess various processing units that have been identified in studies of infants (e.g., sensitivity to grammatical, semantic, and stress cues) and relate them to the acquisition of production units.

In summary, shifts in articulatory variability index multiple aspects of short-term learning, as well as longer term developmental change. Production practice leads to decreased variability, but only when the structure is at the 'edge of learning' (Walsh et al., 2006). Further, it appears that perceptual learning results in similar changes in articulatory variability (Heisler et al., in press). As suggested by Thelen and her colleagues (e.g., Thelen and Smith 1994), variability is an important indicator of learning.

8.3 Theme 2: sizes of articulatory units

Another critical construct in developmental research is the size of the production units. The emergence of segments, syllables, and words has been a topic of discussion in theoretical accounts of early phonological development (e.g., Bernhardt and Stemberger 1998; McCune and Vihman 2001). For example, relying on phonetic transcription, researchers have hypothesized that young children produce broad vocal-motor schemas associated with relatively large production units (McCune and Vihman 2001). That is, infants establish vocal motor patterns in babbling that are phonetically consistent and are used to produce first words. For example, a child who produces [bababa] is especially likely to acquire first words like 'baby' and 'bottle', since these contain the preferred [b] and may easily be produced with a preferred CVCV syllable structure. Segmental detail emerges from these early vocal motor schemes. Levelt and his colleagues also describe first linkages between words and actions, stating that 'word production emerges from a coupling of two initially independent systems, a conceptual system and an articulatory system' (Levelt et al., 1999, p. 1).

While still relying on transcription evidence, the related movement-based hypothesis of MacNeilage and Davis (2000) is consistent with this view. These investigators suggest that the oscillatory movement corresponding with an open–close cycle of jaw movement serves as the organizing frame for early speech production. With time, children fill in the local details, or the content, from which segmental organization emerges. The initial organizing unit is the syllable, or the frame, with the segment emerging later in development.

Acoustic analyses further support that early production units are organized broadly, at the level of the syllable or word (Nittrouer 1993). Young children show more gestural overlap than adults in their production of disyllable sequences (Goodell and Studdert-Kennedy 1993; Nittrouer et al., 1989). Further, children show less precision than adults in their production of fricatives. In fact, some investigators have argued that it is this increased variability, not differences in the size of production units, that differentiate children from adults (Katz et al., 1991; Sereno et al., 1987). Overall, transcription and acoustic studies have revealed that children produce relatively broad speech production units, probably organized at the level of syllables or words rather than segments. With time, smaller segmental units emerge. What is notable is that few if any direct motor analyses have been applied to the assessment of children's production units.

As is evident in the above review, the syllable is considered a prominent production unit early in development. Compatible with the developmental evidence, Levelt and colleagues hypothesize that adult speakers store an inventory of frequently occurring syllables that provide the interface between phonological processing and the motor implementation of speech. Thus, for adults the syllable serves as the predominant unit involved in speech motor aspects of production (Cholin et al., 2006; Levelt and Wheeldon 1994). However, there is little direct evidence assessing the size of the language units that interact with speech motor production. Nittrouer and colleagues have described the gesture and gestural overlap as the relevant units, with coordination of these units changing over the course of development (Nittrouer 1993; Nittrouer et al., 1989). Recently, we have been investigating the breadth of production units in an attempt to assess whether the syllable should be viewed as a privileged unit at the level of speech motor control.

8.3.1 **Segmental units**

Perhaps the most basic approach to assessing the size of production units in speech motor control is to consider the influence of manipulating a single phonetic segment on production characteristics of various units, including syllables. Coarticulation in adults shows whether the manipulation of a single segment influences the motor commands associated with a syllable or with even broader components of a sentence (e.g., Recasens 2002). Developmental studies of coarticulation have focused on acoustic analysis and on the syllable or word as the unit of analysis. Our objective was to assess the breadth of lip rounding across a broader temporal window than included in prior studies (i.e., a sentence) using direct kinematic evidence.

Four- to five-year-old children and adults participated in this study (Goffman et al., 2008). The speakers imitated pairs of sentences that differed only in a medial vowel that did or did not include lip rounding (e.g., 'Mom has the b*oo*t in the box' vs. 'Mom has the b*ee*t in the box'). Because the control sentence only varied with respect to the medial vowel, the extent of the coarticulatory effect could be measured across the entire utterance. Initially, the kinematic trajectory for the entire utterance was extracted, beginning with the word 'Mom' and ending with the word 'box.' Then, the amplitude and the temporal extent of the anterior–posterior motion of the upper lip was assessed across the rounded and the unrounded conditions for the entire utterance. Both children and adults produced lip rounding movements that subsumed approximately 50% of the entire utterance, thus crossing word and phrase boundaries. A comparison of the overall movement patterning for the whole sentence suggested that lip retraction differed across the entire sentence, not just the 50% included in the temporal extent of the rounding movement, because a lip retraction movement preceded and followed the rounded gesture. Coarticulatory effects were far broader than the syllable and perhaps transcended the entire utterance.

These results indicated that speech motor commands are not confined to the segment or the syllable, but cross multiple language units. Very broad effects were observed in both children and adults, suggesting that while movement consistency changed after age four to five years, the breadth of production units did not. Performance factors related to movement variability differentiated children and adults, but the breadth of production units was similar across the developmental periods studied.

8.3.2 **Lexical units**

Manipulating lexical parameters of language also has shown broad effects on speech motor output. In another study, children produced either novel or familiar words in utterance final position (Goffman, Chakraborty, and Schnoor, in preparation). Four-year-old children were asked to produce sentences such as 'Bobby pushed the baby' (familiar word in final position) and 'Bobby pushed the bapa' (novel word in final position; 'bapa' referred to a creature from outer space). Because the phonetic content of the novel and familiar words by necessity differed and we were interested in broad effects, we assessed the influence of familiarity on the variability of articulatory movement for the initial word in the sentence, 'Bobby'. Children produced the word 'Bobby' with more articulatory variability when the word at the end of the sentence was novel compared with when it was familiar. These data again suggest that the breadth of influence of language on speech motor output is temporally extensive. Motor planning and execution for the onset of the sentence was influenced by the novelty of a sentence final lexical item.

8.3.3 **Prosodic units**

Prosodic factors also show differential effects within and across word boundaries. In our previous work, we have demonstrated that children and adults produce more variable movement output in iambic compared with trochaic words (Goffman, 1999, 2004; Goffman and Malin 1999; Goffman et al., 2006). This was initially rather surprising, since trochees occur more frequently and develop early. However, we suggest that children rely on more primitive movement patterns for the production of trochees and devote increased resources to their production of iambs. Recently, we investigated whether more difficult stress patterns (i.e., weak–weak strings vs. easier strong–weak alternations) were produced with more or less articulatory variability when they crossed word boundaries (e.g., in sentences such as 'Emma's baboon' which is SWWS compared with 'Emma's baby' which is SWSW; Goffman and Westover, submitted). Contrary to the within-word effects, utterance medial weak–weak prosodic sequences were more variable across word boundaries. More difficult prosodic sequences were produced with less variability within a word, but more variability between words. That is, the same prosodic sequence was produced with different degrees of articulatory variability as a function of lexical status. It appears that lexical factors were related to changes in the temporal overlap of articulatory movements. Once again, factors beyond the syllable or word influenced speech movement output.

In sum, a more comprehensive model of the development of speech production must account for influences of syntactic, semantic, and phonological processing on speech motor output. It must also address the nature of units that are used in planning and production and how the size of the units changes over development from babbling to first words and in later sentence production. Nittrouer and colleagues (Nittrouer 1993; Nittrouer et al., 1989) have claimed that phonetic transcription neglects the critical components of the acquisition of speech, arguing that gestures and the coordination among gestures more accurately characterize development. We suggest, consistent with aspects of the gestural perspective, that very broad interactions exist between multiple-sized language units and the movement trajectories through which they are implemented.

Overall, the results of studies from children who are normally developing provide empirical support that language production involves multiple interactive units that operate in parallel. These results seem consistent with the parallel and distributed models of neural organization described by Kent (2004), Pulvermuller (1999), and others. That is, multiple levels of language processing have direct effects on motor planning and execution.

8.4 Theme 3: co-occurrence of language and motor deficits in SLI – representational and performance factors

The diagnostic category of SLI provides a strong clinical test-case of interactions between language and motor domains, since this disorder is defined on the basis of language deficits. That is, children with SLI show significant deficits in receptive or expressive language that are not explained by cognitive, auditory, or oral motor limitations (Leonard 1998). There are many accounts of SLI, most focusing on problems with the acquisition of grammatical aspects of language (e.g., Rice et al., 1998; Van der Lely 1998). Processing deficits have also been implicated (e.g., Ellis Weismer 1996; Tallal et al., 1996).

Recently, broader accounts of SLI have been introduced, such as Ullman and Pierpont's (2005) procedural deficit hypothesis. These investigators propose that children with SLI show deficits that may be related to the procedural memory system, the brain system underlying the learning and implementation of skills for the production of motor and language sequences. The procedural deficit hypothesis provides a cohesive explanation for why children with SLI have difficulty with speeded, sequential, and timed movement (e.g., Bishop 2002; Hill 2001), as well as with working memory and with language.

8.4.1 Generalized motor deficits

In fact, children with SLI's difficulties with gross and fine motor tasks have been well documented. For example, children with SLI show difficulties with fine motor skills requiring sensorimotor precision, such as copying shapes (Schwartz and Regan 1996) and with imitating gestures such as brushing teeth and saluting (Hill et al., 1998). What is striking about these findings is the generality of the observations from both language and motor domains (e.g., copying shapes relates in some way to language comprehension; children with language impairment have relative difficulty standing on one foot). Jancke et al. (2006) related difficulties with manual tasks to neuroanatomical differences in children with language impairments. Behaviourally, these children with language impairments had difficulty with manual tasks, such as tapping and peg moving. Critically, structural imaging studies revealed that children with SLI showed decreased white matter in a neural circuit linking structures in the left hemisphere (e.g., motor cortex, premotor cortex, planum polare on the superior temporal gyrus). Thus, motor and language areas are both implicated.

Children with SLI are diagnosed on the basis of poor performance on a standardized test of language function (Leonard 1998). Similarly, children diagnosed with developmental coordination disorder show significantly impaired gross and/or fine motor skills. The data reviewed above indicate that there is a great deal of overlap between these two groups of children; most relevant for the present purposes is that children with SLI also show gross and fine motor impairments. However, to date, the experimental findings are highly descriptive, and we have little understanding of underlying mechanisms that influence the co-development of the language and motor systems.

Studies of the KE family provide further evidence that a genetically based language disorder may involve a motor disorder as well. Investigations of multiple generations of this family reveal that approximately half of its members show language, cognitive, and motor deficits

(Morgan et al., Chapter 6 this volume; Vargha-Khadem et al., 1995). Originally, the morphosyntactic deficits observed in affected members of this family were construed as evidence for a genetic basis of language disorders (Gopnik and Crago 1991). However, further study revealed that these affected family members also showed a significant articulatory impairment along with nonlinguistic orofacial praxis deficits (Shriberg, Chapter 15 this volume; Vargha-Khadem et al., 1995). In summary, concomitant motor disorders are often seen in children with SLI, as well is in other childhood disorders such as attention deficit and hyperactivity disorder and dyslexia. Such linkages across language and motor levels are beginning to be exploited by treatment programmes for adults with aphasia (Buccino et al., 2006). Finally we note that, although the co-occurrence of language and motor deficits has been well established in children with SLI, these findings generally have not been integrated into major accounts of the disorder, with a few exceptions (e.g., Bishop 2002; Hill 2001).

Diamond (2000), Kent (2004), and others suggest that the study of disordered development also informs models of language and motor processing. Children with SLI serve as a strong test-case for language and motor interactions, because their deficits traditionally are defined as specific to language (Leonard 1998; Rice et al., 1998). Of course, in the context of our changing understanding of development, several researchers have more carefully considered the profiles of these children and have observed many other areas of deficit, including gross and fine motor skill (Bishop and Edmundson 1987; Hill 2001). Consistent with these prior studies, we have observed that six- to eight-year-old children with a history of SLI may have resolved their overt difficulties with grammatical morphology, but continue to show significant gross and fine motor deficits (Zelaznik and Goffman in press). That is, their standard scores are lower than those of their age-matched peers on a test of gross and fine motor development – the *The Bruininks-Oseretsky Test of Motor Proficiency* (Bruininks 1978). Similar to earlier investigations, these global measures do little to specify the dimensions of motor skill that are implicated, though sub-tests concerned with bimanual coordination and balance showed the most depressed scores. These gross and fine motor difficulties do not correspond linearly with language scores; so the relationship between language and motor skill is not direct.

8.4.2 **Speech motor skill**

One domain of motor development that may be implicated, of course, is that of speech motor skill. In their production of speech, children with SLI have demonstrated higher oral movement variability in multi-movement sequences in comparison to their age-matched peers (Goffman 1999, 2004; Goffman, Chakraborty, and Schnoor, in preparation). Thus, like younger normally developing children, neuromotor, or background noise (Walsh et al., 2006) appears to influence their speech motor systems. It is unclear if such variability is simply an immaturity reflecting increased flexibility or implies a disordered speech motor system. Regardless of the explanation, speech motor skills are affected in children with SLI.

In the speech motor domain, children with SLI also have difficulties with producing the small and short articulatory movements associated with weak syllables. Indeed, transcription evidence shows that the initial, unstressed syllables in iambs are often omitted by young normally developing children (e.g., Echols 1993; Gerken 1994) and older children with SLI (McGregor and Leonard 1994; Leonard 1998). For example, children will say [lun] for 'balloon'. Importantly, these stress-related error patterns also influence grammatical inflections (e.g., the weak syllable 'the' is omitted in the sentence 'pushes the dog'). Children omit more grammatical inflections in problematic prosodic sequences, especially those involving initial or contiguous (i.e., unfooted) weak syllables. These stress patterns are particularly difficult for children with SLI and with childhood apraxia of speech (CAS) and are often deemed diagnostically important in these disorders (Hall et al., 1993; McGregor and Leonard 1994; Shriberg et al., 1997).

For adults and young children who are normally developing, initial weak syllables in iambs are produced with small and short movements (Goffman 1999, 2004; Goffman and Malin 1999). Unlike their normally developing peers, even once overt productions of initial weak syllables are in place, four- to five-year-old children with SLI produce larger movements with longer durations in these problematic syllables (Goffman 1999, 2004). These findings provide kinematic evidence of 'misplaced or equal stress' (Shriberg et al., 1997), in that these children have difficulty producing the stress modulations associated with iambic sequences. It may be that the production of movements with greater amplitude provide a compensatory, or stabilizing, function, similar to that observed by Van Lieshout and colleagues in their investigation of an adult speaker with AOS (Van Lieshout et al., 2007). It is critical that children with SLI do produce differentiated movement patterns for trochaic (or strong–weak) in contrast with iambic (weak–strong) categories. Their difficulties with the weak syllables in iambs arise from degraded motor performance rather than limitations in the representations of these linguistic categories. Although these children are defined based on their language deficits, in these prosodic tasks they do produce covert contrasts and show motor not language difficulties.

8.4.3 Manual timing

Because of these difficulties with timing in speech (i.e., prosody) in conjunction with gross and fine motor skill, we hypothesized that manual timing may show subtle deficits in children with SLI. We conducted a study of timing based on the classic study of Wing and Kristofferson (1973) in which children performed a repetitive tapping task that supposedly draws upon classic clock-like timing processes involving cerebellar resources. These children also performed a repetitive circle drawing timing task that does not require clock-like timing and does not involve cerebellar timing resources (Ivry et al., 2002; Spencer et al., 2003; Zelaznik et al., 2002). Because the movement of a single finger may be difficult for young children, we included an easier version, in which children tapped with their entire arm. Using the Wing and Kristofferson (1973) paradigm, the children first tapped in beat to a metronome which was turned off after 13 pacing taps. The children were asked to continue to tap for 31 cycles. In these simple rhythmic tasks involving a single effector, the finger or arm, there were no group differences in timing variability or accuracy between children with SLI and their age-matched controls. Contrary to our hypothesis, simple timing tasks do not appear to be problematic for these children. It may be that increasing cognitive load or incorporating coordination across multiple effectors may underlie some of the motor deficits observed in children with SLI. This is an important area of further enquiry.

In sum, children with SLI whose primary deficits are characterized by language problems actually show persistent motor deficits. However, these deficits apparently are not directly tied to more generalized difficulties with timing. Further, 'covert' articulatory analyses demonstrate that speech motor factors often occlude that children with SLI are representing many of the same language categories as their normally developing peers; performance rather than representational factors often interfere. Although it is evident that language and motor factors interact in disordered development, the nature of such interactions remains unspecified.

8.5 Conclusion

While neurophysiological findings have shown a highly interactive organization for language and action, models of normal and disordered development remain modular in their conceptualization of perceptual, language, and motor processing. It was the aim of this chapter to report on empirical findings detailing interactions between language and motor domains in normally developing and language disordered learners. For example, it was shown that speech motor variability may serve as an index of learning, one that changes as a function of both perceptual and production input. Further, articulatory and linguistic production units were found to interact in complex ways, with changes in segmental, lexical, and prosodic variables showing broadly distributed effects on motor output. Finally, as demonstrated in previous studies, language and generalized motor impairments co-occur. However, the specific nature of these interactions was revealed to be complex, with speech motor skills implicated, but no evidence of a generalized timing deficit. Empirical data of this sort will ultimately contribute to a more comprehensive model of language production that incorporates perceptual, language, and speech motor components. Such approaches have major implications not only for developing a full theoretical account of language production, but for designing powerful and empirically driven interventions for young children with communication disorders.

Acknowledgements

This work was supported by the National Institutes of Health, National Institute on Deafness and Other Communicative Disorders, Grant DC04826. I am especially grateful to Anne Smith for her contributions to multiple dimensions of this research.

References

Arbib, M. A. (2006). *Action to Language via the Mirror Neuron System.* Cambridge, MA: Cambridge University Press.

Bernhardt, B. H., and Stemberger, J. P. (1998). *Handbook of Phonological Development from the Perspective of Constraint-Based Nonlinear Phonology.* San Diego, CA: Academic Press.

Bishop, D. V. M. (2002). Motor immaturity and specific speech and language impairment: Evidence for a common genetic basis. *American Journal of Medical Genetics, 114,* 56–63.

Bishop, D. V. M., and Edmundson, A. (1987). Specific language impairment as a maturational lag: Evidence from longitudinal data on language and motor development. *Developmental Medicine and Child Neurology, 29,* 442–459.

Bruininks, R. H. (1978). *The Bruininks-Oseretsky Test of Motor Proficiency.* Circle Pines, MN: American Guidance Service.

Buccino, G., Soldkin, A., and Small, S. L. (2006). Functions of the mirror neuron system: Implications for neurorehabilitation. *Cognitive Behavioral Neurology, 19,* 55–63.

Chakraborty, R., Goffman, L., and Smith, A. (2008). Physiological indices of bilingualism: Oral motor coordination and speech rate in Bengali–English speakers. *Journal of Speech, Language, and Hearing Research, 51,* 321–332.

Cholin, J., Levelt, W. J. M, and Schiller, N. O. (2006). Effects of syllable frequency in speech production. *Cognition, 99,* 205–235.

Deutsch, K. M., and Newell, K. M. (2004). Changes in the structure of children's isometric force variability with practice. *Journal of Experimental Child Psychology, 88,* 319–333.

Diamond, A. (2000). Close interrelation of motor development and cognitive development and of the cerebellum and prefrontal cortex. *Child Development, 71,* 44–56.

Echols, C. H. (1993). A perceptually-based model of children's earliest productions. *Cognition, 46,* 245–296.

Ellis Weismer, S. (1996). Capacity limitations in working memory: The impact on lexical and morphological learning by children with language impairment. *Topics in Language Disorders, 17,* 33–44.

Flege, J. E., Yeni-Komshian, and Liu, S. (1999). Age constraints on second language learning. *Journal of Memory and Language, 41,* 78–104.

Gerken, L. A. (1994). Young children's representation of prosodic structure: Evidence from English-speakers' weak syllable omissions. *Journal of Memory and Language, 33,* 19–38.

Gibbon, F. (1999). Undifferentiated lingual gestures in children with articulation/phonological disorders. *Journal of Speech, Language, and Hearing Research, 42,* 382–397.

Goffman, L. (1999). Prosodic influences on speech production in children with specific language impairment and speech deficits. *Journal of Speech, Language, and Hearing Research, 42,* 1499–1517.

Goffman, L. (2004). Kinematic differentiation of prosodic categories in normal and disordered language development. *Journal of Speech, Language, and Hearing Research, 47,* 1088–1102.

Goffman, L., Ertmer, D., and Erdle, C. (2002). Changes in speech production in a child with a cochlear implant: Acoustic and kinematic evidence. *Journal of Speech, Language, and Hearing Research, 45,* 891–901.

Goffman, L., Heisler, L., and Chakraborty, R. (2006). Mapping of prosodic structure onto words and phrases in children's and adults' speech production. *Language and Cognitive Processes, 21,* 25–47.

Goffman, L., and Malin, C. (1999). Metrical effects on speech movements in children and adults. *Journal of Speech, Language, and Hearing Research, 42,* 1003–1015.

Goffman, L., Smith, A., Heisler, L., and Ho, M. (2008). Speech production units in children and adults: Evidence from coarticulation, *Journal of Speech, Language, and Hearing Research, 51,* 1423–1437.

Gomez, R. L., and Gerken, L. (1999). Artificial grammar learning by 1-year-olds leads to specific and abstract knowledge. *Cognition, 70,* 109–135.

Goodell, E. W., and Studdert-Kennedy, M. (1993). Acoustic evidence for the development of gestural coordination in the speech of 2-year-olds: A longitudinal study. *Journal of Speech and Hearing Research, 36,* 707–727.

Gopnik, M., and Crago, M. (1991). Familial aggregation of a developmental language disorder. *Cognition, 39,* 1–50.

Hall, P., Jordan, L., and Robin, D. (1993). *Developmental apraxia of speech: Theory and clinical practice.* Austin, TX: Pro-Ed.

Hammill, D. D., Brown, V. L., Larsen, S. C., and Weiderholt, J. L. (1994). *Test of Adolescent and Adult Language,* Third Edition. Austin, TX: Pro-Ed Inc.

Heisler, L. (2004). The influence of neighborhood density and phonotactic probability on representational and production factors in word learning. Unpublished doctoral dissertation, Purdue University.

Heisler, L., Goffman, L., and Younger, B. (in press). Lexical and articulatory interactions in children's language production. *Developmental Science.*

Hill, E. L. (2001). Non-specific nature of specific language impairment: A review of the literature with regard to concomitant motor impairments. *International Journal of Language and Communication Disorders, 36,* 149–171.

Hill, E. L., Bishop, D. V. M., and Nimmo-Smith, I. (1998). Representational gestures in developmental coordination disorders and specific language impairment: Error types and the reliability of ratings. *Human Movement Science, 17,* 655–678.

Hollich, G., Golinkoff, R., and Hirsh-Paskek, K. (2007). Young children associate novel words with complex objects rather than salient parts. *Developmental Psychology, 43,* 1051–1061.

Ivry, R., Spencer, R. M., Zelaznik, H. N., and Diedrichsen, J. (2002). The cerebellum and event timing. In S. M. Highstein and W. T. Thach (eds), *The Cerebellum: Recent developments in cerebellar research* (Vol. 978, pp. 302–317). New York: New York Academy of Sciences.

Jancke, L., Siegenthaler, S., Preis, S., and Steinmetz, H. (2006). Decreased white- matter density in a left-sided fronto-temporal network in children with developmental language disorder: Evidence for anatomical anomolies in a motor-language network. *Brain and Language, 102,* 91–98.

Johnson, E. K., and Jusczyk, P. W. (2001). Word segmentation by 8-month-olds: When speech cues count more than statistics. *Journal of Memory and Language, 44,* 1–20.

Jusczyk, P., Houston, D., and Newsome, M. (1999). The beginnings of word segmentation in English-learning infants. *Cognitive Psychology, 39*, 159–207.

Katz, W. F., Kripke, C., and Tallal, P. (1991). Anticipatory coarticulation in the speech of adults and young children: Acoustic, perceptual, and video data. *Journal of Speech and Hearing Research, 34*, 1222–1232.

Kent, R. D. (2004). Models of speech motor control: Implications from recent developments in neurophysiological and neurobehavioral science. In: B. Maasen, R. Kent, H. Peters, P. van Lieshout, and W. Hulstijn (eds), *Speech Motor Control In Normal and Disordered Speech* (pp. 3–28). Oxford: Oxford University Press.

Kleinow, J., Smith, A., and Ramig, L. (2001). Speech motor stability in IPD. *Journal of Speech, Language, and Hearing Research, 44*, 1041–1051.

Leonard, L. B. (1998). *Children with Specific Language Impairment.* Cambridge, MA: MIT Press.

Levelt, W. J. M., Roelofs, A., and Meyer, A. S. (1999). A theory of lexical access in speech production. *Behavioral and Brain Sciences, 22*, 1–75.

Levelt, W. J. M., and Wheeldon, L. (1994). Do speakers have access to a mental syllabary? *Cognition, 50*, 239–269.

MacNeilage, P. F., and Davis, B. L. (2000). On the origin of internal structure of word forms. *Science, 288*, 527–531.

McCune, L., and Vihman, M. M. (2001). Early phonetic and lexical development: A productivity approach. *Journal of Speech, Language, and Hearing Research, 44*, 670–684.

McGregor, K. K., and Leonard, L. B. (1994). Subject pronoun and article omissions in the speech of children with specific language impairment: A phonological interpretation. *Journal of Speech and Hearing Research, 37*, 171–181.

Newell, K. M., Deutsch, K. M., Sosnoff, J. J., and Gottfried, M. (2006). Variability in motor output as noise: A default and erroneous proposition? In K. Davids, K. Newell, and S. Bennett (eds), *Movement System Variability* (pp. 3–24). Champaign, IL: Human Kinetics.

Newman, R., Ratner, N. B., Jusczyk, A. M., Jusczyk, P. W., and Dow, K. A. (2006). Infants early ability to segment the conversational speech signal predicts later language development: A retrospective analysis. *Developmental Psychology, 42*, 643–655.

Nittrouer, S. (1993). The emergence of mature gestural patterns is not uniform: Evidence from an acoustic study. *Journal of Speech, Language, and Hearing Research, 36*, 959–972.

Nittrouer, S., Studdert-Kennedy, M., and McGowan, R. S. (1989). The emergence of phonetic segments: Evidence from the spectral structure of fricative-vowel syllables spoken by children and adults. *Journal of Speech and Hearing Research, 32*, 120–132.

Owen, A. J., and Goffman, L. (2007). Acoustic correlates of inflectional morphology in the speech of children with specific language impairment and their typically developing peers. *Clinical Linguistics and Phonetics, 21*, 501–522.

Plante, E., Gomez, R., and Gerken, L. (2002). Sensitivity to word order cues by normal and language/learning disabled adults. *Journal of Communication Disorders, 35*, 453–462.

Pulvermuller, F. (1999). Words in the brain's language. *Behavioral and Brain Sciences, 22*, 253–336.

Rapp, B., and Goldrick, M. (2006). Speaking words: Contributions of neuropsychological research. *Cognitive Neuropsychology*, 23, 39–73.

Recasens, D. (2002). An EMA study of VCV coarticulatory direction. *Journal of the Acoustical Society of America, 111*, 2828–2841.

Rice, M., Wexler, K., and Hershberger, S. (1998). Tense over time: The longitudinal course of tense acquisition in children with specific language impairment. *Journal of Speech, Language, and Hearing Research, 41*, 1412–1431.

Saffran, J. R., Aslin, R. N., and Newport, E. L. (1996). Statistical learning by 8-month-old infants. *Science, 274*, 1926–1928.

Schwartz, M., and Regan, V. (1996). Sequencing, timing, and rate relationships between language and motor skill in children with receptive language delay. *Developmental Neuropsychology, 12*, 255–270.

Scobbie, J. M., Gibbon, F., Hardcastle, W. J., and Fletcher, P. (2000). Covert contrasts as a stage in the acquisition of phonetics and phonology. In *Papers in Laboratory Phonology, 5*, 194–207. Cambridge, MA: Cambridge University Press.

Seidl, A. (2007). Infants' use and weighting of prosodic cues in clause segmentation. *Journal of Memory and Language, 57*, 24–48.

Sereno, J. A., Baum, S. R., Marean, G. C., and Lieberman, P. (1987). Acoustic analyses and perceptual data on anticipatory labial coarticulation in adults and children. *Journal of the Acoustical Society of America, 81*, 512–519.

Shriberg, L. D., Aram, D. M., and Kwiatkowski, J. (1997). Developmental apraxia of speech I: Descriptive and theoretical perspectives. *Journal of Speech, Language, and Hearing Research, 40*, 273–285.

Smith, A., and Goffman, L. (1998). Stability and patterning of movement sequences in children and adults. *Journal of Speech, Language, and Hearing Research, 41*, 18–30.

Smith, A., and Goffman, L. (2004). Interaction of motor and language factors in the development of speech production. In B. Maasen, R. Kent, H. Peters, P. van Lieshout, and W. Hulstijn (eds), *Speech Motor Control in Normal and Disordered Speech* (pp. 225–252). Oxford: Oxford University Press.

Smith, A., Goffman, L., Zelaznik, H., Ying, S., and McGillem, C. (1995). Spatiotemporal stability and patterning of speech movement sequences. *Experimental Brain Research, 104*, 493–501.

Smith, A., Johnson, M., McGillem, C., and Goffman, L. (2000). On the assessment of stability and patterning of speech movements. *Journal of Speech, Language, and Hearing Research, 43*, 277–286.

Smith, A., and Zelaznik, H. (2004). The development of functional synergies for speech motor coordination in childhood and adolescence. *Developmental Psychobiology, 45*, 22–33.

Spencer, R. M. C., Zelaznik, H. N., Diedrichsen, J., and Ivry, R. B. (2003). Disrupted timing of discontinuous but not continuous movements by cerebellar lesions. *Science, 300*, 1437–1439.

Stathopoulos, E. (1995). Variability revisited: An acoustic, respiratory, and aerodynamic comparison of children and adults during speech. *Journal of Phonetics, 23*, 67–80.

Tallal, P., Miller, S., Bedi, G., Byma, G., Wang, X., Nagarajam, S., Schreiner, C., Jenkins, W., and Merzenich, M. (1996). Language comprehension in language-learning impaired children improved with acoustically modified speech. *Science, 271*, 81–84.

Thelen, E., Corbetta, D., Kamm, K., Spencer, J., Schneider, K., and Zernicke, R. (1993). The transition to reaching: Mapping intention and intrinsic dynamics. *Child Development, 64*, 1058–1098.

Thelen, E., and Smith, L. (1994). *A Dynamical Systems Approach to the Development of Cognition and Action*. Cambridge, MA: The MIT Press.

Thiessen, E. D., and Saffran, J. R. (2003). When cues collide: Use of stress and statistical cues to word boundaries by 7- to 9-month-old infants. *Developmental Psychology, 39*, 143–158.

Ullman, M. T., and Pierpont, E. I. (2005). Specific language impairment is not specific to language: The procedural deficit hypothesis. *Cortex, 41*, 399–433.

Van der Lely, H. (1998). SLI in children: Movement, economy, and deficits in the computational-syntactic system. *Language Acquisition, 7*, 161–192.

Van Lieshout, P. H. H. M., Bose, A., Square, P. A., and Steele, C. M. (2007). Speech motor control in fluent and disfluent speech production in an individual with apraxia of speech and Broca's aphasia. *Clinical Linguistics and Phonetics, 21*, 159–188.

Vargha-Khadem, K., Watkins, K., Alcock, K., Fletcher, P., and Passingham, R. (1995). Praxic and nonverbal cognitive deficits in a large family with a genetically transmitted speech and language disorder. *Proceedings of the National Academy of Sciences, 92*, 930–933.

Walsh, B., and Smith, A. (2002). Articulatory movements in adolescents: Evidence for protracted development of speech motor control processes. *Journal of Speech, Language, and Hearing Research, 45*, 1119–1133.

Walsh, B., Smith, A., and Weber-Fox, C. (2006). Short-term plasticity in children's speech motor systems. *Developmental Psychobiology, 48*, 660–674.

Weber-Fox, C. and Neville, H. (1996). Maturational constraints on functional specializations for language processing: ERP and behavioral evidence in bilingual speakers. *Journal of Cognitive Neuroscience, 8*, 231–256.

Werker, J. F., Fennell, C. T., Corcoran, K. M., and Stager, C. L. (2002). Infant's ability to learn phonetically similar words: Effects of age and vocabulary size. *Infancy, 3*, 1–30.

Wing, A. M., and Kristofferson, A. B. (1973). Response delays and the timing of discrete motor responses. *Perception and Psychophysics, 14*, 5–12.

Wohlert, A. B. (1996). Perioral muscle activity in young and older adults in speech and nonspeech tasks. *Journal of Speech, Language, and Hearing Research, 39*, 761–770.

Zelaznik, H. N., and Goffman, L. (in press). Motor abilities and timing behavior in children with specific language impairment. *Journal of Speech, Language, and Hearing Research.*

Zelaznik, H. N., Spencer, R. M. C., and Ivry, R. B. (2002). Dissociation of explicit and implicit timing in repetitive tapping and drawing movements. *Journal of Experimental Psychology: Human Perception and Performance, 28*, 575–588.

Chapter 9

Lip rounding anticipatory control: crosslinguistically lawful and ontogenetically attuned

Aude Noiray, Marie-Agnès Cathiard,
Lucie Ménard, and Christian Abry

Abstract

The first part of this study reports on a test of the classical rounding anticipatory coarticulation models with adults from two different language backgrounds (American English and Canadian French). Anticipatory movement patterns were described by means of collecting protrusion and constriction data with Optotrak system (flesh-point protrusion) and Lip-Shape-Tracking-System (area constriction). A bite-block condition was added to control the possible neighboring consonantal influence (via the jaw, particularly for coronals) on the time course of rounding anticipation. This study allowed a test of the *Movement Expansion Model* (*MEM*), initially elaborated for French to Canadian French and American English. All speakers displayed a lawful *MEM* anticipatory behavior including English subjects who have been reported to display a different rounding behavior from French or Swedish. We attribute the failure of the preceding studies to a too small protrusion magnitude.

The second part of this study reports on a test of the *MEM* model to account for the evolution of vocalic rounding anticipation in 7 French-speaking children (aged from 3.5 to 8 years). Results showed that the rounding movement timing pattern for the production of the French vowel [y] can be mastered as early as 3.5 years of age, and at least by 5.5 years.

Key-words: Rounding anticipation, coarticulation, speech motor control, emergence of vocalic control, child speech development

9.1 Part 1: a cross-linguistic test of the MEM

9.1.1 Introduction

Anticipatory motor control is a ubiquitous benefit for behavioural efficiency (for a follow-up of the general conceptions about anticipatory behaviour, see Butz et al., 2003; Swarup and Gasser 2007). In speech, coarticulatory aspect of the anticipatory motor control is the binding element for syllable components and for between syllables and words. In the literature on labial anticipatory coarticulation three models based on protrusion are traditionally taken as reference to account for the temporal expansion of the labial rounding movement for vowels in adults. The *Look-ahead Model* developed by Henke (1966) for English, and later tested for French by Benguerel and Cowan (1974), predicts that the rounding gesture would start at the acoustic offset of the unrounded vowel [i], with a movement expansion proportional to the consonant interval between the two vowels in utterances like [iCnu] (see below). A diverging interpretation was proposed by Bell-Berti and Harris (1982), who claimed that (for a defined speech style) the movement onset is time-locked to the acoustic onset of the rounded vowel, regardless of the number of intervocalic consonants (*Time-locked Model*).

Finally, according to a *Hybrid* model (Perkell and Chiang 1986), the rounding gesture would start at the acoustic offset of the unrounded vowel, with an initial slow phase characterized by a rather look-ahead expansion, followed by a more rapid phase with a time-locked acceleration peak.

These three models were tested in a major study carried out by Perkell and Matthies (1992) on four American subjects in [iCnu] sequences, in which Cn corresponded to a varying number of intervocalic consonants. The variability evidenced by Perkell and Matthies led them to conclude that 'data [...] allow us to reject strong versions of all three models' (p. 280). An alternative model, the Movement Expansion Model (MEM) was proposed for French by Abry and Lallouache (1995; for a general presentation of the MEM among the other models, see Farnetani 1999). They tested the extent of anticipatory movement in [iCny] sequences in four French adults. Their results showed that the protrusion movement time (MT) was associated with: (1) a rather incompressible duration (*execution constant*) of about 140 ms for the sequence [iy], approximately the same for [iCy]; (2) a linear expansion of MT from [iCy] to [iCCCCCy]; (3) significant correlation coefficients for all speakers; and (4) speaker-specific slopes for the calculated regression lines. Since the slopes of the French speakers ranged from 0.42 to 0.93, a typical look-ahead pattern could not be generalized to all speakers. However, it was considered as a possible speaker-specific behaviour described in the framework of MEM principles, with a speaker-specific parameterization. Contrary to the intra-subject variability found by Perkell and Matthies (1992), the variability found for the four French speakers was assessed as being lawful (technically by means of significant correlation coefficients together with regression functions). Since the amplitude of upper lip protrusion for one subject was too small to be reliably extracted, MEM model was extended to constriction (between-lip area) to account for rounding patterning in all speakers, including those achieving little protrusion (Abry et al., 1996). The constriction anticipatory behaviour of the four French subjects was found also to be lawful within MEM principles.

Divergence in modelling anticipatory behaviour was recently formulated by Byrd and Saltzman (2003, note 4, p.157) as a language-specific issue. In their control model, the discrepancy between French and American data is solved by the use of 'side constraint' (Rubin et al., 1996). Therefore, shall anticipatory labial coarticulation be considered as a language-specific control? Or is protrusion an unreliable indicator of rounding in languages using small protrusion amplitude such as English? On the other hand, to acoustically achieve rounding, could the constriction gesture be more robust to evidence the anticipatory control pattern?

Our motivation for the present study was both to test the cross-language validity of the MEM and its developmental relevance. In the first part of this study, we tested MEM comparatively between Quebec French and American English speakers. In order to describe the subjects' anticipatory movement patterns, protrusion as well as constriction temporal functions were obtained simultaneously via two motion captures: Optotrak for flesh-point protrusion, together with the ICP-Lip-Shape-Tracking-System (with so-called 'Tahar Lallouache's blue' painted on the lips). This procedure delivers area constriction data as an addition. In the second part of the study, we described the developmental trajectory of French-speaking children aged between three and eight years.

9.1.2 Method

9.1.2.1 Subjects and task

The productions of four French-speaking adults from Quebec (two males: ANT, JER; and two females: ANN, LUC; mean age: 28 years) and four American English-speaking adults (two males: DAN, KAL; and two females: LAU, SAR; mean age: 22 years) were audiovisually recorded with a video camera.

The talkers' principal task consisted of producing a series of [iCnu] sequences (presented) randomly. We manipulated the number of intervocalic consonants between the two vowels in order to observe the evolution of children rounding movement time-span. The rounded vocalic target [u] was selected for comparison purposes since it is phonemic in both languages. The resulting sequences ([iu], [iku], [ikku], [iksku], [ikstku], [ikstsku]; and [ikstski] for control) were embedded into carrier sentences like 'Two keaks cookeek'. These nonsense sentences had the same syntactic structure (Det-Noun-Verb). Each target sequence was repeated 10 to 12 times at least. The presence of intervocalic consonants [k, t, s], in spite of being phonologically neutral with respect to rounding, could induce labial motion due to their coupling with the mandibula especially for coronals (see Perkell and Matthies 1992). Therefore, the whole corpus was duplicated with a 4-mm bite-block clenched between the left molars, in order to address the possibility of consonantal jaw interferences on the rounding pattern.

Prior to the experiment, participants were trained to produce the sequences as naturally as possible, with a constant rate and intonation pattern. They were also asked not to produce any silent pause between the noun and the verb in order to minimize word boundary effects on the timing of the rounding movement. At the end of the experiment, subjects received a compensation for their participation.

9.1.2.2 Audiovisual and kinematic data collection

Speakers were audiovisually recorded at Motor Control Lab (McGill University, Montreal) using a Panasonic AG-DVC30 video. Images were digitized at a 30 Hz rate. Since one video image corresponded to two interleaved frames, we were able to obtain a 60 Hz rate through line interpolation; synchronized with the acoustic signal recorded via a SHURE SM-86 microphone and digitized at 48 KHz. Acquisition of labial shapes was performed with the ICP-Lip-Shape-Tracking-System. Speakers' lips were made up with a waterproof blue lipstick for the accurate acquisition of labial contours via a numerical Chromakey processing. Front lip shape was automatically detected for each sequence with Tacle software developed at ICP.

Upper lip protrusion was simultaneously recorded via an Optotrak system at the Motor Control Lab. We captured the three-dimensional displacement of small infrared light-emitting diodes (IREDS). For the experiment, three diodes were attached with doubled-sided tape to the midline of the upper and lower lip, close to the vermilion border and to the midline of the chin. No attention was given in order not to obstruct the inner labial contours with the infrared diodes threads. In addition, a plexiglass frame with four IREDS diodes was designed for reference measures and attached to the speaker's goggles. The orientation of the occlusal plane was measured by asking the subject to bite on a plexiglass frame to which three IREDS were attached. IREDS' signals were sampled at 175 Hz. A cross-correlation function (Matlab 7) was used to resynchronize the 48 KHz acoustic signal from the camera with the low 10 KHz signal synchronized with the Optotrak. Matlab algorithms were used to perform the rotation of the data with respect to the speaker's occlusal plane and to correct the signals for head movement.

Given the high sensitivity of the Optotrak system, in our analysis we only included protrusion signals with at least 2-mm minimum amplitude. We took this precaution to avoid monitoring any 'tremor' signals instead of rounding gestures reflecting vocalic rounding anticipation control.

9.1.2.3 Articulatory analysis

For the description of rounding anticipatory behaviour, we identified the same acoustic and kinematic events or phases as previously with French adults (Abry et al., 1996).

On the time course of lip area (Fig. 9.1), we detected maximum and minimum area values (events 1 and 4) that are both characterized by a zero value for velocity. The obstruence interval (OI) has been labelled on the acoustic signal, corresponding to the duration between the acoustic offset of the vowel [i] (characterized by the disappearance of the upper formant structure) and onset of [u] (by formants appearing again). Other robust landmarks were selected using the classical 10% and 90% levels describing Time Falling (TF) and Time Rising in the literature on hysteresis curves. We identified the time corresponding to a 10% decrease of area amplitude (event 2), time corresponding to 90% of this range (event 3), and finally time corresponding to a 10% increase of lip area following minimal area of the vowel [u] (event 5). The interval between event

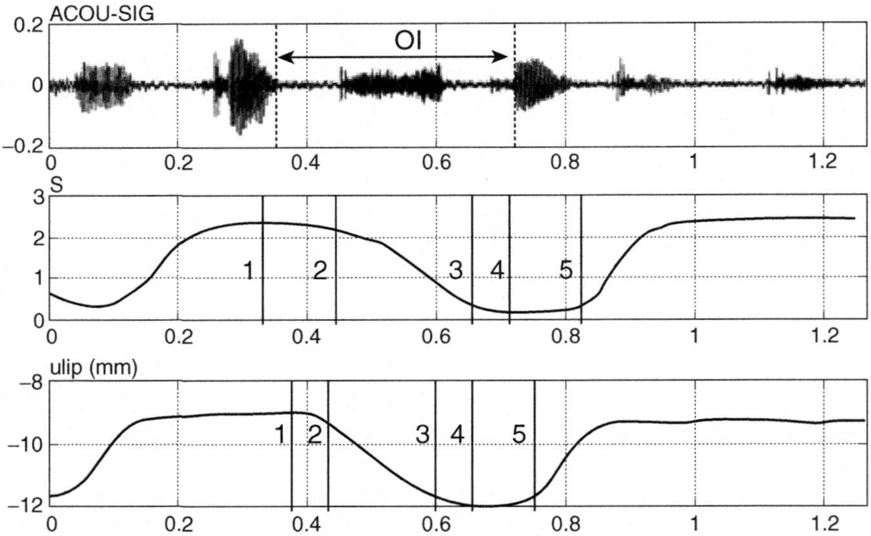

Fig. 9.1 Synchronized on a time scale in seconds: sound wave (upper signal), lip area (middle signal, in cm^2) and upper lip protrusion (bottom signal, in mm referenced to the plexiglass frame; inverted for visual correspondence with area). This sequence [iksku] in the carrier phrase 'Two keaks cookeek' was uttered by a Quebec French speaker (LUC) in a bite-block condition. The obstruence interval (OI) is determined on the spectrogram by the acoustic offset of [i] and the acoustic onset of [u] formants. Identification numbers of events on lip area or constriction: (1) maximal area for [i]; (2) 10% of area difference between [i] and [u]; (3) 90% of area range between [i] and [u]; (4) minimal area for [u]; (5) 10% of lip area difference between [i] and [u] following minimal area of [u]. Interval 2–3 corresponds to Time Falling (TF) and interval 3–5 to the duration of the Hold phase (H). Identification numbers of events on the upper lip protrusion: (1) minimal protrusion for [i]; (2) 10% of protrusion difference between [i] and [u]; (3) 90% of protrusion range between [i] and [u]; (4) maximal protrusion for [u]; (5) 10% of protrusion difference between [i] and [u] following maximal protrusion of vowel [u]. Interval 2–3 also corresponds conventionally to the duration of protrusion TF and interval 3–5 to protrusion H.

2 and 3 was defined as a TF phase and the interval between event 3 and 5 as a Hold (H), corresponding to a phase in which acoustic efficiency of constriction area is ascertained.

On the protrusion time course (Fig. 9.1, bottom signal; inverted for comparison with lip area), we also detected minimum and maximum protrusion, coinciding with a zero velocity (events 1 and 4). We selected the date corresponding to a 10% range between [i] and [u] (event 2), the date corresponding to 90% of this range (event 3), and finally the date corresponding to a 10% range following maximal protrusion of the vowel [u] (event 5). We used the same labels for protrusion phases (TF and H) as for between lip area.

9.1.3 **Results**

9.1.3.1 Upper lip protrusion analysis

Regarding the analysis of rounding anticipation timing, we selected the two main phases, TF and H that best account for the time course of the rounding movement without any part-whole artefact when correlated with OI, (Benoît 1986). The total duration of these two phases (TF+H) was plotted against OI (Fig. 9.2 and Table 9.1). A detailed report on the variability of the two subphases TF and H in relation to OI is provided by Noiray (2007). Note that no overall lawful behaviour was found with TF or H alone compared to TF+H. Each speaker uttered [iu] without any interruption between the two vowels, i.e., with a zero OI value. Linear regression analysis (correlation coefficients and slopes) was performed on data from [iCu] to [iCCCCCu], excluding [iu] sequences.

From the productions of the four Quebec French participants, we obtained significant correlation coefficients ($p < 0.00001$) and speaker-specific slopes. These slopes ranged from 0.24 to 0.65 for the no-bite-block condition and from 0.18 to 0.78 for the bite-block condition. Only one subject (LUC) had a protrusion profile close to a time-locked profile, with data grouped along his regression line. However, the slope corresponding to his anticipatory behaviour was sufficiently distinct from a zero time-locked slope (statistically corresponding to the null hypothesis). The slopes obtained for the four other subjects did not differ from one jaw condition to the other except for speaker JER with a 0.45 slope for the no-bite-block condition and a 0.78 in the

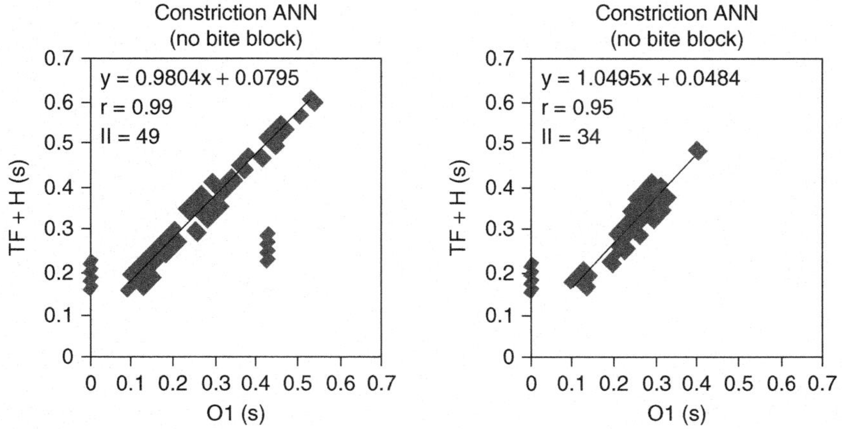

Fig. 9.2 Rounding anticipatory behaviour for a Quebec English speaker (ANN) in bite-block (right) and no-bite-block (left) conditions. Correlations (significant at $p < 0.0001$) between total duration of lip constriction movement (TF+H) and duration of obstruence interval (OI).

Table 9.1 Regression slopes (and correlation coefficients) obtained for American English and Quebec French speakers for upper lip protrusion and constriction data (in bite-block and no-bite-block conditions)

	Regression slopes and correlation coefficients (p<0.0001)			
	Upper lip protrusion		Constriction (lip area)	
American English subjects	Bite block condition	No bite block condition	Bite block condition	No bite block condition
DAN	0.04 (0.57)	0.51 (0.67)	0.75 (0.84)	0.87 (0.88)
KAL	Non protruding speakers		0.90 (0.82)	0.99 (0.94)
LAU			1.08 (0.78)	1.12 (0.72)
SAR			0.95 (0.97)	0.84 (0.93)
Canadian French subjects				
ANN	0.68 (0.85)	0.60 (0.92)	1.05 (0.95)	0.98 (0.99)
ANT	0.63 (0.93)	0.85 (0.93)	0.85 (0.93)	0.86 (0.94)
JER	0.78 (0.65)	0.45 (0.65)	0.94 (0.96)	0.92 (0.95)
LUC	0.18 (0.69)	0.24 (0.75)	0.86 (0.95)	0.88 (0.98)

bite-block condition ($t = 2.76$, $ddl = 67$, $p < 0.01$). This speaker generally displayed small amplitude of protrusion so that a large portion of his data was excluded from analysis in the bite-block condition.

For the English speakers, three out of four participants (KAL, LAU, SAR) displayed a too small protrusion to be reliably processed in the bite-block condition. Indeed, for each speaker we were only able to collect around 20 signals out of 60 possible, with at least 2-mm amplitude (Table 9.1). In the no-bite-block condition, we occasionally collected a greater number of relevant signals but protrusion did not generally exceed the 3-mm amplitude level. Perkell and Matthies had previously reported a similar phenomenon for American English for about half of their subjects (1992,

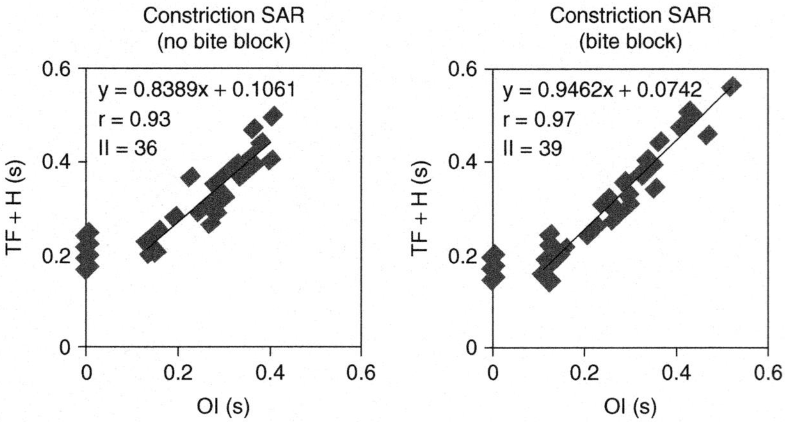

Fig. 9.3 Rounding anticipatory behaviour for an American English speaker (SAR) in bite-block (right) and no-bite-block (left) conditions. Correlations (significant at $p < 0.0001$) between total duration of lip constriction movement (TF+H) and duration of obstruence interval (OI).

p. 2914). Thus for these speakers we decided to rely mainly on constriction, which is an essential geometric parameter in relation to vowel acoustics. Furthermore, a previous study supported that constriction can undoubtedly account for rounding anticipation in a non-protruding French adult (e.g., Abry et al., 1996).

9.1.3.2 Constriction (lip area) analysis

The total duration of constriction movement (TF+H) was also plotted in relation to the OI (for an example, see Fig. 9.3). Linear regression analysis performed on all [iCu] to [iCCCCCu] sequences highlighted significant correlation coefficients ($p < 0.0001$) and speaker-specific slopes for the eight speakers (Table 9.1, Fig. 9.4). For the English participants, slopes ranged from 0.84 to 1.12 in the no-bite-block condition and from 0.75 to 1.08 in the bite-block condition. Significant correlation coefficients ($p < 0.00001$) were also obtained for the Canadian French-speaking participants with idiosyncratic anticipatory profiles giving slopes ranging from 0.86 to 0.98 for the no-bite-block condition and from 0.85 to 1.05 for the bite-block condition. Like for the upper lip protrusion results, constriction slopes were rather similar between the two conditions (no significant difference). Note that the two speakers (LAU and ANN) showed a look-ahead profile, with a slope approximating 1. Again, this type of behaviour could be described in the framework of the speaker-specific MEM model, being a possible case but not a general modelling. Finally, regarding the three 'non-protruding' English speakers, a main finding was that the parameter of constriction could lawfully account for their anticipatory behaviour. As a whole, these results support those previously obtained for French adults.

9.1.4 **Summary**

Over the past few decades, several studies investigated vocalic anticipatory coarticulation in adults. The literature shows that it is still a tricky challenge (i) to accurately track acoustically relevant labial kinematics, (ii) to select relevant events and landmarks for the appropriate modelling of anticipatory strategies. In the first part of our investigation, we extended a speaker-adaptable model initially elaborated to account for vocalic anticipation in French to English and Canadian French. Results showed that each speaker displayed idiosyncratic rounding behaviour, with a personal expansion rate and slope around which data were lawfully grouped.

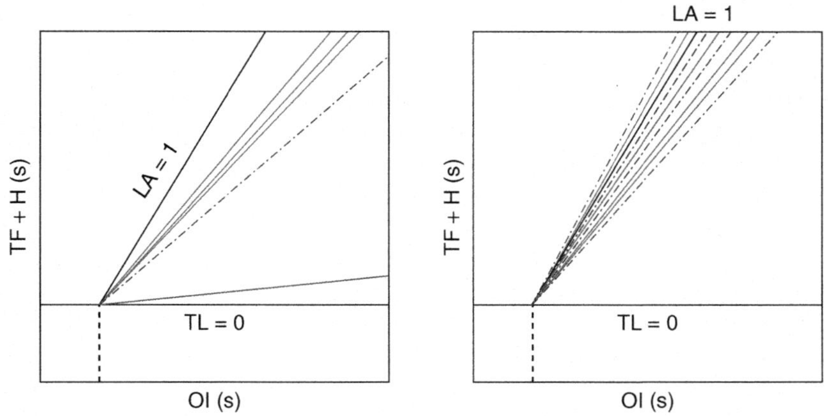

Fig. 9.4 An overview of American English speakers' slopes (broken lines) and Quebec French (solid lines) for protrusion (left) and constriction (right) in the bite-block condition.

Another interesting finding was that upper lip protrusion could not be generalized to the description of rounding control in every speaker of both language backgrounds. The data of three non-protruding English speakers corroborated this weak reliability. It seems reasonable to think that this phenomenon (previously reported by Perkell and Matthies 1992), is related to the fact that protrusion is not as crucial in English as it is in French or other languages such as Swedish, German, Danish, or Norwegian having front and back rounded vowels. However, our results indicate that, even in languages for which rounding is phonemically highly distinctive, some speakers (as evidenced in Abry et al., 1996, for a French subject or in the present study with a Canadian French speaker) may display very small protrusion. On the contrary, it seems that the parameter of labial constriction offers promising perspectives for cross-language explorations of anticipatory rounding control, starting with Continental French, Canadian French, and American English.

9.2 **Part 2: a developmental attunement test of the MEM**

9.2.1 **Introduction**

Our motivation to extend our investigation to the developmental field comes from the fact that little interest has been shown for vowel acquisition with respect to consonants', although vowels are reputedly difficult to master motorically (MacNeilage and Davis 1990). The aim of this second part is specifically to explore the acquisition – or the attunement to the ambient language – of the temporal pattern for this universal dimension of vowel systems, i.e., rounding, and specifically, in this study with French-speaking children, the specific [i] vs. [y] contrast. The concept of *attunement* has been used in different acceptations in various domains including child development. Here, we will point to its recent use by Gallese (2004, 2006: target paper with peer comments), using the learning and imitation paradigms, including vocal imitation.

We studied the articulatory behaviour for vocalic anticipation in French children aged between three and eight years. Lip motion data were collected with a Lip-Shape-Tracking-System developed at ICP to evaluate whether there is a critical age for the acquisition of this motor control. The main questions addressed were: (i) can the anticipatory behaviour be studied in children with the same general paradigm used for French adults, i.e., the MEM; (ii) can we expect their behaviour to resemble that of the adults with similar anticipatory strategies; and finally, (iii) what is the time path of this process?

9.2.1.1 From emulation to imitation of vowel specific coordination

Few articulatory studies have been dedicated to the acquisition of speech production, partly because of the experimental constraints of measuring the articulatory behaviour of young children. Therefore, our knowledge of speech acquisition mainly rests on the acoustic analysis of early productions (e.g., temporal and spectral characteristics of CV productions). These studies shed light on our understanding of the development of speech motor control, from canonical babbling up to adult performance (*cf.* a large-scale study relying only on auditory transcriptions, see James et al., 2001).

Regarding the emergence of motor control, Kent (1976, p. 421; also Kent 2004, for a recent reiteration of this point) argued that 'the accuracy of motor control improves with age until adult-like performance is achieved at about 11 or 12 years, somewhat after the age at which speech sound acquisition usually is judged to be completed'. His review included a substantial section concerning the acquisition of vowel control. Diverging reports are found on the age of correct vowel production. This discrepancy in results is probably due to differences in the type of data collected, transcriptional methods, or acoustical analysis. A review of existing data on vowel production in intelligible words was provided by Stoel-Gammon and Herrington (1990).

They concluded that the cardinal vowels [i a u] are usually acquired by two years of age, and all vowels by three years.

Among the few cross-sectional studies reporting an early acquisition of the point vowels, the most intriguing finding remains that of Kuhl and Meltzoff (1995, p. 149) study on vocal imitation. They reported that the acoustic spacing (contrast) of [i a u] would emerge as early as five months. These results are undoubtedly interesting from an imitation perspective. However, it seems that their conclusions cannot be accepted as complete production of vowels, at the same level as current results on early vowel perception, (see Kuhl and Meltzoff 1995, p. 149) including discrimination, categorization, and prototypization. In our view, the attunement to the ambient language can be seen by the difference between *imitation* and *emulation*. This distinction has been first proposed by Wolfgang Köhler and reformulated by Bard and Russell (1999), and later by Horner and Whiten (2005). They observed two very different behaviours related to ape and child learning: (i) the 'copy' of the goal and the path, i.e., imitation; (ii) versus the copy of final goal solely, that is emulation. In the case of vowel production, the contrast of different [i a u] acoustic goals does not necessarily imply the acquisition of their specific coordination. Various jaw perturbation experiments testing acoustic equivalence in vowel production in adults and children showed that in spite of compensatory behaviours, the jaw contributes to the raising of the tongue for [i] and [u], and its lowering for [a] (Gibson and MacPhearson 1980; Oller and MacNeilage 1983). The jaw–tongue(lip) coordination is fundamental for vowel production. In this view, a main finding from longstanding observations by Koopmans-van Beinum and Van der Stelt (1986, p. 42) was that between 2 months and 4.5 months, 'one articulatory movement per breath unit combined with continuous or interrupted phonation' characterizes most infants' productions. Productions with two or more articulations did not occur before 6 months. Kent (1992, p. 169) supports this view by observing 'Another stage, beginning at about three to four months and extending up to about six months, is one marked accomplishment in supraglottal or articulatory actions. In this stage, phonation often is accompanied by supraglottal constrictions and releases [...] and an impression [our emphasis] of consonant-vowel sequence'. Recent experiments performed in ICP by Serkhane (2005) tested bayesian learning with an articulatory robot model on Kuhl and Meltzoff's data (1995). Results showed that at five months children could only master vowel-like constrictions without any linguo(labio)-mandibular coordination. It is only when babbling occurs at around seven months of age (also evidenced by similar bayesian learning in Davis and MacNeilage's data, 1989) that the jaw is recruited by the baby to distinguish vowels. Therefore, as Kent's suggestion above can be interpreted, it is not simply a matter of late control of accuracy, but an issue of acquiring specific vowel coordination.

9.2.1.2 **Emergence of production coordination of lip closure and rounding**

The development of the coordination controls for the cardinal vowels — from [a], to [i] and [u] – corresponds to the acquisition of two crucial motor controls: the control of lip closure and lip rounding.

MacNeilage's (1998) Frame-then-Content Theory suggests that the jaw would be the first supralaryngeal articulator that is rhythmically controlled, the lips and the tongue remaining passive, simply carried by the jaw during the babbling period. This hypothesis has been supported, first anecdotally by the tracking of two LEDS on the lips of an eight-month-old baby (Munhall and Jones 1998); then, quantitatively by Green and colleagues (2000, 2002, 2003) for one-, two-, and six-year-old children. The consequence of this control is that as long as the tongue is simply carried by the jaw, the vocalic cycle looks a [bəabəa]-like production. In his observations of X-ray films and articulatory modelling, Vilain (2000) showed that in order to achieve an adult-like

[baba] pattern, the tongue must resist to the elevation of the jaw when it carries up the lower lip, 'by-producing' the bilabial closure. This means that instead of achieving a neutral [ə]-like vocal-tract, the tongue needs to be pulled down by the hyoglossus to keep an open [a]-like configuration during the bilabial closure. In their longitudinal acoustic analysis (Locus Equations) of an infant, Sussman et al. (1999) observed that this coproduction control ([a] within [b]) emerges at the end of the first year (13 months, cf. their Fig. 9.2 for [ba]). This finding is important for tongue lowering, i.e., vocal-tract opening 'vocant' control. What about lip closing, 'closant' control? The emergence of an independent lip control (not as a simple by-product of the jaw) for bilabial closure was evidenced in Green et al. (2002)'s measurements on basic [baba] and [papa] productions. They revealed that – compared to the early stability of jaw motion – toddlers from one to two years of age displayed highly variable movements of the upper lip, as compared to adults and even to six-year-old children. It means that the fine control of closure, corresponding to the appropriate coordination of both the jaw and the lips, as achieved by adults in a language-specific temporal window, is not mastered at two years of age. Another interesting finding is that even though upper lip movements of the six-year-old group approximate more the adults' than younger children, they do not match the adults' yet. Unfortunately, no data are presented for the two- to six-year-old period, although it is a crucial period in which, important changes on articulatory control occur.

The acquisition of both tongue and lip control needed for the production of a rounded vowel such as [u], addresses a new challenge. According to MacNeilage and Davis (1990, p. 470) this would require, just for the tongue 'a new movement [...] achieved by the cooperation of two muscles inserting on the styloid process of the cranium, the styloglossus and stylohyoid muscles', plus 'another new movement, that of lip rounding, is also necessary for high back vowels.' Hence 'It is also of interest to note that back vowels, which, according to our analysis, make more demand on new movements, are acquired later than high front vowels.'

Taken as a whole, these findings offer a new fractionation of the different types of control acquired in the course of speech development. Kent (1976, p. 440) states that 'the age of two or three years is assumed as the beginning of a child's extensive speech usage on a daily basis' and concluded that 'the variability of speech motor control progressively diminishes until the age of eight–12 years, when adult like stability is achieved'. Tingley and Allen (1975, in Kent, 1976, p. 439) also suggested that 'motor patterns for speech are largely preplanned rather than feedback controlled even at the age of five years'. Thus exploring formant frequencies, F0 patterns and temporal patterns, the authors conclude 'the declining variabilities for the three types of measurements appear to reflect an increasing precision of motor control over a five-to-eight years' (Tingley and Allen 1975, in Kent, 1976, p. 440). Thus until the age of eight years, vocalic productions could be considered as variable individual templates that are more or less well achieved, depending on the child, the age, and the phonetic context. In addition, the temporal coordination required for segment production would not be finely tuned: in our scope without any stable anticipatory patterning. The final mastering of vowels and the attunement of vocalic timing to the language-specific adults' models should require much more refinement in motor control than those exerted during the babbling period.

The present study does not aim to describe vocalic target acquisition *per se*, but rather the emergence of the control of a language-specific temporal pattern related to vowel production. More specifically, we explored the acquisition of a lawful anticipatory behaviour for vocalic contrast in French, with the expectation that this control would be acquired within a smaller temporal window than the above-mentioned three-to-eight or twelve-year-old period.

In acquisition studies, the different models of rounding anticipation (see Part 1) were not extensively tested mostly because of the difficulty to collect articulatory data with young children. Hence, the only major study was run several years ago by Abelin et al. (1980) on anticipatory lip rounding behaviour for six Swedish children, aged from seven to ten years and a referent adult (Lubker 1981). The EMG activity of the orbicularis oris superior was recorded and processed for detection of rounding onset. While one child displayed the typical pattern corresponding to the Look Ahead behaviour evidenced by Lubker for the referent adult (with a slope value of around 1), the five remaining children showed scattered results. In fact, and contrary to the authors' claim, a plot of these five children's data would demonstrate that the null hypothesis corresponding to a Time-locked behaviour could be supported.

Therefore, in the second part of our investigation, the MEM model was extended from adults to children to account for the control of vocalic rounding gesture in early productions.

9.2.2 Method

9.2.2.1 Subjects and task

Seven children were recruited for the production task: five boys (NP: 3.5 yrs, KV: 4.5, TB: 4.5, JB: 7, DV: 8) and two girls (CA: 4, EC: 4 yrs). The four youngest children (NP, KV, TB, CA) were recorded twice with a year interval. Two female French-speaking adults were recorded as referent speakers. The children recruited were not known to have any schooling problems, or articulatory disabilities. No perceptible French dialectal accents were noticed.

The task consisted in the random repetition of eight items containing the two contrasted vocalic targets [i] and [y]. These items, prompted by the experimenter, were [i(Cn)y] puppet names, in which Cn corresponded to a series of intervocalic consonants varying from 0 to 3. These names ([iy], [isy], [iky], [iksy], [ikRy], [itkRy], [iskRy], [iksty]) were embedded into carrier sentences such as « Le toutou *Iku* est rouge » (Doggie Iku is red).

Surprisingly, it was not necessary to find subtle tricks to record the young subjects as it is often stated in the developmental literature evaluating the child's oromotor skills. However, because of obvious methodological constraints underlying kinetic studies, we paid delicate attention to the experimental design. Children were told they were participating in a work on character voices (comics), so that they would feel confident and interested in the experiment. In a preliminary familiarization phase with the experimenters, children were invited to play with the eight puppets corresponding to the different names. This initial step allowed them to easily assimilate puppet names and understand the task. The anechoic chamber was decorated with sheen material, fairy lights, and luminous stars to create a friendly atmosphere. A snack was organized at the end of the recording session and each child received a present.

9.2.2.2 Audio-visual recording

The seven children have been audio-visually recorded in an anechoic chamber in ICP with the Lip-Shape-Tracking-System developed by Lallouache (1991). Children voice was recorded with an AKV C 1000S microphone. Images were recorded on a Betacam via two cameras (face and profile). A baby seat and a piece of foam rubber slightly dug for the children head were used to limit face or body movements. Since two daylight neons were used to get a correct detection of lip variations, children wore black glasses for protection. Two calibration blue discs were stuck on the glasses and a small blue-painted ruler was fixed on one side of the glasses so that profile references could be obtained. Lips were made up with the same waterproof saturated blue lipstick. This blue was chosen in order to facilitate the acquisition of labial contours with the automatic detection system via numerical Chromakey processing. Since one video image (at 25 Hz rate) corresponded to two interleaved frames, it was possible to obtain a 50 Hz rate through line interpolation, synchronized with the digitized acoustic signal (44.1 kHz, encoded in 32 bits, stored in 24 bits). Lateral (protrusion) and front lip shape and position parameters were automatically detected for each sequence with a software developed in our lab (*Tacle*, Audouy 2000).

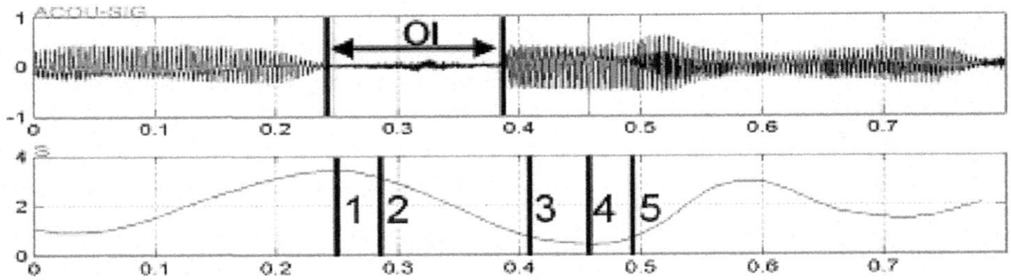

Fig. 9.5 Acoustic signal (above, in seconds) and lip area time course (below, in cm^2) for a sequence [isy] in a carrier phrase 'Le veau *Issu* est blanc' (the calf *Issu* is white) uttered by a 4.5-year-old French child. Identification numbers of events: (1) maximal area for vowel [i]; (2) 10% of area difference between [i] and [y]; (3) 90% of area range between [i] and [y]; (4) minimal area for [y]; (5) 10% of lip area difference between [i] and [y] following minimal area of vowel [y]. Interval 2–3 corresponds to Time Falling (TF) and interval 3–5 to the duration of *Hold* phase (H). The obstruence interval (OI) is determined on the spectrogram by the acoustic offset of [i] and the acoustic onset of [y].

9.2.2.3 Articulatory analysis

In order to study the anticipation timing of rounding, we focused on lip area, i.e., constriction (see Noiray et al., 2004 for protrusion measurements in children). Events on velocity and acceleration derivatives have been used in a preliminary report on two of the children and the two adults investigated (Ménard et al., 2004). In accordance with the analysis performed by Abry and Lallouache (1995), they do not influence the conclusions in favour of the MEM model. In addition to these classic kinetic events, similar landmarks as the ones selected in adults were selected on the constriction temporal function, using the classical 10% and 90% levels describing Time Falling and Time Rising (Fig 9.5).

9.2.3 **Results**

The total duration of constriction movement (TF+H) was plotted against the OI. Five children as well as the two adults females uttered [iy] with a zero OI value, i.e., with no voicing interruption between the two vowels. For these seven subjects, the mean value was calculated, showing that – as compared to adults – the execution constant varied within a larger range: 180–420 ms for children. A separate linear regression analysis was performed for each speaker: on all [iCy], [iCCy], [iCCCy] sequences, [iy] excluded, for these seven speakers; and on all sequences including [iy] for the two other children who realized [i#y], with a glottal stop interval instead of a continuous [iy] voicing.

One of the child participants, a 4.5-year-old boy (KV) exhibited an irregular timing behaviour in the first recording session (Fig. 9.6), while some younger children (NP, 3.5; CA, 4; EC, 4; TB, 4.5 years) had already acquired their lawful regime. However, when comparing his rounding behaviour a year later, we found a significant correlation coefficient with a personal slope around which his data were grouped (Fig. 9.6), displaying a lawful variability like the other 'more precocious' children. Therefore, we observed a later acquisition of his anticipatory regime for this child, i.e., at 5.5 years of age.

For the other six children, significant correlation coefficients corresponded to regression slopes ranging from 0.63 to 1.58 (Figs 9.6 and 9.7). We also discovered stable rounding behaviour for the children recorded twice with a year interval. As a reminder, the data from the two adult control subjects (MA and CL) revealed slope values of 0.60 and 0.81, respectively. The hypothesis corresponding to a time-locked behaviour was supported for all subjects (as well as for KV in the

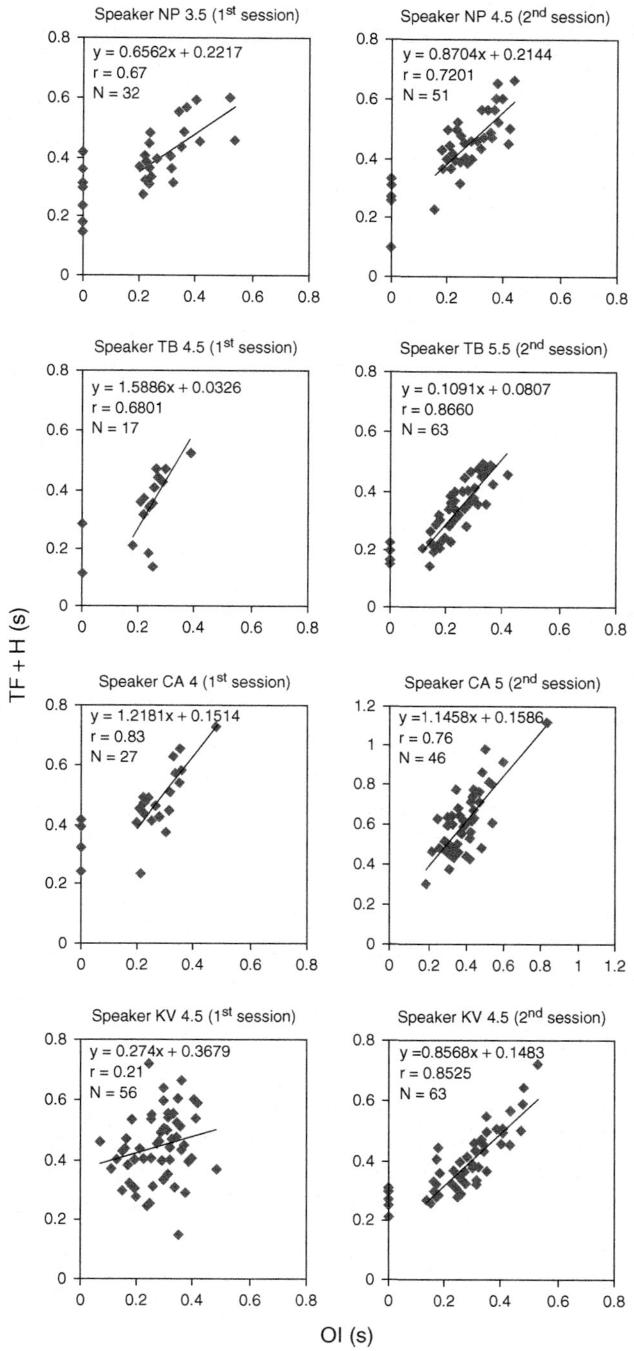

Fig. 9.6 Rounding movement behaviour for the four French-speaking children who have been tested twice with a year interval (1st session at left; 2nd session at right). Correlations between total duration of lip rounding movement (TF+H) and duration of obstruence interval (OI) in seconds (correlation coefficients are significant at $p < 0.01$, except for KV in the 1st session).

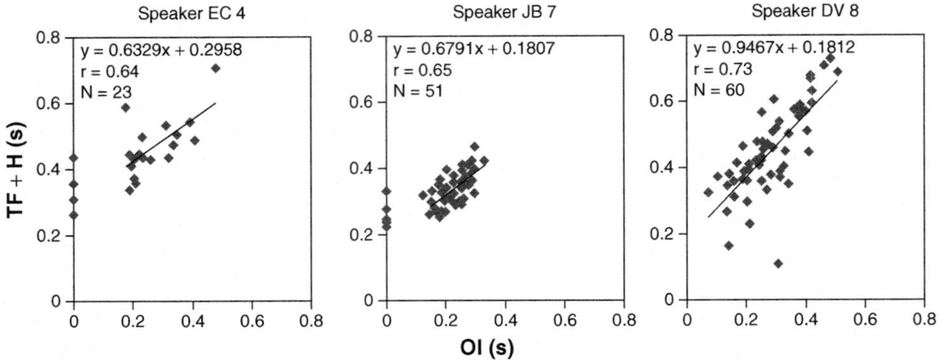

Fig. 9.7 Rounding movement behaviour for the three French-speaking children who have been tested in only one session. Correlations (significant at $p < 0.001$) between total duration of lip rounding movement (TF+H) and duration of obstruence interval (OI) in seconds.

second recording session). These results confirm those previously obtained for French adults (Abry et al., 1996). Indeed, all speakers (except KV for the first session) displayed a linear expansion of movement when the duration of consonants increased in the V-to-V transition, adopting idiosyncratic movement expansion rate. Thus each speaker achieved a personal coefficient of movement expansion (slope) around which data were lawfully grouped (with a significant correlation coefficient).

These results are in contrast with the scattered data obtained for the five Swedish children in Abelin et al. (1980) study. In our study, we found that the control of lip area could be acquired early (as soon as 3.5 years of age) in French children. Individual strategies were observed for the control of vowel timing, strategies that seem as lawful as those of adults belonging to the same linguistic community.

9.2.4 **Summary**

As mentioned above, very few articulatory studies have so far been dedicated to the exploration of anticipatory rounding gesture control in young children. One pioneering challenge overcome in this study was to validate, with children as young as 3.5 years old, an experimental paradigm initially designed for adults, testing a model of speaker-specific lawful variability, the MEM. Children succeeded in producing up to three-element consonant clusters. Thus we could track the evolution of their rounding movement time-span, depending on the variation in intervocalic consonantal string. Totally non-invasive, the Lip-Shape-Tracking-System provided us with accurate information on coarticulatory strategies as cues for the underlying control mechanisms. More precisely, lip-area proved to be a robust parameter to account for vocalic anticipatory behaviour in young children as previously in adults (Abry et al., 1996).

The present findings suggest that in a language like French for which labial constriction is much more crucial for vocalic rounding contrast than in English, we found very regular anticipatory behaviours for six of the seven French children tested. These six young subjects behaved like French adults, as early as 3.5 years old.

What about our seventh French subject? It is important to explore the case of this 4.5-year-old boy (KV) who exhibited a scattered behaviour in the first recording session. At 3 years of age, his motion data were typical of the 3 to 5–8–12 years old period of speech motor control instability as mentioned by Kent. Yet, the 7 children studied were able to achieve sufficiently small controlled lip area for [y] (i.e., without by-producing closure), as small as 20 mm^2 to 2 mm^2. As regards

KV – in spite of acoustically achieving sufficient constriction for the vowel goal achievement – his results may simply mean that he was not yet able to achieve a sufficiently fine timing control over the coordination of his supralaryngeal articulators and conform to the typical French temporal pattern of vocalic anticipation. However, when testing his rounding behaviour just a year later, we found a 0.85 correlation coefficient with a personal slope around which his data were well grouped, i.e., with a personal lawful variability. For this child, his specific anticipatory regime seemed to be simply acquired a bit later than for the others, i.e., at 5.5 years of age. However, notice that some French bilabial productions are not protruded at all (e.g., 'Christophe' in Abry et al., 1996). So regarding more generally individual differences along a child's development path – not simply in variable emulation, but in a language-specific imitation behaviour of a vowel coordination – differences in path are particularly difficult to explain idiosyncratically, except for some obvious retardation cases.

From our point of view, coupled with previous reports (Kent 1976; Green et al., 2002), these results confirm the occurrence of a critical period around three to six years, along which children speech motor control is one step further stabilized, here for the vowel coordination timing pattern.

9.3 **Conclusion**

For more than 40 years, two main anticipation models have been in competition in the context of different languages, mainly on the visible lip rounding anticipation of vowels. The controversy has had no winner, but a compromise was found with a Time-locked Model for English vs. a Look-ahead Model for French or Swedish. The MEM, elaborated at the beginning of the 1990s for French, predicts a lawful anticipation behaviour that can be extended ahead of the vowel target in a VCnV transition, at a speaker-specific rate. A main finding in this contribution is that models have focused on a universally non-reliable parameter, namely lip protrusion. We found that when tested on lip area control, English speakers behave like French speakers with a regular speaker-specific MEM pattern. We found that children could also join French adults and attune their labial rounding behaviour as early as 3.5 and not later than 5.5 years in our study. Hence the MEM seems to reconcile a universal speech motor behaviour principle, proposing a speaker-specific parameterization.

Other languages have yet to (and should) be tested. But as far as children are concerned, the obvious prediction is that if adults are found to display a lawful anticipatory behaviour as described with MEM principles (regardless of their language), children eventually join their older counterparts. Individual attunement seems to be a matter of date, characterizing the passage from a simple goal emulation of the vowel target to the reproduction of this goal and its path (anticipatory imitation).

Acknowledgements

This study was supported by the Quebec's Government (FQRSC and SSHRC grants) and NIHDC-02717. Preliminary parts of this work have been presented first in Jeju (Noiray et al., 2004) and Ubatuba (Noiray et al., 2007). We are grateful to David Ostry, who kindly let us perform the recordings in the *Motor Control Lab* (McGill University, Montreal) with Optotrak system. We are also grateful to Jérôme Aubin for his experimental and data processing support and to Johanna-Pascale Roy for her technical assistance. Regarding the children recording, we would like to thank Christophe Savariaux and Alain Arnal for their technical assistance and Virginie Attina for her data processing assistance. We are also very grateful to Ben Maassen and Dogu Erdener for comments. Finally, we thank all the participants for their interest and patience during the recordings.

References

Abelin A Landberg I and Persson L (1980). A study of anticipatory labial coarticulation in the speech of children. In *PERILUS*, **2**, 2–18.

Abry C and Lallouache T (1995). Le MEM: Un modèle d'anticipation paramétrable par locuteur. Données sur l'arrondissement en français. *Bulletin de la Communication Parlée*, **3**, 85–99.

Abry C Lallouache MT and Cathiard MA (1996). How can coarticulation models account for speech sensitivity to audio-visual desynchronization? In D Stork and M Hennecke, eds. *Speechreading by Humans and Machines*, NATO ASI Series F: Computer and Systems Sciences, 150, pp. 247–255. Springer-Verlag, Berlin Heidelberg New York London Paris Tokyo.

Audouy M (2000). Logiciel de traitement d'images vidéo pour la détermination de mouvements des lèvres. ENSIMA, Grenoble.

Bard KA and Russell CL (1999). Evolutionary foundations of imitation: social, cognitive and developmental aspects of imitative processes in non-human primates. In J Nadel and G Butterworth, eds. *Imitation in Infancy*, pp. 89–123. Cambridge University Press.

Bell-Berti F and Harris KS (1982). Temporal patterns of coarticulation: lip rounding. *Journal of the Acoustical Society of America*, **71**, 449–459.

Benguerel AP and Cowan HA (1974). Coarticulation of upper lip protrusion in French. *Phonetica*, **30**, 41–55.

Benoît C (1986). Note on the use of correlations in speech timing. *Journal of the Acoustical Society of America*, **80(6)**, 1846–1849.

Butz M Sigaud O Gérard P (2003). Anticipatory behavior in adaptive learning systems, foundations, theories, and systems. *Lecture Notes in Computer Science*, 2684, Springer.

Byrd D and Saltzman E (2003). The elastic phrase: modeling the dynamics of boundary-adjacent lengthening. *Journal of Phonetics*, **31**, 149–180.

Farnetani E (1999). Labial coarticulation. In WJ Hardcastle and N Hewlett, eds. *Coarticulation: Theory, Data, and Techniques*, pp.144–163. Cambridge: Cambridge University Press.

Gallese V (2004). Being like me: self-other identity, mirror neurons and empathy. In S Hurley and N Chater, eds. *Perspectives on Imitation: From Cognitive Neuroscience to Social Science*, Boston, MA: MIT Press.

Gallese V (2006). Intentional attunement: the mirror neuron system and its role in interpersonal relations. Interdisciplines. [http://www.interdisciplines.org/mirror/papers/1]

Gibson A and McPhearson L (1980). Production of bite-block vowels by children. *PERILUS*, **2**, 26–43.

Green JR Moore CA Higashikawa M and Steeve RW (2000). The physiologic development of speech motor control: lip and jaw coordination. *Journal of Speech, Language, and Hearing Research*, **43**, 239–256.

Green JR Moore CA and Reilly KJ (2002). The sequential development of jaw and lip control for speech. *Journal of Speech, Language, and Hearing Research*, **45**, 66–79.

Green JR Moore CA and Reilly KJ (2003). Methodological issues in studies of early articulatory development: a response to Dworkin, Meleca, and Stachler (2003). *Journal of Speech, Language, and Hearing Research*, **46**, 1020–1021.

Henke WL (1966). Dynamic articulatory model of speech production using computer simulation. Ph. D. Dissertation MIT, Cambridge.

Horner V and Whiten A (2005). Causal knowledge and imitation/emulation switching in chimpanzees (Pan troglodytes) and children (Homo sapiens). *Animal Cognition*, **8(3)**, 164–181.

James DGH Van Doorn J and McLeod S (2001). Vowel production in mono-, di-and polysyllabic words in children aged 3;0 to 7;11 years. In *Proceedings of Speech Pathology*, Australia Conference, 127–136.

Kent RD (1976). Anatomical and neuromuscular maturation of the speech mechanism: evidence from acoustic studies. *Journal of Speech and Hearing Research*, **19**, 421–447.

Kent RD (1992). The biology of phonological development. In CA Ferguson L Menn and C Stoel-Gammon, eds. *Phonological Development. Models, Research, Implications*, pp. 65–91. Timonium, Maryland, York Press.

Kent RD (2004). Development, Pathology and Remediation of Speech. Proceedings of From Sound to Sense, 50+ years of discoveries in speech communication, Cambridge, B148–162.

Koopmans-van Beinum F and Van der Stelt J (1986). Early stages in the development of speech movements. In L Zetterström, ed. *Precursors of Early Speech*, pp. 37–49. New York, Stockton Press.

Kuhl K and Meltzoff N (1995). Vocal learning in infants: development of perceptual-motor links for speech. In *Proceedings of the XIIIth International Congress of Phonetic Sciences*, Stockholm, **1**, 146–149.

Lallouache MT (1991). Un poste «Visage-parole » couleur. Acquisition et traitement automatique des contours des lèvres. PhD, ENSERG, Grenoble, France.

Lubker J (1981). Temporal aspects of speech production: anticipatory labial coarticulation. *Phonetica*, **38**, 51–65.

MacNeilage PF (1998). The frame/content theory of evolution of speech production. *Behavioral and Brain Sciences*, **21**, 499–511.

MacNeilage PF and Davis BL (1990). Acquisition of speech production: frames, then content. In Jeannerod, ed. *Attention and Performance XIII: Motor Representation and Control*, pp.452–468. Hillsdale, Erlbaum.

Ménard L Cathiard MA and Savariaux C (2004). Le développement de la coarticulation labiale anticipante en français: une étude préliminaire. *25èmes Journées d'Etude sur la Parole*, 373–376.

Noiray A (2007). L'anticipation d'arrondissement vocalique et le Modèle d'Expansion du Mouvement. Deux extensions: du français à L'anglais et de l'adulte à l'enfant. PhD ICP/Stendhal, Grenoble, France.

Noiray A Ménard L Cathiard MA Abry C and Savariaux C (2004).The development of anticipatory labial coarticulation in French: a pioneering study. In *Proceedings of INTERSPEECH, 8th ICSLP*, 53–56.

Oller DK and MacNeilage PF (1983). Development of speech production: perspectives from natural and perturbed speech. In PF MacNeilage, ed. *The Production of Speech*, pp. 91–108. New-York, Springer Verlag.

Perkell JS and Chiang C (1986). Preliminary support for a 'hybrid model' of anticipatory coarticulation. *12th International Conference of Acoustics*, Toronto, A3-6.

Perkell JS (1990). Testing theories of speech production: implications of some detailed analyses of variable articulatory data. In WJ Hardcastle and A Marchal eds. *Speech Production and Speech Modelling*, pp. 263–288. Kluwer Academic Publishers.

Perkell JS and Matthies L M (1992). Temporal measures of anticipatory labial coarticulation for the vowel /u/: within- and cross-subject variability. *Journal of the Acoustical Society of America*, **91(5)**, 2911–2925.

Rubin P Saltzman E Goldstein L McGowan GR Tiede M and Browman C (1996). Casy and extension to the task dynamic model. In *Proceedings of 4th Speech Production Seminar*, pp. 125–128.

Serkhane J (2005). Un bébé androïde vocalisant: Etude et modélisation des mécanismes d'exploration vocale et d'imitation orofaciale dans le développement de la parole. PhD, INPG, Grenoble, France.

Stoel-Gammon C and Herrington P (1990). Vowel systems of normally developing and phonologically disordered children. *Clinical Linguistics and Phonetics*, **4**, 145–160.

Sussman HM Duder C Dalston E and Cacciatore A. (1999). An acoustic analysis of the development of CV coarticulation: a case study. *Journal of Speech and Hearing Research*, **42**, 1080–1096.

Swarup S and Gasser L (2007). The rote of anticipation in the emergence of language. In MV Butz OSigaud, G Pezzulo and G Baldassarre, eds. *Anticipatory Behaviour in Adaptive Learning systems*, pp. 35–56. Berlin/Heidelberg. Springer.

Tingley BM and Allen GD (1975). Development of speech timing control in children. *Child Development*, **46**, 186–194.

Vilain A (2000). Apports de la modélisation des degrés de liberté articulatoires à l'étude de la coarticulation et du développement de la parole. PhD, Language Sciences, Stendhal University, Grenoble, France.

Chapter 10

Some organization principles in early speech development

Jordan R. Green and Ignatius S. B. Nip

Abstract

In early speech development, progressive gains in phonetic ability represent progress in multiple domains (e.g., sensory, perceptual, cognitive, linguistic, and neuromotor) all of which are ultimately conveyed through the speech motor system. Accordingly, the comprehensive understanding of speech development requires knowledge about age-related changes in speech motor performance and about the factors affecting those changes during the various phases of speech development. In this chapter, we consider why motor-based descriptions are essential for addressing long-standing practical and theoretical issues regarding early speech development. We also present a conceptual framework for studying early speech motor development, which guides our current line of research inquiry. The conceptual framework proposes that developmental stages in speech motor behavior are guided by *production constraints* and *catalysts* to speech motor performance: Production constraints are factors that limit speech production abilities in young children and catalysts are factors that engender change toward mature speech. Finally, we consider findings from our studies on early speech motor development that are motivated by the framework.

10.1 Introduction: the need for motor-based descriptions of speech development

To even the most casual observer, it is obvious that infants are capable of producing only a small number of crude, uncoordinated articulatory gestures. Learning to produce speech poses a significant physical challenge to the young child. The motor skills required to produce speech are among the most sophisticated learned by humans. During speech, a large number of muscles are activated to move respiratory, phonatory, and articulatory structures. Because speech is produced very quickly (180 words/minute or 15 sounds/second), speech muscles must be activated rapidly and timed precisely with respect to speech goals. Very little is understood about how young children learn this remarkable ability.

Over the past three decades, a significant amount of research has been directed towards identifying the order in which typically developing children acquire and subsequently master new speech sounds, syllable shapes, and sound combinations (Locke 1983; Roug et al., 1989;

Stoel-Gammon 1985; Vihman et al., 1985). Although this research has provided a rich description of early vocal and speech development, it has not identified the improvements in oromotor skills that underlie those gains. Compared to other aspects of motor control in humans, speech motor control has been notably understudied[1] and the extant corpus of work is particularly modest in size. Research on speech motor development is limited to approximately 30 published studies, which have typically included only small samples of older children (i.e., four and ten years) who have already obtained many fundamental skills for speech production. Moreover, most of these studies have relied on cross-sectional observations even though speech, like all motor behaviours, is known to develop at irregular intervals and at different rates across children (Vihman 1986). One reason for slow scientific progress has been the absence of technologies for directly quantifying articulatory performance in very young children (Kent and Miolo 1995).

Developmental studies of speech kinematics involve the recording of articulatory movements from young children as they learn to produce the segmental and suprasegmental features of their language. Most of the methods (i.e., articulography, x-ray microbeam) currently used to record the movements of the tongue, velum, oropharynx, and larynx during speech in adults are not suitable for use with infants and toddlers. These technologies require placement of sensors or pellets inside the mouth, which is not tolerated by infants and toddlers, and some involve exposure to small doses of radiation. Consequently, investigators have focused their studies primarily on more accessible articulators, such as the lips and jaw. The movement of these articulators has been recorded using video- and optically based motion tracking technologies (Goffman and Smith 1999; Green 1998; Grigos et al., 2005). Knowledge about the development of control over the lips and jaw is crucial because they have a predominant role in early sound production. Obviously, the jaw is involved in the production of all speech sounds because the motion of the lower lip and tongue depend on those of the jaw. Furthermore, data from early phonemic inventories suggest that approximately 40% of the consonants of early speech are typically produced with the lips and jaw as primary articulators (Stoel-Gammon 1985).

10.1.1 **Motion capture technology for noninvasively studying early articulatory development**

Over the past decade, the number of studies on the development of lip and jaw control for speech has increased steadily due to the recent advent of three-dimensional (3D) passive optical motion capture devices. These systems provide a non-invasive method to obtain high-precision tracking (often < 0.10 mm) of small facial movements in three dimensions. High-speed digital cameras are used to register the movements of small (2 mm) retroreflective markers attached to the face, which are illuminated using infrared light. Only two cameras are needed to triangulate the 3D positions of each facial marker; however, in practice more cameras are needed to track movements on both sides of the face. These systems provide the 3D coordinates of each marker as a function of time. Rotational information is derived from the relative orientation of three or more markers. This system is particularly well suited to capture facial movement of very young children, even newborn infants, because the markers can be very small and facial data can be captured while children are comfortably seated in the presence of their parents.

Figure 10.1 depicts the data collection environment in our laboratory. As displayed in Fig. 10.1, the optical motion capture system (Motion Analysis Corp 2007) we use has eight cameras each

[1] One overly simplistic – but nonetheless revealing – demonstration of the paucity of studies on speech physiology is the results from a PubMed database search limited to the past five years of research. While the terms 'grasp and hand' yielded 1882 publications, 'speech and tongue' only yielded 285.

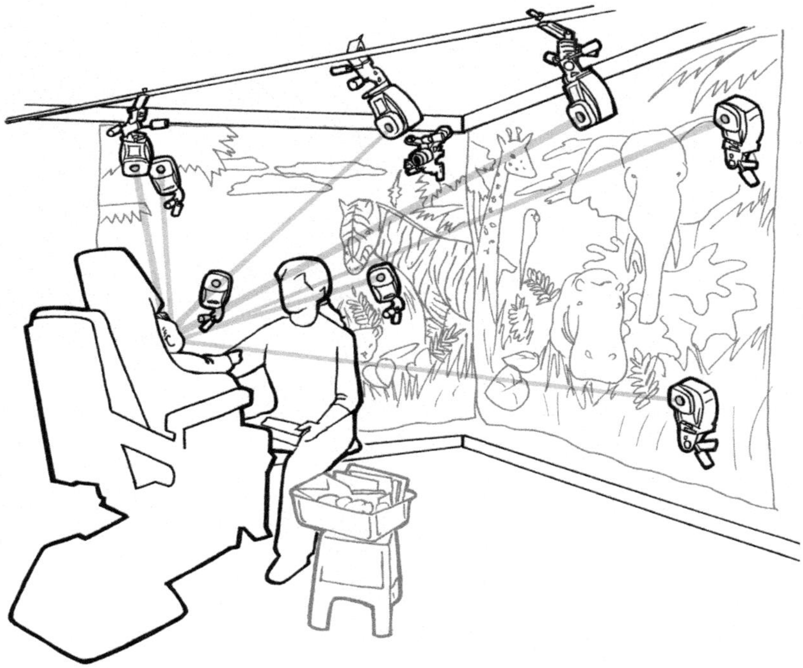

Fig. 10.1 Continuous recordings of facial movements from newborns, infants, and young children are obtained during parent–child interactions using an eight-camera optically-based motion capture system.

with a temporal resolution of 500 fps and a spatial resolution of 4 million pixels. To minimize visual distraction to the child, the cameras are semicamouflaged by a mural depicting an animal scene and the infrared light sources are in the nonvisible spectrum. The cameras are positioned so that parents can sit directly in front of their children without interfering with facial motion tracking. The top right panel of Fig. 10.2 displays a child fitted with the marker array and the reconstructed 3D facial model. During data collection, young children are secured in a car seat using a five-point safety belt system, which helps to minimize extraneous body movement. Speech is recorded using a microphone that is attached to the forehead marker array to maintain a constant mouth-to-microphone distance. The forehead markers are used to subtract extraneous head movements from the movement of the facial markers.

Speech movements are recorded during parent–child play. The data collection session is structured to maximize the ecological validity of our observations and the likelihood of obtaining a representative sample of communicative contexts from each parent and child dyad. During data collection, parents are encouraged to let their children initiate communication and are instructed to select toys from three distinct bins. Each bin contains items that elicit one of three targeted types of communication interactions (Wetherby and Prizant 2002): behavioural regulation, joint attention, social interaction. Recording a large number of speech samples per subject is imperative to ensure that a representative sample of different behaviours is obtained and an appropriate level of statistical power is achieved in the face of high performance variability. Each data collection session results in a permanent recording of the lip and jaw movements from which a large number of quantitative indicators of articulatory performance can be derived.

The recordings of lip and jaw movement can reveal developmental changes in articulation that cannot be detected using transcription or acoustic analyses. Transcription-based characterizations

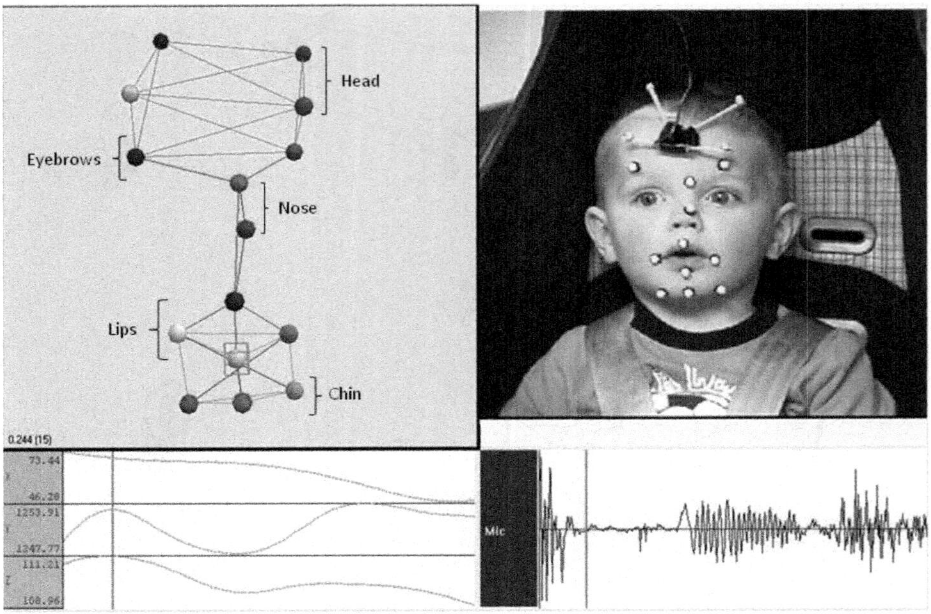

Fig. 10.2 A 2-year-old participant fitted with facial markers.

of speech are biased from listener's auditory and visual processing and linguistic knowledge and context (Cucchiarini 1996; Shriberg and Lof 1991). Consequently, developmental studies are often conducted assuming that children's speech conforms to adult-based phonetic and phonemic categories (Shriberg and Kent 2002). Moreover, obtaining reliable transcriptions of early vocalization and speech can be very difficult (Oller 2000; Stockman et al., 1981). One consequence of these limitations is that important articulatory changes occurring in early speech development may be missed or misclassified.

Acoustic-based characterizations of early speech may also be insensitive to important developmental changes in articulation. Speakers are capable of using a variety of articulatory strategies to achieve a given speech goal (i.e., motor equivalence; Folkins and Linville 1983; Hughes and Abbs 1976; Perkell et al., 1993). Consequently, during speech sound development, changes in articulatory control and coordination may not be evident in speech output. Moreover, during the first several years of life, the relations between articulatory movements and acoustic output are continually changing as a function of vocal tract growth (Ménard et al., 2004; Vorperian et al., 1999). These changes may limit the sensitivity of acoustic variables to developmental changes in articulatory performance.

Kinematic studies, however, are not without limitations. As stated previously, the movements of the tongue during speech cannot be easily recorded in young children and some children (15–20%) object to having markers on their face or to sitting during data collection. Another challenge is the significant time required to reduce the large volume of data obtained from these studies. Transcription of the utterances is also required to provide a behavioural reference for the kinematic data. Finally, small to moderate errors (i.e., approximately 0.81 mm and 7.30%) occur when tracking the jaw because the skin of the chin is loosely coupled to the underlying mandible (Green et al., 2007).

To summarize, a complete description of speech motor development will need to account for the factors that shape the course of speech sound development. Although some developmental changes in articulatory performance may not have perceptual or acoustic consequences, knowledge about these changes is essential for understanding the influence of cognitive, linguistic, and motor factors at different stages of development. Of course, a complete account of speech development will need to consider observations at different levels of analysis, with each level informing the other. For example, changes in articulatory performances will be most meaningful if they are interpreted with respect to information about perceptual and acoustic aspects of speech (see Weismer 2006).

10.2 **Towards an explanatory model of speech motor development**

Although studies on speech development are unified by their search for factors governing the course of phonetic and phonologic development, only a small number of theoretical and empirical frameworks have been advanced that consider speech development in the context of motor development. The empirical framework we use to guide our studies considers articulatory performance as the confluence of changes occurring in multiple developmental domains. The framework assimilates concepts introduced by contemporary motor development theorists such as Bernstein (1967), Newell (1986), and Thelen (1991), who conceptualize early motor development as the interaction between the developing central nervous system and other intrinsic and extrinsic factors. Within our framework, immature speech is viewed as a 'motor adaptation' to two opposing forces: *catalysts* that spur the development of articulatory skills and *production constraints* (Green et al., 2000) that are slow to respond to newly emerging demands on the speech motor system. Thus, catalysts are driving forces that guide and, in some cases, accelerate speech motor learning, and production constraints are developmental factors that limit speech production abilities in the young child.

The concept of motor adaptation is central to our framework – they are young children's solutions for achieving some level of speech proficiency despite their immature articulatory abilities. In early speech, children appear to favour adaptations that use muscle groups and articulators they have the most control over (Green et al., 2000). Adaptations are organized with respect to speech goals and new strategies emerge as speech goals become increasingly complex during development.

10.2.1 **Organizing principles in speech motor development: production constraints, catalysts, and adaptation**

All complex motor skills take years to master and it is therefore not surprising that children typically take up to eight years to master the sounds of their language (Sanders 1972). Production constraints[2] are limitations (e.g., biomechanic, neuromotor, perceptual, or cognitive) in the child's ability to form, store, retrieve, or produce mature speech. For example, presumably limitations in cognitive skills such as slow processing speeds (relative to adult's processing speeds) for message formulation may explain why children speak slower than adults do (Kowal et al., 1975). Similarly, limitations in articulatory coordination and control in early childhood may restrict the number of vocal tract configurations available for sound production (Green et al., 2000). Studies of early infant vocal development focused on identifying production constraints will essentially

[2] The term *constraint* is used to convey a large number of concepts in the scientific literature. In our framework, production constraints refer broadly to developmental factors that limit the young child from producing mature speech, and are consistent with Newell (1986) and Thelen's (1991) concept of organismic constraints, and in some cases, Smith and Thelen's (1993) concept of rate-limiting factors. The result of production constraints is behaviour rigidity.

yield a description of the initial conditions from which speech production emerges. This information is not only essential for explaining the features of immature articulatory control that shape early speech, but also how subsequent changes in articulatory performance depend on earlier stages of development. Thus, within our framework, important steps in furthering our understanding of speech development is to identify the various production constraints at each phase of speech motor development and the functional limitations they impose on the child's sound-producing capabilities.

Catalysts are the neural, cognitive, and environmental supports that predispose a child to progress through the various phases of speech development. Catalysts have a profound influence on early speech learning – without these facilitators a child's vocal repertoire would advance more slowly or not progress beyond primitive vocalizations. Current views on which catalysts moderate or mediate the development of speech are diverse and more studies are needed to understand their significance and critical periods. Although many catalysts have been considered important for normal speech development (e.g., exposure to exaggerated and simplified speech patterns, endogenously generated spontaneous orofacial motility, rapid learning of auditory-visual perceptual aspects of speech, interest in vocal imitation and play, strong attentional bias to moving faces), few causal relations have been firmly established.

One putative catalyst to speech motor development is the rapid increase in expressive linguistic demands during early word learning (Lindblom 1989; Studdert-Kennedy 1991). Like perceptual learning, new word learning is very fast in young children, approximately ten new words per day (Bloom 2000). Strong correlations have been reported between many aspects of early lexical development and phonologic development (see Stoel-Gammon 1998 for review). For example, a study by McCune and Vihman (2001) showed that precocious talkers acquired speech sounds at a greater rate than did typically developing children. Conversely, children with relatively small vocabularies exhibited an impoverished phonologic system relative to typically developing peers of the same age (Paul and Jennings 1992). Collectively, these studies suggest the articulatory practice afforded to children with relatively large expressive vocabularies accelerates the rate of speech motor development. Explanations of early speech motor development will need to account for the varying language abilities exhibited across children.

The characterization of speech motor development in terms of production constraints and catalysts may have implications for several well-known phenomena in speech development including individual and group patterns of speech sound development, rapid progressions and regressions in speech performance, and transient periods of variability and dysfluency in speech abilities. To the extent production constraints represent biologically determined predispositions in behaviour, they may explain why some aspects of typical speech development follow a similar path across individuals. For example, early constraints in vocal tract coordination and control (Green et al., 2000, 2002) may provide a biomechanic or neuromotor explanation for the limited diversity of sounds produced by young children (e.g., Stoel-Gammon 1985), biases in sound co-occurrence patterns (MacNeilage and Davis 2000), and continuity in segmental development from babble to speech (Locke 1989). In contrast, individual variation in speech development is expected due to differences among children in the developmental progression and strength of catalysts. For example, children are expected to vary in the quality and quantity of environmental stimulation, and in the age at which spurts in lexical acquisition occur (e.g., Li et al., 2007).

10.2.2 **Nonmonotonic change in speech motor development**

Several concepts considered in the motor development literature suggest that periods of significant linguistic, cognitive, or social change will be associated with rapid changes in speech behaviour, regressions in speech motor performances, or increases in speech errors. The significance of nonmonotonic change in motor behaviour has been emphasized prominently in Dynamic Systems Theory (DST). The developmental literature shows nonmonotonic changes in motor performance taking several forms including accelerations, decelerations, plateaus, and even regressions (see Fig. 10.3; Wimmers et al., 1998; Thelen and Smith 1994). In other words, motor development rarely proceeds in a straight line but more typically in fits, spurts, intermixed with brief periods of no change.

Dynamic systems theory predicts that a child may revert to old stable forms of motor behaviour or adopt a coordinative strategy to achieve some stable level of performance during periods in development when the demands of the task exceed a child's motor capabilities (Thelen and Smith 1994). Thus, a transient period of reduced motor performance may occur as children transition towards higher levels of motor functioning. For example, at the onset of walking, infants have been observed to revert to using two hands to reach for objects rather than one (Corbetta and Bojczyk 2002). This regression appears to be a coordinative strategy used by children to maintain an effective grasp while they are grappling with new challenges posed by walking.

Plateaus in motor skill development have also been observed. For example, in a study by Hay (1978), pointing accuracy to a visual target plateaued or decreased at around age seven years. In this experiment, the view of the hand was obstructed by a barrier and, therefore, children were not able to see their hand while it was moving towards the target, which was visible. Because children could not use visual information to guide their hand to the target, they were forced to rely on proprioceptive feedback or to plan the trajectory in advance of moving. The author speculated that performance decreased at age seven years because children shifted from using a ballistic guidance system (i.e., movement without online monitoring of proprioceptive feedback) to one that relied on continuous proprioceptive feedback.

There is some evidence for regressions in articulatory motor performance at two years of age, which is when children are rapidly acquiring new words. Specifically, Green and colleagues (2000) observed less-coordinated upper and lower lip movements during speech in two-year-olds than in one-year-olds, six-year-olds, and adults (Green et al., 2000). Another example from the speech literature is the findings from Smith and Zelaznik (2004) on developmental changes in the variability of the lip and jaw movement patterns on repeated productions of a sentence. In this large cross-sectional study of typically developing children and young adults, variability in articulatory performance plateaued between the ages seven and twelve years but was statistically different between the ages of four and five years and between fourteen-year-olds and young adults. The authors speculated about anatomic and physiologic factors that may have engendered nonmonotonic changes in performance variability with age.

Anatomic growth may be an additional factor underlying temporary developmental regressions in articulatory skills. Children must develop articulatory performance stability as vocal tract structures undergo rapid changes in mass and geometry (Kent 1984; Vorperian et al., 1999). Such changes must complicate the infant's attempts to acquire a target acoustic output. It might be anticipated that changes in the absolute or proportional size of the child's articulators would dramatically alter the coordinative organization of speech, or result in regressions in articulatory performance and speech sound development (Callan et al., 2000).

10.2.3 **Performance variability as an indicator of motor development**

Performance variability has long been hypothesized to play an important role in the development of movement control (Thelen and Smith 1994). Like the development of most motor skills, the variability of speech motor performance shows an overall decreasing trend with age that is overlaid with some transient periods of elevated variability (Green et al., 2002; Smith and Zelaznik 2004).

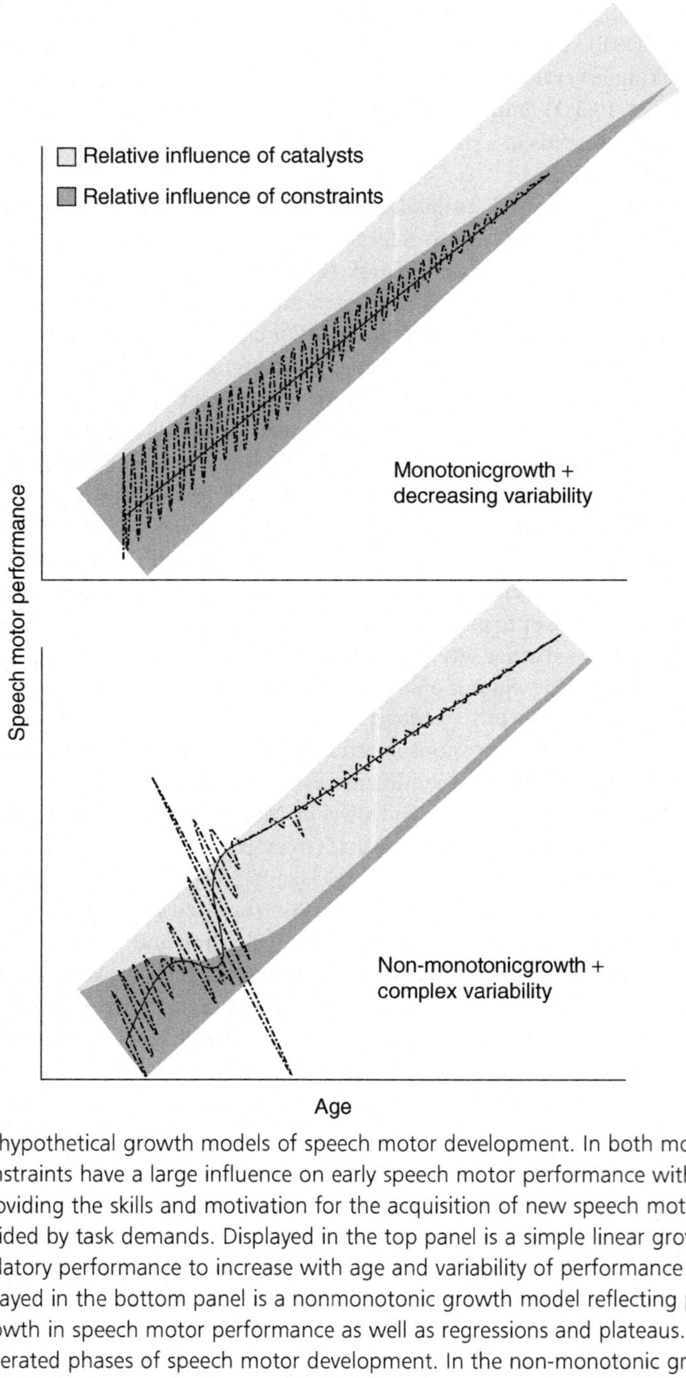

Fig. 10.3 Two hypothetical growth models of speech motor development. In both models, production constraints have a large influence on early speech motor performance with catalysts increasingly providing the skills and motivation for the acquisition of new speech motor skills, which is a process guided by task demands. Displayed in the top panel is a simple linear growth model showing articulatory performance to increase with age and variability of performance to decrease with age. Displayed in the bottom panel is a nonmonotonic growth model reflecting periods of accelerated growth in speech motor performance as well as regressions and plateaus. Catalysts engender accelerated phases of speech motor development. In the non-monotonic growth model, performance variability decreases with age overall, but also varies as a function of the rate of change in performance, with high rates of change in speech motor performance being associated with periods of increased variability.

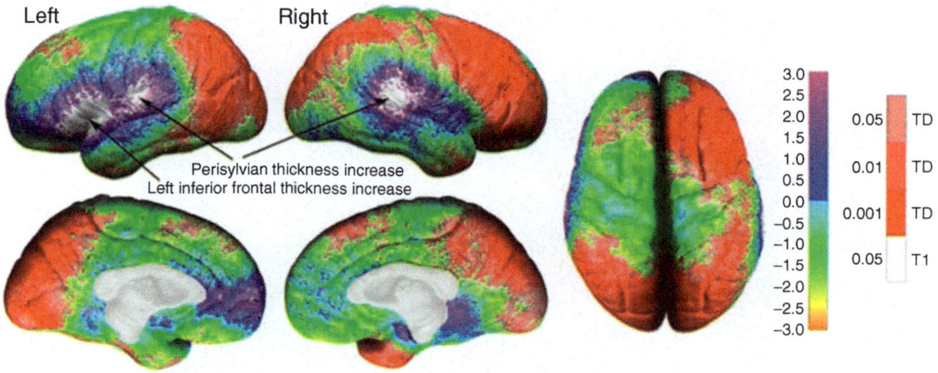

Plate 1 Longitudinal mapping of cortical thickness changes in children between 5 years and 11 years of age. Colour bar to the left shows colour coding corresponding to *t* values at each cortical surface point, and significance values are overlaid in shades of red (significant thickness decreases [TD] and increases [TI]) represented in the colour bar to the right (Sowell et al., 2004. Figure reprinted with permission). (See p.76, Fig. 5.4).

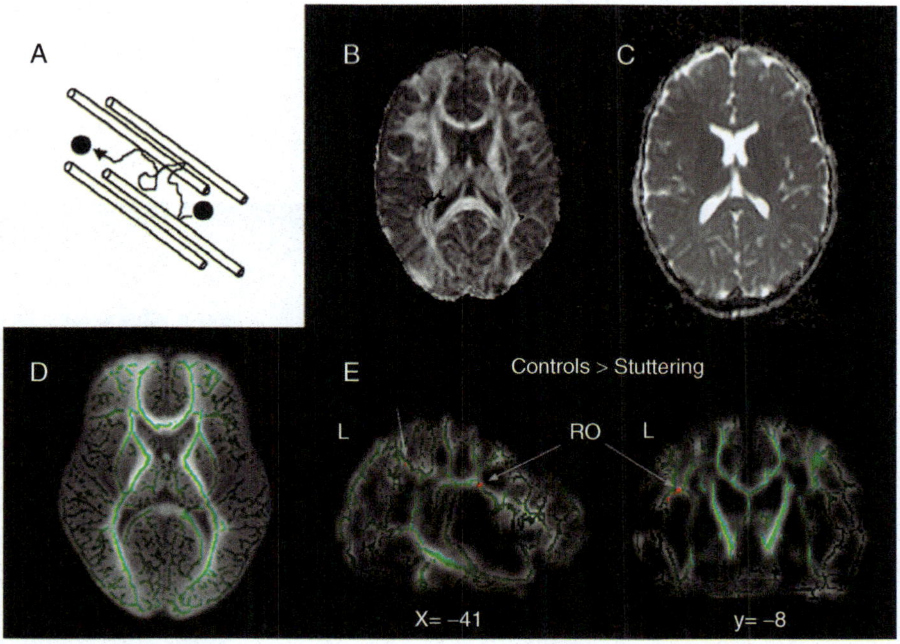

Plate 2 A. Schematic view of water diffusion (water molecule is depicted as a solid sphere) restricted by highly aligned fibres (depicted as poles). B–C. Axial views of a 12-year-old brain scanned with a DTI sequence showing maps of the fractional anisotropy (FA) (B), and mean diffusivity (MD) (C). D. In tract-based spatial statistics (TBSS), individual FA maps are non-linearly aligned voxel-wise to an optimal target FA, typically one of the subjects whose FA map is normalized to a standard brain. An average of all of the aligned FA maps are created, and a 'skeleton' tract that is common to all subjects is created, shown here E. Only those voxels from each subject that are projected onto this skeleton is entered for across-subject statistics. Here, the result of the contrast between control and stuttering children are shown (Chang et al., 2008. Figure modified and reprinted here with permission). (See p.77, Fig. 5.5).

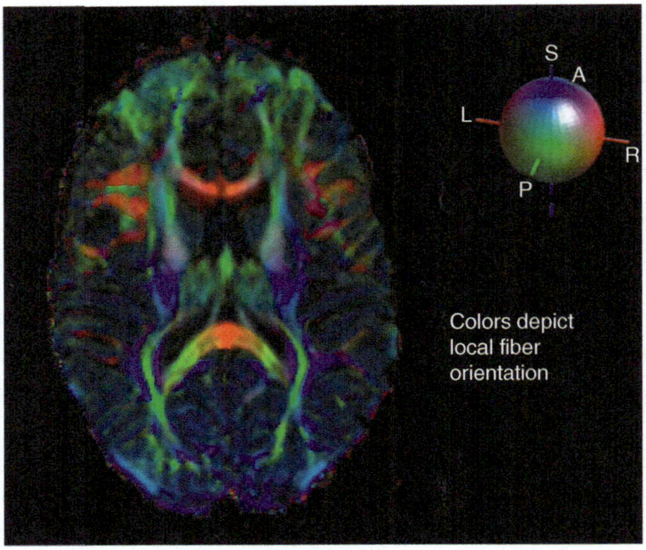

Plate 3 Colour coded map illustrating the direction of fibres in three-dimensional space (See text for more detail). (See p.78, Fig. 5.6).

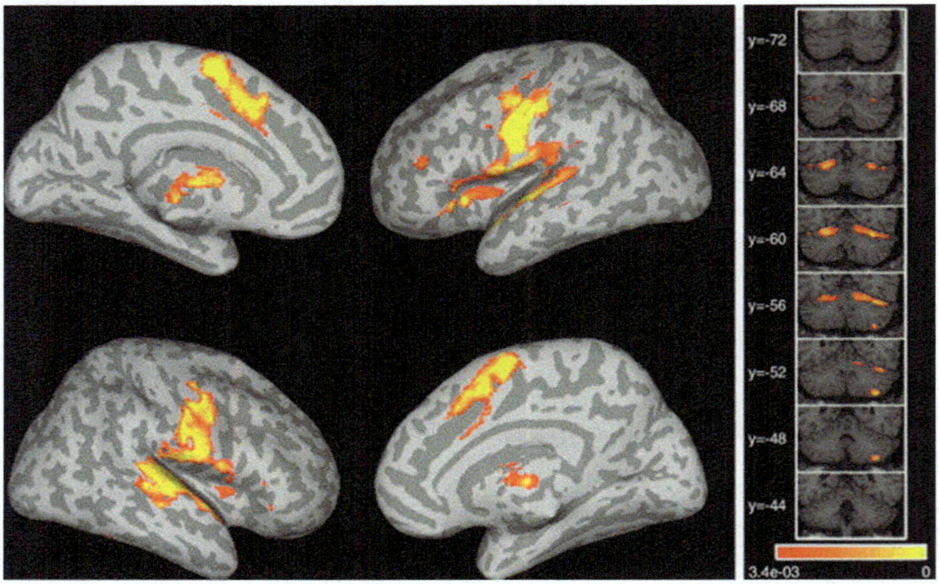

Plate 4 Brain activation associated with overt speech production, captured with fMRI using a sparse sampling paradigm (Bohland and Guenther 2006) (figure reprinted here with permission).
(See p.82, Fig. 5.9).

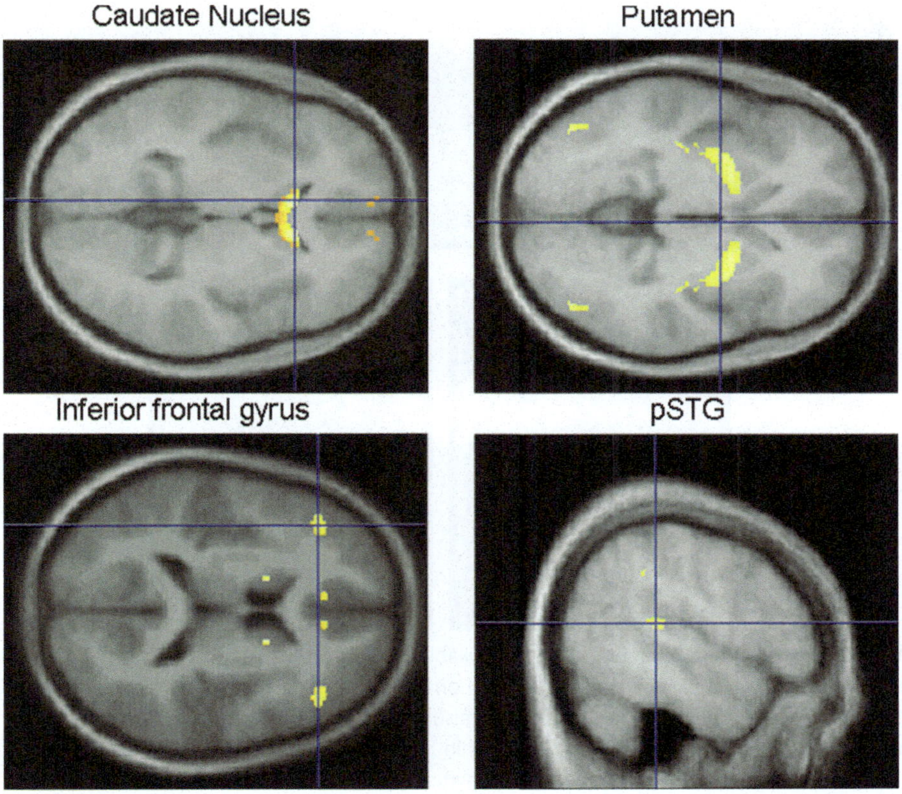

Plate 5 Morphological abnormalities demonstrating regions of reduced (left column) and increased (right column) grey matter density in affected KE family members compared to unaffected members, using VBM. For details see Belton et al., 2003. (See p.98, Fig. 6.2).

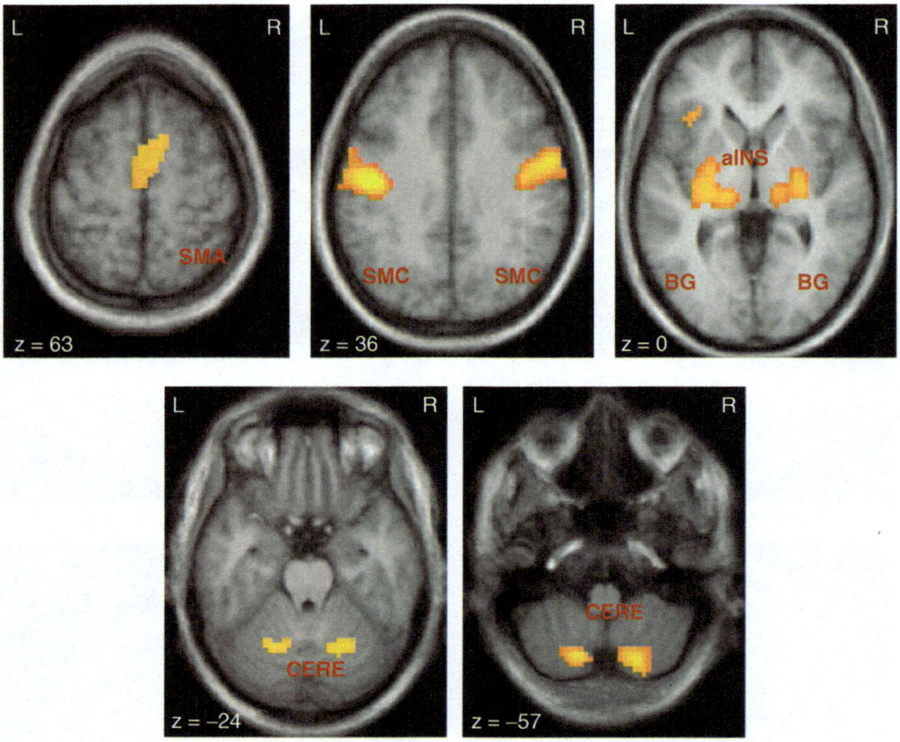

Plate 6 A. Hemodynamic main effects during syllable repetitions computed across all six frequency conditions and subjects (yellow spots), displayed on transverse sections of the averaged anatomic reference images (z = distance to the intercommisural plane; L = left hemisphere, R = right hemisphere). Significant responses emerged within SMA, bilateral sensorimotor cortex, bilateral basal ganglia, left anterior insula, left inferior frontal gyrus, and both cerebellar hemispheres (from left to right). B. Analysis of rate/response relationship: Cerebral areas characterized by a positive linear (red spots) or a negative linear rate/response function (blue spots). C. Group averages of hemodynamic activation across subjects, calculated separately for the six stimulus rates each. Note, no. 1 refers to 2 Hz, 2 = 2.5 Hz etc. (blue columns = right hemisphere, yellow columns = left hemisphere). Bilateral putamen/pallidum and left caudate nucleus show a negative rate/response relationship. By contrast, both cerebellar hemispheres exhibit a positive rate/response function, characterized, most noteworthy, by a step-wise increase of the hemodynamic response at about 3 Hz. (See p.124, Fig. 7.2).

As stated previously, DST predicts that these transient episodes of elevated variability tend to occur at transitional stages in development when task demands greatly exceed a child's capability (Thelen and Smith 1994). During these periods, presumably the child is searching for an optimal coordinative strategy from many possibilities (Sporns and Edelman 1993), a process ensuring successful strategies are repeated more frequently than less successful ones (Sporns and Edelman 1993). Several findings from our cross-sectional studies on early speech development support the existence of increased articulatory performance variability with the emergence of new speech skills. Between the ages of one and two years, children's shifted from an articulatory pattern that relied predominantly on the jaw to achieve oral closure for the /b/ to one that incorporated movements of the lips (Green et al., 2000). A follow-up study showed that this transition was associated with a spike in the variability of upper and lower lip movement patterns (Green et al., 2002). The view of variability as a 'causal prerequisite for learning' (Adolph and Berger 2006, p. 177) continues to be debated.

10.2.4 **A hypothetical framework**

Figure 10.3 shows two hypothetical developmental paths of articulatory performance. The shading in each figure represents the relative influence of production constraints and catalysts at any given time point in development. Thus, production constraints are shown to significantly limit articulatory performance in *early* speech development. As catalysts promote the emergence of new motivations and skills to communicate, the demands on the speech motor system are continually increasing. In the long term, catalysts have a facilitative effect on articulatory skill development; however, catalysts also may have a transient negative effect on performance particularly if their influence is rapid and their demands greatly exceed the child's speech motor abilities.

The purpose of the two panels in Fig. 10.3 is to demonstrate an increasingly complex picture of speech motor development and the variable influence of catalysts on that growth curve. The curve in the top panel represents the simplest scenario: a monotonically increasing growth model where production constraints dominate early motor performance and catalysts gradually increase their influence. In a monotonic growth model, age or time may be a primary independent or explanatory factor. In this simple model, performance variability is modelled as sinusoids overlaid on the growth curves, which represent expected normal variations in performance that regress towards mean performance. Variability is also shown to decrement gradually with age.

The curve in the bottom panel is a complex nonmonotonic curve where articulatory performance responds in a variety of ways to catalysts including an acceleration, deceleration, regression, and plateau. Performance variability varies as a function of the rate of change of the growth trajectory where greater rates of change positive or negative are associated with periods of variable articulatory performance. In a nonmonotonic growth model, variables other than age or time are explanatory factors. Given this simple construct, an important step in furthering our understanding of speech development is to address the following questions: (a) What are the initial conditions (production constraints) from which speech motor control emerges?, (b) How do children get from the initial state to the mature state?, and (c) What factors (catalysts) facilitate the acquisition of speech motor control at various stages of development?

10.3 **Selective review of findings from our laboratory**

Consistent with the framework proposed above, a primary objective of our research has been to identify the articulatory performance constraints (biomechanic and functional) that determine the sound production capabilities during the first four years of life. We have also studied articulatory aspects of infant-directed speech and spontaneous orofacial motility, which are two potentially important factors providing the infant the physiologic and cognitive substrates needed to develop speech.

Our research strategy for identifying articulatory performance constraints has been to quantify the articulatory performance of young children at various stages of development, compare the children's performance to older children and adults, and speculate about the production constraints that may be limiting the child's speech. The adult performance is used to provide a quantifiable developmental endpoint for the movement sequence being studied. One necessary aspect of our work has been to identify developmental 'targets' of articulatory performance that can be used to quantify differences between the articulatory performance of children and adults. An ideal target needs to be within the typical repertoire of young children and to exhibit a relatively low degree of intra- and inter-subject variability in mature talkers. Many of the production constraints we have identified in early articulatory performance have parallels in early limb function and, therefore, may represent characteristic features of immature motor control.

10.3.1 Reliance on jaw movement to produce speech

Several of our findings suggest that young children learning to articulate their first words rely more on the jaw than on the lips. In one of these studies (Green et al., 2000), closure of the mouth for bilabial consonant production was shown to be accomplished primarily using the jaw with little active assistance of the upper and lower lip. This pattern is in contrast to that exhibited by older children and adults who consistently used both the lip and jaw to achieve bilabial closure. In a follow-up study (Green et al., 2002), we tested the hypothesis that control over the jaw would develop earlier than control over the lips. An index of similarity between the jaw, upper lip, lower lip movements of children aged one, two, and six years and those produced by a group of healthy adults. The findings from this study provided strong support for the advanced performance of the jaw in early speech; the jaw movement patterns of one-year-olds were highly similar to those of the adult participants, whereas their lip movements bore little resemblance to the adults. This finding suggests (1) early control over the mandible for speech is essential for producing later appearing sounds, which typically involve the lips and tongue and (2) an essential step in learning to talk requires the coordination of lower lip and tongue with those of the underlying jaw. On the basis of extensive observation of co-occurrence patterns of consonant and vowels in infant speech, MacNeilage and Davis (2000) have argued that young children's dependency on the jaw to produce early speech significantly restricts the variety of sound combinations they can produce.

10.3.2 Limited fine force control over the mandible

Although the jaw appears to have a control advantage in early speech development, fine force control over jaw may be limited in young children. In the Green et al., (2000) study the lower lip tended to collide with the upper lip during oral closure. Consequently, the lower lip tended to move downward as it was pushed against the upper lip by the elevating jaw. Collisions of this magnitude between the upper and lower lip during oral closure were typically not observed in the adult participants. Excessive force generation appears to be a characteristic of immature motor control. For example, overshoot of arm and hand is observed in early grasping (Jeannerod 1988) as is excessive force during the development of a precision grip (Potter et al., 2006). Therefore, as in the development of grasping, the regulation of muscle forces for chewing and speech requires the fine-tuning of force control through practice. For chewing, this process involves a gradual increase in the synchrony between agonist muscles of the mandible for jaw closing and a decrease in the temporal overlap between mandibular antagonists (Green et al., 1997). Less is known about how the mandibular antagonists and agonists are tuned for learning speech (Moore and Ruark 1996);

though studies on adults show a predominant pattern of coactivation of antagonistic muscle pairs (Moore 1993). The limited fine force control over the jaw for speech motor control may partially account for why children have a tendency to master the production of stops prior to fricatives or affricates (Stoel-Gammon and Dunn 1985), which require relatively more fine force control over the mandible than stops.

10.3.3 Dyscoordination between lips and jaw

The developmental course of coordination among the different structures of the vocal tract is protracted and varies among articulators. To produce bilabials, mature talkers simultaneously move the upper lip, lower lip, and jaw to achieve oral closure. This seamless pattern of coordination among orofacial articulators is in stark contrast to the patterns exhibited by infants, whose lip and jaw movements are asynchronous and spatially dissimilar (Green et al., 2000). Because of this constraint, infants should be more proficient at producing sounds and sound combinations that do not require precise timing between articulatory gestures. Studies on infant speech support this assertion at both the sound and syllable level. For example, young children may master voiced consonants earlier than voiceless (Kewley-Port and Preston 1974) because of their limited ability to delay the laryngeal gesture with respect to oral release (Grigos et al., 2005). Similarly, young children may have a tendency to produce adjacent consonants and vowels with similar primary places of vocal tract constriction (i.e., labial-central, coronal consonant-front vowel, dorsal consonant-back vowel) because of their limited ability to coordinate between gesture of consonants and adjacent vowels (MacNeilage and Davis 2000). Adult-like synchrony among the upper lip, lower lip, and jaw movements for simple bilabial utterances appears to be obtained by six years of age (Green et al., 2000). In contrast, development of coordination may be more protracted between the tongue and jaw than the lip and jaw (Cheng et al., 2007).

10.3.4 Obligatory coupling among upper and lower lip

Although spatial and temporal coupling between lips and jaw is poor, upper and lower lip coupling is remarkably strong in young children, particularly at age two (Green et al., 2000). This finding suggests that young children have a limited ability to independently control the upper and lower lips. This pattern of coordination is well suited for producing bilabials, but poorly suited for producing sounds such as labiodentals where the upper lip tends to move little and the lower lip elevates to constrict the vocal tract at the maxillary central incisors. Increases in the ability to independently control functionally linked structures have similarly been observed in the early development of other skilled motor behaviours such as walking and reaching. For example, Thelen and Cooke (1987) observed the movements of the hip, knee, and ankle to be highly synchronous during infant stepping responses. These authors postulated that the development of mature walking requires the differentiation of these functionally coupled joints. Independent control over the arms also emerges as children begin to use the hands for distinct purposes. For example, at this stage of development, children begin to hold an object in one hand, while exploring the object with the other (Fagard and Jaquet 1989; Goldfield and Michel 1986). In a similar way, the acquisition of new words containing new sounds provides the young child the impetus to acquire the ability to move the upper and lower lips independently.

10.3.5 Limited cognitive and linguistic processing

Speaking rate is known to increase with age (Kowal et al., 1975; Walker et al., 1992). One factor that slows children's speaking rate is their tendency to pause frequently. This finding has been interpreted to suggest young children require more time to formulate speech than do older children or adults (Kowal et al., 1975). Slow movement speed in children due to physiologic factors may also contribute to slowed speech. For example, slow neural conduction times in children have been linked to slowed movement of the upper limbs (Müller et al., 1991) and long perioral reflex latencies (Barlow et al., 1993). However, in a recent study, the movement speed of four-year-old children was not significantly slower than were adults' (Nip and Green 2006). In contrast, pausing time and movement displacement decreased significantly with age. Therefore, the observed changes in speaking rate in children appeared to be primarily due to gains in cognitive and linguistic processing (i.e., decreased pause time) and in movement efficiency rather than physiologic-driven increases in articulatory movement speed.

10.3.6 **Variable articulatory performance**

One of the most frequently reported findings in speech motor development research is that children's articulatory performance is more variable than adults' (Goffman and Smith 1999; Green et al., 2002; Grigos et al., 2005; Sharkey and Folkins 1985; Smith and Goffman 1998; Smith and McLean-Muse 1986). During early speech development (i.e., between one and six-years of age), developmental changes in articulatory performance variability are nonmonotonic and vary among the articulators, with the lips exhibiting elevated levels of variability in comparison to the jaw (Green et al., 2002). Interestingly, elevated variability in articulatory performance persists until after 16 years of age (Smith and Zelaznik 2004), which is much longer than was thought previously. For example, classic studies of speech development have long considered speech production to be mastered by eight years of age (Sanders 1972). Variability in the articulatory movement of older children who have already mastered the sounds of their language may be an indication of underlying change. A number of factors could have a destabilizing effect on motor performance including (1) motor immaturity or inexperience, (2) continued remodelling of vocal tract structures, (3) slow rate of speech, and (4) high cognitive-linguistic processing demands. Articulatory movements produced at slower rates are inherently more variable than those produce at typical rates (Adams et al., 1993). Therefore, in comparison to adults, children may exhibit elevated levels of performance variability simply because their movements tend to be relatively slower (Nip and Green 2006; Smith and Goffman 1998). In addition, high cognitive processing demands during early language learning may also engender elevated levels of performance variability in children. Prior research has shown utterances with 'high' cognitive-linguistic demands tend to be produced with greater token-to-token variability of lower lip movements than utterances with 'low' cognitive-demands (see Smith and Goffman 2004 for review).

10.3.7 **Early neuromotor organization through early spontaneous orofacial motility**

The investigation of spontaneous oral movements is motivated by a growing body of evidence suggesting that undirected motor activity in prenatal and postnatal development may be critical for normal anatomic and neuromotor development (Hall and Herring 1990; Thelen 1985). Spontaneous movements are ubiquitous in the developing motor system and thought to be endogenously generated (i.e., an expression of excitatory neuromotor transmitter). A number of investigators have suggested spontaneous motility provides a foundation for later appearing goal-directed behaviours (Bekoff et al., 1986; Thelen and Fisher 1983). From this perspective, endogenously generated spontaneous movements are considered to be the precursors of exploratory movements, which may establish (1) a restricted set of primitives to be later adapted and combined for purposeful movement and (2) learned mappings between articulatory movements and speech sounds required to produce speech.

Spontaneous oral motility has rarely been studied in humans with the exception of the hallmark studies conducted in the 1970s by Humphrey (Humphrey 1971). We recently applied our noninvasive techniques for recording facial movements in infants to identify potential developmental changes in silent, spontaneous oral movement (Green and Wilson 2006). Infants exhibited a remarkable quantity and variety of spontaneous lip and jaw movements. Some age-related changes were observed in spontaneous lip and jaw movement including an increase in the speed of movement, a decrease in the duration of movement epochs, and an increase in the coupling among the movements of different facial regions. These findings suggest early spontaneous facial movements undergo developmental change during the first year of life and provide further impetus for determining the functional role in early oromotor development. From a clinical perspective, several investigators have proposed that the quantity and quality of these movements may serve as useful clinical markers of developmental neuromotor integrity (Roberts et al., 1980). This suggestion raises the possibility that spontaneous oral movements may, in the future, be evaluated for determining the developmental status of nonverbal children and young children before they acquire speech.

10.3.8 **Environmental stimulation: visual aspects of infant-directed speech**

Infant directed speech (IDS), the affective speaking style used by parents to speak to their infants, has been posited to have a number of positive influences on early development including the facilitation of child–parent bonding, attention and affect control, and speech and language development (Bernstein Ratner 1986; Fernald et al., 1989; Kuhl et al., 1997). Although young children rely on both auditory and visual models to learn speech, the characteristics of the visual component of IDS, such as facial and lip movements, have not been identified. In a recent investigation, Green et al. (2007) studied the articulatory modification produced by 24 mothers when speaking to their infants. Lip movements were recorded from the mothers as they interacted with their infants and with an unfamiliar adult. On average, mouth movements were slower and larger during IDS than during adult-directed speech. Parents who exhibited acoustic exaggerations of fundamental frequency also tended to exhibit exaggerated lip movements. These exaggerations in mouth opening during IDS may explain, in part, why children's first utterances are predominantly comprised of consonants in which the primary place of oral constriction is highly visible and why mastery of these same sounds is obtained much earlier than others (Locke 1983).

10.4 **Conclusion**

A comprehensive understanding of speech development will need to account for the factors that shape the course of speech motor development. To this end, direct measures of articulatory performance will be essential. A hypothetical framework is proposed that considers the varying effects of multiple factors on articulatory performance development and thus, speech development. Central to this idea is the expectation for early constraints on articulatory performance and a nonmonotonic growth of articulatory performance. Abrupt changes in articulatory performance with age are considered to reflect fits and spurts in the development of underlying anatomy, sensorimotor control, and linguistic and cognitive skills. The framework motivates further inquiry into (1) defining the features of immature articulatory control, (2) obtaining growth trajectories of articulatory performance variables, and (3) determining longitudinal relations between the development of articulatory performance and other variables (anatomic, physiologic, cognitive, or psychosocial). Findings from our studies on early articulatory development have revealed some characteristic features of early oromotor performance and age-related stages in the development of articulatory control. The results of these studies give the impression that the various components of the vocal tract have a unique developmental course and the immature articulatory system is influenced by multiple production constraints that limit the variety of vocal tract configurations available to the infant. Because our findings are based on cross-sectional studies with only ten or fewer children per age group, the results should be considered tentative until additional large sample and longitudinal studies are conducted. These descriptions will require frequent sampling of articulatory performance to capture potentially rapid change. Of course, this goal will be achieved only through years of research conducted by multiple investigators.

Acknowledgments

This work has been supported by the National Institute of Health, National Institute on Deafness and Other Communication Disorders, Grants R03DC004643 and R01DC006463. The authors would like to thank Chris Moore, Tom Campbell, Gary Weismer, and Erin Wilson for their insights, and Lindsey Fairchild, Kimber Green and Cynthia Didion for preparation of the manuscript.

References

Adams, S. G., Weismer, G., & Kent, R. D. (1993). Speaking rate and speech movement velocity profiles. *Journal of Speech, Language, and Hearing Research, 36*, 41–54.

Adolph, K. E., & Berger, S. A. (2006). Motor development. In W. Damon & R. Lerner (Series Eds.) & D. Kuhn & R. S. Siegler (Vol. Eds.), *Handbook of child psychology: Vol 2: Cognition, perception, and language (6th edn)* (pp. 161–213). New York: Wiley.

Barlow, S. M., Finan, D. S., Bradford, P. T., & Andreatta, R. D. (1993) Transitional properties of the mechanically evoked perioral reflex from infancy through adulthood. *Brain and Language, 623*, 181–188.

Bekoff, M., Kubo, R., & Grey, H. M. (1986). Activation requirements for normal T cells: Accessory cell-dependent and independent stimulation by anti-receptor antibodies. *Journal of Immunology 137*, 1411–1419.

Bernstein, N. A. (1967). *The co-ordination and regulation of movements*. Oxford, UK: Pergamon Press.

Bernstein Ratner, N. (1986). Durational cues which mark clause boundaries in mother–child speech. *Journal of Phonetics, 14*, 303–309.

Bloom, P. (2000). *How children learn the meanings of words*. Cambridge, MA: MIT Press.

Callan, D. E., Kent, R. D., Guenther, F. H., & Vorperian, H. K. (2000). An auditory-feedback-based neural network model of speech production that is robust to developmental changes in the size and shape of the articulatory system. *Journal of Speech, Language, and Hearing Research, 43*, 721–736.

Cheng, H. Y., Murdoch, B. E., Goozée, J. V., & Scott, D. (2007). Physiologic development of tongue-jaw coordination from childhood to adulthood. *Journal of Speech, Language, and Hearing Research, 50*, 352–360.

Corbetta, D., & Bojczyk, K. E. (2002). Infants return to two-handed reaching when they are learning to walk. *Journal of Motivational Behavior, 34*, 83–95.

Cucchiarini, C. (1996). Assessing transcription agreement: Methodological aspects. *Clinical Linguistics & Phonetics, 102*, 131–155.

Fagard, J., & Jacquet, A. (1989). Onset of bimanual coordination and symmetry versus asymmetry of movement. *Infant Behavior and Development, 12*, 229–235.

Fernald, A., Taeschner, T., Dunn, J., Papousek, M., Boysson-Bardies, B., & Fukui, I. (1989). A cross-language study of prosodic modifications in mothers' and fathers' speech to preverbal infants. *Journal of Child Language, 16*, 477–501.

Folkins, J. W., & Linville, R. N. (1983). The effects of varying lower-lip displacement on upper-lip movements: Implications for the coordination of speech movements. *Journal of Speech and Hearing Research, 26*, 209–217.

Goffman, L., & Smith, A. (1999). Development and phonetic differentiation of speech movement patterns. *Journal of Experimental Psychology: Human Perception & Performance, 25*, 649–660.

Goldfield, E. C., & Michel, G. F. (1986). Spatiotemporal linkage in infant interlimb coordination. *Developmental Psychobiology 19*, 259–264.

Green, J. R., (1998). Physiologic development of speech motor control: Articulatory coordination of lips and jaw. (Doctoral dissertation, University of Washington, 1998.)

Green, J. R., Moore, C. A., Higashikawa, M., & Steeve, R. W. (2000). The physiologic development of speech motor control: Lip and jaw coordination. *Journal of Speech, Language, and Hearing Research, 43*, 239–255.

Green, J. R., Moore, C. A., & Reilly, K. J. (2002). The sequential development of jaw and lip control for speech. *Journal of Speech, Language, and Hearing Research, 45*, 66–79.

Green, J. R., Moore, C. A., Ruark, J. L., Rodda, P. R., Morvée, W. T., & VanWitzenburg, M. J. (1997). Development of chewing in children from 12 to 48 months: Longitudinal study of EMG patterns. *Journal of Neurophysiology, 77*, 2704–2716.

Green, J. R., Nip, I. S. B., Mefferd, A. S., Labarge, L., & Wilson, E. M. (2007, November). *Articulatory modifications during infant directed speech.* Paper presented at the meeting of the American Speech-Language Hearing Association, Boston, MA.

Green, J. R., & Wilson, E. M. (2006). Spontaneous facial motility in infancy: A 3D kinematic analysis. *Developmental Psychobiology, 48*, 16–28.

Green, J. R., Wilson, E. M., Wang, Y., & Moore, C. A. (2007). Estimating mandibular motion based on chin surface targets during speech. *Journal of Speech, Language, and Hearing Research, 50*, 928–939.

Grigos, M. I., Saxman, J. H., & Gordon, A. M. (2005). Speech motor development during acquisition of the voicing contrast. *Journal of Speech, Language, and Hearing Research, 48*, 739–752.

Guenther, F. (1995). Speech sound acquisition, coarticulation, and rate effects in a neural network model of speech production. *Psychological Review, 102*, 594–621.

Hall, B. K., & Herring, S. W. (1990). Paralysis and growth of the musculoskeletal system in the embryonic chick. *Journal of Morphology, 206*, 45–56.

Hay, L. (1978). Accuracy of children on an open-loop pointing task. *Perceptual and Motor Skills, 47*, 1079–1082.

Hinton, V. A., & Arokiasamy, W. M. C. (1997). Maximum interlabial pressure in normal speakers. *Journal of Speech, Language, and Hearing Research, 40*, 400–404.

Hughes, O. M., & Abbs, J. H. (1976). Labial-mandibular coordination in the production of speech: Implications for the operation of motor equivalence. *Phonetica, 33*, 199–221.

Humphrey, T. (1971). Development of oral and facial motor mechanisms in human fetuses and their relation to craniofacial growth. *Journal of Dental Research, 50*, 1428–1441.

Jeannerod, M. (1988). The hierarchical organization of visuomotor co-ordination. In *The Neural and Behavioural Organization of Goal-Directed Movements* (15 edn., pp. 55–83). Oxford, UK: |Clarendon Press.

Kent, R. D. (1984). Psychobiology of speech development: Coemergence of language and a movement system. *American Journal of Physiology, 246*, R888–R894.

Kent, R. D., & Miolo, G. (1995). Phonetic abilities in the first year of life. In P. Fletcher & B. MacWhinney (Eds.), *Handbook of Child Language* (pp. 303–334). London: Blackwell.

Kewley-Port, D., & Preston, M. S. (1974). Early apical stop production: A voice onset time analysis. *Journal of Phonetics, 2*, 195–210.

Kowal, S., O'Connell, D. C., & Sabin, E. J. (1975). Development of temporal patterning and vocal hesitations in spontaneous speech. *Journal of Psycholinguistic Research, 4*, 195–207.

Kuhl, P. K., Andruski, J. E., Chistovich, I. A., Chistovich, L. A., Kozhevnikova, E. V., Ryskina, V. L. et al. (1997). Cross-language analysis of phonetic units in language addressed to infants. *Science, 277,* 684–686.

Li, P., Zhao, X., & MacWhinney, B. (2007). Dynamic self-organization and early lexical development in children, *Cognitive Science, 31,* 581–612.

Lindblom, B. (1989). Some remarks on the origin of the phonetic code. In Euler von, Lundberg, & Lennerstrand (Eds.), *Brain and Reading* (pp. 27–44). New York: Stockton Press.

Liu, H. M., Kuhl, P. K., & Tsao, F. M. (2003). An association between mothers' speech clarity and infants' discrimination skills. *Developmental Science, 6,* F1–F10.

Locke, J. L. (1983). *Phonological Acquisition and Change.* New York: Academic Press.

Locke, J. L. (1989). Babbling and early speech: Continuity and individual differences. *First Language, 9,* 191–205.

Locke, J. L. (1993). Learning to speak. *Journal of Phonetics Special Issue: Phonological Development, 21,* 141–146.

MacNeilage, P. F., & Davis, B. F. (2000). Deriving speech from nonspeech: A view from ontogeny. *Phonetica, 57,* 284–296.

McCune, L., & Vihman, M. M. (2001). Early phonetic and lexical development: A productivity approach. *Journal of Speech, Language, & Hearing Research, 44,* 670–684.

Ménard, L., Schwartz, J.-L., & Boë, L.-J., (2004). Role of vocal tract morphology in speech development: Perceptual targets and sensorimotor maps for synthesized French vowels from birth to adulthood. *Journal of Speech, Language, and Hearing Research, 47,* 1059–1080.

Moore, C. A. (1993). Symmetry of mandibular muscle activity as an index of coordinative strategy. *Journal of Speech & Hearing Research, 36,* 1145–1157.

Moore, C. A., & Ruark, J. L. (1996). Does speech emerge from earlier appearing oral motor behaviors? *Journal of Speech & Hearing Research, 39,* 1034–1047.

Motion Analysis Corporation. (2007). Santa Rosa, CA.

Müller, K., Hömberg, V., & Lenard, H. G. (1991). Magnetic stimulation of motor cortex and nerve roots in children: Maturation of cortico-motoneuronal projections. *Electroencephalography and Clinical Neurophysiology, 8,* 163–170.

Newell, K. (1986). Constraints on the development of coordination. In M. G. Wade, & H. T. A. Whiting (Eds.), *Motor Development in Children: Aspects of Coordination and Control* (pp. 341–361). Amsterdam: Martin Nijhoff.

Nip, I. S. B., & Green, J. R. (2006). The development of speaking rate: A kinematic perspective. Paper presented at the Conference on Motor Speech, Austin, TX.

Oller, D. K. (2000). *The Emergence of the Speech Capacity.* Hillsdale, NJ: Lawrence Erlbaum.

Paul, R., & Jennings, P. (1992). Phonological behavior in toddlers with slow expressive language development. *Journal of Speech & Hearing Research, 35,* 99–107.

Perkell, J., Matthies, M., Lane, H., Guenther, F., Wilhelms-Tricarico, R., & Wozniak, J. et al. (1997). Speech motor control: Acoustic goals, saturation effects, auditory feedback and internal models, *Speech Communication, 22,* 227–250.

Potter, N. L., Kent, R. D., Lindstrom, M. J., & Lazarus, J. A. (2006). Power and precision grip force control in three-to-five-year-old children: Velocity control precedes amplitude control in development. *Experimental Brain Research, 172,* 246–260.

Roberts, A. B., Griffin, D., Mooney, R., Cooper, D. J., & Campbell, S. (1980). Fetal activity in 100 normal third trimester pregnancies. *British Journal of Obstetrics and Gynaecology, 87,* 480–484.

Roug, L., Landberg, I., & Lundberg, L. (1989). Phonetic development in early infancy: A study of four Swedish children during the first eighteen months of life. *Journal of Child Language, 17,* 19–40.

Sanders, E. K. (1972). When are speech sounds learned? *Journal of Speech and Hearing Disorders, 37,* 55–63.

Sharkey, S. G., & Folkins, J. W. (1985). Variability of lip and jaw movements in children and adults: Implications for the development of speech motor control. *Journal of Speech & Hearing Research, 28*, 8–15.

Shriberg, L. D., & Kent, R. D. (2002). *Clinical Phonetics (3rd edn).* Boston: Allyn & Bacon.

Shriberg, L. D., & Lof, G. L. (1991). Reliability studies in broad and narrow phonetic transcription. *Clinical Linguistics & Phonetics, 5*, 225–279.

Smith, A., & Goffman, L. (1998). Stability and patterning of speech movement sequences in children and adults. *Journal of Speech, Language, & Hearing Research, 41*, 18–30.

Smith, A., & Goffman, L. (2004). Interaction of motor and language factors in the development of speech production. In B. Maasen, R. Kent, H. Peters, P. van Lieshout, & W. Hulstijn (Eds.), *Speech Motor Control in Normal and Disordered Speech* (pp. 227–252). Oxford, UK: Oxford University Press.

Smith, A., & Zelaznik, H. N. (2004). Development of functional synergies for speech motor coordination in childhood and adolescence. *Developmental Psychobiology, 45*, 22–33.

Smith, B. L., & McLean-Muse, A. (1986). Articulatory movement characteristics of labial consonant productions of children and adults. *Journal of the Acoustical Society of America, 80*, 1321–1328.

Sporns, O., & Edelman, G. M. (1993). Solving Bernstein's problem: A proposal for the development of coordinated movement by selection. *Child Development, 64*, 960–981.

Stockman, E. J., Woods, D. R., & Tishman, A. (1981). Listener agreement on phonetic segments in early infant vocalizations. *Journal of Psycholinguistic Research, 19*, 593–617.

Stoel-Gammon, C. (1985). Phonetic inventories, 15–24 months: A longitudinal study. *Journal of Speech and Hearing Research, 28*, 505–512.

Stoel-Gammon, C. (1998). Sounds and words in early language acquisition: The relationship between lexical and phonological development. In P. Rhea (Ed.), *Exploring the Speech-Language Connection. Communication and Language Intervention Series, Volume 8* (pp. 25–52). Baltimore: Paul H. Brookes Publishing Co.

Stoel-Gammon, C., &. Dunn, C. (1985). *Normal and Disordered Phonology in Children.* Austin, TX: Pro-Ed.

Studdert-Kennedy, M. (1991). Comment: The emergent gesture. In I. G. Mattingly, M. Ignatius & M. Studdert-Kennedy (Eds.), *Modularity and the Motor Theory of Speech Perception: Proceedings of a Conference to Honor Alvin M. Liberman* (pp. 85–90). Hillsdale, NJ: Lawrence Erlbaum.

Thelen, E. (1985). Developmental origins of motor coordination: Leg movements in human infants. *Developmental Psychobiology, 18*, 1–22.

Thelen, E. (1991). Motor aspects of emergent speech: A dynamic approach. In N. A. Krasnegor, D. M. Rumbaugh, R. L. Schiefelbusch, & M. Studdert-Kennedy (Eds.), *Biological and Behavioral Determinants of Language Development* (pp. 339–362). Hillsdale, NJ: Lawrence Erlbaum.

Thelen, E., & Cooke, D. W. (1987). Relationship between newborn stepping and later walking: A new interpretation. *Developmental Medicine & Child Neurology, 29*, 380–393.

Thelen, E., & Fisher, D. M. (1983). From spontaneous to instrumental behavior: Kinematic analysis of movement changes during very early learning. *Child Development, 54*, 129–140.

Thelen, E., & Smith, L. (1994). *A Dynamic Systems Approach to the Development of Cognition and Action.* Cambridge, MA: MIT Press.

Vihman, M. M. (1986). Individual differences in babbling and early speech: Predicting to age three. In B. Lindblom, & R. Zetterstom (Eds.), *Precursors of Early Speech* (pp. 95–112). Basingstroke, UK: MacMillan.

Vihman, M. M., Macken, M., Miller, R., Simmons, H., & Miller, J. (1985). From babbling to speech: A re-assessment of the continuity issue. *Language, 61*, 397–445.

Vorperian, H. K., Kent, R. D., Gentry, L. R., & Yandell, B. S. (1999). Magnetic resonance imaging procedures to study the concurrent anatomic development of vocal tract structures: Preliminary results. *International Journal of Pediatric Otorhinolaryngology, 49*, 197–206.

Walker, J. F., Archibald, L. M. D., Cherniak, S. R., & Fish, V. G. (1992). Articulation rate in 3- and 5-year-old children. *Journal of Speech, Language and Hearing Research, 35*, 4–13.

Weismer, G. (2006). Philosophy of research in motor speech disorders, *Clinical Linguistics & Phonetics, 20*, 315–349.

Wetherby, A., and Prizant, B. (2002). *Communication and Symbolic Behavior Scales- Developmental Profile* (First Normed Edition). Baltimore: Paul H. Brookes Publishing.

Wimmers, R. H., Savelsbergh, G.-J. P., Beek, P. J., & Hopkins, B. (1998). Evidence for a phase transition in the early development of prehension. *Developmental Psychobiology, 32*, 235–248.

Section 4

Fluency disorders

Chapter 11

Speech motor variability in people who stutter

Pascal van Lieshout and Aravind K. Namasivayam

Abstract

Variability in oral motor control has been an important topic in the literature for many years. The typical view is that motor output can be interpreted as a mixture of an invariant control signal (e.g., motor command) contaminated by a degree of random variation or neuromotor noise. This variation is supposed to originate somewhere along the pathway from the central nervous system where the command was generated to the peripheral structures responsible for its execution. In this chapter, different concepts on variability in speech production are explored in more detail using examples of speech kinematic data from people who stutter and normal speaking individuals. The data indicate that popular indices of variability when applied to the same dataset are at odds with each other in terms of identifying specific trends for an individual or groups of individuals. Beyond these data examples, this chapter presents a new approach (for speech) to confront the challenging question if (and how) it is possible to identify the nature of movement variability and its potential relevance for speech motor control.

11.1 **Introduction**

For people who stutter (PWS) and other individuals with speech motor problems, it is often assumed that the underlying patho-physiology increases the amount of variability in their control system, making it harder for them to produce a stable output. In this chapter, we present a general discussion of the concept of variability; how it can be defined, the typical ways of measuring it and their limitations, the alternatives that exist and how we could, and perhaps should, move beyond a mere quantification of variability as a random (i.e., stochastic) influence. In order to make our case, we will question the view that typically attributes a negative role to variation in speech motor output by presenting some recent findings from studies that utilize concepts and methods based on dynamical systems theory or DST (see Van Lieshout 2004, for a basic introduction on this topic). There are obviously other views on variability (e.g., Howell et al., Chapter 12 this volume; Smith et al., 2000; Van Galen and van Huygevoort 2000) and some of these will be discussed as well. However, the focus of this chapter will be on the DST perspective, which highlights that variability may actually serve an important role in that it can enhance the motor control system's adaptability to respond to both short- and long-term changes in demands imposed on the motor system (e.g., Kelso 1995; Newell and Slifkin 1998). On the basis of some recent studies in limb control, we will take this notion a bit further in highlighting that variability comes in different flavours, ranging from truly stochastic to quasi-deterministic. Where possible, we will illustrate these concepts with examples from our own laboratory including data from studies on speech motor variability in stuttering. In conclusion, we will argue in line with DST that the presence of (non-random) variability in the coordination of speech gestures may highlight specific and important aspects of motor control that would be overlooked with more traditional approaches.

11.2 The concept of variability in (speech) motor control

Variability in general can be defined as the fluctuation of a value over repeated measurements (Chau et al., 2005). Figure 11.1 shows some of the main potential sources of measured signal output variation, categorized as subject, task specific, and external factors. Its main goal is to illustrate that output variation(s) as measured from the actual behaviours and which are often labelled in the singular term 'variability', show a wide disparity with respect to their potential nature, origin, and temporal dependencies (e.g., compare variations within a single trial versus variations over time in specific movement characteristics; Alfonso and Van Lieshout 1997).

In the case of speech production, different sources of variability can add and interact in the chain of processes starting at the cortical level and ending with the actual implementation at the articulator level. In the end, the influences of these different sources of variability (normal and/or pathological) converge on the same output mechanism. Uniquely identifying these sources seems a near impossible task as the nature of their interaction is basically unknown. Just imagine a person who stutters, talking about an emotional topic while dividing attention between talking and writing a note for the person he/she is communicating with in a restaurant with background music and people talking. Though extreme, it is nonetheless a realistic scenario that is obvious to all of us who experience on a daily basis many of such real-life situations.

For the sake of argumentation, the discussion around the concept of variability in (speech) motor control will be framed in a overtly simple dichotomy of two opposing views, one labelled the traditional view and the other, the dynamical systems view (Van Lieshout 2004). Although these

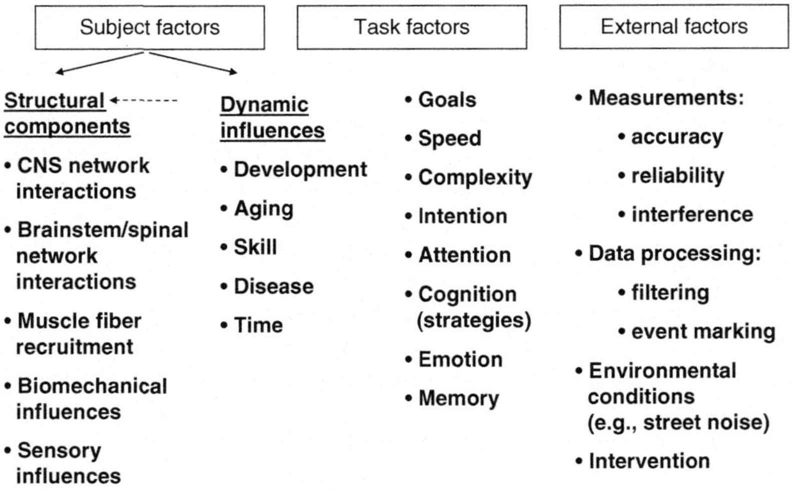

Fig. 11.1 Simplified overview of some of the main potential sources of variation in measured signal output, categorized as subject, task specific, and external factors (see text for more details).

two views do characterize a real contrast in the speech literature (Newell 2003), there is a lot of grey area between them. The following paragraphs will provide more detail on the traditional view, followed by Section 11.3 on methods of measuring variability, which mostly derive their meaning from this view. Section 11.4 will then elaborate on the DST view and provide some further illustrations of how its concepts can be translated into specific measures of variability.

In the traditional view, motor output is interpreted as the resultant of an invariant control signal (e.g., the motor command) which typically is (implicitly or explicitly) assumed to be contaminated by some random variation somewhere along the pathway from the central nervous system where the command was generated to the peripheral structures responsible for its execution. In line with this interpretation, variation in motor output is often labelled neuromotor noise and regarded as a 'nuisance' that interferes with a smooth and accurate implementation of the original motor command (e.g., Walsh et al., 2006; Van Galen and van Huygevoort 2000; see also Newell 2003 for a discussion on this topic). From a modelling perspective, the traditional view can be interpreted as separating a movement signal into two independent components, viz. a deterministic part and a random noise part (Riley and Turvey 2002). A deterministic signal displays a predictable relationship among changes over time that (in principle) can be simulated by unique solutions to a mathematical set of equations. A simplified version of this can be found in the often used model for a mass-spring system (equation 11.1) which describes a single dimension motion as a function of a position variable (x_i) and its derivatives (*v*elocity and *a*cceleration) influenced by mass (m), damping (d), and stiffness (s) parameters as well as the target position (x_0) of the system in motion (e.g., Ostry and Munhall 1985):

$$F(x) = ma + dv + s(x_i - x_0) \qquad (11.1)$$

Equation 11.1 describes a situation where an effector moves to a particular target position, but it is fairly simple to make such a system continuous (cyclic) by adding a forcing function that provides energy to sustain the movement (compare to someone pushing a child in a swing once versus repeatedly at specific intervals). A possible output of the latter system in terms of changes in position over time can be seen in the top panel of Fig. 11.2. This highly deterministic output can be contrasted with a signal that is created by a truly random mechanism, where prior and future states are completely independent from each other. This type of random behaviour can be modelled using a white noise generator, as shown in the second panel of Fig. 11.2. The two component model of movement control is simply the addition of these two parts as shown in the third panel. For a less abstract depiction of movement signals, it is important to incorporate some characteristics of biological systems, like the ones used for speech. For such systems, it has been suggested that neuromotor noise at the muscular level may be low-pass filtered or integrated through the complex multi-system interactions between neural circuitries and effector biomechanics (Prinz 2006), which not only changes the nature of noise at the periphery but may also provide a mechanism to reduce its overall impact on movement accuracy (Van Galen and van Huygevoort 2000). The integrated white noise over time is referred to as a random walk and panel 4 shows the random walk signal based on the white noise signal depicted in panel 2, the original deterministic control signal from panel 1 and their combination. To illustrate that this depiction of a traditional model has some merit, panel 5 shows actual tongue body data over time from a subject repeating the nonword 'api', showing a strong similarity to the combined synthetic signal depicted in panel 4.

Also within the context of the traditional view on variability, is the suggestion that variability is controlled in a task-specific manner, the purpose of which is to reduce variability as a source of instability. For example, jaw perturbation studies carried out by Ostry and co-workers (e.g., Shiller et al., 2005) suggests that articulatory stiffness of the jaw may be actively modified in

1

2

3

4

5

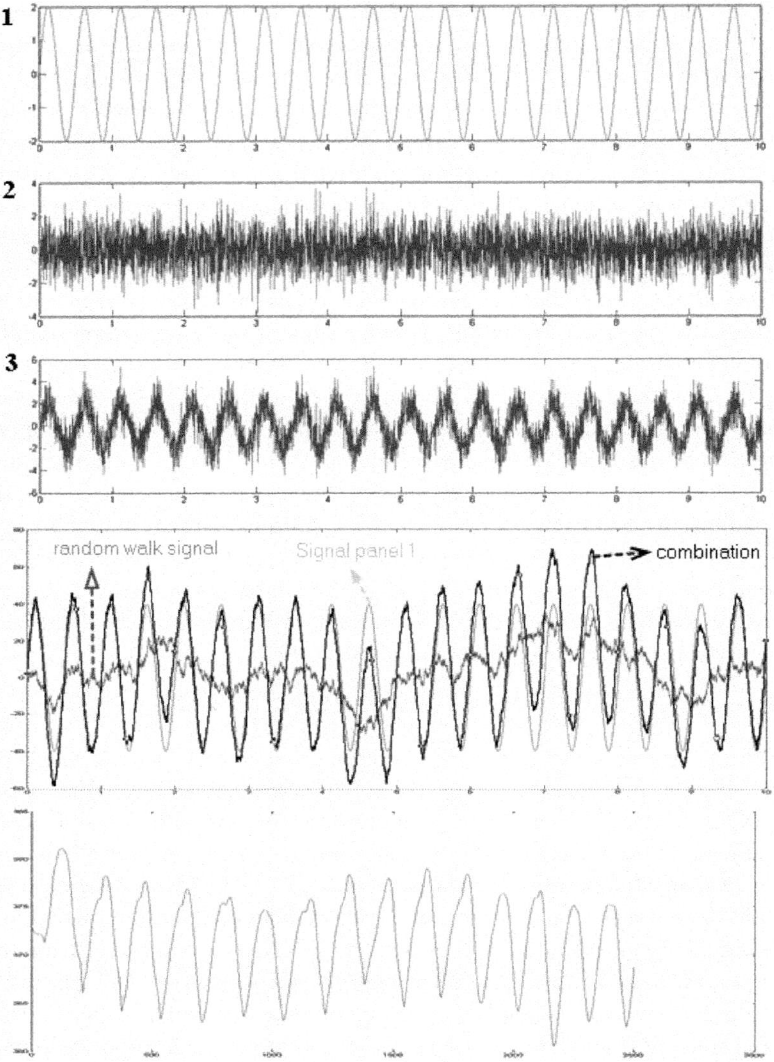

Fig. 11.2 Illustration of a deterministic signal (panel 1), random noise signal (panel 2), their combination (panel 3), combination of deterministic signal with random walk signal (panel 4), actual tongue body signal (panel 5) (see text for more details).

specific directions to reduce variability in speech production that arises from interaction forces generated by articulators. Specifically, the manner in which jaw stiffness was modified in their study was related to the direction of the applied perturbation. When perturbing forces were applied in 16 directions spaced equally along a circle in the mid-sagittal plane using a robot arm firmly attached to the lower jaw, they observed increased jaw stiffness in the vertical as compared to lateral or horizontal directions. Increased stiffness was associated with decreased variability and so these results indicate that articulatory variability in the mandible is reduced for the dimension that is critical for accurate speech production, viz. vocal tract constriction degree. However, it has to be noted that these findings were found for both speech and non-speech tasks, so it likely reflects a more basic adaptation in the oral control system. Further support for directional control of variability can be found for other articulators as well. For example, it has been demonstrated that for high front vowels (e.g., /i/) variability of tongue movements is greater in the front–back (constriction location) dimension of the vocal tract than in the up–down (constriction degree) dimension (Beckman et al., 1995; see Nieto-Castanon et al., 2005 for a similar finding in American English /r/ production). Together, such findings suggest that constriction degree for a given articulator is more tightly controlled than constriction location to prevent large (non-linear) changes in speech acoustics associated with variations in cross-sectional area and resulting aerodynamic consequences (Stevens 1989).

This task-specific control of variability is an important concept and is closely related to optimality control principles in sensory motor control (Todorov and Ghahramani 2004). Optimality control theory suggests that control mechanisms do not correct deviations in movement behaviours unless those deviations affect task performance (commonly referred to as the 'minimal intervention' principle). That is, if we presume articulatory configurations are vectors within a multi-dimensional state space, then according to the optimality control principle a state vector for a particular task is free to vary in directions that do not interfere with the task goal ('uncontrolled manifold'; Scholz and Schöner 1999). For speech, the dimension associated with constriction degree is an important dimension as it has immediate aerodynamic (and thus acoustic) consequences (Catford 1977), and reducing variability in this dimension seems a sensible strategy as discussed above. This does not mean that constriction location for a particular articulator is not important, but apparently in terms of emergent acoustic consequences less sensitive to variations away from a (assumed) target position (see also Hoole 1999). However, despite these insightful observations regarding the task-specific nature of variability control, the basic tenet of controlling (or rather, reducing) variability remains in line with the notion that variability is a random intrusion to an otherwise supposedly invariant specific movement target. A contrasting view based on DST principles will be presented in Section 11.4. This is not to say that according to DST random noise influences do not exist and may not be a source of instability; rather, in DST variability becomes a more qualified concept, allowing for a wider range of options in which variability plays a useful role to enhance flexibility (see also Walsh et al., 2006 for a discussion on this topic in the context of speech motor development), as well as to include a more in-depth investigation into the actual characteristics of variability, in particular, whether it being truly random or not (and why this would matter).

11.3 **How to assess variability in (speech) motor control**

Regardless of one's view on the nature and relevance of variability, it is critical that the phenomenon as such can be captured, summarized, and compared across conditions in a reliable and quantifiable way. Many of these phenomena are defined around discrete events in time like movement onset/offset and peak velocity, and include conventional measures to quantify variability like the standard deviation of a distribution, or its normalized version, called the coefficient of variation (CV = SD/Mean). For such measures, it is assumed that variations around a central moment (e.g., mean) are randomly distributed. These measures tend to be very sensitive to individual outliers (Chau et al., 2005). Although such outliers can be detected, removed, and replaced using statistical software, the application of such techniques is less straightforward with disordered speech data as the true range of that distribution is often unknown. Thus, what seems an outlier may actually be a relevant feature of their behavioural repertoire. An alternative is to use measures that are less sensitive to outliers like the interquartile range (IQR) and the median absolute deviation (MAD), or to determine multi-modal characteristics in data distributions (Chau et al., 2005). IQR is the difference between the 75 and 25 percentile scores, whereas MAD is the median value of the absolute difference between the original value minus the median for a particular dataset. For MAD and IQR, the number of outliers would have to exceed 25% of the sample set before biasing the estimates (Chau et al., 2005).

A different approach towards measuring variability in speech-related movements was proposed by Anne Smith and colleagues (Smith et al., 1995). Their argument is that traditional kinematic measurements sample only one particular discrete aspect (e.g., peak velocity) of an entire motion trajectory and hence are insufficient to assess more general properties of movement control. To address this issue, they proposed a measure that captures variability in the patterning of a movement trajectory that corresponds to a predetermined analysis unit (e.g., a sentence like 'buy bobby a puppy'). This measure is called the spatio-temporal index (STI) and typically uses amplitude and time normalized segments of motion trajectories of single articulators, although one could also use a trajectory that reflects the net result of combined activity, like for example, the distance between the lips (Smith and Zelaznik 2004). These normalized segments are then evaluated in terms of how well they converge on a single pattern, as indexed by a summed series of standard deviations at selected points in normalized time. The underlying assumption of the STI measure is that speech is highly practiced and stable, hence the expectation that amplitude and time normalized movement trajectories of repeated utterances should fall upon a single core template (i.e., the original manifestation of the intended motor plan). The lower the STI value the lesser the deviation from a core template. In the area of stuttering research, Kleinow and Smith (2000) found that for PWS more complex syntactic structures, regardless of utterance length, reduced the stability (higher STI) of lower lip movements. Accordingly, they suggested that movement variability might not be a general characteristic of PWS but rather is triggered by linguistic demands. Similar results have been found in adult fluent speakers, showing that changes in cognitive and/or linguistic demands influenced variability of speech motor performance as indexed by STI and other variables (Dromey and Benson 2003; Van Lieshout et al., 1995).

The STI technique in more general terms is referred to as registration (Ramsay and Silverman 2005). In the case of STI, the registration is linear, stretching and/or compressing an entire part of a trajectory in a uniform way. A recent study compared different methods of registration using synthetic wavelet data, showing that a non-linear method provides the most accurate estimates of true variability (Lucero 2005). Unlike STI, this method has the additional benefit that it can separate temporal and spatial sources of variability. There are also other methods, like the piece-wise technique which uses a linear normalization between kinematic events of interest within the unit of analysis, as identified by for example, peaks in lower lip displacement (Ward and Arnfield 2001). A simplification of the latter technique can be achieved in restricting the unit of analysis to a smaller (i.e., more basic) motor unit like a motion cycle (Van Lieshout and Moussa 2000). In the latter approach, rhythmic movement cycles are assumed to be the underlying unit of speech (syllabic) production roughly corresponding to gestural units (Goldstein and Fowler 2003). Gestures are considered basic building blocks for speech production (and perception) and therefore the consistency of their production may represent a basic feature of core stability in the speech motor system. Using the same calculations as STI, the resultant measure is dubbed c(yclic) STI (Van Lieshout and Moussa 2000).

To illustrate the use of different types of variability measures, we took tongue body gesture data[1] from a single subject, producing the nonword 'api' repeatedly for about 10–12 seconds at different rates (slow, normal, and fast) under both self-paced and metronome conditions (because

[1] A gesture at the kinematic level is defined as the distance travelled by a particular articulator in a two-dimensional space (Van Lieshout et al., 2007).

timing relationships might differ for these two manipulations). For practical purposes, we picked three representational measures from the ones discussed above: (1) CV, (2) MAD, and (3) cSTI. CV represents a widely used measure of variability for discrete kinematic measures but one that is sensitive to outliers. MAD is an alternative that can capture variability in discrete events but is less sensitive to outliers. The cSTI measure can be used to index the consistency of producing individual movement cycles and unlike CV and MAD reflects characteristics of the entire cycle, not just a selection of discrete points within it, as explained above. As shown in Fig. 11.3 in the left upper panel (average movement cycle duration), this subject succeeded in making a systematic and reliable distinction between the three rate conditions, with or without a metronome (the latter was set to match the self-paced rates produced by this subject for the three rate conditions). Upon inspection of the data it is clear that the different variability measures are not consistent with each other. Indicated in the upper right panel of Fig. 11.3, CV data show a decrease in relative variability from slow to fast rates in metronome-paced trials, whereas for self-paced trials both slow and fast rates show lower values compared to preferred rate. For MAD data (Fig. 11.3, bottom left panel) a systematic decrease in values from slow to fast rates is seen for both self-paced and metronome trials. For cSTI, (Fig. 11.3, bottom right panel) both self-paced and metronome trials show the same pattern as that of self-paced trials in CV data (i.e., highest values for preferred speech rate condition). In short, depending on which variability measure is used the data can tell a different story for this individual and there is no clear reason why one measure should be 'better' or 'preferred', except for the statistical arguments mentioned above (e.g., less sensitivity to outliers).

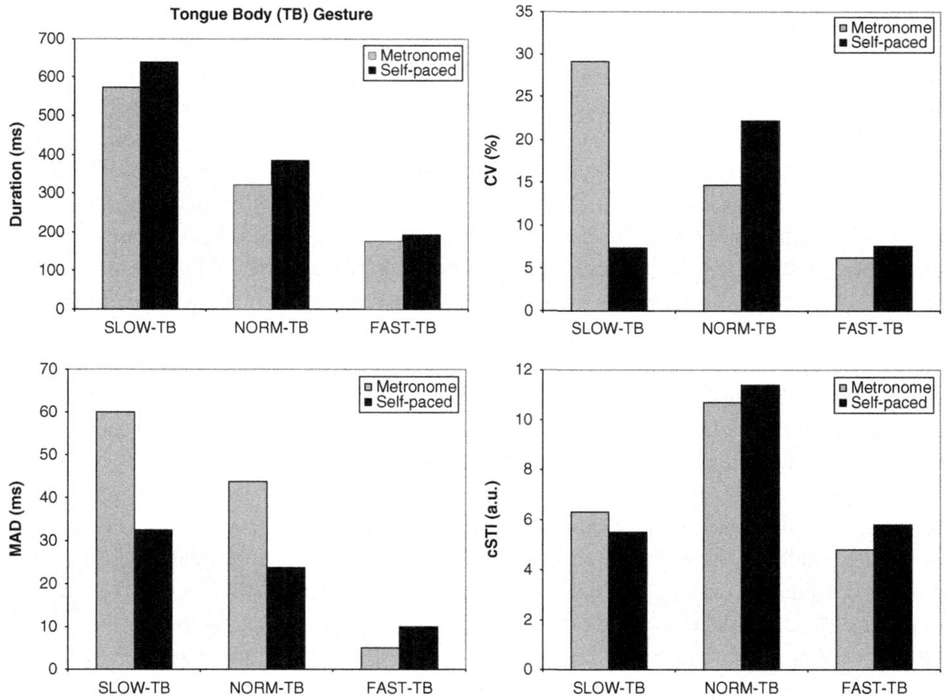

Fig. 11.3 Single subject data on kinematic variability for tongue body gesture motion in the production of the nonword /api/ under self-pacing and metronome conditions. Shown are average cycle duration (upper left panel), coefficient of variation (CV) in upper right panel, MAD data in bottom left panel, and cSTI values in bottom right panel (See text for more details).

With regards to the stuttering literature, initial efforts failed to find consistent group differences between PWS and people who do not stutter (PNS) for discrete movement parameters and their variability (e.g., displacement, velocity, duration, displacement–velocity ratios). This forced researchers to look for other measures that were more promising for distinguishing between these two groups, in particular with respect to movement coordination (for a review see Alfonso 1991; Peters et al., 2000). Early attempts to study coordination in multi-articulate systems focused on the relative contribution of various articulators towards a speech target, for example during bilabial closure (Alfonso and Van Lieshout 1997; Caruso et al., 1988). However, PWS and PNS demonstrated equal amounts of variability in the relative contribution of articulators towards a particular task goal (e.g., bilabial closure) within and across sessions (Alfonso and Van Lieshout 1997), confirming the presence of an inherent (normal) variability in the speech motor system (see also Packman et al., 1996; Peters et al., 2000; Van Lieshout et al., 2004). Similar results were found for other measures in this area, for example with respect to the temporal sequencing and timing of discrete articulatory events (e.g., Alfonso and Van Lieshout 1997; De Nil and Abbs 1991; but see Van Lieshout et al., 1994). For these studies, variability was interpreted as being random in nature, reflecting the presence of neuromotor noise in line with the traditional view mentioned in Section 11.2. One of the problems associated with relative timing measures of the sort discussed so far is that they may be strongly biased by individual differences in movement duration and/or movement amplitude as for example, induced by changes in speech rate (Kelso et al., 1986).

A potential solution to the latter problem can be found in a measure of relative timing (i.e., the degree of synchronization between events in motor control) that is independent of absolute changes in movement duration and amplitude, namely relative phase (Kelso et al., 1986; Van Lieshout et al., 1997). This measure fits well with the concept of coordinative structures (aka functional synergies) in motor control which are typically modelled as (non-linear) oscillatory systems (Kelso 1995). For such systems, relative phase captures how two structures mutually engaged in performing a certain task are synchronized with each other, as expressed in a phase lag. Phase refers to the portion of a movement cycle (defined by normalized position and velocity values in a polar coordinate system) relative to a specified reference point (e.g., onset of movement). The phase lag then shows the difference in phase between two movements at any given point of time. This can be done at discrete events (e.g., peak velocities) or it can be done quasi-continuously, estimating the phase lag for every point on the unit circle. To give an example, if upper and lower lip are engaged in a bilabial closure gesture, they move in opposite directions which will be shown in a phase lag close to 180° or π radians (= out-of-phase).

Relative phase measurements provide information on movement coordination that can be tracked over time in order to study their evolving dynamics, for example within a single trial of reiterated speech (Van Lieshout 2004). For speech, relative phase can be measured at two levels, namely between (inter-gestural) and within (intra-gestural) gestures (e.g., Browman and Goldstein 1992; Van Lieshout et al., 2007). The intra-gestural level of coordination indicates how individual articulators within a functional synergy work cooperatively to achieve a task goal (e.g., how upper and lower lip work as a unit towards a common task goal for bilabial closure). Inter-gestural coordination on the other hand indicates the phase relationship between two independent gestures (e.g. bilabial closure and tongue body constriction), which is typically influenced by higher order linguistic constraints (Goldstein et al., 2007). As continuous relative phase measurements can only be used for relatively uniform cyclic events, it is important to identify those frequency components that correspond closely to the main neural drive that shapes these patterns, assuming an oscillatory origin at the gestural level (Goldstein and Fowler 2003; Van Lieshout 2001; Van Lieshout and Goldstein 2008). These frequency components are referred to as motion primitives because they are considered to form the underlying control elements of the composite motion trajectory and they can be identified using cross-spectral analysis (Namasivayam and Van Lieshout 2008). On the basis of the identified motion primitives one can band-pass filter the movement signals for the dominant frequency and calculate a clean estimate of relative phase (Van Lieshout et al., 2007). The relative phase analysis does not need to be limited to the dominant primitive, as the nature and variability of secondary motion primitives can be equally important in the overall stability of speech motor control (Van Lieshout et al., 2004). From the spectral analysis, one can also derive another measure of coordination, namely cross-spectral mean coherence (Namasivayam and Van Lieshout 2008). This is a measure that quantifies the average degree of frequency coupling between frequency components across two signals and provides an estimate of entrainment (i.e., degree of frequency synchronization between coupled structures). As frequency and phase are independent components of the movement cycle, cross-spectral coherence and relative phase reflect different aspects of the coupling relationship between individual articulators (intra-gestural) or gestures (inter-gestural). For example, two articulators can show a high level of entrainment (spectral coherence) but a variable degree of consistency in their relative phase.

To illustrate the use of coordination measures like relative phase and cross-spectral mean coherence Fig. 11.4 shows data related to the inter-gestural coupling between tongue body constriction gestures for /i/ and /a/ and the biliabial closure gesture for /p/ in the nonword /api/. These are based on the same single subject data as shown in Fig. 11.3. The top panel illustrates that there is no difference in relative phase values for self-paced and metronome paced trials, but there is an overall tendency for relative phase values to increase from slow to fast rates in both pacing conditions.

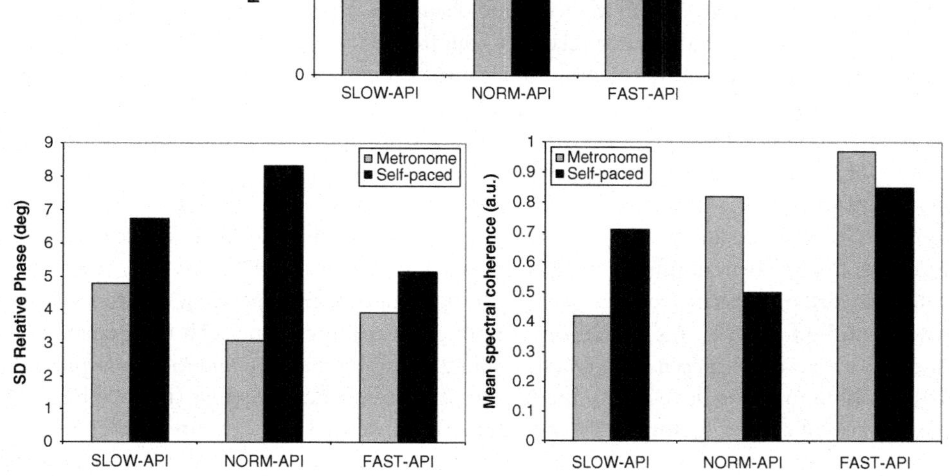

Fig. 11.4 Relative phase (top panel), SD relative phase (left bottom panel), and mean cross-spectral coherence values (right bottom panel) for tongue body gesture and lip closure gesture coordination based on the same subject and conditions as presented in Fig. 11.3 (see text for more details).

The within-trial standard deviation (SD) of relative phase (lower left panel in Fig. 11.4) is less variable for metronome speech, which fits well with other motor studies, where auditory pacing signals were found to stabilize motor coordination (Fink et al., 2000). In the study by Fink and colleagues, it was found that for a bimanual coordination task where participants had to move their left and right index finger in either an in- or out-phase pattern, subjects showed less temporal and spatial variation at reversal points (flexion and extension) when they were synchronized with a auditory metronome signal. In addition, this condition delayed phase shifts as typically found in the out-of-phase pattern. In modelling their findings the authors introduced an environmental parameter to the original Haken-Kelso-Bunz (HKB) model of dynamic coupling (Haken et al., 1985). This parameter represents an extra periodic drive to the internal coupling of effectors, which essentially strengthens the ongoing oscillatory behaviour of that coupling making it less sensitive to an increase in variability at points of phase transitions. Thus, it preserves the system's capability to produce different phase patterns in a relatively stable manner across a wider range of movement parameters. One could argue, that this is tantamount to a mechanism that reduces the impact of neuromotor noise at specific points in the movement cycle while at the same time allowing for variability elsewhere, including in the type of coupling behaviours. As such, it has some similarity to the uncontrolled manifold concept discussed above (Scholz and Schöner 1999) and fits well with the notion of piecewise determinism discussed in Riley and Turvey (2002). In the latter theory, certain regions in the phase plot (position versus velocity) of trajectories corresponding to rhythmic movements show reduced variability, and these regions are assumed to 'play a role in the perceptual regulation of coordinated movements' (p. 112; Riley and Turvey 2002).

Further inspection of the SD relative phase values in Fig. 11.4, reveals an opposite trend for self-paced and metronome-paced trials with respect to rate variations. For self-paced trials variability is lower in both slower and faster rates compared to normal rate. This increase in variability for self-paced speech at normal rates parallels the increase in kinematic variability of CV and cSTI found for these data (Fig. 11.3). In contrast, for metronome-paced trials the lowest variability is found for normal rate. Notice also that for both metronome and self-paced conditions the slower rate shows a more variable phase coupling compared to faster rates.

With respect to cross-spectral coherence (lower right panel in Fig. 11.4), fast rates for both metronome and self-paced speech show the highest values. This fits well with the expectation that at faster rates motion signals tend to show a more simplified harmonic spectrum with fewer (but clearly defined) peaks resulting in a relatively high frequency entrainment for those frequencies (Peper et al., 1995). For self-paced trials, normal speech rate conditions show the lowest coherence, which aligns with the higher values for SD relative phase. This combination of reduced frequency entrainment and increased phase variability provides a control system with more flexibility to adapt to changes in demands on coordination. One could argue that the speed at which one habitually speaks is optimized for maintaining flexibility while preserving a certain degree of stability to implement and preserve the ongoing coupling relationship. This is nicely detailed in the concept of 'relative coordination' as described by Scott Kelso (1995).

Recent work on speech errors has also shown that in producing speech at different rates, the system employs mechanisms to stabilize coupling relationships. One such mechanism that is especially active at fast speech rates, when coupling strength is reduced and more complex ratios are difficult to maintain, is to reduce the complexity of frequency couplings (indexed by the frequency ratio of coupled gestures). This is achieved by inserting extra gestures (called intrusion gestures) to create a more basic and more stable, but also less flexible 1:1 coupling ratio (Goldstein et al., 2007). This means that at fast speech rates, flexibility is reduced to the extent that one can perform a task fast and stable only if it can be done in a fairly stereotypical manner (i.e., with a 1:1 coupling ratio). For the metronome-paced speech data shown in Fig. 11.4, normal rates also show less coherence, but in contrast to self-paced trials, the variability of relative phase is lower compared to the other conditions. As mentioned above, the extrinsic timing is likely to stabilize coordination (Fink et al., 2000). In metronome speech, it is the slow rate condition that shows the lowest coherence and highest relative phase variability. This can partly be explained by the increase in spectral components, creating more complex coupling ratios. Furthermore, unlike other rates, the benefit of an extrinsic timing signal is less obvious at this slow rate condition (see Jirsa et al., 2000 for a discussion on this topic). This echoes with the findings from a study by Boutsen et al. (2000), who found that for slower than habitual speech PWS did not show the expected decrease in temporal variability under speaking with a metronome, as was found in other studies when subjects were speaking at a faster rate (Janssen and Wieneke 1987).

There are only a few studies in the stuttering literature that report the use of coordination measures like relative phase. For example, Ward (1997) compared relative phase differences to other relative timing measures. There were no group differences between PWS and PNS in articulator sequencing, but they did appear for relative phase (between upper lip and jaw). Specifically, PWS showed greater variability in the relative phase measure than PNS at fast rates of speech and when altered stress patterns had to be produced. In contrast, a study by Jäncke and colleagues (Jäncke et al., 1995) measured relative phase between jaw and lip movements across speaking rates with two different stress patterns but failed to elicit any group differences in phase angle or phase angle variability. This was also the case for a more recent study using oral articulatory perturbations (bite-block), where PWS and PNS were found to be similar in their variability of intragestural (between upper and lower lip) relative phase values at either normal or fast rates of speech (Namasivayam et al., 2008).

In order to provide some tentative explanations for these differences across studies, we introduce the concept of a motor control strategy (Van Lieshout et al., 1993; Van Lieshout 1995). A motor control strategy in this context is defined as a sub-conscious task-specific control mechanism that induces a more stable performance at the cost of reduced flexibility. The example of intrusion gestures mentioned above (Goldstein et al., 2007) can be seen as one particular instantiation of a motor control strategy of this type. In our work we have found evidence for the use of motor control strategies that provide a way to strengthen coordination patterns in the context of reduced overall stability due to limitations in motor skill as assumed to underlie stuttering behaviours (Van Lieshout et al., 2004). For example, the Namasivayam et al. (2008) study revealed a significant increase in upper lip movement amplitude in PWS relative to PNS in the presence of a bite-block and at fast speech rates. This increase in movement amplitude was associated with a decrease in upper lip cSTI values in PWS in comparison to PNS. Interestingly, no such amplitude differences between the groups were found for lower lip data and in fact, PWS were found to have higher cSTI values than PNS for this articulator especially at normal speech rates (see also Smith and Kleinow 2000). In line with the suggestion that the upper lip may have less importance in the expression of linguistic contrasts during speech production (Barlow and Netsell 1986) it is speculated that its main function is to ensure stability of lip closing in bilabial tasks through the entrainment of kinesthetic feedback at the level of the neural oscillators that control the articulators (see Van Lieshout 2004; Van Lieshout et al., 2007 for more details on this notion). In a different study, we have also found the opposite to be true in that a physical limitation in the use of the upper lip (due to scarring resulting from surgery to repair an upper lip cleft) was associated with a more variable upper lip movement and bilabial coordination pattern (Van Lieshout et al., 2002). Further support for the use of this motor control strategy and extending it beyond the use of lips was found in a study with a patient suffering from acquired apraxia of speech (AOS), where it was shown that the amplitude of tongue body and bilabial closure gestures involved in a simple speech task seem to have a direct impact on the stability of their coordination (Van Lieshout et al., 2007).

A recent study from our laboratory adds another dimension to this issue, namely on the role of sensory information in coordination. In this study, we perturbed both auditory and kinesthetic sensory systems using masking noise and tendon vibration either in isolation or combined (Namasivayam et al., 2009). To further increase the demands on motor control a bite-block was also used, either on its own or with different combinations of feedback perturbations while speech rate was varied for a group of PWS and matched PNS. Subjects produced VCV nonwords, two of which required lip closure with tactile contact between the lips (/ipa/ and /api/) while the third was produced with no midsagittal tactile contact between the lips (/awi/). Findings from the study suggest that when sensory systems were perturbed at fast speaking rates, PNS had significantly higher variability for intra-gestural relative phase than PWS. The latter group also showed a significantly greater upper lip movement under these circumstances, which again, may suggest the use of a motor control strategy as described above. However, at the inter-gestural level, the combined (masking noise + tendon vibration) presence of perturbation increased variability of relative phase at fast speech rates for both groups of speakers in comparison to no perturbation or tendon vibration alone conditions, but only for nonword /awi/ (which has less tactile lip contact). Contrary to the popular notion that sensory information may not be used at fast rates of speech, these results suggest that sensory information might play a role in maintaining coordination stability (at both intra- and inter-gestural levels) at higher speech rates. Interestingly, the data also suggest that PWS and PNS may differ in the use of sensory information at the intra- versus inter-gestural level of coordination.

From the above examples, it is clear that coordination variability provides an interesting window on the underlying dynamics of the speech motor control system. The mechanisms described above, in particular with respect to the use of specific motor control strategies, do not necessarily entail the concept of neuro-motor noise. The level of entrainment and hence stability between an effector and neural oscillator can directly vary as a function of feedback gain itself, as elegantly demonstrated in a robot model (Williamson 1998). However, interpretation of variability in coordination is a complex topic. High variability of relative phase does not necessarily depict a system that is unstable. It may actually reflect a system that is multi-stable and therefore flexible at the same time (Davids et al., 2003). However, low variability may reflect a stable performance for relatively simple and well-defined tasks, but in more demanding conditions it may indicate a rigid or stereotypical (and therefore inflexible) pathological mode of coordination (e.g., Newell et al., 2002). Thus, a simple quantification of variability of coordination may not be sufficient to understand its true nature and significance. As shown in this section, the problem of quantifying variability is compounded by a lack of consistency among the various measures used for that purpose. In general, it seems wise (until a firmer grasp has been obtained on this issue) to select a mixture of variables to evaluate patterns of change that may reveal underlying control mechanisms or at least select a group of variables that pertain to a particular theoretical framework (like coherence and relative phase measures fit well with concepts of DST). In addition, it seems useful to supplement quantification of variability with information on the nature of variability. This can be achieved with other techniques such as Hurst analysis and Visual Recurrence Analysis (VRA), detailed in the following section. The use of the latter two analyses will be illustrated on kinematic data from a small group of PWS and PNS.

11.4 New approaches towards assessing the nature of variability in speech motor control

In Section 11.2 we discussed a typical representation of noise, depicted as a random perturbation which contaminates an otherwise 'invariant' control signal, affecting the speaker's ability to perform a motor action in a stable and/or predictable manner. This claim entails three independent assumptions:

1. variability means random
2. variability means instability
3. control signal is 'invariant' (i.e., purely deterministic)

Each of these assumptions can been questioned, as exemplified in the following statement by Riley and Turvey (2002): 'More variable does not mean more random, and more controllable does not always mean more deterministic' (p. 100). To illustrate the issue that Riley and Turvey raised, two synthetic signals are shown in Fig. 11.5. One is a one-dimensional chaotic signal (defined below), the other is pure white noise. At first glance, both look 'noisy' in the time display (left panels), but if one plots their phase trajectories (right panels) with position on the *x*-axis (x) and its time delayed version (x+1) on the *y*-axis, differences become apparent. True white noise (bottom right panel) has no obvious deterministic structure (each point in time is completely independent from preceding and following points), but the chaotic system has a deterministic underlying process where specific points in phase space as shown on the parabola (top right panel) are revisited in a consistent manner. This system, called the logistic model, is governed by the following equation:

$$x_{n+1} = 3.95\, x_n\, (1 - x_n) \qquad (11.2)$$

Because each sample is a function of previous samples, such systems are referred to as recurrence systems.

When faced with noisy data (e.g., Fig. 11.5), the challenge is to find ways to quantify the nature of the time-based variations for that particular output. Is it truly random or does it arise from a deterministic process such as shown in the logistic model? One popular method to provide an answer to this question is the Hurst rescaled range or R/S analysis (R being the amplitude range of time series, S being its standard deviation, measured over time windows with different length), which is typically applied to fractal time series (e.g., Amoud et al., 2007). Fractal time series are

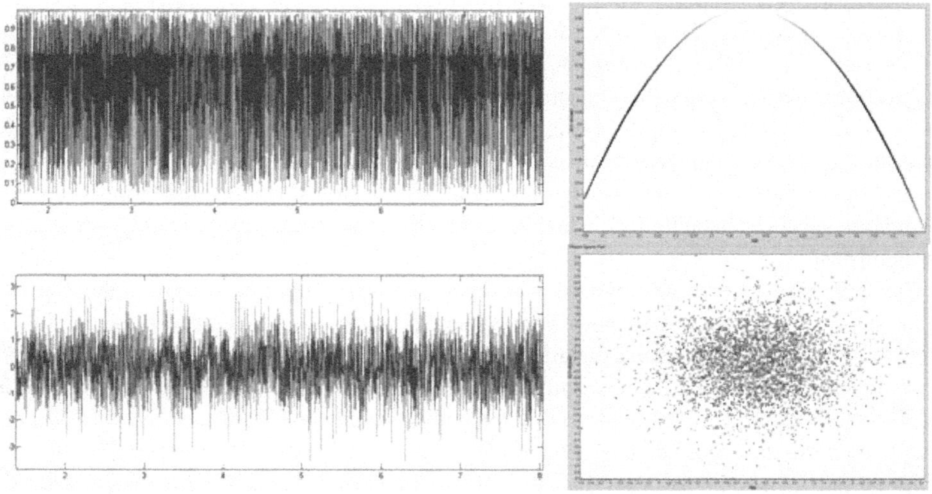

Fig. 11.5 Time series of low dimensional chaotic signal (based on logistic model) and corresponding phase space reconstruction (top two panels) and white noise signal with corresponding phase space reconstruction (bottom two panels) (see text for more details).

characterized by self-similarity, meaning that small variations over small time windows look similar to larger variations in larger time windows, past values correlate with future values or in terms of spectral characteristics, energy varies with frequency (Liebovitch 1998). Essentially, to derive the Hurst exponent for a given time series, one determines the variation in values (dispersion expressed in R/S) for different window sizes along the time dimension and then calculates the slope of the log–log relationship between dispersion and window size. In other words, one determines how variance depends on temporal resolution (Liebovitch 1998). The Hurst exponent provides an index of whether the system is controlled by a truly random process or if there are underlying trends that create short- or long-term correlations over time among the samples. The following interpretations hold for different values of the Hurst exponent (Treffner and Kelso 1999):

- $H = 0.5$ applies to true Brownian motion (Shvindlerman et al., 2006) for which past and future samples are uncorrelated (random). In the power spectrum, energy is equally distributed across frequencies.
- $0.5 < H < 1$ applies to fractal Brownian motion, showing a positive correlation between past and future samples (an increase is likely to be followed by an increase, a decrease in value by a decrease etc.). The differences between consecutive values are called persistent. In the power spectrum, low frequency noise dominates.
- $0 < H < 0.5$ applies to fractal Brownian motion, showing a negative correlation between past and future samples, called anti-persistence. In the power spectrum, high frequency noise dominates.

In order to illustrate the characteristics of these fractal time series, Fig. 11.6 shows examples of synthetic Brownian motion signals with different Hurst exponent values. Only the middle one ($H = 0.5$) is based on a truly random process. Notice how signals with lower Hurst exponent values show more jaggedness due to the influence of higher frequencies in the spectrum, whereas the signals with Hurst exponent values above 0.5 show relatively slow variations, indicative of a more dominant presence of low frequencies in the spectrum. Fractal Brownian motion has been demonstrated in limb motor systems (e.g., Riley and Turvey 2002; Treffner and Kelso 1999) but to our knowledge, for speech motor control such data have not been published yet. In order to illustrate the feasibility of this approach, Fig. 11.7 shows an example of a relative phase time series for the gestural pair bilabial closure (BC) and tongue body constriction (TB) for a subject repeating the nonword 'ipa' (top panel) together with a synthetic fractal time series (bottom panel) with an nearly equal H-exponent value (around 0.7; indicating a persistent type of relationship among the samples). The data for relative phase shown here have a remarkable similarity with data presented in the paper by Riley and Turvey (2002) for postural fluctuation time series (with H-exponent values close to 0.7), which may suggest some similarities in underlying control mechanisms.

However, what does it mean when a signal shows fractal properties? In principle, we cannot make simple assumptions about the origin of these fluctuations. A deterministic signal does not have to be invariant (e.g., when generated by a chaotic system as shown in Fig. 11.5). In this conceptualization, variability becomes an important element of the control system and not just something that is added somewhere along the pathways involved in motor execution (see Riley and Turvey 2002 for more details). One way to quantify this mix of deterministic and (fractal) noise properties is to perform a VRA, also known as recurrence quantification analysis or RQA (Eckmann et al., 1987; Webber and Zbilut 1994). Originally, this is a graphical method used to detect recurring patterns and non-stationarities in data. On the basis of its relative ease of use (not necessarily ease of interpretation) and forgiveness for 'flaws' in data sets (related to size, stationary,

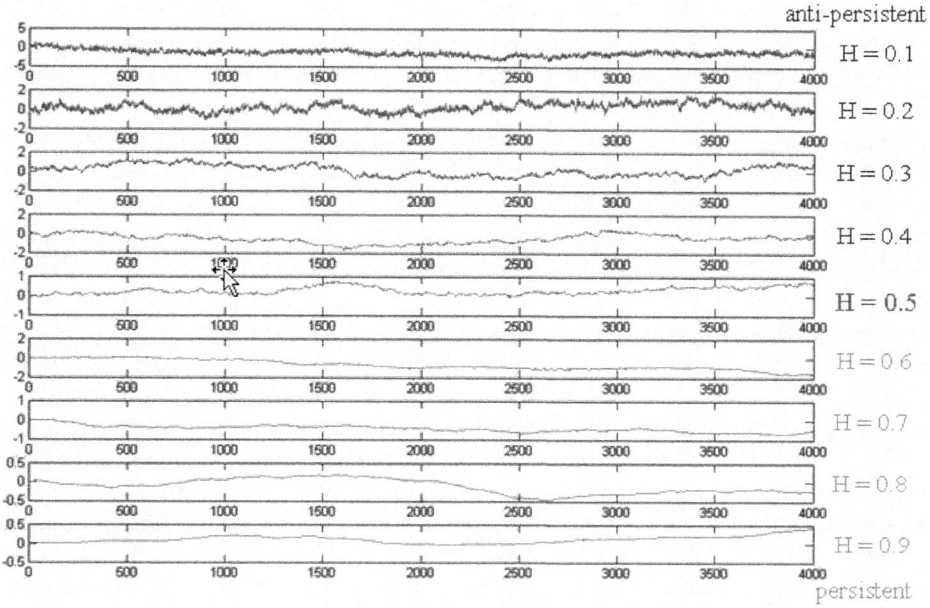

Fig. 11.6 Examples of Brownian motion signals with different Hurst exponent values (see text for more details).

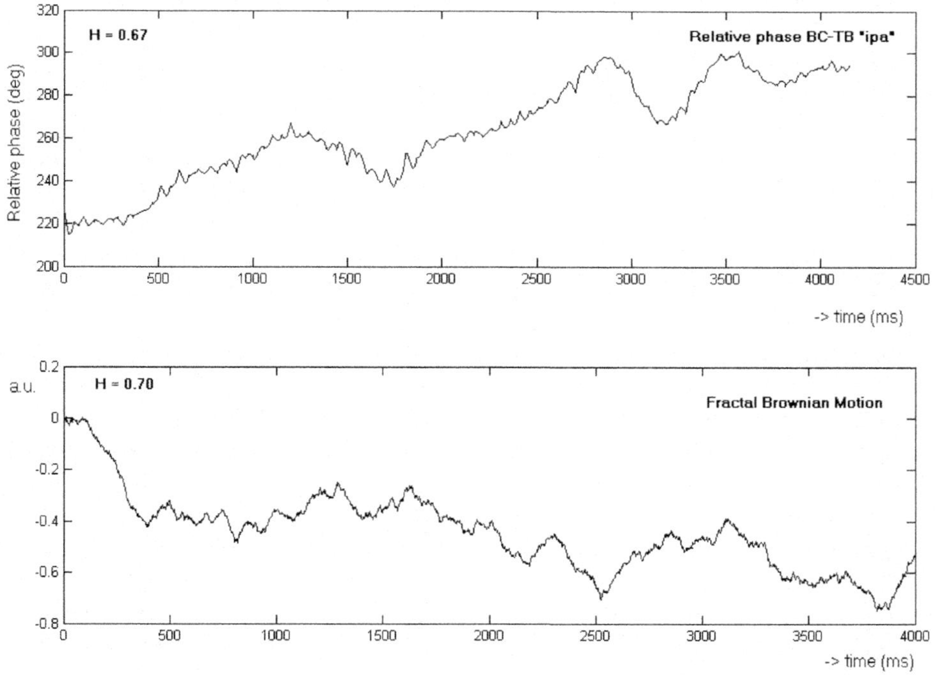

Fig. 11.7 Example illustrating fractal properties in the relative phase signal of inter-gestural coordination between bilabial closure (BC) and tongue body constriction (TB) gestures for a subject repeating the nonword 'ipa'. This is compared to a synthetic fractal time series with a similar H(urst)-exponent value (around 0.7).

and/or statistical properties), it has been deemed very useful for studying patterns over time in data sets of all sorts, including voice and speech (Little et al., 2007), limb movements (Richardson et al., 2007), and postural control (Riley et al., 1999). The behaviour of complex systems (like speech) is determined by many different (and interacting) control levels that eventually converge on the output of a single time series, like the movements of a lip or tongue. A technique called delayed coordinate embedding (Takens 1981) is used to determine the minimum number of dimensions needed to describe the internal structure of these time series (i.e., the degrees of freedom needed to unfold the system's control or phase space). If this embedding is done correctly, the reconstructed dynamics are qualitatively identical to the true dynamics of the system (Bradley 1999). In this technique, a single value at time *t* in the original signal is replaced with a vector consisting of multiple preceding values, as determined by the signal's embedding dimension and time delay (see Liebovitch 1998 for an illustration of this technique). The recurrence analysis then calculates the (Euclidean) distance between pairs of (all) constructed vectors and can use for example, colour coding to display this information. The stronger the amount of determinism (i.e., the more values repeat themselves over time), the more structured (i.e., more points forming line patterns) the VRA plot will be. This can be quantified in per cent determinism, a measure of temporal dependency among samples of a given time series. It is important to note the distinction between the Hurst and the VRA analysis; the former can tell us if noise is random or not (i.e., fractal) while the latter can tell us more specifically if and how much of the signal is generated by a deterministic (as opposed to a truly random) process. This is perhaps easiest to illustrate in the data shown in Fig. 11.8 for a highly deterministic signal (sinusoid) versus a completely stochastic signal (white noise). Delays and embedding dimensions are typically determined using specific procedures (see below) that are explained in more detail elsewhere (Webber and Zbilut 2005). Clearly, the sinusoid shows a highly patterned structure with long diagonal lines, indicating that for this type of signal specific values are repeated over time and future values can be predicted from past values. No such pattern is visible for white noise.

To illustrate the use of recurrence analysis, Fig. 11.9 shows per cent determinism for the same tasks discussed in Section 11.3 (see Figs 11.3 and 11.4). Slow speech rates (regardless of whether this was self-paced or using a metronome) show much higher per cent determinism values (i.e., less randomness) as compared to normal and fast rates. Data on postural control (Riley et al., 1999) suggested that the presence of external feedback lowers variability but at the same time, increases the random influence. This perhaps reflects the shift from (more deterministic relatively long-term) internal feedback control loops to a stronger reliance on on-line externally guided control with low correlations between data points across different time scales. This also fits well with our findings for the metronome data showing lower determinism values for normal and fast rates compared to self-paced speech. That slow speech does not show this difference fits with the assumption stated above in Section 11.3 that for slow rate external pacing effects would be diminished (Jirsa et al., 2000). In the following paragraph we will provide a more detailed illustration of the Hurst and recurrence analysis as applied to a dataset from a small group of PWS and PNS to highlight some of the possibilities and limitations for research in this area.

In this study we examined five PWS and five PNS on their ability to produce two reiterant speech tasks using the nonwords /api/ and /ipa/ at their preferred or normal rate and at a fast rate (for more details see Namasivayam et al., 2009). For the purpose of this illustration we analysed the relative phase patterns of the coupling between the tongue body constriction gesture and bilabial closure gesture (i.e., inter-gestural coordination) as described in Section 11.3. For these signals, we determined the Hurst exponent value and the per cent determinism (using the VRA software, v.5.01, E. Kononov, May 2007) to get an estimate of the nature of variability in gestural coordination patterns as they unfold over time within a single trial (see also Fig. 11.7).

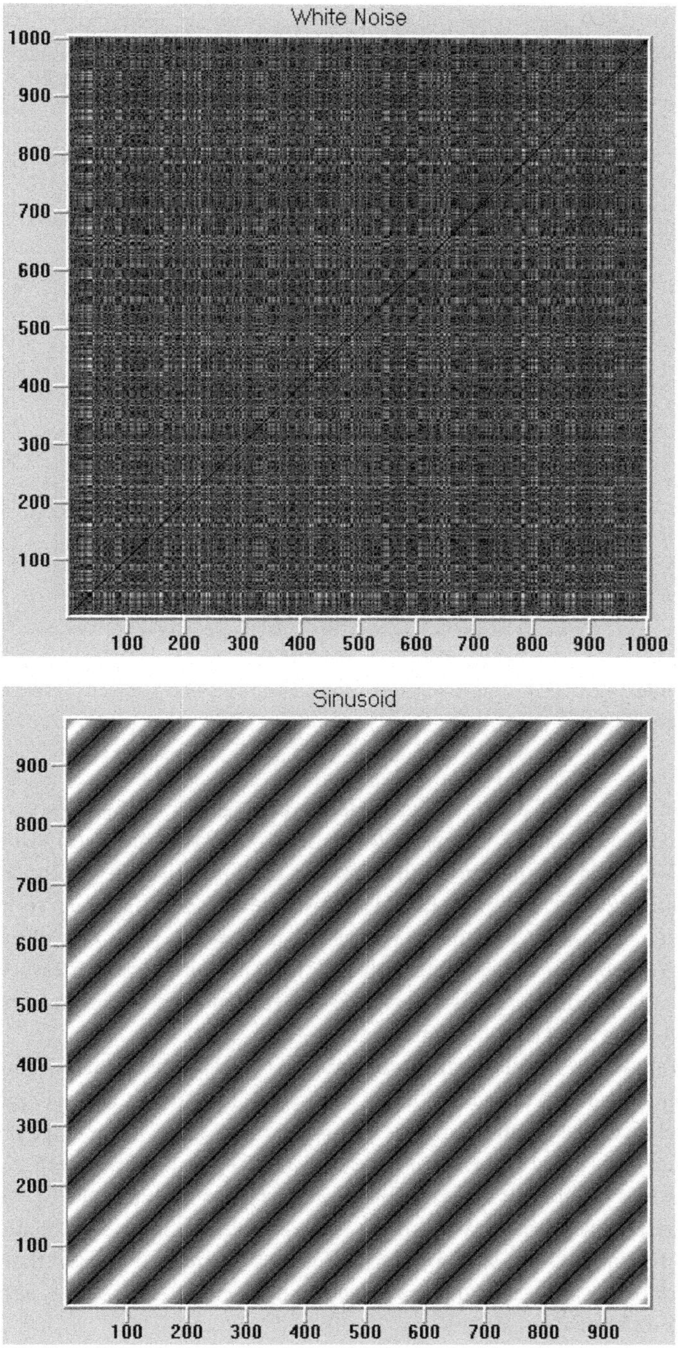

Fig. 11.8 Example of Visual Recurrence Analysis (VRA) plots for a deterministic signal (sinusoid; delay = 25 samples; embedding dimension = 2; % determinism = 100) and a truly random signal (white noise; delay = 1, embedding dimension = 1, % determinism = 0). Note that for white noise, the delay time and embedding dimension are typically chosen to be 1 as no true estimate can be determined given the fact that there is no repeat pattern. The grey scales indicates Euclidian distance between corresponding points on the x and y axes (difference in values), with lighter colours showing greater differences (e.g., diagonal indicates each point onto itself, hence values are identical).

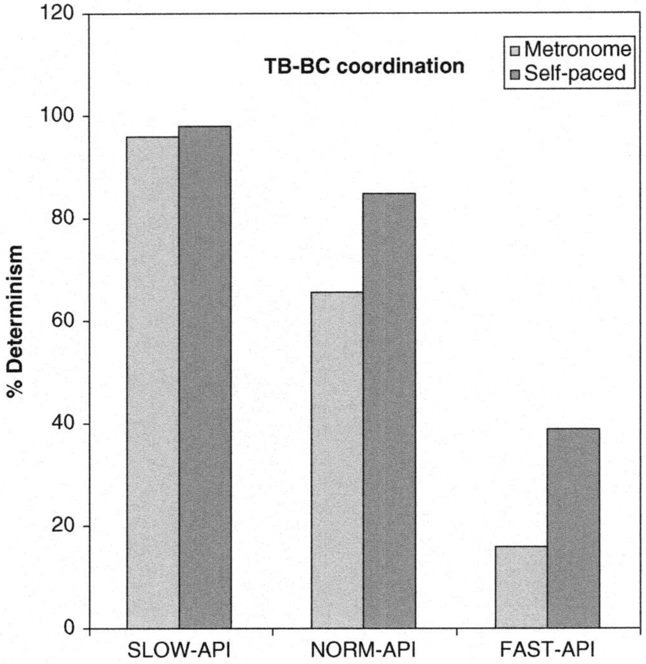

Fig. 11.9 Estimates of per cent determinism for the same tasks and subject presented in Fig. 11.4 (see text for more details).

The selection of appropriate delays and embedding dimension for the analyses was based on recommended techniques, namely mutual information for delay (Fraser and Swinney, 1986) and False Nearest Neighbors to determine the appropriate dimensionality (Kennel and Abarbanel 2002). The radius (i.e., the maximum Euclidean distance at and below which recurrent points are defined) was set to 4%, which is within the range recommended for our type of data (Webber and Zbilut 2005). We tested for effects using a mixed ANOVA with repeated measures with group as between-subject factor, task (/api/ versus /ipa/) and rate (normal versus fast) as within-subject factors with a p-value set at 0.05 for significance.

Figure 11.10 shows the results for the inter-gestural relative phase data. We found a significant task effect for inter-gestural coordination [$F(1,8) = 16.65$, $p < 0.01$], which depicts the expected difference in relative phase values for /api/ versus /ipa/. For the SD of relative phase we found a significant main effect for group [$F(1,8) = 14.07$, $p < 0.01$], task [$F(1,8) = 16.22$, $p < 0.01$] and, most importantly, a group x task interaction effect [$F(1,8) = 10.17$, $p < 0.05$]. The latter reflects that PWS showed higher variability in tongue body – bilabial closure coordination compared to PNS, but only for /ipa/. Other studies from our laboratory have indicated that /ipa/ is a more demanding task in this respect than /api/ (Van Lieshout et al., 1997, 2007), although the exact reasons for this difference remain unclear.

Figure 11.11 shows the findings for the Hurst exponent analysis and per cent determinism. Regarding the Hurst values, there is a trend for PWS to have slightly smaller values (except for /ipa/ at normal rates) compared to PNS, but overall the data for both groups show values in the 0.6–0.7 range. As mentioned in Section 11.3, this indicates a persistent type of fractal Brownian motion, as also found for other types of motor behaviour (Riley et al., 1999). We found a significant group x rate interaction [$F(1,8) = 5.58$, $p < 0.05$), which indicated that for normal rates both

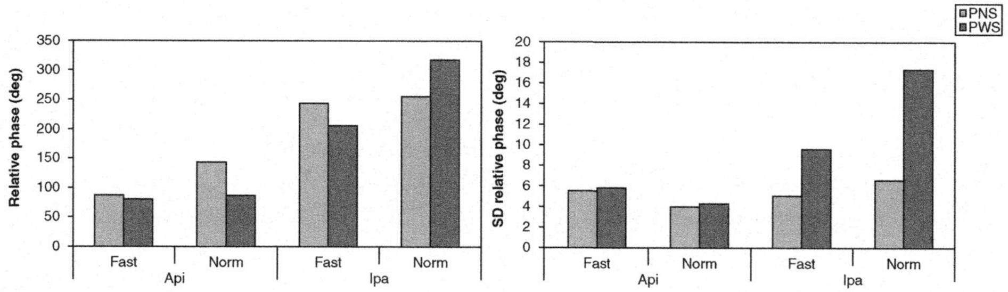

Fig. 11.10 Relative phase values (mean and SD) for tongue body gesture and lip closing gesture coordination in a group of PWS and matched controls for /api/ and /ipa/ and two self-paced rates (normal and fast) (see text for more details).

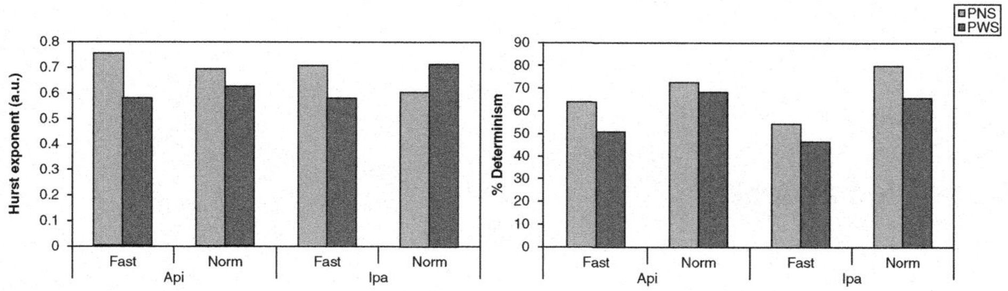

Fig. 11.11 Hurst exponent and per cent determinism values for the same subjects and tasks as shown in Fig. 11.8 (see text for more details).

groups showed comparable values, but at fast rates, PWS showed a decrease (closer towards 0.5) whereas PNS showed an increase in Hurst exponent values. The latter is quite contrary to what we would expect, if indeed higher Hurst values can be associated with a stronger influence of long delay feedback loops (dynamic stabilization; Treffner and Kelso 1999), which would normally be expected to become less relevant at faster rates. However, it does correspond to other findings from our laboratory mentioned above, which showed that PNS (in comparison to PWS) are more sensitive to feedback perturbations in fast rate conditions only (Namasivayam et al., 2009). For per cent determinism, we found a significant main effect for rate [$F(1,8) = 12.03$, $p < 0.01$], showing a decrease for fast rates (i.e., fluctuations in relative phase showed a stronger random contribution).

Summarizing these preliminary results, it was found that PWS showed no difference in the nature of phase coupling (relative phase values), but they did show a task-specific effect for coordination variability (higher in /ipa/). This did not seem to be related to apparent differences in 'randomness' of the relative phase signal. At fast rates only, PNS showed an unexpected increase in Hurst values, but no corresponding increase in per cent Determinism values. In general, these data do not support the view that PWS are more reliant on feedback control compared to normal speakers for this type of task as has been suggested earlier (Neilson and Neilson 1991; Van Lieshout et al., 1993; see also Namasivayam et al., 2009).

Conclusions and future directions

To support (or refute) the notion that PWS have limitations in speech motor control requires new tools that are better able to reflect dynamical aspects of a control system's organizational principles.

This information may help researchers to get closer to understanding what factors drive changes in a system, how the system performs under different task demands, and what leads to a breakdown at the overt behavioural level (Van Lieshout et al., 2004). At present, the traditional approach in treating variability in motor control as 'unwanted noise' may be too limited, and neglects potential differences in its origin, nature and significance for motor control. Thus, future work needs to be directed towards not only quantifying variability but also understanding its nature in the context of stuttering and motor control, complementing (robust) measures of variability with non-linear techniques. This information will no doubt force us to revisit the current concept of (speech) motor variability. These techniques (like any other tool) however, have their challenges in terms of ease of use, relative dependency on stationary signals, and the complexity of their interpretation. Further, as shown in Section 11.3, different measures of variability can depict conflicting stories and it is important not to rely on a single method and to seek expertise in using and interpreting such variables. Variability may be a hallmark of healthy systems, whereas the lack of such could indeed be a sign of (serious) impairment (e.g., Goldberger et al., 2002). Finally, variability in single articulator data needs to be interpreted in the context of its impact on coordination, since coordination and its stability are main features that determine efficiency and skill in speech production (Van Lieshout 2004).

Acknowledgements

This work was supported in part by the Connaught Scholarship, University of Toronto, granted to the second author, and research grants from the Natural Sciences and Engineering Research Council (NSERC) and the Canadian Research Chair program, awarded to the first author. A part of the data from this manuscript was presented at the 4th World Congress on Fluency Disorders, Montreal, Canada and at the 5th International Speech Motor Conference, Nijmegen, The Netherlands.

References

Alfonso, P. J. (1991). Implications of the concepts underlying task-dynamic modeling on kinematic studies of stuttering. In H. F. Peters, W. Hulstijn & C. W. Starkweather (Eds.), *Speech Motor Control and Stuttering* (pp. 79–100). Amsterdam: Elseviers Publishers.

Alfonso, P. J., & Van Lieshout, P. H. H. M. (1997). Spatial and temporal variability in obstruent gestural specification by stutterers and controls: Comparisons across sessions. In W. Hulstijn, H. F. M. Peters & P. H. H. M. Van Lieshout (Eds.), *Speech Production: Motor Control, Brain Research and Fluency Disorders* (pp. 151–160). Amsterdam, The Netherlands: Elsevier Publishers.

Amoud, H., Abadi, M., Hewson, D. J., Michel-Pellegrino, V., Doussot, M., & Ne, J. (2007). Fractal time series analysis of postural stability in elderly and control subjects. *Journal of NeuroEngineering and Rehabilitation, 4*(12). [on-line]

Barlow, S. M., & Netsell, R. (1986). Differential fine force control of the upper and lower lips. *Journal of Speech and Hearing Research, 29*(2), 163–169.

Beckman, M. E., Jung, T., Lee, S., De Jong, K., Krishnamurthy, A. K., Ahalt, S. C., et al. (1995). Variability in the production of quantal vowels revisited. *Journal of the Acoustical Society of America, 97*(1), 471–490.

Boutsen, F. R., Brutten, G. J., & Watts, C. R. (2000). Timing and intensity variability in the metronomic speech of stuttering and nonstuttering speakers. *Journal of Speech, Language, and Hearing Research, 43*(2), 513–520.

Bradley, E. (1999). Analysis of time series. In M. Berthold & D. J. Hand (Eds.), *Intelligent Data Analysis: An Introduction* (pp. 199–227). New York: Springer-Verlag.

Browman, C. P., & Goldstein, L. M. (1992). Articulatory phonology: An overview. *Phonetica, 49*(3–4), 155–180.

Caruso, A. J., Abbs, J. H., & Gracco, V. L. (1988). Kinematic analysis of multiple movement coordination during speech in stutterers. *Brain; a Journal of Neurology, 111 (Pt 2)*, 439–456.

Catford, J. C. (1977). *Fundamental Problems in Phonetics.* Edinburgh, UK: Edinburgh University Press.

Chau, T., Young, S., & Redekop, S. (2005). Managing variability in the summary and comparison of gait data. *Journal of NeuroEngineering and Rehabilitation, 2*(22). [On-line]

Davids, K., Glazier, P., Araújo, D., & Bartlett, R. (2003). Movement systems as dynamical systems: The functional role of variability and its implications for sports medicine. *Sports Medicine, 33*(4), 245–260.

De Nil, L. F., & Abbs, J. H. (1991). Influence of speaking rate on the upper lip, lower lip, and jaw peak velocity sequencing during bilabial closing movements. *The Journal of the Acoustical Society of America, 89*(2), 845–849.

Dromey, C., & Benson, A. (2003). Effects of concurrent motor, linguistic, or cognitive tasks on speech motor performance. *Journal of Speech, Language, and Hearing Research, 46*(5), 1234–1246.

Eckmann, J. P., Kamphorst, S. O., & Ruelle, D. (1987). Recurrence plots of dynamic-systems. *Europhysics Letters, 4*(9), 973–977.

Fink, P. W., Foo, P., Jirsa, V. K., & Kelso, J. A. S. (2000). Local and global stabilization of coordination by sensory information. *Experimental Brain Research. Experimentelle Hirnforschung. Experimentation Cerebrale, 134*(1), 9–20.

Fraser, A. M., & Swinney, H. L. (1986). Independent coordinates for strange attractors from mutual information. *Physical Review. A, 33*(2), 1134–1140.

Goldberger, A. L., Amaral, L. A. N., Hausdorff, J. M., Ivanov, P. C., Peng, C. K., & Stanley, H. E. (2002). Fractal dynamics in physiology: Alterations with disease and aging. *Proceedings of the National Academy of Sciences of the United States of America, 99*, 2466–2472.

Goldstein, L. M., & Fowler, C. (2003). Articulatory phonology: A phonology for public language use. In A. S. Meyer, N. O. Schiller & (Eds.), *Phonetics and Phonology in Language Comprehension and Production: Differences and Similarities* (pp. 159–207). Berlin: Mouton de Gruyter.

Goldstein, L. M., Pouplier, M., Chen, L., Saltzman, E. L., & Byrd, D. (2007). Dynamic action units slip in speech production errors. *Cognition, 103*, 386–412.

Haken, H., Kelso, J. A. S., & Bunz, H. (1985). A theoretical model of phase transitions in human hand movements. *Biological Cybernetics, 51*(5), 347–356.

Hoole, P. (1999). Articulatory-acoustic relations in German vowels. *Proceedings of the XIVth International Congress of Phonetic Sciences*, San Francisco. 2153–2156.

Jäncke, L., Kaiser, P., Bauer, A., & Kalveram, K. T. (1995). Patterns of interarticulator phasing relations in stutterers and nonstutterers. In C. W. Starkweather, & H. F. M. Peters (Eds.), *Stuttering: Proceedings of the first world congress on fluency disorders* (pp. 23–26). Nijmegen, The Netherlands: University of Nijmegen Press.

Janssen, P., & Wieneke, G. (1987). The effect of fluency inducing conditions on the variability in the duration of laryngeal movements during stutterers' fluent speech. In H. F. M. Peters & W. Hulstijn (Eds.), *Speech Motor Dynamics in Stuttering* (pp. 337–344). Wien: Springer-Verlag.

Jirsa, V. K., Fink, P., Foo, P., & Kelso, J. A. S. (2000). Parametric stabilization of biological coordination: A theoretical model. *Journal of Biological Physics, 26*(2), 85–112.

Kelso, J. A. S. (1995). *Dynamic Patterns. The Self-Organization of Brain and Behavior.* Cambridge, MA: A Bradford Book (MIT Press).

Kelso, J. A. S., Saltzman, E. L., & Tuller, B. (1986). The dynamical theory in speech production: Data and theory. *Journal of Phonetics,14*, 29–60.

Kennel, M. B., & Abarbanel, H. D. (2002). False neighbors and false strands: A reliable minimum embedding dimension algorithm. *Physical Review E – Statistical, Nonlinear, and Soft Matter Physics, 66*(2), 026209.

Kleinow, J., & Smith, A. (2000). Influences of length and syntactic complexity on the speech motor stability of the fluent speech of adults who stutter. *Journal of Speech, Language, and Hearing Research, 43*(2), 548–559.

Liebovitch, L. (1998). *Fractals and Chaos: Simplified for the Life Sciences.* New York, NY: Oxford University Press.

Little, M. A., McSharry, P. E., Roberts, S. J., Costello, D. A. E., & Moroz, I. M. (2007). Exploiting nonlinear recurrence and fractal scaling properties for voice disorder detection. *BioMedical Engineering Online, 6*(23). [on-line]

Lucero, J. C. (2005). Comparison of measures of variability of speech movement trajectories using synthetic records. *Journal of Speech Language and Hearing Research, 48*(2), 336–344.

Namasivayam, A. K., & Van Lieshout, P. H. H. M. (2008). Investigating speech motor practice and learning in people who stutter. *Journal of Fluency Disorders, 33*, 32–51.

Namasivayam, A. K., Van Lieshout, P. H. H. M., & De Nil, L. F. (2008). Bite-block perturbation in people who stutter: Immediate compensatory and delayed adaptive processes. *Journal of Communication Disorders, 41*(4), 372–394.

Namasivayam, A. K., van Lieshout, P., McIlroy, W. E., & De Nil, L. (2009). Sensory feedback dependence hypothesis in persons who stutter. *Human Movement Science, 28*, 688–707.

Neilson, M. D., & Neilson, P. D. (1991). Adaptive model theory of speech motor control and stuttering. In H. F. M. Peters, W. Hulstijn & C. W. Starkweather (Eds.), *Speech Motor Control And Stuttering* (pp. 149–156). Amsterdam: Elsevier Science Publishers B.V.

Newell, K. M. (2003). Schema theory (1975): Retrospectives and prospectives. *Research Quarterly for Exercise and Sport, 74*(4), 383–388.

Newell, K. M., Challis, J. H., Boros, R. L., & Bodfish, J. W. (2002). Further evidence on the dynamics of self-injurious behaviors: Impact forces and limb motions. *American Journal on Mental Retardation, 107*(1), 66–68+74

Newell, K. M., & Slifkin, A. B. (1998). The nature of movement variability. In J. P. Piek (Ed.), *Motor Behavior and Human Skill: A Multidisciplinary Approach* (pp. 143–160). Champaign, IL: Human Kinetics.

Nieto-Castanon, A., Guenther, F. H., Perkell, J. S., & Curtin, H. D. (2005). A modeling investigation of articulatory variability and acoustic stability during American English /r/ production. *Journal of the Acoustical Society of America, 117*(5), 3196–3212.

Ostry, D. J., & Munhall, K. G. (1985). Control of rate and duration of speech movements. *The Journal of the Acoustical Society of America, 77*(2), 640–648.

Packman, A., Onslow, M., Richard, F., & van Doorn, J. (1996). Syllabic stress and variability: A model of stuttering. *Clinical Linguistics & Phonetics, 10*(3), 235–264.

Peper, C. E., Beek, P. J., & van Wieringen, P. C. W. (1995). Frequency-induced phase transitions in bimanual tapping. *Biological Cybernetics, 73*(4), 301–309.

Peters, H. F. M., Hulstijn, W., & Van Lieshout, P. H. H. M. (2000). Recent developments in speech motor research into stuttering. *Folia Phoniatrica et Logopaedica, 52*(1–3), 103–119.

Prinz, A. A. (2006). Insights from models of rhythmic motor systems. *Current Opinion in Neurobiology, 16*(6), 615–620.

Ramsay, J. O., & Silverman, B. W. (2005). *Functional Data Analysis.* New York: Springer.

Richardson, M. J., Schmidt, R. C., & Kay, B. A. (2007). Distinguishing the noise and attractor strength of coordinated limb movements using recurrence analysis. *Biological Cybernetics, 96*(1), 59–78.

Riley, M. A., Balasubramaniam, R., & Turvey, M. T. (1999). Recurrence quantification analysis of postural fluctuations. *Gait & Posture, 9*(1), 65–78.

Riley, M. A., & Turvey, M. T. (2002). Variability of determinism in motor behavior. *Journal of Motor Behavior, 34*(2), 99–125.

Scholz, J. P., & Schöner, G. (1999). The uncontrolled manifold concept: Identifying control variables for a functional task. *Experimental Brain Research. Experimentelle Hirnforschung. Experimentation Cerebrale, 126*(3), 289–306.

Shiller, D. M., Houle, G., & Ostry, D. J. (2005). Voluntary control of human jaw stiffness. *Journal of Neurophysiology, 94*(3), 2207–2217.

Shvindlerman, L. S., Wynblatt, P., Mehrer, H., Philibert, J., & Bokstein, B. (2006). Einstein's theory of brownian motion. *Diffusion and Defect Data. Pt A Defect and Diffusion Forum, 249*, 7–16.

Smith, A., Goffman, L., Zelaznik, H. N., Ying, G. S., & McGillem, C. (1995). Spatiotemporal stability and patterning of speech movement sequences. *Experimental Brain Research, 104*(3), 493–501.

Smith, A., Johnson, M., McGillem, C., & Goffman, L. (2000). On the assessment of stability and patterning of speech movements. *Journal of Speech Language and Hearing Research, 43*(1), 277–286.

Smith, A., & Kleinow, J. (2000). Kinematic correlates of speaking rate changes in stuttering and normally fluent adults. *Journal of Speech, Language, and Hearing Research, 43*(2), 521–536.

Smith, A., & Zelaznik, H. N. (2004). Development of functional synergies for speech motor coordination in childhood and adolescence. *Developmental Psychobiology, 45*(1), 22–33.

Stevens, K. N. (1989). On the quantal nature of speech. *Journal of Phonetics, 17*(1–2), 3–45.

Takens, F. (1981). Detecting strange attractors in turbulence. In D. A. Rand, & L. -. Young (Eds.), *Dynamical Systems and Turbulence, Lecture Notes in Mathematics, volume 898* (pp. 366–381). Berlin: Springer Verlag.

Todorov, E., & Ghahramani, Z. (2004). Analysis of the synergies underlying complex hand manipulation, *Annual International Conference of the IEEE Engineering in Medicine and Biology – Proceedings, 26*(VI), 4637–4640.

Treffner, P. J., & Kelso, J. A. S. (1999). Dynamic encounters: Long memory during functional stabilization. *Ecological Psychology, 11*(2), 103–137.

Van Galen, G. P., & van Huygevoort, M. (2000). Error, stress and the role of neuromotor noise in space oriented behaviour. *Biological Psychology, 51*(2–3), 151–171.

Van Lieshout, P. H. H. M. (1995). Motor planning and articulation in fluent speech of stutterers and nonstutterers. Doctoral Thesis, University of Nijmegen, The Netherlands; also NICI Technical Report 95–07.

Van Lieshout, P. H. H. M. (2001). Coupling dynamics of motion primitives in speech movements and its potential relevance for fluency. *Society for Chaos Theory in Psychology & Life Sciences Newsletter, 8*(4) 18.

Van Lieshout, P. H. H. M. (2004). Dynamical systems theory and its application in speech. In B. Maassen, R. D. Kent, H. Peters, P. H. H. M. van Lieshout & W. Hulstijn (Eds.), *Speech Motor Control in Normal and Disordered Speech* (pp. 51–82). Oxford, UK: Oxford University Press.

Van Lieshout, P. H. H. M., Alfonso, P. J., Hulstijn, W., & Peters, H. F. (1994). Electromagnetic midsagittal articulography (EMMA). In F. J. Maarse, A. E. Akkerman, A. N. Brand, L. J. M. Mulder & M. J. Van der Stelt (Eds.), *Computers in Psychology: Applications, Methods, and Instrumentation* (pp. 62–76). Lisse: Swets & Zeitlinger.

Van Lieshout, P. H. H. M., Bose, A., Square, P., & Steele, C. (2007). Speech motor control in fluent and dysfluent speech production of an individual with apraxia of speech and broca's aphasia. *Clinical Linguistics and Phonetics, 21*(3), 159–188.

Van Lieshout, P. H. H. M., & Goldstein, L. M. (2008). Gestural phonology and speech impairments. In M. J. Ball, M. Perkins, N. Müller & S. Howard (Eds.), *Handbook of Clinical Linguistics* (pp. 467–479). Oxford, UK: Blackwell Publishing.

Van Lieshout, P. H. H. M., Hulstijn, W., Alfonso, P. J., & Peters, H. F. (1997). Higher and lower order influences on the stability of the dynamic coupling between articulators. In W. Hulstijn, H. F. Peters & P. H. H. M. van Lieshout (Eds.), *Speech Production: Motor Control, Brain Research and Fluency Disorders* (pp. 161–170). Amsterdam: Elsevier Science Publishers.

Van Lieshout, P. H. H. M., Hulstijn, W., & Peters, H. F. M. (2004). Searching for the weak link in the speech production chain of people who stutter: A motor skill approach. In B. A. M. Maassen, R. D. Kent, H. F. M. Peters, P. H. H. M. van Lieshout & W. Hulstijn (Eds.), *Speech Motor Control in Normal and Disordered Speech* (pp. 313–356). Oxford, UK: Oxford University Press.

Van Lieshout, P. H. H. M., & Moussa, W. (2000). The assessment of speech motor behaviors using electromagnetic articulography. *The Phonetician, 81*(1), 9–22.

Van Lieshout, P. H. H. M., Peters, H. F. M., Starkweather, C. W., & Hulstijn, W. (1993). Physiological differences between stutterers and nonstutterers in perceptually fluent speech – Emg amplitude and duration. *Journal of Speech and Hearing Research, 36*(1), 55–63.

Van Lieshout, P. H. H. M., Rutjens, C. A. W., & Spauwen, P. H. M. (2002). The dynamics of interlip coupling in speakers with a repaired unilateral cleft-lip history. *Journal of Speech Language and Hearing Research, 45*(1), 5–19.

Van Lieshout, P. H. H. M., Starkweather, C. W., Hulstijn, W., & Peters, H. F. M. (1995). Effects of linguistic correlates of stuttering on emg activity in nonstuttering speakers. *Journal of Speech and Hearing Research, 38*(2), 360–372.

Walsh, B., Smith, A., & Weber-Fox, C. (2006). Short-term plasticity in children's speech motor systems. *Developmental Psychobiology, 48*(8), 660–674.

Ward, D. (1997). Intrinsic and extrinsic timing in stutterers' speech: Data and implications. *Language and Speech, 40*(3), 289–310.

Ward, D., & Arnfield, S. (2001). Linear and nonlinear analysis of the stability of gestural organization in speech movement sequences. *Journal of Speech, Language, and Hearing Research, 44*(1), 108–117.

Webber, C. L., & Zbilut, J. P. (2005). Recurrence quantification analysis of nonlinear dynamical systems. In M. A. Riley, & G. C. Van Orden (Eds.), *Tutorials in Contemporary Nonlinear Methods for the Behavioral Sciences* (pp. 26–94) Retrieved March 1, 2005, from http://www.nsf.gov/sbe/bcs/pac/nmbs/nmbs.jsp.

Webber, J., & Zbilut, J. P. (1994). Dynamical assessment of physiological systems and states using recurrence plot strategies. *Journal of Applied Physiology, 76*(2), 965–973.

Williamson, M. M. (1998). Neural control of rhythmic arm movements. *Neural Networks, 11*, 1379–1394.

Chapter 12

Speech motor timing and fluency

Peter Howell, Andrew Anderson, and Jorge Lucero

Abstract

Smith's spatio-temporal index (STI) is widely used to assess variability in motor timing performance in various speaking conditions. STI has been shown to be a sensitive index of developmental changes and as a way of assessing performance differences between speakers with fluency disorders and controls. STI typically takes records obtained from an articulator (e.g., the lower lip) for repeated attempts at the same utterance. STI aligns the set of records linearly, normalizes the amplitude axis, and obtains the standard deviation at 50 points along the aligned time axis which are then averaged to give the index. This chapter uses the functional data analysis (FDA) method that aligns features on the time axis (it is a non-linear method). FDA allows separate estimates of timing and amplitude deformations. When two or more signals are obtained concurrently on utterances (here the lower lip and speech energy are used), the timing deformations can be compared to estimate their degree of inter coordination. The method is described and applied to see whether a group of speakers who stutter have poorer inter coordination than a group of fluent speakers.

12.1 Introduction

This chapter describes work on speech motor timing and fluency. Its main aims are: (1) to describe a newly developed method for measuring interarticulator coordination (inter coordination); and (2) to apply these methods to see whether a group of speakers who stutter have poorer inter coordination than a group of fluent speakers. The methods are a development of functional data analysis (FDA), which can be used to measure the variability across a set of records when a speaker attempts to repeat the same utterance a number of times (Lucero et al., 1997; Ramsay and Silverman 1997).

12.1.1 Estimating timing variability using FDA

To estimate timing variability in speech, usually ten or more records that represent repetitions of the same articulatory movement are obtained. Due to natural variation in speech, similar events are likely to be misaligned in their relative timing. FDA is used to manipulate the time lines of records nonlinearly to bring their features into alignment across the set. Variation in the degree of adjustment necessary to bring the records into alignment provides an estimate of temporal variability over the course of the records. After the set of records has been aligned, differences on the amplitude axis provide an estimate of amplitude variability over time. This allows separate statistics to be formulated indexing temporal and amplitude variability in an analogous way to that in Smith's spatio-temporal index (STI) (Smith et al., 1995). Phase variability can be indexed by estimating the standard deviation (*sd*) in phase adjustments over the normalized time axis and averaging across the extract. The *sd* of the amplitudes can be processed in a similar way to index amplitude variability (see also Lucero 2005). The procedure for obtaining the STI score is basically the same as that described for FDA except that the adjustments to the time base are linear (proportional stretching or squeezing) for STI rather than aligned according to features in the signal. Consequently, the amplitude variability cannot be separated from the timing variability. STI is a statistic that reflects joint temporal and amplitude variation.

Fluent speech requires a set of quasi-autonomous articulatory systems to work in coordination. For example, when a voiceless plosive is produced, the speaker has to control the pulmonary and laryngeal systems to ensure there is a transition from aspirated to voiced excitation and this has to be coordinated with the vocal tract opening gesture. If a speaker repeated a phrase involving voiceless plosives, as described above, and records associated with the laryngeal, pulmonary, and vocal tract systems were obtained, each record could be processed independently by FDA. If the three components were exactly coordinated, the time deformations would be the same. When coordination is poor (as would occur when a speaker is dysfluent or when materials are selected which are hard to produce), there will be some departure from this situation. The analysis procedure described here uses the time deformations to obtain a statistic that indicates the inter coordination between different articulators.

As has been seen, multiple records associated with a single activity (speech or otherwise) are required to apply the procedures necessary to obtain inter coordination. Here we used a lower lip (L) kinematic record obtained directly by using a movement transducer and a record derived from the audio waveform, the amplitude of the energy envelope (E). The lower lip record does not require further introduction as it is widely used in contemporary studies of speech variability (Smith and Goffman 2004). The amplitude envelope is computed from an audio recording obtained concurrently. It is a continuous signal that mainly represents the pulmonary system, but also includes the activity of the laryngeal and vocal tract systems. Because of its integrated nature, it incorporates aspects of all the major structures that must be controlled in order to produce speech, so if problems in control of any articulator occur across ages or clinical groups, it should be present in this record.

12.1.2 **Inter coordination ability in speakers with fluency problems**

In this section, we outline how articulatory coordination has featured in some perspectives about stuttering. Several authors have hypothesized that speakers with fluency problems, such as stuttering, have difficulty with inter coordination compared to fluent speakers. For instance, Alfonso and van Lieshout (1997) reported that speech gestures are not coordinated appropriately for production by speakers who stutter. Max and Caruso (1997) also used syllable- and phrase-level estimates for assessing temporal performance in detail. However, in a study of the relative timing of acoustic measures of stop gap and voice onset time, stuttering and fluent individuals were not found to differ significantly (Max and Gracco 2005).

Other groups have also hypothesized that speakers who stutter have inter coordination problems that lead to difficulties (Packman et al., 1996). Recently, some of these authors in their syllable initiation hypothesis of stuttering (Packman et al., 2007) proposed that fluency-enhancing techniques such as syllable-timed speech reduce levels of linguistic stress, which is thought to trigger stuttering in speakers who stutter. Support for these hypotheses was drawn from studies that showed that decreasing speech motor variability reduced stuttering in adults (Packman et al., 1994) and preschool children (Packman et al., 1992).

All the above hypotheses focus on variability in the motor system. Howell's (2002, 2004) EXPLAN model includes linguistic and motor factors and predicts that there are specific things the motor system does that cannot be performed by the linguistic system (such as inter coordination). Some general details about EXPLAN are required before the hypothesis that inter coordination would affect fluency in this model is discussed.

EXPLAN maintains that linguistic processing (PLAN) and motor programming (EX) are involved during speech production. These operate together and have to be synchronized in time for speech to proceed fluently. An utterance starts with the speaker planning the first element. When the PLAN is complete, it is input to EX where a fluent motor programme is generated and the speech is output. While the first element is being programmed for output, PLAN of the next element occurs. As we have said, speech is fluent when the successive plans are sent for motor programming on time, so that the sequence can proceed continuously. This process is most likely to fail and speech to be dysfluent when there is a sequence where the element currently being executed is programmed for output rapidly, and/or the next element takes a long time to plan. Sequences like this only allow a short planning-time and can arise because PLAN is slow and/or EX is rapid.

A single junction where planning is slow and prior execution is rapid occurs in a prosodic word (PW) in which the obligatory content word is preceded by at least one function word (Selkirk 1984), as in a sequence such as 'the swing'. The properties of the elements at the quick-to-execute/slow-to-plan junctures determine whether speech is fluent or not. When problems arise, they can be dealt with in one of two ways: (1) Stalling, where speech before the juncture is interrupted by pausing or repeating one or more of the preceding, already planned, words; (2) Advancing speech and using the completed part of the linguistic plan on the difficult word coming up to generate motor output. This leads to dysfluencies on parts of words, such as part-word repetitions, prolongations, and word breaks.

According to EXPLAN, the major questions to address are what affects: (1) language planning timing; and (2) motor programming timing. To date, most work has been conducted on factors affecting language planning. Here we look at inter coordination of lip movement (L) with the speech amplitude envelope (E) in speakers who stutter or who are fluent. Next we describe a method we have developed to assess inter coordination. We then apply this procedure to assess inter coordination between lip and energy records and to see whether this differs between people who stutter and fluent controls. We consider a number of specific questions about the temporal variability measures for L and E signals. First, do the speakers with high temporal variability for L also tend to have high temporal variability on E? This would be the case if variability affects all speech systems, not any particular one. We addressed this question by examining whether temporal variability indices in L and E (temporal quantities like these indices use the term 'phase') correlate for each of the participant groups. Second, we asked whether temporal variability in L or E differed between the participant groups. Third, we explored whether inter coordination between L and E differs between the participant groups.

12.2 **Method**

12.2.1 **Participants**

There were 24 participants who were secondary referrals to a specialist stuttering clinic in London. They were confirmed as stuttering by a speech-language pathologist. There were 12 participants who stuttered, with a mean age of 14 years 9 months (*sd* was 3 years 3 months). Two were female and the rest were male. Stuttering Severity Instrument version three, SSI-3, (Riley 1994), scores ranged from very mild to severe. There were 12 fluent participants (seven females and five males), with a mean age of 16 years 11 months (*sd* was 6 years 7 months).

12.2.2 **Procedure**

Participants repeated the phrase 'buy Bobby a puppy' 20 times at their normal speech rate in a quiet room. At least ten fluent repetitions were made. Participants repeated the phrase as exactly as possible, paying attention to timing and amplitude control. Participants adopted their most comfortable rate and level. Lip movement and speech records were obtained concurrently. The microphone-to-mouth distance was monitored for each participant by the experimenter to ensure it was kept at a constant distance of approximately 20cm. Any amplitude fluctuations due to slight differences in microphone-to-mouth distance or because of different voice levels of participants were removed when *z*-transformations were made. Phrases that contained word repetition, phrase repetition, pause, prolongation, part-word repetition, and word break were omitted from the analysis.

12.2.3 **Lower lip movement and energy envelope data processing**

The lower lip movement signal (L) was obtained by a cantilever/strain gauge transducer arrangement. The transducer was suspended from a headcage that consisted of an adjustable low-mass tubular aluminum assembly (Barlow et al., 1983). The apparatus matched that described by Abbs and Gilbert (1973) and the headcage superstructure and transducers were positioned and stability checks were made in the same way as reported by Barlow et al. (1983).

The strain gauge output was connected to an integrated circuit socket whose output was passed through an amplifier and low-pass filtered (four-pole Butterworth with a cut-off of 10 Hz) and then captured by a PC for signal processing. An extra channel on the converter recorded speech (transduced by a Sennheiser K6 microphone). The output from the microphone was low-pass filtered at 3.5kHz through a four-pole Butterworth filter. The strain gauge and speech signals were each sampled at 8kHz.

The original audio oscillogram and L track were uploaded into Speech Filing System (SFS) files (http://www.phon.ucl.ac.uk/resource/sfs/). The audio record was processed after capture to obtain the energy over time envelope (E). E was obtained by rectifying and low-pass filtering the signal at 15 Hz. The track of E over time was calculated at every millisecond along the waveform as the average of the sum of the amplitude values within that millisecond frame.

The oscillogram, L and E records can be displayed in alignment, one beneath the other in SFS. The onset of the first /b/ in the phrase was located on the oscillogram and the point where voicing ceased in 'puppy' was marked, again using the oscillogram. These start- and end-points were used as pointers to the L and E tracks in order to select the appropriate section of the respective record for analysis. Subsequently each L and E records were amplitude normalized by transforming to z-scores (as is standard for the STI).

12.2.4 **FDA Registration**

Non-linear time normalization (also termed registration) using FDA is described before the extension, which allows inter articulator coordination to be estimated. Readers who are already familiar with FDA procedures can go directly to the section entitled 'Phase and amplitude deformations and inter coordination'.

It is assumed that variability in speech motor control can be decomposed into independent components of amplitude and time, and that the difference between observed and expected articulation patterns can be determined in terms of amplitude-time deviations across the length of the observed records. Thus, an observed pattern $O_i(t)$, $i = 1,2,...,N$, can be modelled as:

$$O_i(t) = E[t + \phi_i(t)] + \beta_i(t) \tag{12.1}$$

Where t is the closed interval $[0,1]$ (records were linearly normalized in time to satisfy this requirement, as is done with the STI), $\phi_i(t)$ is the expected (estimated) target pattern, and $\beta_i(t)$ and $\phi_i(t)$ are the set of temporal and amplitude deformations between the observed and the expected pattern.

$E(t)$, $\phi_i(t)$, and $\beta_i(t)$ can be estimated by optimizing a set of non-linear time transformations (or warps) $h_i(t)$ that best align the set of observed records, whilst satisfying the constraints that transformed time: (1) is smooth (parts of records are not unreasonably stretched or squashed); and (2) increases monotonically (i.e., parts of records are not reordered).

The degree of alignment can be measured in terms of the variance in the amplitude displacement pattern across the set of aligned records. An aligned record is obtained from $O_i[h_i(t)]$) and the form of $h_i(t)$ can be constrained by expressing it in terms of the second order differential equation:

$$\frac{d^2 h_i(t)}{dt^2} = w_i(t)\frac{dh_i(t)}{dt} \tag{12.2}$$

The terms in the equation can be rearranged and it can then be seen that $w_i(t)$ is the ratio of the curvature of the transform to its incline. Therefore, manipulation of $w_i(t)$ allows control over smoothness (and by penalizing large values in the optimization, unwanted undulations in the time transformation can be restricted).

The standard approach to solving equation 12.2 is to integrate it twice giving:

$$h_i(t) = C_0 + C_1 \int_0^t [\exp \int_0^u w_i(v)dv]du \tag{12.3}$$

C_0 and C_1 are set so they keep $h_i(t)$ in the range $[0,1]$.

With this solution, records can be aligned by optimizing $h_i(t)$ to minimize the cost function given in equation 12.4. This function is formed from the variance in amplitude of the aligned records and a roughness penalty $\lambda \int_0^1 w_i(t)^2$. λ stipulates the penalty (large λ inhibits undulation in the time transform). λ was set at 0.001 as done by Lucero et al. (1997).

$$Cost = \sum_{i=1}^{N} \int_0^1 [O_i[h_i(t)] - E(t)]^2 dt + \lambda \int_0^1 w_i(t)^2 dt \tag{12.4}$$

The expected pattern is the mean of the aligned records as follows:

$$E(t) = N^{-1} \cdot \sum_{i=1}^{N} O_i[h_i(t)] \tag{12.5}$$

As cost is defined by $E(t)$, which is estimated using $h_i(t)$ minimization must follow an iterative process with the following two steps repeated until the differences between successive costs is negligible: (1) recalculate $E(t)$; (2) re-optimize $h_i(t)$. To make optimization tractable, the standard approach is to represent $\int_0^u w_i(v)dv$ in equation 12.3 in terms of a linear summation of B-splines. For further information, see Ramsay and Silverman (1997) and Lucero et al. (1997).

MATLAB functions that perform all processing discussed are available at ftp://ego.psych.mcgill.ca/pub/ramsay/FDAfuns/.

12.2.5 **Phase and amplitude deformations and inter coordination**

After the records have been non-linearly aligned, the phase and amplitude deformations of each record from the target can be calculated ($\phi_i(h_i(t))$ and $\beta_i(h_i(t))$ respectively). The phase deformation is given by the difference in actual time and transformed time as in equation 12.6 (see Lucero 2005).

$$\phi_i(h_i(t)) = t - h_i(t) \tag{12.6}$$

The amplitude deformation for two kinematic signals is obtained by differencing the amplitude of each aligned record and the expected record as shown in equation 12.7:

$$\beta_i(h_i(t)) = O_i[h(t)] - E(t) \tag{12.7}$$

The amplitude deformation for these signals is not reported in this study as our focus is on timing.

If records are available for two signals p and q, then if each is aligned independently, the temporal inter coordination can be estimated by comparing their phase deformations. Temporal inter coordination (also termed asynchrony) may be estimated as the difference between phase deformations (equation 12.8):

$$\alpha_i(h_i(t)) = \phi_{i,p}(h_i(t)) - \phi_{i,q}(h_i(t)) \tag{12.8}$$

where a positive value indicates that an event occurs relatively later than planned in p than q. ($\alpha_i(h_i(t))$ is the temporal offset necessary to bring into synchrony with p.

12.2.6 **Indices of variability**

The statistic that summarizes variability in timing or asynchrony is denoted here by the function *IV*. This corresponds to the average variability in the respective measure over the time line. Variability in phase is indicated in equation 12.9, and variability in amplitude would be given by replacing ϕ with α. $IV(\phi)$ is equivalent to the Index of Phase Variability (IPV) in Lucero (2005) and is similar to the STI (Smith et al., 1995)

$$IV(\phi) = (N-1)^{-1} \cdot \sum_{i=1}^{N} \int_{t=0}^{1} [\phi_i(h_i(t)) - \bar{\phi}(h_i(t))]^2 \tag{12.9}$$

Figure 12.1 shows an example of FDA registration for the E (left) and lip displacement (right) signals. The panels are the same for the two signals and are described for the E signal on the left. The superimposed tracks are given in the first row and these same tracks after non-linear registration are given in the second row. Phase variability is shown in the third row. Here, the x-axis represents a linear scaling of time so that all records fit on the same (arbitrary) time frame. The y-axis is the non-linear deformation of the x-axis resulting from FDA registration. If the records were identical, this would be a single line with a slope of one. The width of the stripe gives a visual impression of phase variability across records. Phase variability is quantified as the average stripe width as indicated in equation 12.9. The last row gives the mean of the aligned records over transformed time with +/− 1 *se* indicated.

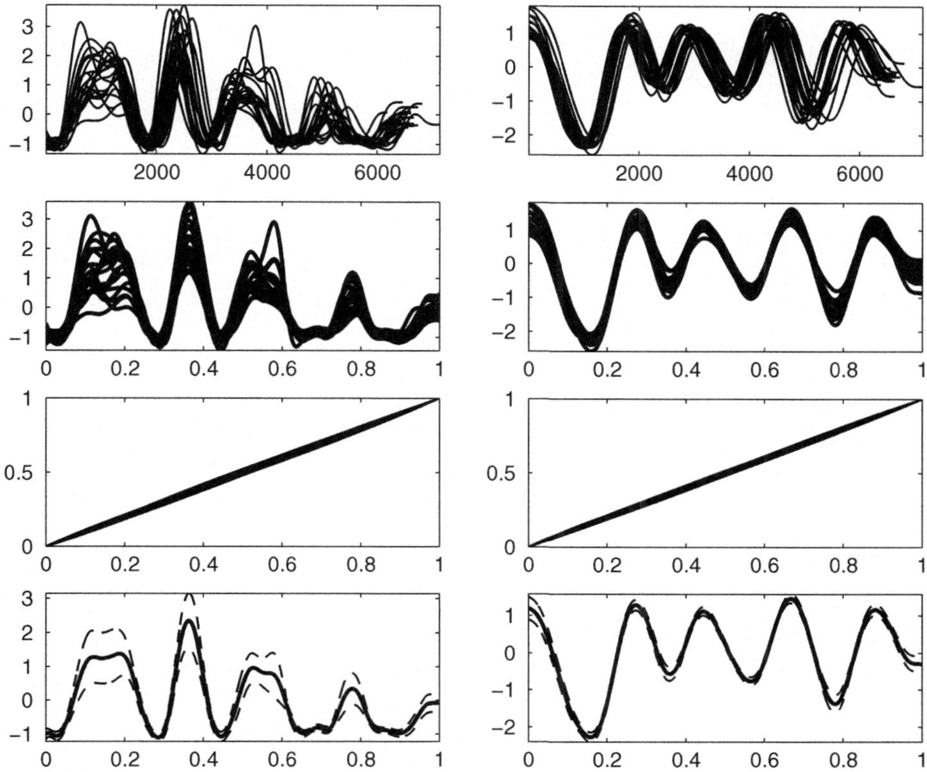

Fig.12. 1 Example results for FDA registration. The left column corresponds to speech energy and the right column to lower lip displacement. The first row are the observed records overlaid (low pass filtered at 15Hz and amplitude transformed to z-scores). Units on the x-axis correspond to sample number (frequency 8 kHz). The second row shows the same records post registration $[O_i h(t)]$. Units on the x-axis correspond to the artificial time line [0,1] as for the bottom two rows. The third row plots the new time lines $[h_i(t)]$ on the y-axis against t. If there were no warping the transform would be a straight diagonal line gradient 1. The bottom row shows the mean of the aligned records $[E(t)]$ +/− standard deviation in amplitude. Units on the y-axis are z-scores.

12.3 **Results**

The results reported are: (1) correlation of phase variability in L against E; (2) the differences in L and E phase variability indices for the participant groups; and (3) inter coordination between L and E for the participant groups.

12.3.1 **Correlation of phase variability in lips and energy across participants**

Figure 12.2 gives plots of phase variability for E (abscissa) against phase variability for L (ordinate). Each point represents one participant, and the participant group can be identified from the caption in the inset. The correlations were significant for fluent participants ($r = 0.79$, df = 10, $p = 0.002$, 2-tail) and participants who stutter ($r = 0.64$, df = 10, $p = 0.03$, 2-tail). Participants who have high temporal variability on one measure also tend to have higher temporal variability on the other.

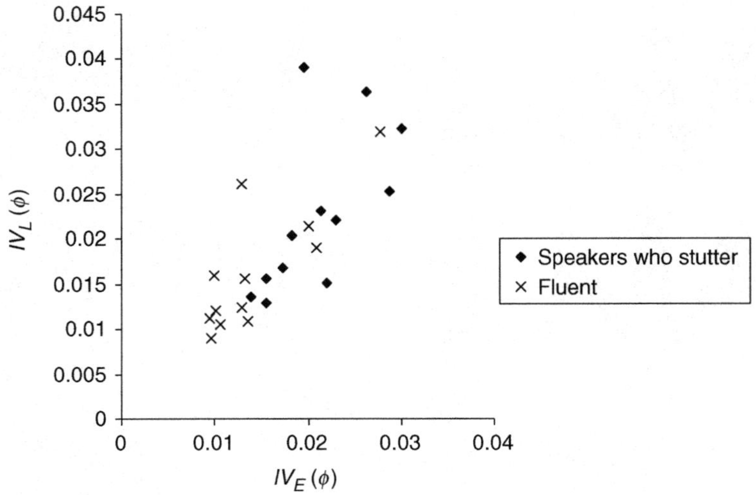

Fig. 12.2 Correlation between phase variability in energy and lips.

12.3.2 Differences between fluency groups in phase variability between L and E

The L phase variability of the participants who stuttered differed by t-test from the participants who were fluent ($t = 1.938$, df = 22, $p = 0.03$, 1-tail). Similarly, the mean E phase variability of the participants who stuttered differed by t-test from the participants who were fluent ($t = 2.92$, df = 22, $p < 0.005$, 1-tail). These results are shown in Fig. 12.3 where group mean and +/− 1 *se* are plotted for E (abscissa) and L (ordinate).

12.3.3 Inter coordination differences between fluency groups

The mean phase inter coordination scores between L and E for each participant group and +/−1 *se* are plotted on the abscissa of Fig. 12.4. A *t*- test showed that the participant groups differed

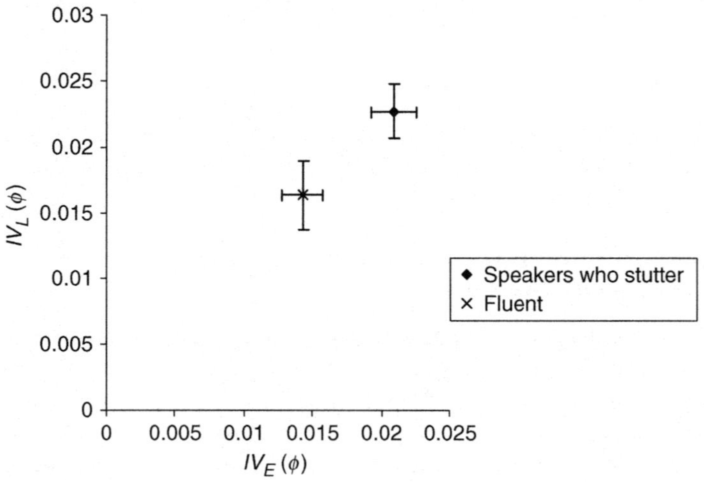

Fig. 12.3 Comparison of mean +/− *se* (top) phase variability in energy vs. lips.

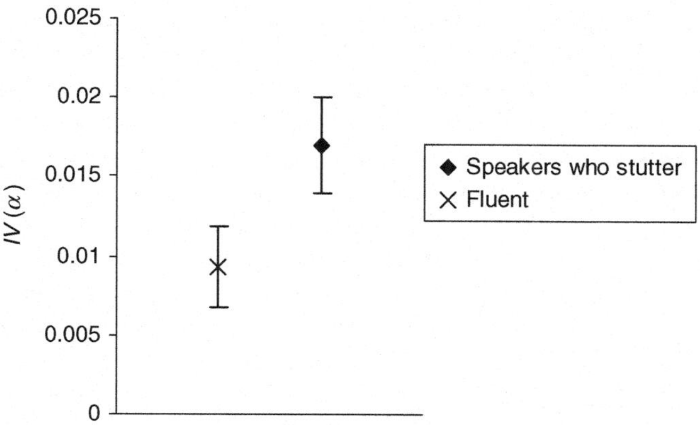

Fig.12.4 Comparison of mean +/− *se* phase asynchrony.

significantly in their ability to inter coordinate the temporal component of FDA ($t = 2.278$, df = 22, $p = 0.02$, 1-tail).

12.4 **Discussion**

Three results were reported: (1) Phase variability in L and E correlated (both for the groups of participants who stuttered and controls); (2) Phase variability was significantly different across participant groups; and (3) Inter coordination between L and E differed between the participant groups.

The first finding may be interpreted as showing that when a participant's timing is variable, it affects diverse structures (L and E) not specific ones (L or E). Second, the higher variability in people who stutter than in controls indicates that the control of the lower lip and the mechanisms that generate the amplitude envelope are more problematic for participants who stutter than for fluent controls. Third, the novel method for assessing inter coordination (here between L and E) shows that participants who stutter are more variable in the way they coordinate lip and pulmonary control. The latter finding, in particular, offers support for theories which propose that a motor deficit alone (Alfonso and van Lieshout 1997; Max and Caruso 1997; Packman et al., 1992, 1994, 1996), or in conjunction with a language system deficit (Howell 2002, 2004), occurs in people who stutter. The latter view allows language factors (which are well documented) to affect stuttering as well as motor ones like inter coordination. This comprehensiveness comes at the price of: (1) specifying how the independent language and motor systems link together; and (2) how variability in motor performance could affect fluency. The EXPLAN account of these matters is considered briefly.

Howell (in press) addressed the first of these issues. He argued that gestures serve as output from the PLAN system and that they drive the programming in the EX system. According to this view, gestures are symbolic representations in the language planning system and specifications of the goals of motor programming. In EXPLAN, motor-programming time has been treated as proportional to language planning time for simplicity. For example, in Howell's (2007) spreading activation version of EXPLAN, motor programming is directly related to planning time. In this account, time for activation to build up represents planning, and this activation decays at the same rate over the time that the word was executed. Function and content words had different decay and activation rates. The goal of this work was to show how serially organized inputs representing the words in a PW could lead to elements being triggered out of order and how this could lead to stalling and advancing dysfluency patterns. A threshold activation level was stipulated which automatically specified when a motor programme had to be initiated and what programme from the elements in the current PW should be selected. The selection procedure allows an entire past word, or part of the next word, to be selected for motor programming which gives rise to stalling and advancing behaviour depending on parameter settings such as number of function words prior to the content word and relative activation rates of the function and content words. The model also allowed motor factors to influence fluency by varying speech rate (e.g., when there is a long sequence of function words, rate will accelerate). The current results suggest that motor timing may fluctuate more in speakers who stutter. This could be incorporated into the model by treating execution as a stochastic process (the variability of which must be taken into account in planning) and examining how word sequencing is affected by modifying motor variability. This would also offer insight into whether motor timing impairments alone serve as a possible explanation for the symptoms of stuttering.

Turning to some general issues about the procedure, comparison across kinematic and audio records is possible providing the temporal signal can be obtained separately. In turn, this commends use of FDA registration (decomposition of temporal and amplitude information is not possible with STI). Further justification for use of FDA registration is that it gives more accurate estimates of amplitude variability for synthetic kinematic sequences where the outcome is known (Lucero 2005). Average articulator trajectories calculated from non-linearly aligned records also appear closer to the pattern seen in original records than those aligned linearly (Lucero et al., 1997). FDA and possibly the inter coordination statistic are useful for looking at other fluency problems. For example, Anderson et al.(2008) have used FDA coordination to examine McHenry's (2003) hypothesis that Parkinson Disease and ataxic patients are more variable on different dimensions. Anderson et al. (2008) found Parkinson Disease patients had more variability on the amplitude domain, and ataxic patients more on the temporal domain, relative to controls.

The method needs to be generalized to estimate inter coordination for other articulatory and acoustic measures of speech control. Strictly speaking, the current results favour a motor contribution to problems of speech control in participants who stutter and they rule out theories which exclude such a possibility. As no examination has been made of linguistic processing, they are neutral about whether there is a linguistic problem that co-occurs with the motor problem (Howell 2002, 2004). However, Smith has investigated language-speech motor interactions in her work using a similar paradigm as was employed here (Smith and Goffman 2004). Language factors and motor factors can be manipulated factorially. For instance, the 'buy Bobby a puppy' phrase can be inserted in phrases which differ in syntactic complexity, and participants required to speak them at different rates. Such studies would help inform interaction theories like EXPLAN, which admits a contribution to fluency control for both of these levels.

Acknowledgements

This work was supported by grant 072639 from the Wellcome Trust to Peter Howell.

References

Abbs, J.H., & Gilbert, B. (1973). A strain gauge transduction system for lip and jaw motion in two dimensions: Design criteria and calibration data. *Journal of Speech and Hearing Research*, 16, 248–256.

Alfonso, P.J., & van Lieshout, P.H.H.M. (1997). Spatial and temporal variability in obstruent gestural specification by stutterers and controls: Comparisons across sessions. In W. Hulstijn, H.F.M.

Peters & P.H.H.M. van Lieshout (Eds), *Speech Production: Motor Control, Brain Research and Fluency Disorders* (pp.151–160). Amsterdam: Elsevier.

Anderson, A., Lowit, A., & Howell, P. (2008). Temporal and spatial variability in speakers with Parkinson's Disease and Friedreich's ataxia. *Journal of Medical Speech Language Pathology*, 16, 173–180.

Barlow, S.M., Cole, K.J., & Abbs, J.H. (1983). A new head-mounted lip-jaw movement transduction system for the study of motor speech disorders. *Journal of Speech and Hearing Research*, 26, 283–288.

Howell, P. (2002). The EXPLAN theory of fluency control applied to the treatment of stuttering by altered feedback and operant procedures. In E Fava (Ed.), *Pathology and Therapy of Speech Disorders.* (pp. 95–118). Amsterdam: John Benjamins.

Howell, P. (2004). Assessment of some contemporary theories of stuttering that apply to spontaneous speech. *Contemporary Issues in Communicative Sciences and Disorders*, 39, 122–139.

Howell, P. (2007). A model of serial order problems in fluent, stuttered and agrammatic speech. *Human Movement Science*, 26, 728–741.

Howell, P. (in press). Language processing in fluency disorders. In J. Guendouzi, F. Loncke and M. Williams (Eds). *The Handbook on Psycholinguistics and Cognitive Processes: Perspectives on Communication Disorders.* London: Taylor & Francis.

Lucero, J.C. 2005. Comparison of measures of variability of speech movement trajectories using synthetic records. *Journal of Speech, Language and Hearing Research*, 48, 336–344.

Lucero, J.C., Munhall, K.G., Gracco, V.L., & Ramsay, J.O. (1997). On the registration of time and the patterning of speech movements. *Journal of Speech, Language and Hearing Research*, 40, 1111–1117.

Max, L., & Caruso, A. J. (1997). Acoustic measures of temporal intervals across speaking rates: Variability of syllable- and phrase-level relative timing. *Journal of Speech, Language and Hearing Research*, 40, 1097–1110.

Max, L., & Gracco, L. V. (2005). Coordination of oral and laryngeal movements in the perceptually fluent speech of adults who stutter. *Journal of Speech, Language and Hearing Research*, 48, 524–542.

McHenry, M. A. (2003). The effect of pacing strategies on the variability of speech movement sequences in dysarthria. *Journal of Speech, Language, and Hearing Research*, 46, 702–710.

Packman, A., Code, C., & Onslow, M. (2007). On the cause of stuttering: Integrating theory with brain and behavioral research. *Journal of Neurolinguistics*, 20, 253–262.

Packman, A., Onslow, M., & van Doorn, J. (1994). Prolonged speech and the modification of stuttering: Perceptual, acoustic, and electroglottographic data. *Journal of Speech, Language and Hearing Research*, 37, 724–737.

Packman, A., Onslow, M., Richard, F., & van Doorn, J. (1996). Syllabic stress and variability: A model of stuttering. *Clinical Linguistics and Phonetics*, 10, 235–263.

Packman, A., van Doorn, J., & Onslow, M. (1992). Stutteirng treatments: What is happening to the acoustic signal? *Proceedings of the Fourth Australian International Conference on Speech Science and Technology*, Brisbane, Australia.

Ramsay, J.O., & Silverman, B.W. (1997). *Functional Data Analysis.* New York: Springer-Verlag.

Riley, G.D. (1994). *Stuttering Severity Instrument for Children and Adults, Third Edition.* Austin, TX: Pro-Ed.

Selkirk, E. (1984). *Phonology and Syntax: The Relation Between Sound and Structure.* Cambridge, MA: MIT Press.

Smith, A., & Goffman, L. (2004). Interaction of motor and language factors in the development of speech production. In B. Maasen, R. Kent, H. Peters, P. van Lieshout, & W. Hulstijn (Eds), *Speech Motor Control in Normal and Disordered Speech* (pp. 227–252). Oxford: Oxford University Press.

Smith, A., Goffman, L., Zelaznik, H. N., Ying, G., & McGillem, C. (1995). Spatiotemporal stability and the patterning of speech movement sequences. *Experimental Brain Research*, 104, 493–501.

Section 5

Clinical impact

Chapter 13

Classification and taxonomy of motor speech disorders: what are the issues?

Gary Weismer and Yunjung Kim

Abstract

This paper presents a historical overview of the Mayo Clinic perspective on motor speech disorders, and argues that this perspective has served its purpose and should be abandoned in favor of a different approach. The Mayo Clinic perspective assumes a tight coupling between 'classic' neurological symptoms of the various diseases causing dysarthria and the associated speech symptoms; there is little or no empirical support for this assumption. Moreover, the Mayo Clinic perspective has fostered a scientific concern with oromotor, nonverbal performance of persons with motor speech disorders, but there is little evidence that such a concern has produced insights to the *speech production* disorder in dysarthria or apraxia of speech. The scientific literature on dysarthria and apraxia of speech has been very concerned with the differences between the dysarthria types originally identified in the Mayo Clinic studies, and between dysarthria and apraxia of speech, yet a careful examination of the literature reveals many speech production phenomena that are similar across these speech disorders. We argue for a speech production and perception program that identifies these commonalities as 'core' phenomena of motor speech disorders. Knowledge of these core phenomena will permit a more specific identification of the speech production and perception factors that truly distinguish different kinds of motor speech disorder. Motor speech disorders should be pursued scientifically by a focus on speech research, rather than work on oromotor, nonspeech behaviors.

13.1 **Prologue**

Classification of motor speech disorders was systematized by the work of Grewel (1957) and Darley et al. (1969a, b; 1975). The classification system developed by Darley et al. (1975) hereafter referred to as the Mayo Clinic System, has been slightly modified as described by Duffy (2005) and continues to be the gold standard among clinicians and scientists interested in motor speech disorders. The Mayo Clinic System is based on the assumption of a straightforward relationship between the classic symptoms of different neurological diseases and the speech production symptoms observed in those diseases. The classic symptoms of neurological disease referred to here are mostly signs and symptoms from limb behaviour, including deficits of tone, reflex, posture, and movement speed, range, and rhythm. As reviewed in an earlier paper (Weismer 2006), these signs and symptoms were co-opted by Darley et al. (1975) for application to the performance of the orofacial, laryngeal, and respiratory system in speech production. More specifically, these classic signs and symptoms were regarded as likely explanations for the disease-specific speech production deficits inferred by Darley et al.(1975) from their perceptual measurements.

Because Darley et al.'s(1975) presentation of the Mayo Clinic System emphasized the uniqueness of the different dysarthria types (as well as of apraxia of speech [AOS] as a separate category), dysarthria studies since the 1970s have tended to document the characteristics of individual dysarthria types. Dysarthria types are typically defined in terms of speakers who share a disease type. Independent perceptual judgments of dysarthria type may be made, but rarely with the judges blinded to disease type. The close link between disease and dysarthria type follows from the assumption that the classical signs of a particular disease will produce a specific kind of dysarthria for speakers having that disease, with variations in the observed speech symptoms resulting from (perhaps) variations in severity of involvement and/or idiosyncratic adaptations (compensations) to the speech motor dysfunction.

This perspective on the nature of dysarthria emphasized *classification* as the primary objective of dysarthria research. This emphasis is, for the most part, still with us, as the majority of published work in motor speech disorders seeks answers to, for example, what makes hypokinetic dysarthria different from spastic dysarthria, or either of these different from, say, AOS. From this perspective, studies of single disease groups of speakers with dysarthria make sense. The collection of data from many such studies should, in theory, lead to a substantial knowledge base of characteristics of the different dysarthrias and AOS, making the classification more precise and complete.

There is another approach to understanding motor speech disorders, however, one that has not enjoyed a lot of popularity but (in the present opinion) makes a good deal of sense from a scientific perspective. It seems reasonable to expect that the variety of neurological diseases resulting in dysarthria and AOS would produce a core of *similar* speech symptoms across the many diseases, along with whatever differences are assumed to distinguish the various types of motor speech disorders. This perspective would add a taxonomical approach to the study of motor speech disorders, in addition to the dominant classification approach described above. As summarized by Balint et al. (2006), taxonomy focuses on similarities, classification on differences. The application of a taxonomical approach to the scientific investigation of motor speech disorders requires studies in which speakers with different disease and dysarthria types are evaluated for their performance in a speech production task or tasks. If substantial similarities are observed across many such studies, scientists may be in a position to identify a core set of deficits common to most (if not all) motor speech disorders. That core, if identified, could serve as the basis for the development of an effective model (one that would make specific predictions), or if we want to be really ambitious, a well-developed theory of motor speech disorders. Focusing on such a core does not rule out potentially important differences between different types of motor speech disorders. To use a statistical metaphor, these differences may be considered as the residuals of the model fit to the core symptoms. Perhaps it is these residuals that permit us to hear, not always with great success (Bunton et al., 2007; Zeplin and Kent 1996; Zyski and Weisiger 1987) the different dysarthria types identified in the Mayo Clinic System.

This prologue sets up a more detailed consideration of the history of classification in motor speech disorders, and of the consequences to the recent four-decade history of the scientific treatment of dysarthria and AOS. We would like to ask the more specific question, 'Where did the current gold standard come from, and how has that dominant system affected progress in the understanding of motor speech disorders?'

13.2 The Grewel/Mayo Clinic approach: it's origins and consequences

Grewel (1957, p. 327), in specifying his conceptual framework for an understanding of dysarthria, said, '. . . the definition of dysarthria as a neurological speech disorder compels us to a neurological analysis of every dysarthria'. As pointed out in Weismer and Liss (1991), such a statement is tautologous, and therefore has little logical or inferential truth value. Saying that something is *x*, and that only *x* techniques can therefore illuminate *x*, is completely circular. Grewel (1957, pp. 328–329) follows his premise with, '. . . dysarthria . . . is the expression of the muscular disease, and the specific traits of such a dysarthria are readily explained by the characteristics of the neurological disease as such, manifesting themselves in the arthric functions'. This quote is consistent with, and the likely origin of, the Mayo view that the speech symptoms in dysarthria are the classic symptoms of neurological disease as filtered through the speech mechanism (see Weismer 2006).

Grewel (1957) offered a classification system for dysarthria that was largely anatomical. Nine of his fourteen categories – such as cortical dysarthria, subcortical dysarthria, cerebellar dysarthria – were based on the location of a more or less circumscribed lesion. An assumption behind this classification, not unlike the Mayo System, was that these anatomical lesion locations would translate to neurological signs and symptoms and therefore to speech function (dysarthria symptoms) in a fairly direct way. Given what we know about speaker variability in dysarthria, even within a group of patients with a well-documented disease process, this assumption seems very wrong. In particular, it fails to capture any aspect of severity, which is a major shortcoming of the Grewel/Mayo classification systems.

The remainder of Grewel's classification system included categories for 'diffuse' pathologies of the nervous system, such as head injury, epilepsy, and myasthenia gravis. The Mayo System does not recognize these as separate dysarthrias, but there is a history of using the original dysarthria labels (e.g., spastic, ataxic, and so forth, as well as various combinations (mixed dysarthrias) of the primary categories) to classify patients with these disorders. This is especially pertinent to the wide variety of dysarthrias heard in adults and children with head injury (for examples of this variety, see Wang et al., 2005, Table 1; and Cahill et al., 2005, Table I).

13.3 The Mayo Clinic System: its role and impact on the study of motor speech disorders

The Mayo Clinic System for the classification of motor speech disorders had its genesis in the 1969 two-part report of Darley et al. (1969a, b). That report described clusters of perceptually measured speech symptoms that appeared to be unique to the different disease groups selected by the authors for study. Those disease groups included persons with lower motor neuron, upper motor neuron, cerebellar, Parkinson, and basal ganglia disease. Within any one of these groups, there was variation in aetiology, but the assumption was made that the essentials of the underlying pathophysiology were more or less homogeneous. In addition to the five major groups of flaccid, spastic, ataxic, hypokinetic, and hyperkinetic dysarthria, Darley et al. (1975) also identified 'mixed' types in which damage was known or assumed to be located in two or more of the major type locations. For example, multiple sclerosis (MS) was said to involve both cerebellar and upper motor neuron damage, and hence was associated with a spastic-ataxic type of mixed dysarthria. The mixed types showed how much the Mayo Clinic System relied, like Grewel (1957), on presumed correspondences between *location* of damage and presumed perceptual outcome. No reasons were given, however, for why combined upper and lower motorneuron damage, as seen (for example) in amyotrophic lateral sclerosis (ALS), should produce the additive effect of a spastic-plus-flaccid sounding speech disorder, rather than some integrated effect that produced a different perceptual impression. The same can be said for any other mixed type of dysarthria identified in the Mayo Classification System.

It is not an exaggeration to say that the Mayo Clinic System dominates the field of motor speech disorders, both in the clinical and research domains. This enormous research effort, in which a team of clinical scientists combined their skills to make careful perceptual ratings of close to forty perceptual dimensions for well over 200 speakers with neurological disease, stands as a monument in the literature on speech disorders. The Mayo Clinic System attained the rare status of a 'gold standard' for the description and diagnosis of motor speech disorders (see Duffy 2005, p. 9). In the first edition of Duffy's outstanding text, he said, 'The work of Darley, Aronson, and Brown . . . is nearly universally accepted by speech-language pathologists and many neurologists' (Duffy 1995, p. 4). This is quite an accolade when so many other areas of the discipline of clinical and research speech-language pathology have failed to converge on a single, universally understood and employed system.

The Mayo Clinic System was the catalyst for a world-wide research effort to understand the nature and manifestations of different motor speech disorders. Over the last forty years or so, many studies either directly or indirectly guided by the Mayo Clinic System have been published in leading scientific journals (see Duffy 2005; and Murdoch 1998, for good reviews of this work). Clearly, the Mayo Clinic System had a beneficial influence on the science of speech production disorders.

In the present opinion, however, the dominance of the Mayo Clinic System has also produced some undesirable influences on the understanding of motor speech disorders. In fact, our argument is that these undesirable influences are holding back the improvement of the scientific knowledge base, and ultimately the construction of a theory of motor speech disorders.

Currently, there is no empirically based theory of motor speech disorders. There is, however, a theoretical vantage point offered by the Mayo Clinic System, one very much like that proposed by Grewel. In the Mayo Clinic System view, the speech production deficit in motor speech disorders can be understood as the effect of the classic signs of the various underlying diseases (e.g., Parkinson disease, ALS) as 'filtered' or 'expressed' through the speech mechanism. Know the disease and its classical pathophysiology, and the speech symptoms are revealed as the outcome of such pathophysiology. This is what Darley et al. (1975) meant when they said the speech symptoms of a person with neurological disease had a localizing value. That claim simply inverted the forward link between underlying pathophysiology and speech production effects. For example, a stenotic voice quality was thought to be the logical outcome of hypertonicity and possibly hyperreflexia, both of which are classical symptoms of upper motor neuron disease. Thus the perception of a stenotic voice quality, perhaps in combination with certain other impressions, is a localizing sign to upper motor neuron damage.

The impact of this dominant view on the science of motor speech disorders cannot be minimized. In some cases, this impact is obvious, in others it is more subtle. For example, the Mayo Clinic System promoted a focus on diagnosis of *disease*, not the speech production deficit. This follows directly from the (unproven, to this point in time) assumption that if you know the disease and its associated neuropathology, you know the speech production deficit. A careful reading of Darley et al. (1969b, p. 496) suggests that at one level they understood this as *hypothesis* concerning unique speech physiology characteristics in the different dysarthria types. The evaluation of that hypothesis, however, often took the form of attempts to measure classical neuropathological signs in orofacial structures (Hunker et al., 1982; Hunker and Abbs 1984), rather than a careful investigation of speech production characteristics in speakers with dysarthria. When such 'neurological sign' measures were developed and related to phoneme-specific speech movements in unnatural utterances (and in the absence of acoustic or perceptual measures), the results were typically equivocal (compare Caligiuri 1987, to Hunker et al., 1982). Moreover, in the single example of connected speech examined for evidence of a straightforward connection between an assumed underlying neuropathophysiology and speech production phenomena, the results were unequivocal but in the *opposite* direction predicted by the Mayo Clinic perspective. Neilson and O'Dwyer (1984) showed that electromyograms obtained from orofacial structures in adult speakers with athetoid cerebral palsy and dysarthria were as stable across repetitions as data obtained from neurologically normal speakers. This result – largely ignored in the literature on motor speech disorders – is not consistent with the expectation of constantly fluctuating tone in athetosis causing abnormal variability in the speech production of persons with hyperkinetic dysarthria (see full discussion of this issue in Weismer 2006).

The Mayo Clinic System has had a very direct effect on research design and the publication of experimental results. These issues are very difficult to document in the traditional way, because the proper documentation (grant reviews and reviews of papers submitted for publication) is confidential. This being said, it seems unlikely that scientists would argue with the *presumed* research design requirement of homogeneous dysarthria types (or, perhaps, type of neurological disease) in studies concerned with speech production characteristics in motor speech disorders. An assumption of many reviewers and editors seems to be that a group of persons with motor speech disorders is not properly constituted unless dysarthria type and disease are specified as 'controlled' (that is, the same) for however many participants are included in the group of persons studied. This is, however, nothing more than a premise from the Mayo System perspective. To our knowledge, there is no evidence in the literature – indeed, not even an experimental attempt to demonstrate the fact – that dysarthria type (or disease type) is a proper blocking variable in experimental designs or descriptive data bases dealing with motor speech disorders. Recent experimental evidence (Kim 2007) suggests, in fact, that a variable such as speech severity (indexed by speech intelligibility scores) explains at least as much variance in speech production measures as dysarthria type. The legacy from the Mayo Clinic System of dysarthria type as a meaningful blocking variable must be recognized as unproven, and more specifically, as a hindrance to the development of an adequate theory of speech production in motor speech disorders.

The claim that the broad acceptance of the Mayo Clinic System in clinical and scientific arenas has inhibited the development of a theory of speech production deficits in motor speech disorders is not a trivial, armchair issue. Theories are developed and refined as part of the process of seeking explanations for phenomena. Presumably, the primary explanandum in a theory of motor speech disorders is why persons with neuromotor disease experience problems with their *speech* intelligibility. Theory development was, and continues to be, inhibited by the Mayo Clinic System because the theory is already assumed to be known. As pointed out above, however, the failure to link classical, disease-specific pathophysiologies with specific aspects of speech production deficits shows the assumption to be a bad one. Moreover, the theoretical assumptions have directed the attention and efforts of clinicians and scientists primarily to the mechanism, and away from other areas that should enter into theory-building efforts in motor speech disorders. For example, large-scale studies of the acoustic characteristics of motor speech disorders, and especially of how they are *similar or different* (see above) within and across dysarthria or disease types, have not been undertaken. Of greater concern is the absence, until recently, of any concern with how the unusual speech signal produced by a person with a motor speech disorder might be processed by a human listener. The Mayo Clinic System, with its theoretical vantage point focused exclusively on the production mechanism and its assumed disabilities, ignores the role of the listener in speech intelligibility. Work by Liss and her colleagues (Liss et al., 1998, 2000, 2002; Mattys and

Liss 2008) shows why speech perception issues are a critical component of an adequate theory of motor speech disorders.

The focus of the Mayo Clinic System on classical neuropathophysiology and its presumed direct link with speech symptoms of various dysarthrias, is nowhere more obvious than in the fascination of our field with oromotor, nonverbal behaviours as a window to speech motor control. Weismer (2006) has reviewed the 40-year history of empirical work in this area, and concluded that there is no evidence that evaluation of an articulatory structure or structures in nonspeech behaviours provides insight to *speech* motor control processes. Weismer (2006) also presents theoretical arguments, consonant with those offered by Ziegler (2003; but see Ballard et al., 2003), against a concerted research effort on oromotor nonverbal behaviours that takes as its purpose the elucidation of *speech* motor control processes. This theoretical position is derived from (1) the lack of empirical evidence for a link between the two behaviours, (2) the contemporary view of many motor control theorists, including speech motor control theorists (Guenther et al., 1998; Tourville et al., 2008), that control strategies depend in significant ways on the nature of the task, and (3) the wholly arbitrary nature of oromotor, nonverbal tasks chosen to 'represent' speech motor control capabilities. Weismer (2006) points out that research in motor speech disorders has been dominated by studies of oromotor, nonverbal behaviours, or repeated-syllable strings that bear little relationship to actual speech production behaviours. That paper concludes with a call for a concerted effort to describe speech production behaviours in motor speech disorders, and to formulate hypotheses concerning speech behaviour, rather than nonspeech behaviors.[1]

13.4 Speech production behaviours in Motor Speech Disorders: a preliminary theoretical perspective

Despite the focus on oromotor, nonverbal behaviours in persons with motor speech disorders, there is a literature that allows some preliminary theoretical considerations concerning speech production characteristics in motor speech disorders. One component of these considerations is a small set of operating principles and assumptions. First, and most importantly, we assume that the speech acoustic signal is an integral part of speech motor control. Eliminate the speech acoustic signal and the control task is no longer speech; it is rather another type of motor control. This assumption is consistent with the role of task specificity in general motor control theories, and was originally postulated by Netsell (see collection of papers in Netsell 1986) as a requirement for understanding the specific case of speech motor control. Contemporary statements of the task-specific nature of speech motor control can be found in Ziegler (2003) and Weismer (2006). The speech acoustic signal is an integral part of the computational model of speech motor control described and under refinement by Guenther and his associates (Guenther et al., 1995; Tourville et al., 2008).

This major assumption of speech motor control as task specific, and more precisely the role of the speech acoustic signal as an integral component of the control style and strategy of producing speech, drives the second operating principle. This principle relates to the empirical content of theory development in motor speech disorders. Specifically, a large-scale descriptive and

[1] The emphasis on *speech* is meant to highlight the specific issue of relating oromotor nonverbal behaviours to speech motor control. We are not arguing against basic studies of orofacial control, as they may bear on interesting issues, but against the specific claim that, for example, the steadiness of tongue or lip force or the ability to follow a varying signal with tongue motions has something to do with speech motor control. These propositions are very difficult to defend empirically or theoretically.

experimental effort focused on speech production in persons with motor speech disorders must be undertaken to understand what must be explained by a theory of motor speech disorders. The data base on speech movement characteristics in motor speech disorders, for example, is very limited, and studies in which movement characteristics are related to speech acoustic and perception characteristics are even more scarce. If a useful theory of motor speech disorders is developed, it will require such multiple-level data, including analyses of the transforms between speech movements, the speech acoustic signal, and perception of that signal. This means that descriptive work and experiments (in which variables are manipulated – such as rate, stress, speaking style – and analysed in 'true' experimental designs) must include collection and analysis of at least these three levels of data.[2]

The final operating principle revisits the distinction, made in the Prologue and elaborated in the middle section of this essay, of the difference between diagnosis and taxonomy. The motivation for the large-scale studies suggested above should be the abandonment of the Mayo Clinic System, and rejection of the idea of differences between dysarthria types as a primary assumption or expectation. We should seek to discover *similarities*, not differences, across speakers with different neuromotor diseases and varying speech severities (as indexed by measures of speech intelligibility). The discovery of these similarities will point to the differences, the 'residuals' of the model.

Why should this be done? Why abandon a long-standing and widely accepted classification system for motor speech disorders? Several reasons have been given above, but the issue can be pushed even further within the framework of the current discussion of how to begin model and theory development in motor speech disorders. First, the Mayo Clinic System virtually ignores the contribution from severity of involvement to speech production variation in persons with motor speech disorders. The Mayo Clinic System does not explicitly reject the idea of severity as a major player in the speech symptoms of motor speech disorders, it simply pays no attention to it in the classification scheme.[3] As noted above, Kim (2007) has shown that when severity is defined by speech intelligibility scores, the measure is equally or more explanatory of variation in acoustic measures of speech as is dysarthria type. Second, the existing literature on speech production characteristics in persons with motor speech disorders suggests some notable similarities across speakers with different disease and dysarthria types. Some of these similarities are discussed briefly here.

13.4.1 **Speaking rate**

A survey of the literature suggests that the majority of speakers with motor speech disorders have slower-than-normal speaking rates. The tendency for speaking rates to be slower than normal can be inferred from studies in which actual speaking rates of phrase-level material are

[2] This kind of statement is open to the criticism of infinite regress, because there are other worthy levels of analysis (for example, electromyographic, imaging of brain regions) that could (and will) enter into a complete theoretical account of speech production in motor speech disorders. We keep the focus on movement, acoustics, and perception here as most immediately relevant to models that relate different levels of analysis to an index of the communication impairment.

[3] It can be argued that severity played a role in the original specification of types, because multiple covariations among perceptual dimensions that varied along a scale of severity (the 7-point rating scale) were the basis of the perceptual clusters that differentiated the types. We mean to say the Mayo Clinic System pays no attention to severity variation within any one dysarthria type. For example, mild and severe hypokinetic dysarthria are the same entity, varying in 'how extensive' the symptoms are. There are no data to support such an assertion, and preliminary data to suggest that the assertion is at least not quite correct (Kim 2007).

reported (Liss et al., 2006; Turner and Weismer 1993) or from studies of segment (and especially vowel) duration in which longer vowel durations imply slower speaking rates. An exception to this rule is sometimes said to be hypokinetic dysarthria, in which speaking rates may be faster than normal, but even this notion is arguable (see Weismer 1984). In one of the only studies to compare speaking rate across different types of dysarthria (associated with different disease types), Nishio and Niimi (2001) found slower-than-normal speaking rates for a reading passage in persons with flaccid, spastic, ataxic, hypokinetic, hyperkinetic, mixed, and unilateral upper motor neuron dysarthrias.

13.4.2 Compressed vowel space

Compressed vowel spaces, typically demonstrated with the American English corner vowels, also seem to be an almost universal characteristic of motor speech disorders, regardless of dysarthria type. Lehiste (1965) was the first to report the relative collapse of the vowel space in a small number of speakers with varying neuromotor diseases and presumably different-sounding dysarthrias, and others (Jeng 2000; Liu et al., 2005; Weismer 1991; Weismer et al., 2001; Ziegler and Von Cramon 1983) have reported the same thing for speakers with head injury, Parkinson disease, ALS, and cerebral palsy. Speakers with dysarthria apparently have restricted mobility of the articulators for vowel production, regardless of the dysarthria or disease type.

13.4.3 Reduced formant transitions and articulatory speeds

There is also compelling evidence for reduced formant transitions (either in extent – range of frequencies covered – or rate) in speakers with motor speech disorders, especially when diphthongs and perhaps vowel-to-vowel sequences are the object of study. These findings have been reported for speakers with Parkinson disease, ALS, and Multiple Sclerosis (Weismer 1991; Weismer et al., 2001; Rosen et al., 2008). A related finding in the literature, summarized by Weismer (1997) and supported by more recent work (e.g., Ackermann et al., 1997; and see review in Yunusova et al., 2008), is that speech movements of individual articulators are slower in speakers with dysarthria, as compared to neurologically normal speakers.

13.4.4 Reduced phonetic contrasts

A final commonality reported for several different dysarthria types is a reduction of certain phonetic contrasts when measured acoustically, as compared to those contrasts measured in the speech of neurologically normal speakers. These contrast reductions have been observed for voice-onset time among speakers with a variety of dysarthria types (Auzou et al., 2000; Jeng 2000), for Mandarin and Cantonese tone types in speakers with cerebral palsy (Jeng et al., 2006; Whitehill et al., 2000), and for the spectral characteristics of selected obstruents in speakers with ALS and cerebral palsy (Jeng 2000; Tjaden and Turner 1997). These contrast reductions are consistent with the vowel space compression reviewed here; taken together, these effects seem to reflect a general reduction of articulatory behaviour likely to be observed in almost any motor speech disorder. This reduced articulatory behaviour yields reduced acoustic contrasts that are a key part of intelligible speech.

The phenomena discussed above suggest that there is already good evidence for common characteristics in motor speech disorders, regardless of dysarthria or disease type. Data such as these should serve as one impetus to initiate a taxonomic approach to the study of motor speech disorders. Future theoretical efforts would feature these similarities, and others discovered in the course of research, as the core of neuromotor disruption of speech production processes. Whatever differences emerge from a programme of study devoted to understanding these core features of motor speech disorders may eventually be the basis for the occasional ability of *blinded* listeners to identify type of dysarthria/type of disease.

As the science currently stands, we should make no demands on authors of journal articles or grant proposals to specify dysarthria type as a blocking variable in experimental designs; there is simply no empirical evidence to support such a demand, and sufficient evidence that the dysarthria types and their underlying perceptual dimensions are not judged reliably (Bunton et al., 2007; Zyski and Weisinger 1987; Zeplin and Kent 1996). Moreover, there are no *a priori* reasons for using the Mayo Clinic System as a set of premises for subject selection in experiments having particular purposes. A good example of this latter issue is the notion that investigations of articulatory incoordination in motor speech disorders may be best served by speakers with cerebellar disease (and, presumably, ataxic dysarthria), because classic cerebellar symptoms include coordination difficulties. There is no empirical evidence to support the presence of articulatory incoordination in speakers judged to have ataxic, as compared to (for example) hypokinetic dysarthria, or no evidence to the contrary, in fact. *A priori* assumptions concerning which dysarthria types (which disease type) will be associated with which particular articulatory problems are obstacles, rather than good starting points, for the development of an adequate theoretical treatment of motor speech disorders (see for example, Spencer and Slocumb (2007) on expectations of articulatory discoordination as a defining characteristic of ataxic dysarthria, and presumably the absence of such an expectation in at least some other types of dysarthria). An example of this from the nonspeech literature is the demonstration of gait incoordination in patients with ALS but also with Parkinson disease (Hausdorff et al., 2000). We should not allow our empirical efforts to be constrained by unproven assumptions with historical, but no laboratory, cachet.

13.5 **Indices of speech motor control: is there direction?**

As reviewed by Weismer (2006), oromotor, nonverbal tasks were designed as a way to assess the integrity of speech motor control in persons with neuromotor disorders.[4] A reasonable question is, if we do not evaluate integrity of speech motor control using oromotor, nonverbal tests, how then can it be done? One attraction of oromotor, nonverbal tests is that they are highly controllable, can be instrumented with a certain degree of sophistication, and eliminate the messy side effect of interspeaker variability so common in the production of actual speech sequences. We argue here that these are not reasons to reject the use of speech production behaviours to evaluate speech motor control integrity. The ability to instrument a behaviour does not make it attractive in the absence of a rationale for the particulars of the measurement, and the choice to eliminate

[4] There are some interesting historical oddities in the assumption that these kinds of evaluation would reveal the underlying, subsytem pathophysiology of the articulatory mechanism, and, having these data, generate some meaningful statements concerning the expected speech motor control deficit. One oddity is the failure to pose any interesting questions about how these oromotor, nonpeech measures might vary *across* the different dysarthria/disease types, especially because the types are assumed to be determined by very different neuropathologies. As reviewed by Weismer (2006), speakers with a variety of motor speech disorders (defined either by dysarthria or disease type) have been evaluated using such measures, but always in *separate* studies with the question of how the performance *for that one group* differs from *normal* performance. The more obvious and relevant question, given the assumption of a mapping of classical neuropathological signs on to speech production behaviour via nonspeech evaluations, is how oromotor, nonspeech performance differs across the types of dysarthria/neuromotor disease. To the best of our knowledge, such an experiment has never been published, nor have relevant hypotheses concerning the outcome of such an experiment been posed in the literature. To report data from such tasks in which speakers with one form of neuromotor disease and dysarthria perform differently from normal is to report the obvious.

the speech signal leads, as discussed above, to an evaluation of motor control of behaviour that is not speech. We propose a concerted effort to establish knowledge of how speech motor control varies in word and sentence productions, and offer here a preliminary starting point for how such work might be initiated.

The approach suggested here is in the form of a hypothesis. The hypothesis is that some *normal* bounds of variability can be determined for selected movement and/or acoustic measures from word and/or sentence productions, and that when the measure is made for a speaker with dysarthria, its *distance* from this normal range of variability will have some meaning. That distance is hypothesized to index something about the speaker's speech motor control capabilities.

An example of this kind of analysis is shown in Fig. 13.1. The figure shows data on F2 slope (*x*-axis) for the word *wax*. F2 slope is a measure known to be sensitive to the presence of neuromotor disease, as discussed above and originally demonstrated by Weismer et al. (1988) and Weismer (1991). Moreover, several studies have shown that F2 slope varies systematically with speech intelligibility in speakers with dysarthria (Kent et al., 1989; Weismer et al., 2001). The word *wax* has an extensive F2 transition from the relatively low value associated with the [w] to the value associated with the following low-front vowel. In other words, the word requires a fairly extensive and rapid change in vocal tract configuration, which would seem to provide an optimal setting for the expression of speech motor control problems, if they are present. Figure 13.1 has two *y*-axes, the left one showing cumulative probability of F2 slope values for *wax* collected from neurologically normal speakers, the right one speech intelligibility scores from a small set of speakers with neurological disease and dysarthria. Normal productions of *wax* were collected from ten speakers (five males, five females), in a task requiring multiple productions of the word. From the string of repeated words, the middle eight were chosen for analysis and are the basis for the cumulative probability distribution shown in Fig. 13.1. The plotted curve shows how the

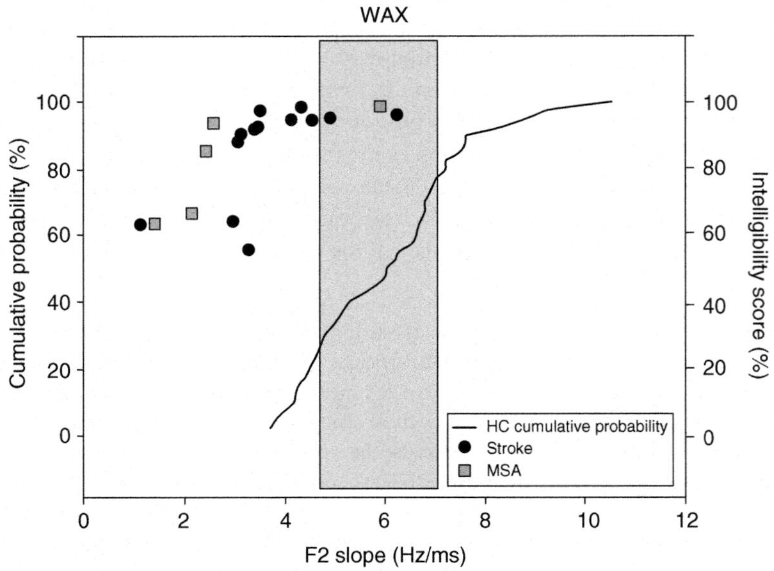

Fig. 13.1 Cumulative probability function (solid line, referred to left *y*-axis) showing distributional characteristics of F2 slope for neurologically normal speakers producing the word *wax*, and individual speaker averages of F2 slope for the same word produced by speakers with MSA and Stroke, plotted as a function of single word speech intelligibility scores (right *y*-axis). See text for additional description.

value of F2 slope grows from lowest to highest across these eighty repetitions, and the shaded box superimposed on this distribution depicts the interquartile range – 4.7 to 7.0 Hz/ms – for these eighty values. The individual points plotted in Fig. 13.1 are average F2 slopes produced in the same task by thirteen speakers with Multiple System Atrophy (MSA; boxes) and five with Stroke (circles). These data are plotted as a function of single-word speech intelligibility scores (right *y*-axis) to illustrate the main point of this speculative demonstration of how one might approach the issue of indexing speech motor control capabilities using speech production data. Note, for example, how the majority of plotted points for speakers with neurological disease fall outside the interquartile range for normal speakers, a finding consistent with reduced F2 transitions in speakers with dysarthria, regardless of type or disease. Note further how there are a group of points between roughly 90% and 100% intelligibility that vary by relatively large degrees in their distance from normal-range values of F2 slope. Here we have similar intelligibilities, at least as measured using a single word test, but widely varying 'severities' of the F2 slope for the word *wax*. A similar group of points is seen for five speakers in the 60% intelligibility range. Do these varying speech production 'severities' for this specific measure, at a given level of speech intelligibility, mean anything? Do they predict other aspects of speech motor control? Or more functional estimates of speech intelligibility?

Our concluding argument is not that these measures are the right ones. It is that there are ways to use actual speech production data to explore variations in speech motor control capabilities in persons with dysarthria. There are challenges in such a research programme, however. Just as in the case of oromotor, nonverbal tasks, where the choice of task has typically not been rationalized, or has been rationalized in a way that is an infinite regress (e.g., making the oromotor, nonverbal task as speech-like as possible; see Weismer 2006), the choice of words or sentences for indices of speech motor control cannot proceed without a good rationale. The choice of the word *wax* for the demonstration data in Fig. 13.1 was rationalized in terms of the large articulatory movements required to produce the word in a successful way. But other words with the same characteristics of relatively large-scale changes in vocal tract configuration have been shown to produce a different pattern of results as those shown in Fig. 13.1 (Kim 2007). And clearly, F2 slope is merely one measure among many that could be used in the development of such indices.

The point is, if research efforts over the next thirty or forty years focus on speech production in persons with motor speech disorders, in a manner parallel to the research effort in oromotor, nonspeech control for the past forty-some years, we are likely to learn a great deal about *speech* motor control and its vulnerabilities in motor speech disorders. In our opinion, it is time to drop classification for taxonomy, and allow taxonomy to generate theory.

References

Ackermann, H., Hertrich, I., Daum, I., Scharf, G., & Spieker, S. (1997). Kinematic analysis of articulatory movements in central motor disorders. *Movement Disorders*, **12**, 1019–1027.

Auzou, P., Özsancak, C., Morris, R.J., Jan, M., Eustache, F., & Hannequin, D. (2000). Voice onset time in aphasia, apraxia of speech and dysarthria: A review. *Clinical Linguistics and Phonetics*, **14**, 131–150.

Balint, G.P., Buchanan, W.W., & Dequeker, J. (2006). A brief history of medical taxonomy and diagnosis. *Clinical Rheumatology*, **25**, 132–135.

Ballard, K.J., Robin, D.A., & Folkins, J.W. (2003). An integrated model of speech motor control: A response to Ziegler. *Aphasiology*, **17**, 37–48.

Bunton, K., Kent, R.D., Duffy, J.R., Rosenbek, J.C., & Kent, J.F. (2007). Listener agreement for auditory-perceptual ratings of dysarthria. *Journal of Speech, Language, and Hearing Research*, **50**, 1481–1495.

Cahill, L.M., Murdoch, B.E., and Theodoros, D.G. (2005). Articulatory function following traumatical brain injury in childhood: A perceptual and instrumental analysis. *Brain Injury*, **19**, 55–79.

Caligiuri, M.P. (1987). Labial kinematics during speech in patients with Parkinsonian rigidity. *Brain*, **110**, 1033–1044.

Darley, F.L., Aronson, A.E., and Brown, J.R. (1969a). Differential diagnostic patterns of dysarthria. *Journal of Speech and Hearing Research*, **12**, 246–269.

Darley, F.L., Aronson, A.E., and Brown, J.R. (1969b). Clusters of deviant speech dimensions in the dysarthrias. *Journal of Speech and Hearing Research*, **12**, 462–496.

Darley, F.L., Aronson, A.E., and Brown, J.R. (1975). *Motor Speech Disorders*. Philadelphia, PA: Saunders.

Duffy, J.R. (1995). *Motor Speech Disorders*. St. Louis, MO: Mosby.

Duffy, J.R. (2005). *Motor Speech Disorder* (2nd Edn.). St. Louis, MO: Mosby.

Grewel, F. (1957). Classification of dysarthrias. *Acta Psychiatrica Neurologica Scandinavica*, **32**, 325–327.

Guenther, F.H., Hampson, M., & Johnson, D. (1998). A theoretical investigation of reference frames for the planning of speech movements. *Psychological Review*, **105**, 611–633.

Hausdorff, J.M., Lertratanakul, A., Cudkowicz, M.E., Peterson, A.L., Kaliton, D & Goldberger, A.L. (2000). Dynamic markers of altered gait rhythm in amyotrophic lateral sclerosis. *Journal of Applied Physiology*, **88**, 2045–2053.

Hunker, C.J., & Abbs, J.H. (1984). Physiological analyses of Parkinsonian tremors in the orofacial system. In M.R. McNeil, J.C. Rosenbek, and A.E. Aronson (Eds.), *The Dysarthrias* (pp. 69–100). San Diego, CA: College-Hill Press.

Hunker, C., Abbs, J.H., & Barlow, S.M. (1982). The relationship between Parkinsonian rigidity and hypokinesia in the orofacial system: A quantitative analysis. *Neurology*, **32**, 749–754.

Jeng, J-Y. (2000). *The speech intelligibility and acoustic characteristics of Mandarin speakers with cerebral palsy*. Unpublished Ph.D. dissertation, University of Wisconsin-Madison.

Jeng, J-Y., Weismer, G., & Kent, R.D. (2006). Production and perception of Mandarin tone in adults with cerebral palsy. *Clinical Linguistics and Phonetics*, **20**, 67–87.

Kent, R.D., Kent, J.F., Weismer, G., Martin, R., Sufit, R.L., & Brooks, B.R. (1989). Relationships between speech intelligibility and the slope of second formant transitions in dysarthric subjects. *Clinical Linguistics and Phonetics*, **3**, 347–358.

Kim, Y-J. (2007). *Patterns of speech abnormality in a large dysarthria database: Interactions between severity, acoustic features, and dysarthria type*. Unpublished Ph.D. dissertation, University of Wisconsin-Madison.

Lehiste, I. (1965). Some acoustic characteristics of dysarthric speech. *Bibliotheca Phonetica*, **2**, 1–124.

Liss, J.M., Spitzer, S., Caviness, J.N., Adler, C., & Edwards, B. (1998). Syllabic strength and lexical boundary decisions in the perception of hypokinetic dysarthric speech. *Journal of the Acoustical Society of America*, **104**, 2457–2466.

Liss, J.M., Spitzer, S., Caviness, J.N., Adler, C., & Edwards, B. (2000). Lexical boundary error analysis in hypokinetic and ataxic dysarthria. *Journal of the Acoustical Society of America*, **107**, 3415–3424.

Liss, J.M., Spitzer, S., Caviness, J.N., & Adler, C. (2002). The effects of familiarization on intelligibility and lexical segmentation in hypokinetic and ataxic dysarthria. *Journal of the Acoustical Society of America*, **112**, 3022–3030.

Liss, J.M., Krein-Jones, K., Wszolek, Z.K., & Caviness, J.N. (2006). Speech characteristics of patients with pallido-ponto-nigral degeneration and their application to presymptomatic detection in at-risk relatives. *American Journal of Speech-Language Pathology*, **15**, 226–235.

Liu, H-M., Tsao, F-M., & Kuhl, P. (2005). The intelligibility of reduced vowel working space on speech intelligibility in Mandarin-speaking young adults with cerebral palsy. *Journal of the Acoustical Society of America*, **117**, 3879–3889.

Mattys, S., & Liss, J.M. (2008). On building models of spoken-word recognition: When there is as much to learn from natural 'oddities' as artificial normality. *Perception & Psychophysics*, **70**, 1235–1242.

Murdoch, B.E. (Ed.) (1998). *Dysarthria: A Physiological Approach to Assessment and Treatment*. Cheltenham, UK: Stanley Thornes.

Neilson, P.D., & O'Dwyer, N.J. (1984). Reproducibility and variability of speech muscle activity in normal and cerebral palsied subjects: EMG findings. *Journal of Speech and Hearing Research*, **27**, 502–517.

Netsell, R. (1986). *A Neurobiologic View of Speech Production and the Dysarthrias*. San Diego, CA: College-Hill Press.

Nishio, M., & Niimi, S. (2001). Speaking rate and its components in dysarthric speakers. *Clinical Linguistics and Phonetics*, **15**, 309–317.

Rosen, K.M., Goozée, J.V., & Murdoch, B.E. (2008). Examining the effects of multiple sclerosis on speech production: Does phonetic structure matter? *Journal of Communication Disorders*, **41**, 49–69.

Spencer, K.A., & Slocumb, D.L. (2007). The neural basis of ataxic dysarthria. *The Cerebellum*, **6**, 58–65.

Tjaden, K., & Turner, G.S. (1997). Spectral properties of fricatives in amyotrophic lateral sclerosis. *Journal of Speech, Language, and Hearing Research*, **40**, 1358–1372.

Tourville, J.A., Reilly, K.J., & Guenther, F.H. (2008). Neural mechanisms underlying auditory feedback control of speech. *NeuroImage*, **39**, 1429–1443.

Turner, G.S., & Weismer, G. (1993). Characteristics of speaking rate in the dysarthria associated with amyotrophic lateral sclerosis. *Journal of Speech and Hearing Research*, **36**, 1134–1144.

Wang, Y.T., Kent, R.D., Duffy, J.R., & Thomas, J.E. (2005). Dysarthria in traumatic brain injury: A breath group and intonational analysis. *Folia Phoniatrica et Logopaedica*, **57**, 59–89.

Weismer, G. (1984). Articulatory characteristics of Parkinsonia dysarthria: Segmental and phrase-level timing, spirantization, and glottal-supraglottal coordination. In M.R. McNeil, J.C. Rosenbek, & A. Aronson (Eds.), *The Dysarthria: Physiology, Acoustics, Perception, Management* (pp. 101–130). San Diego: College-Hill Press.

Weismer, G. (1991). Assessment of articulatory timing. In J. Cooper (Ed.), *Assessment of Speech and Voice Production: Research and Clinical Applications*. NIDCD Monograph Vol.1 (pp. 84–95). Bethesda: NIH.

Weismer, G. (2006). Philosophy of research in motor speech disorders. *Clinical Linguistics and Phonetics*, **20**, 315–349.

Weismer, G. (1997). Motor speech disorders. In W.J. Hardcastle and J. Laver (Eds.), *The Handbook of Phonetic Sciences* (pp. 191–219) London: Blackwell.

Weismer, G., Jeng, J-Y., Laures, J.S., Kent, R.D., & Kent, J.F. (2001). Acoustic and intelligibility characteristics of sentence production in neurogenic speech disorders. *Folia Phoniatrica et Logopaedica*, **53**, 1–18.

Weismer, G., Kent, R.D., Hodge, M., & Martin, R. (1988). The acoustic signature for intelligibility test words. *Journal of the Acoustical Society of America*, **84**, 1281–1291.

Weismer, G., & Liss, J.M. (1991). Reductionism is a dead end in speech research: Perspectives on a new direction. In C.A. Moore, K. Yorkston, and D. R. Beukelman (Eds.), *Clinical Dysarthria: Perspectives on Management* (pp. 15–27). Baltimore: Brookes.

Whitehill, T.L., Ciocca, V., and Chow, D.T.Y. (2000). Acoustic analysis of lexical tone contrasts in dysarthria. *Journal of Medical Speech-Language Pathology*, **8**, 337–344.

Yunusova, Y., Weismer, G., Westbury, J.R., & Lindstrom, M. (2008). Articulatory movements during vowels in speakers with dysarthria and healthy controls. *Journal of Speech, Language, and Hearing Research*, **51**, 596–611.

Zeplin, J., & Kent, R. D. (1996). Reliability of auditory perceptual scaling of dysarthria. In D. Robin, K. Yorkson, & D. R. Buekelman (Eds.), *Disorders of Motor Speech: Recent Advances in Assessment, Treatment, and Clinical Characterization* (pp. 145–154) Baltimore: Paul H. Brookes.

Ziegler, W. (2003). Speech motor control is task-specific: Evidence from dysarthria and apraxia of speech. *Aphasiology*, **17**, 3–36.

Ziegler, W., & Von Cramon, D.R. (1983). Vowel distortion in traumatic dysarthria. *Phonetica*, **40**, 63–78.

Zyski, B. J., & Weisiger, B. E. (1987). Identification of dysarthria types based on perceptual analysis. *Journal of Communication Disorders*, **20**, 367–378.

Chapter 14

Developmental models of childhood apraxia of speech

Ben Maassen, Lian Nijland, and Hayo Terband

Abstract

Childhood Apraxia of Speech (CAS) is a highly controversial clinical entity with respect to both clinical signs and underlying neuro-motor deficit. This chapter is an attempt to analyse the origin of these controversies and offer an alternative clinical approach and direction for research based on a review of the literature and studies conducted in our own laboratory. The review of a series of studies shows evidence for a deficit at each of the psycholinguistic and neuro-motor stages from lexical retrieval to motor execution as the primary, proximal origin of CAS. This lack of convergence together with the reported associations rather than dissociations between psycholinguistic and neuro-motor functions during development forms a serious challenge for the modular view on the cognitive architecture of the infant speech production system. An alternative view on clinical classification, the issue of co-morbidity, and research in speech pathology are discussed based on longitudinal analyses of developmental trajectories. By way of example, a computational modelling study is presented in which characteristics of CAS are simulated by manipulating parameters of the DIVA (Directions Into Velocities of Articulators) model.

14.1 Introduction

Since the critical review by Guyette and Diedrich (1981) on Developmental Apraxia of Speech (DAS) or Childhood Apraxia of Speech (CAS)[1] as a diagnostic entity, many approaches have been suggested to solve the diagnostic problem of differentiating CAS from other childhood speech disorders (see also Chapter 15 by Shriberg in this volume). The different diagnostic features that have been proposed since and the theoretical perspectives on which these features are based, have been discussed extensively by Shriberg et al. (Shriberg et al., 1997a, b, c; 2003). The discussion comprises two fundamental issues: first, the attribution of speech symptoms to deficits in the underlying speech production model and second, the developmental trajectory of infants and children moving toward the adult speech production model. The first issue concerns the deficits

[1] Terminology has changed over the last decades. In this text we use childhood apraxia of speech (CAS), a synonym for developmental apraxia of speech (DAS) and the older term developmental verbal dyspraxia (DVD).

in the speech production model that can describe (and explain) speech phenomena distinguishing between normal, skilled speech production, and speech disorders. Although researchers seem to agree that acquired apraxia of speech (AOS) in adults is a speech motor disorder, no agreement exists with respect to the differential diagnostic symptoms. McNeil and colleagues (2004) argue that: '. . . it is not a lack of theory or the inability to select the correct theory from the known alternatives that limits understanding of AOS' but that '[the] most important impediment to theoretical and clinical advancement in AOS is [. . .] the lack of a comprehensive and clear definition that leads to an agreed-upon set of criteria for subject selection' (pp. 389–390). Thus, McNeil and colleagues do not question that AOS should be attributed to motor rather than linguistic levels of processing. Instead, they argue that we lack criteria to distinguish between speech motor and linguistic (i.e., phonological) symptoms.

Theoretically, the distinction between speech motor and phonological symptoms is based on a modular view of the speech production process, which stems from the speech production model of Levelt (Levelt 1989; Levelt et al., 1999). According to this model, the phonological encoding module takes word forms or lexemes as input, and produces a phonetic plan as output. Subsequently, the phonetic plan is transferred to the articulator module for execution. Based on models proposed by Sternberg et al. (1978) and Klapp (2003) the motor processes that are supposed to take place in the articulation stage were further explicated by Van der Merwe (1997). Van der Merwe distinguished three processing components, speech motor planning, speech motor programming, and speech motor execution, which function in a cascade-like architecture. According to Levelt et al. (1999) and Van der Merwe (1997), phonological encoding is a qualitatively different process than speech motor planning, programming, and execution. Phonological encoding produces a *representation* as output (the phonetic code), whereas motor processes are executed. This description of AOS, however, contains a significant presupposition, namely that the speech production process is modular in nature in that for each processing level or 'module' a specific domain can be determined.

In this chapter, we challenge the strict modularity of phonological encoding and speech motor processes. In a recent overview, Kent (2004) questioned the modularity of motor control processes in general, arguing that: '. . . speech, or any motor behavior, is best viewed as a cognitive–motor accomplishment' (p.3). Although, strictly speaking, this only questions whether speech motor processes can be clearly distinguished from cognitive processes, and does not question the modularity of motor control processes as such, still, it seems applicable to speech because of the interaction with higher order psycholinguistic and lexicalization processes. Section 14.2 describes a series of studies that attributed the underlying deficit of CAS each to a different level of processing, ranging from lexical storage, to phonological encoding, motor planning, motor programming, and motor execution. The lack of convergence on a specific level of processing between studies forms a major theoretical and practical challenge, which goes beyond 'the lack of a comprehensive and clear definition that leads to an agreed-upon set of criteria for subject selection' (McNeil et al., 2004, pp. 389–390).

The second fundamental issue, to be discussed in Section 14.3, concerns the developmental trajectory infants and children go through in order to build up the adult speech production model. Bishop (1997) drew attention to a fundamental distinction in cognitive neuropsychological reasoning applied to acquired disorders in adults as compared to developmental (or very early in life acquired) disorders in children. In contrast to the neuropsychology of acquired disorders, in which the focus is on *dissociation*, in developmental disorders *associations* are the rule rather than the exception. The argument is that modules develop in interaction. In contrast to the sequential architecture of the adult production system, in which a particular deficit in the production system has only down-stream effects, in the developing system effects of subsystems spread in both directions.

Along the same line of reasoning, Karmiloff-Smith and Thomas (2003) refer to a gradual emergence of the adult modular system. Processes become modular only after a phase of automation.

14.2 **Processing level**

To date, many studies have been conducted to delineate precisely at which processing level the underlying deficit in CAS is localized. From a theoretical point of view, the results are puzzling since the processing levels at which deficits have been found, comprise nearly the whole speech production chain, ranging from lexical storage and retrieval to motor execution. These results put the specificity of the symptoms and deficits in CAS seriously into question, thus weakening the theoretical basis for delineating the core processing deficit, and thereby the clinical basis for differentiating CAS from other speech disorders in children (see also Chapter 15 by Shriberg in this volume). In the following sections, we will review a number of studies on CAS that have been reported in the literature, some of which were conducted in our own laboratory, and discuss what the speech symptoms may tell us about the underlying speech motor control deficits and the global architecture of the production system.

14.2.1 **Lexical representation**

The highest level at which the underlying deficit of CAS has been localized is at the level of lexical representation. In a series of papers, Shriberg et al. (Shriberg et al., 1997a, b, c) reported on a comprehensive study of speech symptoms in children diagnosed with 'suspected' CAS. The studies started from the premise that the speech characteristics of children with CAS are different from those of children with Speech Delay (SD), such that these differences allow for diagnostic differentiation. Note that this is not a trivial assumption. Despite clinical studies to further characterize CAS (Aram and Horwitz 1983; Blakeley 1980), Guyette and Diedrich (1981) had concluded that: '... No pathognomonic symptoms or necessary and sufficient conditions were found for the diagnosis ...' (p.44).

In the first study by Shriberg and colleagues, a total of 148 children who were referred to the phonology clinic were examined. The authors found that clinicians tend to use the label 'suspected' CAS primarily for children who make (too) little progress despite intensive therapy (Shriberg et al., 1997a). Fourteen children were diagnosed as 'suspected' CAS. In the second study (Shriberg et al., 1997b), it turned out that the prosody-voice profiles of these 14 children, as well as an additional 20 children, were similar to that of children with SD, except for 'inappropriate stress', which distinguished about 50% of the children with 'suspected' CAS from the remaining children with SD. This finding was confirmed in the third study (Shriberg et al., 1997c). Summed across the three studies, 25 out of 48 children with 'suspected' CAS had inappropriate stress, compared to 10% of children with speech delay of unknown origin. A deficit in phonological representational processes was proposed as the underlying mechanism that causes inappropriate stress (Shriberg et al., 1997c). This hypothesis was based on two findings. First, their results showed that – regarding stress – children with CAS do not show many self-corrections. As self-monitoring does not reveal many errors, this suggests that the representations are incorrect and thus are not detected as errors by the monitoring system. Second, they found that the production of inappropriate stress does not tend to decrease with speech development, which also suggests a deficit at the representational level.

Marquardt et al. (2002) further elaborated on the involvement of lexical representation with rhyming studies. In an earlier study, it was shown that children with CAS, aged 5–7 years, were not only poor in generating rhymes, but also in judging rhymes (Marion et al., 1993). In their subsequent study, Marquardt et al. addressed the issue whether or not children with CAS exhibit a metalinguistic awareness of the syllable that is appropriate for their age. Three children with CAS performed tasks in which they identified the number of syllables in words, judged intrasyllabic sound positions, and constructed syllable shapes within monosyllabic frames. The results suggested that the children with CAS were poor in their ability to perceive syllabic features, and to access and compare syllable representations with regard to phoneme position and structure. From this, the authors concluded that CAS goes well beyond a purely articulatory-based motor control deficit. Instead, according to Marquardt et al. (2002), CAS should be characterized at a deeper level of linguistic competence, namely an impoverished phonological/lexical representation system.

14.2.2 **Phonological encoding**

According to the speech production model of Levelt (Levelt 1989; Levelt et al., 1999), phonological encoding starts with retrieval of the word-form ('lexeme'). The process uses a stored phonological repertoire and stored phonological rules. In normal infant and childhood speech acquisition, the gradual development of phonological knowledge is reflected in the increase of the phonological repertoire and the reduction of so called 'phonological processes'. The information processing that takes place during phonological encoding entails the selection of segments (typically phonemes) from the phonological repertoire, sequencing these according to the phonological rules, and inserting the segments within syllable frames. Many speech characteristics found in children with CAS have been hypothesized to originate from the phonological encoding stage, although in many cases it is disputed whether particular characteristics should be attributed to either the storage (i.e., lexical representation and phonological repertoire) or the process (i.e., retrieval) component of the phonological encoding. Among these characteristics are: poor or very restricted production of consonants and vowels (as assumed due to an incomplete phonemic repertoire), high rates of consonant and vowel substitution errors, sequencing difficulties of phonemes and syllables, and the inability to produce complex phonemic sequences such as consonant clusters (Hall et al., 1993; Pollock and Hall 1991; Stackhouse and Snowling 1992; Velleman and Strand 1994; Walton and Pollock 1993). For other characteristics, however, such as complications (i.e., productions of consonant clusters or syllables that are more complex than the target clusters or syllables), inconsistent error patterns, and 'groping' or searching articulation, it has been suggested that they specifically originate from deficits in processing, with the phonological repertoire and rule system being intact (or poorly developed but not causing the particular characteristic) (Davis et al., 1998; Hall et al., 1993; McNeil et al., 1997; Stackhouse and Snowling 1992; Velleman and Strand 1994).

Only very few studies have aimed to quantify error patterns of phonological encoding in children with CAS as compared to other speech disorders. Almost all of these studies have restricted their scope to very crude measures, such as overall percentage consonants correct (PCC) or percentages correct for particular phonemes or phoneme classes. Assessment of a phonological encoding deficit, however, requires an analysis that takes phonotactic context into account, which is not captured by simple error counts.

The only rather comprehensive study that used a quantitative analysis of segmental error patterns in relation to phonotactic context was published by Thoonen et al. (1994). In this study, the authors conducted a paradigmatic and syntagmatic feature value analysis of the consonant substitution and omission errors in the speech of 11 children with CAS as compared to age-matched controls. Phonetic transcriptions of consonants produced in a word and pseudo-word imitation task revealed overall high substitution and omission rates for the children with CAS; almost all error types were increased in comparison to children with normal speech. Furthermore, the children with CAS showed a particularly low percentage of retention of place of articulation in words, an inconsistency with respect to feature realization and feature preference, and a high syntagmatic error rate. Because errors were quantified, it was possible to correct for overall error rate, thus yielding profiles of relative error rates. Applied to the effect of context on error types, it turned out that the clinical impression that children with CAS produce relatively many syntagmatic errors was not substantiated. That is, although children with CAS produce a higher rate of phoneme anticipations, perseverations, and metatheses (i.e., syntagmatic errors) as compared to controls, after correction for the overall higher error rate, the relative number of syntagmatic and paradigmatic errors appeared identical for both groups. In general, the error profiles showed only very few differences between groups, which suggests that the speech of children with CAS can be characterized by a high rate of 'normal' slips of the tongue. We will come back to the issue of lack of specificity of speech symptoms in Section 14.3, where we present different models of speech production and speech development.

14.2.3 **Speech motor planning**

Motor planning is a process aimed at defining motor goals. According to Van der Merwe (1997), this should be distinguished from the abstract linguistic choice of the speech sound that is to be uttered. Motor planning can be compared to phonetic planning in Levelt's model (1989). At this stage, the spatial and temporal goals of the articulatory movements are collected from a sensorimotor storage, presumably in chunks of the size of syllables, the so-called 'syllabary' (e.g., Aichert and Ziegler 2004; Cholin, et al., 2005, 2006; Levelt and Wheeldon 1994; Ziegler et al., this volume). Varley and Whiteside (2001) argued that the core deficit in adults with acquired AOS consists of missing or insufficiently stable syllable storage, forcing these speakers to make use of the 'indirect route', where syllables must be assembled from the phonological plan. This would explain the reduced coherence of apraxic speech, resulting in reduced coarticulation and reduced prosodic structure. Although Aichert and Ziegler (2004) have found effects of syllabic complexity and syllable frequency on error rate in patients with AOS, indicating that syllabic representations can be accessed to some degree, still a deficiency in speech motor planning could consist of a deficiency in the planning of syllables. Assuming that in normal speech the use of syllable-sized chunks has the effect of preserving the coherence of the spatial, temporal, and other scaling aspects of speech movements, a deficiency in speech motor planning could cause deviant coarticulation and durational patterns. This idea was explored with respect to CAS in a study (Nijland et al., 2003b) in which syllable structure was manipulated in an otherwise unchanged phonetic context (resulting in Dutch phrases like 'zus giet' /zʌs-xit/, meaning: sister pours, versus 'ze schiet' /zɘ - sxit/, meaning: she shoots; note that the sequence of speech sounds is very similar in the two phrases; compare the English phrases 'ice cream' versus 'I scream'). It was hypothesized that syllable structure would have an effect on coarticulation and durational structure. Specifically, stronger anticipatory coarticulation was expected from the second vowel ([i] in the example above, which was compared to [a] and [o]) on the preceding consonant in intra-syllabic context ([s] in /zɘ - sxit/) than in inter-syllabic context ([s] in /zʌs-xit/). This was assessed by comparing the acoustic signal in the trajectories of the second formant in the first vowel and both fricatives as they occurred in the utterances with [i], [a], and [o].In addition, because of the coherence of the syllable structure, more stable relative durations of the consonants [s] and [x] were expected in intra- as compared to inter-syllabic context. In the English example, this would mean that the [s] would show stronger coarticulation with the [i] and show less variable relative duration in the intra-syllabic context 'I scream' than in the inter-syllabic context 'ice cream'. In contrast to these expectations, no effects of syllable structure were found on coarticulation, neither in the normally speaking children, nor in the children with CAS. Children with CAS did show an overall larger variability of vowel and consonant quality, irrespective of syllable structure. However, systematic durational adjustments to syllabic structure were found in the segments of the stressed syllable in normally speaking children (both [s] and the second vowel were shorter in / zə - sxit/ as compared to /zʌs-xit/). In children with CAS, such systematic durational patterns were missing. Furthermore, in normally speaking children inter-syllabic effects were found in durational structure, in the form of prosodic differences between the phrases. Again this effect was absent in the speech of children with CAS. The lack of a consistent intra- and inter-syllabic temporal structure in the speech of children with CAS, which is clearly present in normal speech, suggests that motor planning in children with CAS is poorly organized at the syllabic level.

14.2.4 Speech motor programming

The acoustic variability in the speech of children with CAS (as reported in measurements of repeated utterances) suggests high variability in the amplitude and velocity of speech movements. According to speech production models, these kinematic parameters are controlled at the level of motor programming. In our laboratory, a possible deficit in motor programming was further evaluated by determining formant trajectories and segment durations in a bite-block speech condition. The normal speaking children were not able to completely compensate for the bite-block, although it did not affect the extent of anticipatory coarticulation. A surprising result was that in the children with CAS vowel quality had improved in the bite-block speech condition, which suggests that children with CAS were actually helped by the bite-block. Probably, the restriction in degrees of freedom of the articulators facilitated articulation in children with CAS in that fewer aspects of the articulatory movements have to be controlled. Namasivayam et al. (2008) found larger movement amplitude after insertion of a bite-block in people who stutter as well as people who do not stutter. Larger movement amplitude could explain the vowel quality improvement found in the above-mentioned study in children with CAS. In contrast to Namasivayam et al. (2008), who found a stabilizing effect of the bite-block, the children with CAS in our study showed an increase of within-subject variability in the bite-block condition, indicating that the children with CAS did experience difficulty in the articulatory process while speaking with a bite-block. These results were interpreted as a demonstration of deficient motor programming in CAS, that is a less automated and controlled processing mode (Nijland et al., 2003a). Further studies are needed, especially to account for differential effects of speech rate

14.2.5 Speech motor execution

In order to investigate a possible involvement of motor execution in children with CAS, articulation is the ultimate study object. In our laboratory, we collected kinematic data of the articulation in children with speech output disorders (among others in children with CAS). From these data, discrete kinematic (displacement and peak velocities) parameters and the stiffness coefficient (peak velocity over amplitude) of the articulations of mono-, bi-, and trisyllabic sequential and alternate motion utterances (pa, pata, pataka) were determined. Results showed that the pathological groups showed larger lip closing movements and faster velocities than the control group. The pathological groups, especially the children who were not able to produce the alternate motion task with 'pataka', produced more variability in closing movements and velocities, but less variability in the stiffness coefficient as compared to controls.

Variability in kinematics seems to indicate the inability to generate a stable pattern that will facilitate (repetitive) speech (Hulstijn et al., 1991). The stiffness coefficient represents flexibility, or lack of flexibility, which is related to adaptive articulatory behaviour needed for demanding speech situations (Alfonso and van Lieshout, 1997; Kelso et al., 1985). Higher stiffness means less variability, as shown by Nasir and Ostry (Chapter 3 this volume). The pathological groups showed a fairly rigid pattern of stiffness over time, which may indicate that underlying control processes are less flexible as required for skilful articulatory movements and, therefore, less able to adapt to demanding speech tasks. Likewise, Namasivayam et al. (2008) showed that speakers fall back on a more simplified but stable pattern under demanding speaking conditions. See also Van Lieshout and Namasivayam (Chapter 11 this volume) on the role of variability in flexibility and learning versus pathology.

Concluding this section (Section 14.2), results of a variety of studies seem to suggest that the underlying deficit in CAS cannot be confined to one particular psycholinguistic stage or one particular level of speech motor control, which forms the primary motivation to explore alternative models of speech pathology and developmental issues in the next section (Section 14.3).

14.3 **Speech production models**

In this section, we question the theoretical demarcation of speech motor and phonological levels of processing in CAS. Bishop (1997) drew attention to a fundamental distinction in cognitive neuropsychological reasoning applied to acquired disorders in adults as compared to developmental (or very early in life acquired) disorders in children. In classic, clinical neuropsychological studies, the diagnostic reasoning of *double dissociation* is used to demonstrate mutual independence of functions. That is, if patients can be found who are defective in function A (e.g., lexical retrieval) but not B (e.g., speech motor control), and other patients who are defective in function B but not A, then one can conclude that both functions operate independently, and are subserved by partly non-overlapping neurological structures. In contrast, in developmental neuropsychology associations rather than dissociations are the rule. Therefore, the traditional logic of cognitive neuropsychology is not applicable to define the deficits that underlie developmental disorders. Bishop (1997) was concerned with defining Specific Language Impairment (SLI), where the difficulty is to find the *specific* symptoms that distinguish SLI from language delay due to diverse or unknown etiology (see also de Jong 2004). Over the years, several specific deficits have been suggested to underlie SLI [i.e., poor discrimination of rapid or brief auditory stimuli (Tallal et al., 1996)], limitations in phonological short-term memory (Gathercole and Baddeley 1990), and impairment of specialized mechanisms for grammar acquisition, but these underlying deficits are not transparent. Many factors influence the symptoms that a child with SLI shows at a particular moment in time. Not only the developmental stage and developmental history of the child obviously determine the expression of the deficit, but also environmental factors. The conclusion is that SLI is a diagnostic category in search for an underlying deficit. CAS on the other hand, is defined as a speech motor planning disorder, of which the diagnostic criteria are lacking ('in search of a population').

We can take this line of argument a step further. Evidence from developmental studies shows that the phonology of the first words mastered at age 1–1.5 years builds on babbling experience in the preceding months. McCune and Vihman (2001) followed infants from age 9 to 16 months going through the transition from babbling to producing referential words. One of the interesting observations was that the children varied in the specific consonants they produced consistently, and that these same consonants characterized nearly all consonant-based words produced by each child at the end of the observation period. Thus, there is evidence for a continuous progression to the adult system, both in normal development as in developmental disorders. Cognitive modules are the outcome of development, not its starting point and the 'gradual process of ontogenetic development' comprises interactions between emerging modules (Karmiloff-Smith and Thomas 2003; Karmiloff-Smith 2006).

Edwards et al. (1999) explored two components of non-symbolic phonological competence, namely acoustic-perceptual performance and articulatory-motor performance. Results showed that children with a phonological disorder need more redundant acoustic information to perform a perception task, and produce less precise and less controlled (more ballistic) speech movements in a production task, as compared to age-matched controls and adults. These results are interpreted as evidence for the view that phonological knowledge not only reflects the level of categorical lexical contrasts, but also comprises the incremental acquisition of representations at different levels, among those the acoustic-perceptual and articulatory-motor level.

Green et al. (2000) made systematic observations of jaw and lip movements in1-, 2-, and 6-year-olds and adults, and showed that early articulations are produced with relatively rapid or 'ballistic' movements, and that precise control of jaw movements precedes lip-control, control over jaw and lip coupling, and independence of upper- and lower-lip movement. General consequences for the sequence of phonological development can be derived from these observations, such as the observation that plosives develop earlier than fricatives. This is promising research, waiting for applications in developmental motor speech disorders. These results from normal speech development suggest that phonological development may be disrupted due to poor motor control (See also Davis et al., 2002; Ruark and Moore 1997; Smith 2001; Westerman and Reck-Miranda 2004). Due to space limitations, we cannot go into accounts of speech development based on Gestural Phonology, but see for instance Goldstein and Fowler (2003).

To conclude by referring to Bishop (1997), 'The problem with developmental disorders is that, although one may see fractionation along the lines of major domains of functioning (e.g., language, spatial perception, motor co-ordination, social cognition, numeracy) within any one domain, the typical observation is one of a complex pattern of associated impairments rather than the highly selective deficits that may be found in acquired disorders' (Bishop 1997, p. 904). Although selective deficits in adult patients might justify claims about cognitive modularity, seemingly similar deficits found in children cannot be used to argue that such cognitive modules are pre-specified in the infant brain. What is needed then, are developmental studies to determine how the patterns of deficits and proficiencies change over time.

14.3.1 **How does this apply to CAS?**

With respect to clinical diagnosis, the main issues are *sensitivity* and *specificity*. In Section 14.2, we showed that symptoms of CAS have been interpreted at different levels of speech production, respectively lexical representation and retrieval, phonological encoding, motor planning, motor programming, and motor execution. At the level of lexical representation, inappropriate stress might be a specific symptom for diagnosing CAS, but it has low sensitivity. Due to the lack of a golden standard exact sensitivity and specificity figures cannot be determined, but the clinical sensitivity was estimated to be around 50% (Shriberg et al., 1997a, b, c). For errors at the level of phonological encoding, results suggest that measures like high relative frequency of syntagmatic as compared to paradigmatic consonant production errors and particular errors relating to syllabic structure are not very specific for CAS. Frequencies of these error types are increased in comparison with normal speech, thus yielding an overall quantitative measure of severity of involvement of the speech disorder. However, after correction for the total number of errors, these error types do not distinguish CAS from other speech disorders in children. Also at the level of motor planning/programming, research did not yield symptoms that are both specific and sensitive. Studies by Thoonen et al. (1994) and Maassen (2004) have indicated that in a diverse group of children with speech disorders, frequency of place-of-articulation errors is highly correlated with sequencing difficulty in a sequential and alternate motion task. However, Forrest and Morrisette (1999) challenged the interpretation of place errors as specific symptom for CAS because they found high place-of-articulation error rates in children with speech delay as well.

Unfortunately, Forrest and Morisette did not collect sequential and alternate motion data, but we can conclude that the sensitivity and specificity of the relatively high rate of place-of-articulation errors as a diagnostic marker for CAS is poor. Apparently, many children with diverse speech disorders show dyspraxic symptoms to some extent (Maassen 2004).

A crucial assumption underlying the search for a diagnostic marker that is seldom discussed explicitly is the assumption that different disorders lead to different symptoms. However, rather than expecting to find single diagnostic markers for specific disorders, it seems more realistic to aim for diagnostic profiles of strengths and weaknesses. See also Duffy (Chapter 16, this volume) on issues related to diagnostic profiles for dysarthria. In a different domain, Cornish et al. (2007) recently made a similar suggestion: 'We propose a new approach to the study of attentional deficits in genetic disorders, arguing for tracing cross-syndrome developmental trajectories from infancy through childhood to adulthood' (p.672). A methodological issue that arises here is the sensitivity and validity of our measurement instruments. Of course, if we understood the whole mechanism of speech production, and were able to measure all variables that are of relevance (including neurological processes), then for any two disorders some symptoms or symptom complex must emerge that distinguishes between the two. If two disorders cannot be distinguished in any measurable aspect at any stage of development, then it makes no sense to distinguish the two and the diagnostic categories should better be merged. This is precisely the issue Guyette and Diedrich (1981) raised with respect to CAS in their provocative article referred to at the onset of this chapter, and it is also the reason why we try to improve measurement techniques: not only phonemic transcription of speech but also acoustic measures of coarticulation, distortion, speech rate, and kinematic measures of coordination and movement parameters such as amplitude, velocity and their ratio (kinematic stiffness), as well as the indices of variability such as the spatial–temporal index (STI) developed by Smith and Goffman (2004).

However, there is good reason to support the idea that different underlying disorders may lead to similar symptoms; precisely because of the developmental aspect. A child that is unable to practice speech motor skills (because of hearing loss, dysarthria, dyspraxia of speech, mental retardation, and social isolation) may develop poor phonological skills at a later developmental stage. This child will also have problems in vocabulary and grammar, and possibly in reading and spelling skills as well. Many examples have shown that different underlying disorders may lead to similar symptoms. The high overlap in symptoms frustrates attempts to find single diagnostic markers for differential diagnosis, and necessitate an approach aiming at describing *profiles* of symptoms to characterize disorders. As an alternative for the dominant classification approach, Weismer (Chapter 13, this volume) argues for a taxonomical approach to the study of motor speech disorders, expressing the clinical observation that dysarthria and AOS produce a core of similar speech symptoms across the many diseases. The same reasoning applies to developmental speech disorders.

14.3.2 **Programme for future research**

In recent years, neural network models of speech production have been introduced from the field of motor control. One of the most advanced neural network models, that shows overlap with the model of Kröger, Birkholz, and Lowit (Chapter 2, this volume), is the DIVA model (Directions Into Velocities of Articulators, Guenther 1995; Guenther et al., 2006). The DIVA model consists of a computationally implemented neural network controller detailing feedforward and feedback control loops that are involved in early speech development and mature speech production, whose components are associated with regions of the cerebral cortex and cerebellum. The model focuses on the sensorimotor transformations underlying the control of articulator movements. In order to produce an acoustic signal, DIVA controls the movements of an articulatory synthesizer

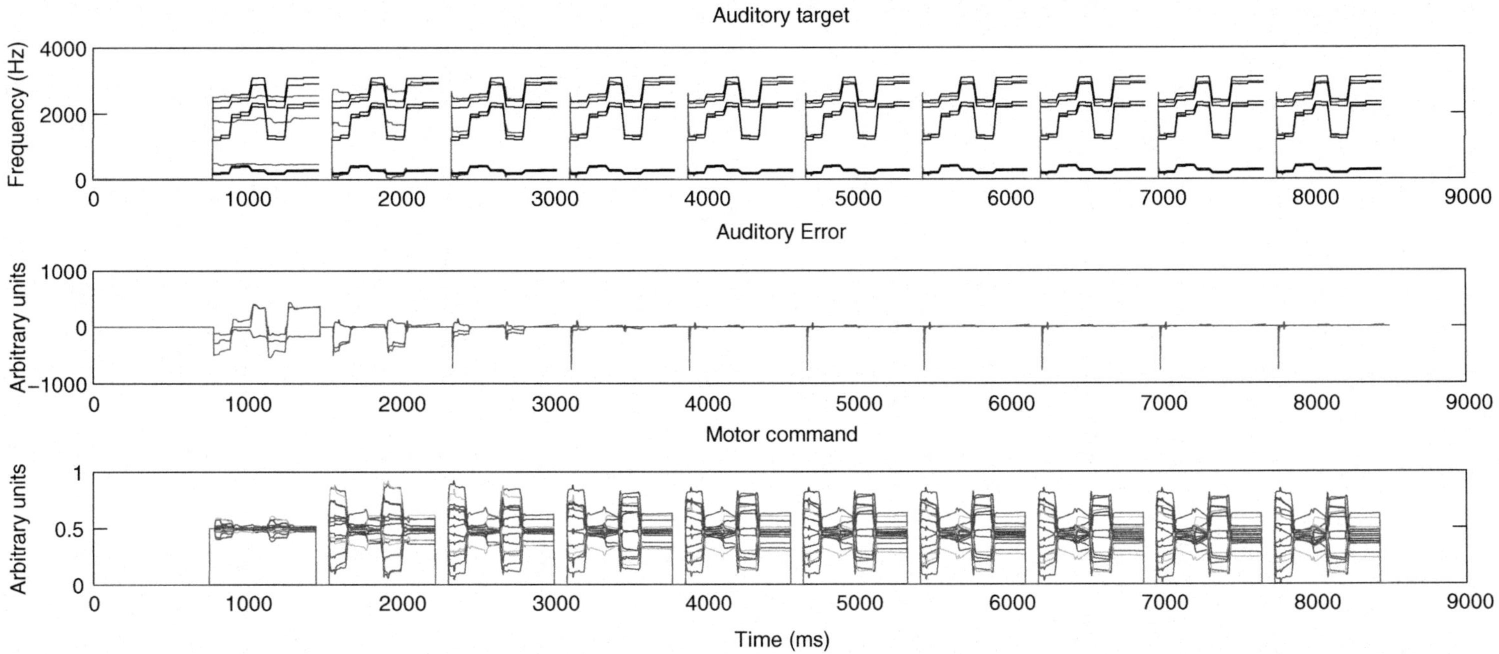

Fig. 14.1 The DIVA model learning the word 'baby'. The top-panel shows the target regions for F1, F2, and F3 (black) and the models auditory realization (grey lines top left; starting in neutral position as horizontal lines). On the basis of the information provided by the auditory feedback control subsystem (middle-panel), the feedforward command (bottom-panel) is updated with each attempt, thus becoming more accurate. After approximately five iterations, learning has become asymptotic.

(Maeda 1990). The acquisitional process comprises three stages. In the first stage, semi-random articulatory movements (resembling the babbling stage) are used to learn the neural relations between motor commands and their auditory and somatosensory consequences (systemic mapping). In the second stage, the model is presented with sample speech sounds and learns an auditory target region for each sound. The targets can consist of a single phoneme, a syllable, a word, or a small phrase. In the final stage, feedforward commands are acquired by the model iteratively attempting to produce the auditory target region (Fig. 14.1). For a detailed description we refer to Guenther (1995) and Guenther et al. (2006).

The search of the underlying deficit of CAS did not yield clear-cut results thus far. In psycholinguistic terms, the core deficit of CAS is thought to reside at the phonetic programming level (Schmidt and Lee 1999; Van der Merwe 1997), but, as was argued in Section 14.2 of this chapter, CAS has been interpreted at various levels: lexical representation, phonological planning, assembly of a phonetic program, and motor implementation. A solution might be to change to a different type of analysis, and focus on neurolinguistic information processing involved in speech motor control, for which neural models like DIVA can provide a valuable reference frame for the speech motor control part of the process. Furthermore, being computationally implemented, DIVA allows for computer simulations of the speech acquisition and production processes.

In collaboration with Frank Guenther and colleagues, we are conducting a series of studies that attempts to trace back the evolving symptoms of CAS to particular deficits of information processing by using computational modelling with the DIVA model. A first study tested the hypothesis that the speech production system in CAS suffers from weak feedforward control and consequently an increased reliance on the feedback control subsystem (Terband et al., 2007; 2009). In terms of psychomotor function, the deficit CAS can be summarized as a deficit of generating motor speech commands. In the DIVA model, the motor commands for different speech sounds are stored in feedforward projections that specify articulatory trajectories, which will produce the desired auditory target. A problem in generating motor speech commands can thus be simulated by poor feedforward control in the DIVA model. In our study, we conducted a series of computer simulations in which the reliance on feedback control was systematically varied during production attempts in the acquisition of forward commands. The simulations accounted for four key-characteristics of speech production in CAS: stronger coarticulation, distorted productions of speech sounds, searching articulatory behaviour, and increased variability between productions. Two possible core deficits of degraded forward control in CAS were discussed: reduced somatosensory information and increased levels of neural noise (Terband et al., 2007; 2009)

The latter hypothesis was subsequently tested in a simulation study (Terband et al., 2008). A noise generator was implemented in the DIVA model and the noise level was systematically varied, again during production attempts in the acquisition of forward commands. The simulations showed an increase in coarticulation, speech sound distortion, searching articulatory behaviour, and variability as the noise level increased. These results suggest that CAS may be caused by an altered level of neural noise.

An important issue to be further investigated is the specificity of the results. Are these the only symptoms resulting from neural noise, or do increased levels of neural noise also have other consequences that do not correspond with CAS? Furthermore, can these symptoms also be explained by other motor control deficits, such as the other hypothesis that was posed – an increased reliance on feedback due to reduced somatosensory information? We are currently working on the implementation of this deficit in DIVA and expanding the results with movement data. Furthermore, we are planning experiments to verify the observations in children with CAS, as compared to speech sound disorders in general.

Although these are modelling studies, they show a clear correspondence with observational and experimental data. The studies confirm that theoretical accounts and simulation studies can give valuable insights into the developmental and neurological mechanisms and deficits that underlie speech disorders.

14.4 Concluding remarks

Returning to our diagnostic dilemma, if a developmental speech motor disorder can lead to deficits at different levels of speech production, such as poor phonological processing and lexical representation, one could argue that CAS and phonological disorder more often than not occur in combination. This would imply that a phonological disorder (i.e., the presence of the marker signalling a phonological disorder) should not be an exclusion criterion for the diagnosis CAS, but rather be accepted as co-morbidity. From the theoretical perspective outlined above, a dissociation of underlying deficits is unlikely, forcing us to accept this type of co-morbidity. Thus, there are interactions between levels of processing that makes that speech motor control and speech motor symptoms may be influenced by difficulties in phonological encoding. This is not only due to degraded input that leads to degraded output, but also because the process itself is likely to adapt to the deviant circumstances. For instance, a general, non-specific feature of speech motor control disorders, irrespective of the underlying deficit, is low speech rate, whether or not as primary symptom or as compensatory response. The fact that this symptom occurs also in other speech disorders than CAS does not exclude it as a symptom of CAS. After all, if we manage to find the underlying deficit(s) of CAS, we should also be able to explain why speech rate is slowed down.

Many authors have claimed that focusing on pure cases by following the double dissociation logic is the one and only solid way to proceed to find the core characteristics or diagnostic marker of a disorder. In contrast, clinicians must reckon with co-morbidity, because in clinical practice the pure cases are a minority (see Bishop 2004, for a balanced discussion on this issue). By restricting research to pure cases, for methodological considerations, we risk throwing out the baby with the bathwater. Why would dyspraxia in the minority of pure cases of CAS be representative for all children with CAS, including those with an additional phonological disorder, auditory processing disorder, dysarthria, etc.? Moreover, we know that AOS disrupts the development of the lexicon, the phonological system, and auditory processing (Crary et al., 1984; Ekelman and Aram 1984; Marion et al., 1993).

The upshot is that there is a specific, intricate relationship between development of speech motor control and phonology, and thus a strong association between deficits within the two domains. To put it more precisely, phonological representations are dynamical, multilayered structures, comprising auditory, motor, and lexical information.

Reference

Aichert, I., & Ziegler, W. (2004). Syllable frequency and syllable structure in apraxia of speech. *Brain and Language, 88*, 148–159.

Alfonso, P. J., & van Lieshout, P. (1997). Spatial and temporal variability in obstruent gestural specification by stutterers and controls: comparisons across sessions. In W. Hulstijn, H. F. Peters, & P. H. H. M. van Lieshout (Eds.), *Speech Production: Motor Control, Brain Research, and Fluency Disorders* (pp. 151–160). Amsterdam: Elsevier Publishers.

Aram, D. M., & Horwitz, S. J. (1983). Sequential and non-speech praxic abilities in developmental verbal apraxia. *Developmental Medicine and Child Neurology, 25*, 197–206.

Bishop, D. V. M. (1997). Cognitive neuropsychology and developmental disorders: Uncomfortable bedfellows. *The Quarterly Journal of Experimental Psychology, 50A*, 899–923.

—— (2004). Specific language impairment: Diagnostic dilemmas. In L.Verhoeven & H. Van Balkom (Eds.), *Classification of Developmental Language Disorders: Theoretical Issues and Clinical Implications* (pp. 309–326). London: Lawrence Erlbaum Associates, Publ.

Blakeley, R. W. (1980). *Screening Test for Developmental Apraxia of Speech.* Austin (USA): Pro-ed.

Cholin, J., Levelt, W. J., & Schiller, N. O. (2006). Effects of syllable frequency in speech production. *Cognition, 99,* 205–235.

Cholin, J., Schiller, N. O., & Levelt, W. J. M. (2005). The preparation of syllables in speech production. *Journal of Memory and Language, 50,* 47–61.

Cornish, K., Scerif, G., & Karmiloff-Smith, A. (2007). Tracing syndrome-specific trajectories of attention across the lifespan. *Cortex, 43,* 672–685.

Crary, M. A., Landess, S., & Towne, R. (1984). Phonological error patterns in developmental verbal dyspraxia. *Journal of Clinical Neuropsychology, 6(2),* 157–170.

Davis, B. L., Jakielski, K. J., & Marquardt, T. P. (1998). Developmental apraxia of speech: Determiners of differential diagnosis. *Clinical Linguistics and Phonetics, 12,* 25–45.

Davis, B. L., MacNeilage, P. F., & Matyear, C. L. (2002). Acquisition of serial complexity in speech production: A comparison of phonetic and phonological approaches to first word production. *Phonetica, 59,* 75–107.

de Jong, J. (2004). Grammatical impairment: An overview and a sketch of Dutch. In L.Verhoeven & H. Van Balkom (Eds.), *Classification of Developmental Language Disorders: Theoretical Issues and Clinical Implications* (pp. 261–282). London: Lawrence Erlbaum Associates, Publ.

Edwards, J., Fourakis, M., Beckman, M. E., & Fox, R. A. (1999). Characterizing knowledge deficits in phonological disorders. *Journal of Speech, Language, and Hearing Research, 42,* 169–186.

Ekelman, B. L., & Aram, D. M. (1984). Spoken syntax in children with developmental verbal apraxia. In D. M. Aram (Ed.), *Seminars in Speech and Language: Assessment and Treatment of Developmental Apraxia* (5 ed., pp. 97–110). New York: Thieme-Stratton Inc.

Forrest, K., & Morrisette, M. L. (1999). Feature analysis of segmental errors in children with phonological disorders. *Journal of Speech, Language, and Hearing Research, 42,* 187–194.

Gathercole, S. E., & Baddeley, A. (1990). Phonological memory deficits in language disordered children: Is there a causal connection? *Journal of Memory and Language, 29,* 336–360.

Goldstein, L., & Fowler, C. A. (2003). Articulatory phonology: A phonology for public language use. In N.O. Schiller & A. S. Meyer (Eds.), *Phonetics and Phonology in Language Comprehension and Production: Differences and Similarities* (6 ed.), Berlin: Mouton de Gruyter.

Green, J. R., Moore, C. A., Higashikawa, M., & Steeve, R. W. (2000). The physiologic development of speech motor control: Lip and jaw coordination. *Journal of Speech, Language, and Hearing Research, 43,* 239–255.

Guenther, F. H. (1995). Speech sound acquisition, coarticulation, and rate effects in a neural network model of speech production. *Psychological Review, 102,* 594–621.

Guenther, F. H., Ghosh, S. S., & Tourville, J. A. (2006). Neural modeling and imaging of the cortical interactions underlying syllable production. *Brain and Language, 96,* 280–301.

Guyette, Th., & Diedrich, W. M. (1981). A critical review of developmental apraxia of speech. In N. J. Lass (Ed.), *Speech and Language. Advances in Basic Research and Practice* (pp. 1–49). New York: Academic Press Inc.

Hall, P. K., Jordan, L. S., & Robin, D. A. (1993). *Developmental Apraxia of Speech: Theory and Clinical Practice.* Austin, TX: Pro-ed.

Hulstijn, W., Van Lieshout, P. H. H. M., & Peters, H. F. M. (1991). On the measurement of coordination. In H. F. M. Peters, W. Hulstijn, & C. W. Starkweather (Eds.), *Speech Motor Control and Stuttering* (pp. 211–230). Amsterdam: Excerpta Medica.

Karmiloff-Smith, A. (2006). The tortuous route from genes to behaviour: A neuroconstructivist approach. *Cognitive, Affective and Behavioural Neuroscience, 6,* 9–17.

Karmiloff-Smith, A. & Thomas, M. (2003). What can developmental disorders tell us about the neurocomputational constraints that shape development? The case of Williams syndrome. *Development and Psychopathology, 15*, 969–990.

Kelso, J. A. S., Vatikiotis-Bateson, E., Saltzman, E. L., & Kay, B. (1985). A qualitative dynamic analysis of reiterant speech production: Phase portraits, kinematics, and dynamic modeling. *Journal of the Acoustical Society of America*, 77(1), 266–280.

Kent, R. D. (2004). Models of speech motor control: Implications from recent developments in neurophysiological and neurobehavioral science. In B. Maassen, R. D. Kent, H. F. M. Peters, P. H. H. M. Van Lieshout, & W. Hulstijn (Eds.), *Speech Motor Control in Normal and Disordered Speech* (pp. 1–28). Oxford: Oxford University Press.

Klapp, S. T. (2003). Reaction time analysis of two types of motor preparation for speech articulation: Action as a sequence of chunks. *Journal of Motor Behavior, 35*, 135–150.

Leonard, L. B. (1998). *Children with Specific Language Impairment.* Cambridge, MA: MIT Press.

Levelt, W. J. M. (1989). Speaking: From intention to articulation. In (pp. 406–411 & 446–457). Cambridge, Massachusetts: The MIT Press.

Levelt, W. J. M., Roelofs, A., & Meyer, A. S. (1999). A theory of lexical access in speech production. *Behavioral and Brain Sciences, 22*, 1–75.

Levelt, W. J. M. & Wheeldon, L. (1994). Do speakers have access to a mental syllabary? *Cognition, 50*, 239–269.

Maassen, B. (2004). Speech output disorders. In L. Verhoeven & H. Van Balkom (Eds.), *Classification of Developmental Language Disorders: Theoretical Issues and Clinical Implications* (pp. 175–190). Mahwah, NJ: Lawrence Erlbaum Associates, Publ.

Maeda, S. (1990). Compensatory articulation during speech: Evidence from the analysis and synthesis of vocal tract shapes using an articulatory model. In W. J. Hardcastle & A. Marchal (Eds.), *Speech Production and Speech Modeling* (pp. 131–149). Boston: Kluwer Academic Publishers.

Marion, M. J., Sussman, H. M., & Marquardt, T. P. (1993). The perception and production of rhyme in normal and developmentally apraxic children. *Journal of Communication Disorders, 26*, 129–160.

Marquardt, T. P., Sussman, H. M., Snow, T., & Jacks, A. (2002). The integrity of the syllable in developmental apraxia of speech. *Journal of Communication Disorders, 35*, 31–49.

McCune, L. & Vihman, M. M. (2001). Early phonetic and lexical development: A productivity approach. *Journal of Speech, Language, and Hearing Research, 44(3)*, 670–684.

McNeil, M. R., Pratt, S. R., & Fosset, T. R. D. (2004). The differential diagnosis of apraxia of speech. In B. Maassen, R. D. Kent, H. F. M. Peters, P. H. H. M. Van Lieshout, & W. Hulstijn (Eds.), *Speech Motor Control in Normal and Disordered Speech* (pp. 389–414). Oxford: Oxford University Press.

McNeil, M. R., Robin, D. A., & Schmidt, R. A. (1997). Apraxia of speech: Definition, differentiation, and treatment. In M. R. McNeil (Ed.), *Clinical Management Of Sensorimotor Speech Disorders* (pp. 311–344). New York: Thieme Medical Publishers Inc.

Namasivayam, A. K., Van Lieshout, P. H. H. M., & De Nil, L. F. (2008). Bite-block perturbation in people who stutter: Immediate compensatory and delayed adaptive processes. *Journal of Communication Disorders, 41*, 372–394.

Munson, B., Bjorum, E. M., & Windsor, J. (2003). Acoustic and perceptual correlates of stress in nonwords produced by children with suspected developmental apraxia of speech and children with phonological disorder. *Journal of Speech, Language, and Hearing Research, 46*, 189–202.

Nijland, L., Maassen, B., & Van der Meulen, Sj. (2003a). Evidence of motor programming deficits in children diagnosed with CAS. *Journal of Speech, Language, and Hearing Research, 46*, 437–450.

Nijland, L., Van der Meulen, Sj., & Maassen, B. (2003b). Subprofiles of auditory processing disorders in children. In M. J. Solé, D. Recasens, & J. Romero (Eds.), (pp. 1393–1396). Barcelona: Universitat Autònoma de Barcelona.

Odell, K. H. & Shriberg, L. D. (2001). Prosody-voice characteristics of children and adults with apraxia of speech. *Clinical Linguistics and Phonetics, 15*, 275–307.

Ozanne, A. E. (1995). The search for developmental verbal dyspraxia. In B. Dodd (Ed.), *Differential Diagnosis and Treatment of Children with Speech Disorders* (pp. 91–109). London: Whurr Publishers Ltd.

Peter, B. & Stoel-Gammon, C. (2005). Timing errors in two children with suspected childhood apraxia of speech (sCAS) during speech and music-related tasks. *Clinical Linguistics and Phonetics, 19*, 67–87.

Pollock, K. E. & Hall, P. K. (1991). An analysis of the vowel misarticulations of five children with developmental apraxia of speech. *Clinical Linguistics and Phonetics, 5*, 207–224.

Ruark, J. L. & Moore, C. A. (1997). Coordination of lip muscle activity by 2-year-old children during speech and nonspeech tasks. *Journal of Speech, Language, and Hearing Research, 40*, 1373–1385.

Shriberg, L. D., Aram, D. M., & Kwiatkowski, J. (1997a). Developmental apraxia of speech: I. Descriptive and theoretical perspectives. *Journal of Speech and Hearing Research, 40*, 273–285.

—— (1997b). Developmental apraxia of speech: II. Toward a diagnostic marker. *Journal of Speech, Language, and Hearing Research, 40*, 286–312.

—— (1997c). Developmental apraxia of speech: III. A subtype marked by inappropriate stress. *Journal of Speech, Language, and Hearing Research, 40*, 313–337.

Shriberg, L. D., Green, J. R., Campbell, T. F., Mcsweeny, J. L., & Scheer, A. R. (2003). A diagnostic marker for childhood apraxia of speech: The coefficient of variation ratio. *Clinical Linguistics and Phonetics, 17*, 575–595.

Smith, A. (2001). Dynamic interaction of motor and language factors in the development of speech production. In B. Maassen, W. Hulstijn, R. D. Kent, H. F. M. Peters, & P. H. H. M. Van Lieshout (Eds.), *Speech Motor Control in Normal and Disordered Speech. Proceedings of the 4th International Speech Motor Conference, Nijmegen, June 13–16, 2001* (pp. 351–354). Nijmegen: Uitgeverij Vantilt.

Smith, A. & Goffman, L. (2004). Interaction of motor and language factors in the development of speech production. In B. Maassen, R. D. Kent, H. F. M. Peters, P. H. H. M. Van Lieshout, & W. Hulstijn (Eds.), *Speech Motor Control in Normal and Disordered Speech* (pp. 225–252). Oxford: Oxford University Press.

Stackhouse, J. & Snowling, M. (1992). Developmental verbal dyspraxia, I: A review and critique; II: a developmental perspective on two case studies. *European Journal of Disorders of Communication, l27*, 19–54.

Sternberg, S., Monsell, S., Knoll, R. L., & Wright, C. E. (1978). The latency and duration of rapid movement sequenccs: Comparisons of speech and typewriting. In G.E.Stelmach (Ed.), *Information processing in motor control learning.* (pp. 117–152). New York: Academic Press.

Tallal, P., Miller, S. L., Byma, G., Bedi, G., Wang, X., Nagarajan, S. S., et al. (1996). Language comprehension in language-learning impaired children improved with acoustically modified speech. *Science, 271*, 81–84.

Terband, H., Maassen, B., & Brumberg, J. (2007). Computational neural modeling of childhood apraxia of speech, poster at the ASHA Convention 2007, Boston, November 15–17, 2007.

Terband, H., Maassen, B., Brumberg, J., & Guenther, F. H. (2008). Increased levels of neural noise as the core deficit in Childhood Apraxia of Speech (CAS), poster at the Conference on Motor Speech 2008, Monterey, CA, March 6–9, 2008.

Terband, H., Maassen, B., Guenther, F. H., & Brumberg, J. (2009). Computational neural modeling of speech motor control in childhood apraxia of speech. *Journal of Speech, Language, and Hearing Research, 52*, 1595–1609.

Thoonen, G., Maassen, B., Gabreëls, F., & Schreuder, R. (1994). Feature analysis of singleton consonant errors in developmental verbal dyspraxia (DVD). *Journal of Speech and Hearing Research, 37*, 1424–1440.

Schmidt, R. and Lee, T. (1999). *Motor Control and Learning: A Behavioral Emphasis.* Champaign, IL: Human Kinetics.

Van der Merwe, A. (1997). A theoretical framework for the characterization of pathological speech sensorimotor control. In M. R. McNeil (Ed.), *Clinical Management of Sensorimotor Speech Disorders* (pp. 1–25). New York: Thieme Medical Publishers Inc.

Varley, R. A. & Whiteside, S. P. (2001). Forum: What is the underlying impairment in acquired apraxia of speech. *Aphasiology, 15*, 39–84.

Velleman, S. L. & Strand, K. (1994). Developmental verbal dyspraxia. In J. E. Bernthal & N. W. Bankson (Eds.), *Child Phonology: Characteristics, Assessment, and Intervention with Special Populations* (pp. 110–139). New York: Thieme Medical Publishers Inc.

Walton, J. H. & Pollock, K. E. (1993). Acoustic validation of vowel error patterns in developmental apraxia of speech. *Clinical Linguistics and Phonetics, 7*, 95–111.

Westerman, G. & Reck-Miranda, E. (2004). A new model of sensorimotor coupling in the development of speech. *Brain and Language, 89*, 393–400.

Chapter 15

A neurodevelopmental framework for research in childhood apraxia of speech

Lawrence D. Shriberg

Abstract

We describe rationale, methods, and genetic findings for a neurodevelopmental framework for research in Childhood Apraxia of Speech (CAS). The proposed framework is motivated by the consensus perspective that despite considerable research and clinical attention, the core speech processing features of idiopathic CAS and its clinical signs remain unknown. The goal of the research framework is to obtain this information from comparative studies of adults with acquired apraxia of speech (AOS), children with CAS as a sequelae of a neurological disorder, children with CAS secondary to complex neurodevelopmental disorders, and the putative clinical entity—children suspected to have CAS of unknown (i.e., idiopathic) origin. Discussion begins with an overview of terms and issues underlying CAS as a speech sound disorder, followed by rationale and methods for the proposed research framework. The final section summarizes findings and issues from 18 studies reporting CAS in the context of genetically based neurodevelopmental disorders.

15.1 Etiological subtypes of speech sound disorders

15.1.1 Terms

Speech Sound Disorders (*SSD*), a classification term recently adopted by the American Speech-Language-Hearing Association, provides a welcome solution to the nosological challenges associated with prior attempts to classify children's speech disorders based on *articulatory* versus *phonological* explanatory processes. *Speech* subsumes all articulatory and phonological mechanisms, *sound* separates this class of speech disorder from speech fluency disorders, and *disorder* is the public health construct required for access to diagnostic and treatment services. Thus, SSD provides a unified term for research and clinical practice in childhood SSD of both known origin (e.g., cleft palate, Down syndrome) and of currently unknown origin, the latter historically termed *functional*, *developmental*, or *idiopathic* speech disorders. Elsewhere, *Speech Delay* (*SD*) and *Speech Errors* (*SE*) are delineated as cover terms for two subordinate classifications of SSD of currently unknown origin (Shriberg 2009). In comparison to children with SE, for whom transient or persistent speech sound distortions may be of negligible to moderate socio-educational significance, children with SD have speech processing deficits that place them at risk for literacy,

Table 15.1 Working terms, distal origins, and proximal processes affected in five putative subtypes of SD

Working Term	Abbreviation	Primary origin	Processes affected
Speech Delay–Genetic	SD-GEN	Polygenic/environmental	Cognitive-linguistic
Speech Delay–Otitis media with effusion	SD-OME	Polygenic/environmental	Auditory-perceptual
Speech Delay–Developmental psychosocial involvement	SD-DPI	Polygenic/environmental	Affective-temperamental
Speech Delay–Apraxia of speech	SD-AOS	Monogenic? Oligogenic?	Speech-motor control
Speech Delay–Dysarthria	SD-DYS	Monogenic? Oligogenic?	Speech-motor control

learning, social, and vocational challenges. The subtype of SD termed Childhood Apraxia of Speech (CAS), one of five proposed subtypes of SD and the focus of this paper, clearly places a child at elevated risk for such challenges (ASHA 2007b).

Table 15.1 is a list of five subtypes of SD posited to have different etiological (*distal*) origins, with each origin having implications for speech processing (*proximal*) constraints. For research needs, a set of working terms and their abbreviations are used to reference children whose SD may be caused or significantly mediated by one or more of these five proposed distal-proximal constraints. As listed in Table 15.1, the five proposed subtypes of SD are defined by (a) cognitive-linguistic processing constraints associated with genetic risk factors (*SD-GEN*); (b) auditory-perceptual processing constraints due to mild-moderate fluctuant conductive hearing loss consequent to early recurrent otitis media with effusion (*SD-OME*); (c) affective, temperamental constraints associated with developmental psychosocial involvement (*SD-DPI*); (d) speech motor planning/programming deficits consistent with apraxia of speech (*SD-AOS*; elsewhere termed *CAS* or Developmental Verbal Dyspraxia [*DVD*]); and (e) speech motor execution constraints consistent with subtypes of dysarthria (*SD-DYS*). For clinical concerns, these five proximal speech-processing constraints presumably are associated with prognosis and treatment, with each constraint comprising a potential focus of treatment. It is important to underscore that the division of SD into these five interim classifications and their abbreviated working terms is used as a heuristic for research. A significant proportion of children who have SD likely have involvement in more than one putative subtype.

A central concept in the classification system proposed in Table 15.1 is that both genetic and environmental sources confer risk and protective elements to the expression, severity, and persistence or normalization of each subtype of SD. As shown in the third column, genetic sources are divided into contributions from *monogenic* (one), *oligogenic* (a few), or *polygenic* (many) genes or genomic regions. For SD-GEN, estimated to be the most prevalent subtype of SD and predicted to have polygenic/environmental origins, *susceptibility loci* (regions of interest) have been reported on four autosomes: chromosomes 1, 3, 6, and 15 (Lewis et al., 2006). The Lewis et al. review of speech-genetic studies includes discussion of the candidate genes within each susceptibility locus that have been linked to verbal trait disorders (i.e., impairments in language, reading, and spelling). Reports by two research groups indicate that at least part of the association of SSD with reading disability is likely due to common genes in regions of interest on chromosomes 5p22 and 15q21 (Smith et al., 2005) and in the centromeric region of chromosome 3 (Stein et al., 2004).

As indicated in Table 15.1, polygenic and environmental origins are posited for SD-OME and SD-DPI. For the subtypes of SD with the working terms SD-AOS and SD-DYS, however, their considerably lower prevalence, marked severity of expression, and involvement of specific motor systems suggest monogenic or oligogenic, rather than polygenic origins, with few or no significant environmental contributions. The third section of this paper returns to genetic issues and findings for SD-AOS in non-idiopathic contexts.

15.1.2 **Differential diagnosis of CAS**

The classification terms in Table 15.1, together with an additional term for speakers with normal or normalized speech (*Typical Speech, TS*), provide three diagnostic challenges for research and practice in CAS (i.e., SD-AOS). The following classification challenges are made more or less difficult as mediated by a child's age (toddler, preschooler, school-age, adolescent) and relative severity of expression (mild, moderate, severe) of CAS.

Differentiate CAS from Typical Speech (TS). The earliest diagnostic/prognostic challenge for children suspected to have CAS occurs before two years of age when a child with moderate to severe CAS may be producing a limited amount of speech. Unlike the histories of children with the other four subtypes of SD in Table 15.1, case histories of children suspected to have CAS indicate that they are late to begin talking. With only limited speech output to evaluate, it is difficult to determine if the delayed onset of speech in such children is due entirely or partially to cognitive-language constraints (i.e., a *Late-Talker*) or to a deficit in *praxis*, the construct from which CAS takes its name. The latter may be suspected if excessive articulatory efforts are apparent in a child's attempt to imitate speech models, compared to the absence of such difficulties in well-practiced, spontaneous speech forms (Velleman 2002).

Differentiate CAS from SD-GEN, SD-OME, and SD-DPI. Once a child of any age is producing a sufficient amount of speech for perceptual, acoustic, and other types of instrumental analyses, the assessment challenge is to differentiate CAS from three of the four other subtypes of SD listed in Table 15.1. Differential diagnosis requires quantitative analyses of SE patterns, including close description of prosodic and vocal features. As noted previously, a primary constraint on such analyses is the lack of research consensus on the speech, prosodic, and vocal signs that are pathognomonic (definitive) for CAS. A Position Statement on CAS by the American Speech-Language-Hearing Association (ASHA 2007a) includes the following three signs for which, as concluded in the position paper, there is consensus in both the adult AOS and child CAS communities: '(a) inconsistent errors on consonants and vowels in repeated productions of syllables or words, (b) lengthened and disrupted coarticulatory transitions between sounds and syllables, and (c) inappropriate prosody, especially in the realization of lexical or phrasal stress' (p. 2). Notice that such behaviours provide only the starting point for development of the methods and quantitative criteria required to translate such observations into reliable diagnostic markers that meet psychometric requirements for research and clinical decision-making.

Differentiate CAS from SD-DYS. Differentiating CAS from SD-DYS, a third diagnostic specificity need, is less widely discussed in the CAS literature than in the adult AOS literature. At present, the criterial speech and non-speech signs of childhood dysarthria draw heavily from the descriptions available in research on acquired dysarthria in adults (e.g., Duffy 2005). Other than descriptions of speech in subtypes of cerebral palsy, there is a notably sparse literature on clinical or subclinical childhood dysarthria. As with SD-AOS, SD-DYS is often a provisional diagnosis (i.e., '*suspected* to have dysarthria' or '*dysarthria cannot be ruled out*') in children who do not have a frank neuromotor disorder.

15.1.3 **Definitional alternatives**

The diversity of definitional perspectives in CAS has been deliberated most recently at an international research symposium (Shriberg and Campbell 2003), at the miniseminar that included the present chapter, and in an American Speech-Language-Hearing Association position paper and accompanying technical report (ASHA, 2007a, b). Rationale for the definitional perspectives outlined in the present paper is based on an affirmative answer to each of the following questions:

Should apraxia of speech be defined by one or more core speech processing features (i.e., as identified by behavioural markers) that are generally similar:

(1) in congenital and acquired forms?

(2) in idiopathic versus non-idiopathic forms?

(3) at all levels of severity?

(4) in the same speaker at different points in development?

On the first question, there are many reasons to suspect that the core speech processing deficit in CAS – constraints in the planning of gestures that subserve speech – might differ in congenital compared to acquired forms. Although both forms have praxis impairment, relevant sensorimotor processes likely vary considerably in children developing speech compared to those with an acquired disorder. Notwithstanding differences in genetic and epigenetic expression and other risk factors that may mediate error severity and error topography, it is parsimonious to posit a common core deficit in speech processing. From a similar perspective, we take the position on the second question that the core speech processing features of idiopathic CAS and non-idiopathic CAS (i.e., whether apraxia occurs as the sole disorder or as a secondary sign in complex neurodevelopmental disorders) should be similar or generally equivalent.

The third and fourth questions above clearly seem to require affirmative answers because severity of expression at any one or more developmental period is a secondary rather than core feature of disease and disorder. Again, a parsimonious view would posit that although severity of expression may be significantly attenuated over time, hopefully with appropriate treatment, core praxic features of CAS as manifest in their behavioural signs and age/severity adjusted diagnostic markers should be stable over even long time periods.

15.2 A neurodevelopmental framework for research in CAS

15.2.1 Rationale and description

Figure 15.1 illustrates a four-phase neurodevelopmental framework for research in CAS. Rationale for this proposal is that the only way to obviate the 'circularity' (Guyette and Diedrich 1981) or 'tautology' (McNeil et al., 1997) problem in subject selection for research in idiopathic CAS is by programmatic study of CAS occurring in forms with known neurogenic origins. Accordingly, the first of the four phases depicted in Fig. 15.1 is to conduct studies to identify and validate the linguistic domains (e.g., vowels, consonants, prosody) in which the core speech processing features of CAS can be quantified as they occur in adult AOS, in children following a neurological disorder (e.g., infection, trauma), and in complex neurodevelopmental disorders. Some examples of complex neurodevelopmental backgrounds reporting CAS as a secondary disorder include the autism spectrum, chromosome translocations, Coffin-Sirus syndrome, Down syndrome, Fragile X syndrome, Joubert syndrome, galactosemia, Rett syndrome, Rolandic epilepsy, Russell-Silver syndrome, Velocardiofacial syndrome, and duplication of the Williams-Beuren locus. As indicated in Fig. 15.1, this phase is increasingly being informed by knockout, knockdown, and knockin avian and mammalian studies of FoxP2 and other genes (e.g., the FMRP gene in Fragile X syndrome).

In the second phase, findings from the studies of non-idiopathic CAS and children suspected to have idiopathic CAS can be used to inform the inclusional/exclusional criteria to classify

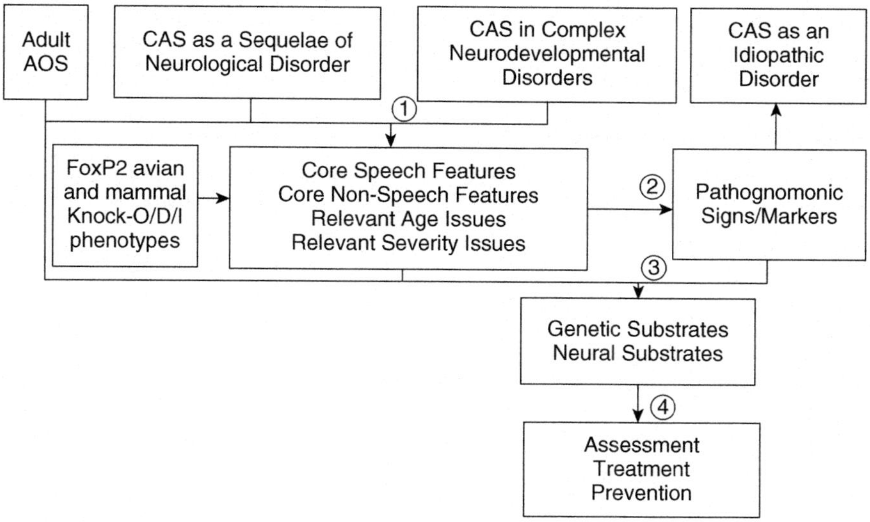

Fig. 15.1 A neurodevelopmental framework for research in CAS.

participants as true positives for idiopathic CAS. Findings from these four forms of CAS can provide the information base needed for third-phase studies of the genetic and neural substrates underlying the pathophysiology of apraxia. Last, in the fourth phase, investigators from a number of disciplines can use aggregate findings to develop optimum methods for assessment, treatment, and ultimately, prevention.

15.2.2 **Method**

The second element required for the research framework shown in Fig. 15.1 is a lifespan assessment protocol for each of the four contexts for CAS. Table 15.2 is an overview of the assessment and analysis framework. As shown in the two left-hand columns, speech targets are organized by three linguistic domains (vowels/diphthongs, consonants, prosody-voice), each subordinated under three analytic constructs reflecting a participant's speech competence, precision, and stability. For each of these nine domains, prior studies in our laboratory and elsewhere have suggested segmental and suprasegmental indices (i.e., signs) that may meet accuracy criteria as diagnostic markers of apraxia, one of several subtypes of dysarthria, or for a classification termed motor speech disorder-not otherwise specified (i.e., a cover term non-specific for apraxia or dysarthria).

Potential diagnostic markers for apraxia (e.g., *unstable planar area, unstable vowel duration, overstressed lexical stress*) are interrogated using a high-throughput computer platform for acoustic-aided transcription and transcription-aided acoustics (Shriberg 2008). Multiple data sources are used to examine contextual influences on each index obtained from a 1-hour assessment protocol that includes 15 speech tasks (e.g., vowel repetition tasks, challenging word tasks, conversational sample). Comparison databases are used to derive age x sex z-scores for each index/variable from each speech task. As shown in Table 15.2, clinical classification information on the resulting profiles of z-scores is consolidated and tabulated within a 27-cell matrix. Shriberg (2008) summarizes findings from four studies of CAS in complex neurodevelopmental disorders using the matrix in Table 15.2.

Table 15.2 Assessment and analyses framework of perceptual and acoustic findings from speakers' responses to the Madison Speech Assessment Protocol. All analyses, including perceptual coding for the Prosody-Voice Screening Profile (PVSP), are completed in the PEPPER environment (Shriberg 2008)

Assessment and analyses framework		**Clinical classification**		
Construct	**Domain**	**Apraxia**	**Dysarthria**	**Motor speech disorder – not otherwise specified**
Competence	Vowels/diphthongs			
	Consonants			
	Prosody-Voice			
Precision	Vowels/diphthongs			
	Consonants			
	Prosody-Voice			
Stability	Vowels/diphthongs			
	Consonants			
	Prosody-Voice			

15.3 **Genetic research in childhood apraxia of speech**

Table 15.3 is a summary of findings from 18 studies reporting behaviours consistent with CAS in the context of genetically based, complex neurodevelopmental disorders. Entries in Table 15.3 were restricted to those appearing in peer-reviewed, English language publications; additional case studies have been reported at conferences and on internet forums. As shown in the source information column, three research groups have provided data for 41 of the 55 (75%) cases of reported CAS included in Table 15.3, with affected members of the KE family (Lai et al., 2001) accounting for 15 (27%) of the cases. Only 5 of the 18 (28%) studies include data for more than one affected family member. Although most reports lack detailed or even basic information on how CAS was assessed, the thesis is that these studies provide the precedent literature for programmatic study of CAS in genetically based neurodevelopmental disorders. Space constraints prohibit discussion of methods and speech findings in each study. The following sections briefly contrast trends in these genetic case reports with those reported for idiopathic CAS (e.g., ASHA 2007b).

15.3.1 **Age and sex**

Patient age in Table 15.3 ranged from three years to older adults, compared with the idiopathic CAS literature which is almost exclusively limited to preschool and school-aged children, with some follow-up studies of adolescents (ASHA 2007b). The nearly equal (0.9:1) ratio of males-to-females in these 18 studies also differs from the sex ratios for idiopathic CAS reported in case-control studies. The latter have routinely reported considerably higher boys-to-girls ratios, approximating 100% boys in some literature reviews (e.g., Hall et al., 1993; Shriberg et al., 1997). Such sex ratio differences in idiopathic CAS compared to CAS in known neurodevelopmental contexts may have significant implications for genetic transmission models. Notice that many cases of reported CAS in Table 15.3 were based on sporadic genetic events (e.g., chromosome translocations), rather than from polymorphisms segregating in families, as is the case in the KE family.

Table 15.3 Patient information, phenotype summaries, and genetic findings for 18 papers providing molecular genetic information for 55 children and adults reported to have speech impairments consistent with CAS

Source		Case information			Phenotype summaries[a]				Genetic findings		
Authors	**Group[b]**	**Case(s)**	**Age (yrs)**	**No. of cases**	**Orofacial Apraxia**	**Cognitive impairment**	**Language impairment**	**Dysmorphology**	**Description**	**Loci**	**Gene**
Sarda et al. (1988)	–	Boy	7	1		X	X	X	Interstitial deletion	7q31.2-q32.3	*FOXP2*
Weistuch and Shiff-Myers (1996)	–	Boy	5	1	X	X	X		Balanced translocation	1q;2q	
Tan-Sindhunata et al. (2000)	–	Boy Girl Mother	4 3 37	3		X		X	Supernumerary ring chromosome	r (7)	
Lai et al. (2000)	A	'CS' boy	5	1	X	X	X		Balanced translocation	5q22; 7q31.2	*FOXP2*
Lai et al. (2001)	A	'KE' 6 males; 9 females	3 generations	15	X	X	X		Point mutation	7q31	*FOXP2*
Liégeois et al. (2001)	A	'AA' Man		1	X	X	X		Deletion	7q31	*FOXP2*
Velagaleti et al. (2002)	–	Boy	12	1		X	X	X	Supernumerary ring chromosome	r (7)	
Tyson et al. (2004)	B	Boy	14	1		X	X	X	Deletion	7q31	*FOXP2*
MacDermot et al. (2005)	A	1 boy; 1 girl; Mother	4 2	3	X	X	X		Point mutation	7q31	*FOXP2*

[a] Patients reported as 'affected' in each report differ in the type and severity of impairments, and for reports with multiple patients, the number of affected patients for each of the three phenotypes. Data are based on varying levels of observational and clinical data. Blank cells typically indicate no information.

[b] Location of research group with two or more table entries: A: London-Oxford; B: Toronto; C: Madison: Other

(Continued)

Table 15.3 (Cont.) Patient information, phenotype summaries, and genetic findings for 18 papers providing molecular genetic information for 55 children and adults reported to have speech impairments consistent with CAS

Source		Case information			Phenotype summaries[a]				Genetic findings		
Authors	**Group[b]**	**Case(s)**	**Age (yrs)**	**No. of cases**	**Orofacial Apraxia**	**Cognitive impairment**	**Language impairment**	**Dysmor-phology**	**Description**	**Loci**	**Gene**
Somerville et al. (2005)	B	Boy		1		X	X	X	Duplication	7q11.23	(Williams-Beuren locus)
Lichtenbelt et al. (2005)	–	Girl	4	1		X	X		Supernumerary ring chromosome	7q	
Zeesman et al. (2006)	B	Girl	5	1	X	X	X	X	Interstitial deletion	7q31.2-q32.2	*FOXP2*
Shriberg et al. (2006)	C	'TB' Mother; daughter	 50 19	2		X	X		Balanced translocation	7q;13q	*FOXP2* (*RFC3*)
Feuk et al. (2006)	B	4 males; 8 females (1 no information)	children	13	X	X	X		Paternal deletion (5); translocation (1); maternal uniparental disomy (7)	7q31	*FOXP2*
Lennon et al. (2007)	–	Boy	7	1		X	X	X	Deletion	7q31	*FOXP2*
Cody et al. (2007)	–	3 boys; 2 girls	2–7	5		X	X	X	Interstitial deletions	18q	
Battini et al. (2007)	–	Boy	9	1	X	X	X		de novo mutation	X-linked	*SLC6A8*
Shriberg et al. (2008)	C	1 boy; 2 girls	11–17	3		X	X	X	Unbalanced translocation	4q;16q	

15.3.2 Cognitive-language impairment

Unlike the idiopathic CAS literature, which frequently reports children whose only sign is a significant speech involvement, all 18 of the studies in Table 15.3 report cognitive-language involvement ('X') in at least one patient. As indicated previously, most of the studies in Table 15.3 provide little information on the assessment procedures and criteria used to classify patients as positive for cognitive, language, or speech impairment, orofacial apraxia, or dysmorphisms. Some of these cases are likely false positives, including patients who have (a) typical speech, (b) SD due to a non-motor etiology (SD-GEN, SD-OME, SD-DPI), or (c) a different motor speech disorder (SD-DYS). Such sensitivity/specificity constraints notwithstanding, the routine finding of language and especially cognitive impairments in these cases compared to findings in the idiopathic CAS literature warrants close research examination.

15.3.3 Orofacial apraxia, dysmorphisms, and dysarthria

Approximately half of the cases reported in Table 15.3 were classified as having orofacial apraxia. This total is heavily weighted by the 15 affected members of the KE family for whom orofacial apraxia was the basis for classifying family members as affected (Vargha-Khadem et al., 1998; see also Chapter 6 Morgan et al., this volume). Again, many studies provide only minimal methodological information and not all studies appear to have reported information for this variable. Of considerable interest is the finding that orofacial apraxia was not found in many cases of *FOXP2* impairments, including two family members whose speech and non-speech characteristics were tested with an extensive battery of speech and non-speech measures (Shriberg et al., 2006). Orofacial apraxia is also reported for only some cases of idiopathic CAS, with implications for an eventual understanding of pathophysiological substrates.

A variety of craniofacial and other dysmorphisms were also reported in approximately half of the cases in Table 15.3. By definition, such findings do not appear in the idiopathic CAS literature. Of interest is an observation in Zeesman et al. (2006), indicating that their patient had dysmorphic features similar to those described in the child reported in both Sarda et al. (1988) and the patient described in Lai et al. (2000). Similarly, Somerville et al. (2005, p. 1700) reported a 'subtle but recognizable facial phenotype' in their patient similar to the phenotype described in Lichtenbelt et al. (2005), Tan-Sindhunata et al. (2000), and Chantot-Bastaraud et al. (2004).

Finally, as shown in Table 15.3, several studies report speech behaviours consistent with dysarthria, whereas few studies of idiopathic CAS report signs of dysarthria. An important research question is whether there may be genomic loci that confer shared risk for either or both of these sensorimotor speech disorders.

15.3.4 Genetic findings

The most frequent genetic finding in Table 15.3 is a disruption in regions of interest or genes on chromosome 7 within or near the *FOXP2* gene. Emphasis on chromosome 7 and *FOXP2* in Table 15.3 is, of course, in part a consequence of the widespread influence of the genetic findings for the KE family, with its implications for study of the neurological substrates and evolutionary biology of speech (see Morgan et al., Chapter 6, this volume). The number of case reports implicating *FOXP2* deficits in Table 15.3 in addition to affected members of the KE family increases its attributable risk for CAS. As noted at the outset of this discussion, however, the KE family remains the only pedigree in which reported CAS has been associated with a point mutation segregating in a large, multigenerational family (Tomblin et al., 2009). In contrast, most of the reports in Table 15.3 are associated with sporadic cytogenetic events in one or a few family members in which copy number variations (i.e., deletions and duplications of genomic material) resulted from chromosome translocations. As chromosome translocations have been associated with a large number of neurodevelopmental syndromes, they would appear to be a productive source for research addressing the genetic origins of CAS.

15.4 **Research directions**

The entries in Table 15.3 sample only some of the possible contexts in which research in genetically based neurodevelopmental disorders can be informative for apraxia of speech. This chapter has suggested that advances in identifying the core motor control processes, speech signs, and diagnostic markers of the idiopathic form of CAS may be possible using a comparative research framework. Some emerging examples of this framework include Shriberg and Potter (2008), Shriberg et al. (2006), Shriberg et al. (2008). Studies in process will focus on genotype-phenotype associations in CAS, with the potential of eventually identifying a biomarker for the early detection of this challenging childhood SSD.

References

American Speech-Language-Hearing Association (ASHA). (2007a). *Childhood apraxia of speech* [Position Statement]. Available at: www.asha.org/policy.

American Speech-Language-Hearing Association (ASHA). (2007b). *Childhood apraxia of speech* [Technical Report]. Available at: www.asha.org/policy.

Battini R, Chilosi A, Mei D, et al. (2007). Mental retardation and verbal dyspraxia in a new patient with de novo creatine transporter (*SLC6A8*) mutation. *American Journal of Medical Genetics*, 143A, 1771–74.

Chantot-Bastaraud S, Muti C, Pipiras E, et al. (2004). Clinical findings and cytogenetic analysis of small supernumerary ring chromosomes 7: report of 2 new cases. *Annales de Génétique*, 47, 241–49.

Cody JD, Sebold C, Malik A, et al. (2007). Recurrent interstitial deletions of proximal 18q: a new syndrome involving expressive speech delay. *American Journal of Medical Genetics*, 143A, 1181–90.

Duffy JR (2005). *Motor Speech Disorders: Substrates, Differential Diagnosis, and Management* (2nd edn). Mosby, Missouri.

Feuk L, Kalervo A, Lipsanen-Nyman M, et al. (2006). Absence of a paternally inherited *FOXP2* gene in developmental verbal dyspraxia. *The American Journal of Human Genetics*, 79, 965–72.

Guyette TW and Diedrich WM (1981). A critical review of developmental apraxia of speech. In NJ Lass, ed. *Speech and Language: Advances in Basic Research and Practice*, pp. 1–49. Academic Press, New York.

Hall PK, Jordan LS, and Robin DA (1993). *Developmental Apraxia of Speech: Theory and Clinical Practice*. Pro-Ed, Texas.

Lai CSL, Fisher SE, Hurst JA, et al. (2000). The SPCH1 region on human 7q31: genomic characterization of the critical interval and localization of translocations associated with speech and language disorder. *The American Journal of Human Genetics*, 67, 357–68.

Lai CSL, Fisher SE, Hurst JA, et al. (2001). A forkhead-domain gene is mutated in a severe speech and language disorder. *Nature*, 413, 519–23.

Lennon PA, Cooper ML, Peiffer DA, et al. (2007). Deletion of 7q31.1 supports involvement of *FOXP2* in language impairment: clinical report and review. *American Journal of Medical Genetics*, 143A, 791–98.

Lewis BA., Shriberg LD, Freebairn LA, et al. (2006). The genetic bases of speech sound disorders: evidence from spoken and written language. *Journal of Speech, Language, and Hearing Research*, 49, 1294–1312.

Lichtenbelt KD, Hochstenbach R, van Dam WM, et al. (2005). Supernumerary ring chromosome 7 mosaicism: case report, investigation of the gene content, and delineation of the phenotype. *American Journal of Medical Genetics*, 132A, 93–100.

Liégeois FJ, Lai CSL, Baldeweg T, et al. (2001). Behavioural and neuroimaging correlates of a chromosome 7Q31 deletion containing the SPCH1 gene. *Society for Neuroscience Abstracts*, 27, Program No. 529.17

MacDermot KD, Bonora E, Sykes N, et al. (2005). Identification of FOXP2 truncation as a novel cause of developmental speech and language deficits. *American Journal of Human Genetics*, 76, 1074–80.

McNeil, MR, Robin, DA, and Schmidt, RA (1997). Apraxia of speech: definition, differentiation, and treatment. In MR McNeil, ed. *Clinical Management of Sensorimotor Speech Disorders*, pp. 311–44. Thieme, New York.

Sarda P, Turleau C, Cabanis MO, et al. (1988). Deletion interstitielle du bras long du chromosome 7. *Annals of Human Genetics*, 31, 258–61.

Shriberg, LD (2008, November). *Toward the Phenotype for Childhood Apraxia of Speech.* Paper presented for the ASHA 2008 Seminar on Genetic, Neuroimaging, and Motor Control Research in Childhood Apraxia of Speech: Annual Convention of the American Speech-Language-Hearing Association, Chicago, IL.

Shriberg LD (2009). Childhood speech sound disorders: from post-behaviorism to the postgenomic era. In R Paul & P Flipsen, eds. *Speech Sound Disorders in Children: Essays in Honor of Lawrence D. Shriberg*, pp. 1–34. Plural Publishing, Inc., California.

Shriberg, LD, Allen, CT, McSweeny, JL, et al. (2001). *PEPPER: programs to examine phonetic and phonologic evaluation records* [Computer software]. Madison, WI: Waisman Center Research Computing Facility, University of Wisconsin–Madison.

Shriberg LD, Aram DM, and Kwiatkowski J. (1997). Developmental apraxia of speech: I. Descriptive perspectives. *Journal of Speech, Language, and Hearing Research*, 40, 273–85.

Shriberg LD, Ballard KJ, Tomblin JB, et al. (2006). Speech, prosody, and voice characteristics of a mother and daughter with a 7;13 translocation affecting *FOXP2. Journal of Speech, Language, and Hearing Research*, 49, 500–25.

Shriberg LD and Campbell TF (Eds). (2003). *Proceedings of the 2002 childhood apraxia of speech research symposium.* Carlsbad, CA: The Hendrix Foundation.

Shriberg LD, Jakielski KJ, and El-Shanti H (2008). Breakpoint localization using array-CGH in three siblings with an unbalanced 4q;16q translocation and Childhood Apraxia of Speech (CAS). *American Journal of American Genetics: Part A*, 146A, 2227–33.

Shriberg LD and Potter NL (2008, June). *Speech characteristics of children with galactosemia and persistent speech disorder.* Paper presented at the 12th Congress of the International Clinical Phonetics and Linguistics Association, Istanbul, Turkey.

Smith SD, Pennington BF, Boada R, et al. (2005). Linkage of speech sound disorder to reading disability loci. *Journal of Child Psychology & Psychiatry*, 46, 1057–66.

Somerville MJ, Mervis CB, Young EJ, et al. (2005). Severe expressive-language delay related to duplication of the Williams-Beuren locus. *New England Journal of Medicine*, 353, 1694–1701.

Stein CM, Schick JH, Taylor HG, et al. (2004). Pleiotropic effects of a chromosome 3 locus on speech-sound disorder and reading. *The American Journal of Human Genetics*, 74, 283–97.

Tan-Sindhunata G, Castedo S, Leegte B, et al. (2000). Molecular cytogenetic characterization of a small, familial supernumerary ring chromosome 7 associated with mental retardation and an abnormal phenotype. *American Journal of Medical Genetics*, 92, 147–52.

Tomblin JB, O'Brien M, Shriberg LD, et al. (2009). Language features in a mother and daughter of a chromosome 7;13 translocation involving *FOXP2. Journal of Speech, Language, and Hearing Research, 52*, 1157–74.

Tyson C, McGillivray B, Chijiwa C, et al. (2004). Elucidation of a cryptic interstitial 7q31.3 deletion in a patient with a language disorder and mild mental retardation by array-CGH. *American Journal of Medical Genetics*, 129A, 254–60.

Vargha-Khadem F, Watkins KE, Price CJ, et al. (1998). Neural basis of an inherited speech and language disorder. *Proceedings of the National Academy of Sciences*, 95, 12695–700.

Velagaleti GVN, Jalal SM, Kukolich MK, et al. (2002). *De novo* supernumerary ring chromosome 7: first report of a non-mosaic patient and review of the literature. *Clinical Genetics*, 61, 202–06.

Velleman SL (2002). *Childhood Apraxia of Speech Resource Guide.* Singular, California.

Weistuch L and Schiff-Myers NB (1996). Chromosomal translocation in a child with SLI and apraxia. *Journal of Speech and Hearing Research*, 39, 668–71.

Zeesman S, Nowaczyk MJM, Teshima I, et al. (2006). Speech and language impairment and oromotor dyspraxia due to deletion of 7q31 that involves *FOXP2*. *American Journal of Human Genetics*, 140A, 509–14.

Chapter 16

Distinguishing among motor speech disorders is important: the role of speech pathology in neurologic diagnosis

Joseph R. Duffy

Abstract

The contribution that distinguishing among motor speech disorders (MSDs) can make to the localization and diagnosis of neurological disease is frequently ignored by medicine and, at the least, underappreciated by speech-language pathology. This is of no small consequence because speech abnormalities can be the presenting or most prominent sign of neurologic disease. This chapter addresses the relationship between the differential diagnosis of acquired MSDs and the localization and diagnosis of neurologic disease. The clinical reality of the relationship is highlighted through five case illustrations and a summary of the specific lessons they provide that illustrate the sometimes crucial importance of recognizing the meaning of speech signs in clinical diagnostic settings. The foundations on which such clinical contributions have been built, and a few examples of recent studies of dysarthria or apraxia of speech associated with neurodegenerative disorders (paraneoplastic cerebellar degeneration, tauopathies) that are helping to refine those abilities, are reviewed. Finally, some thoughts are offered about how future clinical practice and training, and clinical and more basic research, can improve the contributions that MSD diagnosis can make to medical diagnostic efforts in clinical practice.

16.1 Introduction

Clinicians working with people who have motor speech disorders (MSDs) readily recognize that a specific MSD diagnosis can influence management decision making. They know, for example, that speech therapy for the dysarthrias differs from therapy for apraxia of speech (AOS), and therapy strategies that can reduce impairment or disability associated with some dysarthria types can be ineffective or contraindicated for others. In contrast, the value of distinguishing among MSDs in localizing and diagnosing neurological disease has largely been ignored by medicine and, at the least, underemphasized by speech-language pathology. This circumstance is of no small consequence because speech abnormalities can be the presenting or most prominent sign of neurologic disease.

This chapter will address the contributions that differential diagnosis of acquired MSDs can make to the localization and diagnosis of neurologic disease. The clinical reality of such contributions will be highlighted through brief case illustrations. The foundations on which such clinical contributions have been built, and a few examples of recent work with neurodegenerative disorders that is helping to refine those abilities, will be reviewed. Finally, some thoughts about how future clinical practice and research, and more basic research activities, can improve the contribution that MSD diagnoses can make to medical diagnostic efforts will be offered.

16.2 **MSD diagnosis can contribute to the localization and diagnosis of neurologic disease – Some illustrative cases and their lessons**

The following brief vignettes are based on actual clinical practice. Inconsequential facts have been altered to mask patient identity. Some aspects of each case have been modified for the sake of brevity and clarity. Each will review the context in which the patients were seen, the evidence provided by speech examination, the speech diagnosis, and the eventual medical diagnosis.

Case 1

A 74-year-old man presented to neurology with a history of progressive speech and swallowing problems. Evaluations elsewhere raised the possibility of stroke or myasthenia gravis, but workups for those conditions were negative. Head MRI examinations were normal. Neurologic examination revealed only dysarthria. The neurologist requested speech pathology consultation stating, 'we will then decide what additional studies are appropriate'.

During speech evaluation, the patient reported 10 months of gradually progressive difficulty 'saying different letters', and more recent problems with chewing and swallowing. Non-speech oral mechanism examination revealed mild lower facial weakness and moderate bilateral lingual weakness, but without lingual fasciculations or atrophy. Speech was characterized by: strained-hoarse-groaning voice quality; monopitch and monoloudness; hypernasality and weak pressure consonant sounds; and slow rate. Vowel prolongation was strained-harsh, with equivocal vocal flutter. Speech alternating motion rates (AMRs; e.g., rapid repetition of /pʌpʌpʌ/) were slow but regular. Subjectively, intelligibility was mildly reduced.

The clinician concluded and reported that the patient had a moderately severe spastic dysarthria that was strongly suggestive of bilateral upper motor neuron (UMN) dysfunction affecting the bulbar speech muscles. The possibility of a lower motor neuron (LMN) component was also raised. Dysphagia evaluation was recommended. Strategies for managing his dysarthria were addressed, as were alternative and augmentative means of communication.

Based on the speech evaluation, the neurologist proceeded with electromyography (EMG) and nerve conduction studies which showed changes in limb muscles consistent with motor neuron disease (MND). The patient was subsequently seen for management of his dysarthria on a periodic basis through an interdisciplinary amyotrophic lateral sclerosis (ALS) team.

Case 2

A 63-year-old man presented to neurology with a one-month history of slurred speech that his referring physician felt was due to a stroke. Clinical neurology examination was normal with the exception of speech. Subsequent head MRI showed a small cerebellar infarct that was not felt to explain the speech symptom. The neurologist nonetheless felt the most likely cause of the dysarthria was a posterior circulation stroke, on the basis of multiple vascular risk factors that included hypertension, hypercholesterolemia, and previously untreated sleep apnea. Additional tests were ordered, including speech pathology consultation.

During the speech evaluation, the patient said his problems began while eating breakfast, when he had difficulty moving food in his mouth and his speech became abnormal. He subsequently had similar episodes of speech and chewing difficulty. During the evaluation, his speech was initially normal, but after several minutes he developed lingual articulatory imprecision and marked hypernasality. Following 15–30 seconds of rest from speaking, his speech improved nearly to normal. This pattern of deterioration with speaking and speech improvement following rest was replicated several times.

The clinician concluded and reported that the patient had a flaccid dysarthria in which the rapid onset of speech difficulty associated with continuous speaking, followed by significant recovery after a short period of rest, was strongly suspicious for myasthenia gravis. The referring neurologist was immediately contacted and the subsequent neurologic workup was modified. EMG and acetylcholine receptor antibody tests were indicative of myasthenia gravis. The patient was placed on Mestinon and, later, prednisone. His swallowing and speech difficulties subsequently resolved, except during prolonged physical activity, when his weakness would become apparent.

Case 3

A 67-year-old man presented to neurology with a three-year history of progressive gait and balance difficulties, weakness, changes in speech, and occasional choking on saliva. Neurologic examination revealed weakness in the upper and lower extremities, and decreased vibration and joint position sense. It was felt that the patient might have a length dependent peripheral neuropathy, in addition to MND, a cervical myelopathy, or a motor-greater-than-sensory polyradiculoneuropathy; however, the speech and swallowing findings were felt to be unusual for the latter two conditions.

Subsequent speech consultation observed equivocal lower facial weakness during lip retraction and rounding. His speech was characterized by non-specific hoarseness; equivocal strained voice quality; monopitch and monoloudness; irregular articulatory breakdowns; and equivocally slowed rate. The clinician concluded that the patient had a mixed spastic-ataxic dysarthria, without any clear evidence of a flaccid or LMN component. It was explicitly stated that the speech pattern was suggestive of bilateral UMN and cerebellar control circuit dysfunction, that it was not explainable by weakness alone, and that the speech pattern would be quite unusual in MND.

Subsequent EMG failed to reveal evidence of MND. MRI showed abnormalities in multiple areas, including periventricular white matter, the medulla and the cerebellum, and the cervical and thoracic spinal cord. It was concluded that the most likely diagnosis was primary progressive multiple sclerosis.

Case 4

A 69-year-old right-handed woman presented to neurology with a two-year history of progressive speech difficulty that included occasional mispronouncing of words and substitution of sounds. She denied difficulty with memory, thinking, or activities of daily living. She was active socially, read and wrote for pleasure, and travelled independently. Clinical neurologic examination was normal with the exception of the speech difficulty and some slowness of eye movements. Subsequent EEG, MRI, and a variety of laboratory tests were unremarkable. SPECT scan showed marginally decreased profusion in the left and perhaps right temporal lobe. Neuropsychological assessment was normal.

Speech-language assessment revealed normal verbal comprehension. Her spoken language contained infrequent self-corrected function word errors and very infrequent semantic errors. Reading comprehension and writing were normal, and no other language difficulties were apparent. Her speech was characterized by reduced rate; occasional segmentation of syllables; distorted substitutions; and occasional articulatory groping. Her speech AMRs were equivocally rapid. She had a mild non-verbal oral apraxia.

The clinician concluded that the patient had a mild AOS that was more pronounced than a subtle aphasia. The report for the medical record stated that progressive AOS, when it is a prominent manifestation of degenerative neurologic disease, and worse than any accompanying aphasia, is frequently associated with tauopathies such as progressive supranuclear palsy (PSP) or corticobasal degeneration (CBD) (Duffy 2006; Josephs et al., 2006).

She was followed over the next five years, during which the AOS worsened, eventually leaving her unable to produce more than a word or two intelligibly, and ultimately mute and reliant on an augmentative-alternative communication (AAC) system with synthesized speech. One year before her death she was unable to read e-mail because of visual difficulties, and she had difficulty using her AAC device secondary to visual and upper extremity motor difficulties. Shortly before her death, she continued to comprehend reasonably well and enjoyed hearing from people by phone, even though she could not communicate verbally. Autopsy revealed pathology consistent with PSP.

Case 5

A 34-year-old man presented to neurology and neurosurgery for evaluation for deep brain stimulation (DBS) surgery for generalized dystonia, which he had developed five years earlier. Initial clinical neurologic examination was notable for what appeared to be dystonia in all limbs, although with some unusual features. He was also seen by a neurosurgeon who felt that DBS surgery would be appropriate, pending the results of a comprehensive baseline workup, which included speech-language assessment.

During speech consultation, the patient said his speech was normal until two years ago when, during worsening of his other dystonic symptoms, his voice faded to a whisper. He had several subsequent episodes in which his speech was problematic. Two months prior to examination, he had an episode in which he was unable to speak, and he had sporadic similar episodes since that time. His voice had been abnormal for two or three months, without remission. He said his voice would worsen if he counted aloud or was exposed to cold air.

Oral mechanism examination was normal, except that the thyrohyoid space narrowed considerably during phonation. Conversational voice was consistently moderately strained-harsh-raspy. Pitch and loudness variability were moderately reduced, and speaking rate was equivocally slow. Strained voice quality increased markedly during reading. When counting aloud, by the time he reached 30, his voice was a strained, aphonic whisper.

The clinician was uncertain about the nature of the patient's voice problem, but did not think it was consistent with dystonia or any other recognizable dysarthria type. During the diagnostic session, symptomatic therapy was undertaken and within ten minutes the patient's voice improved considerably and the strained component was eliminated. He was able to maintain his improved voice throughout the remainder of the examination, including during conversation and in his wife's presence. He felt his voice was 90% normal after this symptomatic therapy, compared to a baseline of about 20%.

The clinician concluded that the patient's voice and speech difficulty were most likely a reflection of musculoskeletal tension and not any underlying dystonia. The referring neurologist was contacted about these findings and conclusions, after which a second neurologic opinion was sought about his generalized dystonia. Subsequent EMG and evaluation by a neurologist specializing in movement disorders concluded that the patient's dystonia was functional (psychogenic). DBS was not recommended. The patient and his wife were reluctant to accept a diagnosis of a non-organic movement disorder. A rehabilitation programme was offered, but the patient declined.

16.3 **Lessons learned**

The preceding stories contain several lessons. Some of the most important, in the context of this chapter, include:

1. Speech abnormalities (with or without dysphagia) can be the first or predominant manifestation of neurologic disease.
2. Recognizing the meaning of neurologic speech abnormalities (i.e., recognizing a specific MSD type) often can localize the underlying causal disorder. It can sometimes provide strong evidence for a specific neurologic diagnosis, or can provide confirmatory (or non-confirmatory) or converging evidence for neurologic localization and diagnosis.
3. Recognizing the meaning of neurologic speech abnormalities can help to narrow (or sometimes expand) neurologic diagnostic possibilities and, therefore, focus subsequent neurologic investigation.

4. Recognizing patterns of speech abnormality that are not compatible with neurologic disease (i.e., that violate recognized patterns of neurologic speech disorders) can expand, focus, or redirect medical diagnostic and treatment efforts, and sometimes help avoid unnecessary or inappropriate medical and surgical treatments.

The gestalt lesson that speech abnormalities offer a window on the localization and diagnosis of neurologic and other diseases is well known to some. Nonetheless, it often has escaped or has been ignored or forgotten by many clinicians whose practices demand primary attention to management, and by many who teach and prepare new clinicians or engage in research on MSDs. In spite of this, however, there are medical practices (perhaps mostly in tertiary care centres) in which there is an *expectation* from physicians that differential diagnosis among MSDs can contribute to localizing neurologic disease within the context of day-to-day clinical practice. Take, for example, this statement from a neurologist who had just completed the initial examination of a patient with prominent speech complaints and yet undiagnosed neurologic disease[1]:

> *'If the speech consultant determines that there is evidence of ataxia in his speech, then we may be dealing with MSA [multiple system atrophy], in which case it would be reasonable for the patient to undergo thermoregulatory sweat test and an autonomic reflex screen. However, if his speech is in keeping with motor neuron disease then I will have the patient undergo EMG as I suspect we may be dealing with a form of motor neuron disease… I think the diagnosis here will rest on the speech consultation'.*

In at least some settings, scenarios like these should arise frequently, in part because MSDs occur frequently, at least in large medical practices. For example, in the Mayo Clinic speech pathology adult practice (based within a department of neurology, but receiving referrals from many medical subspecialties), MSDs make up 41% of all acquired communication disorders of any etiology, and 59% of all acquired neurologic communication disorders (Duffy 2005a). More than half of the outpatients I see for clinical assessment who are referred by a neurologist do not yet have a firmly established neurologic diagnosis, and many of them have degenerative diseases whose localization is not detected by conventional neuroimaging. I estimate that the speech diagnosis for people with acquired MSDs could make a corroborating or definitive contribution to as yet unestablished neurologic localization and diagnosis in 50–65% of those cases.

The emphasis here on diagnosis is not intended to minimize the importance of management and therapy. However, it is essential to recognize that many people with degenerative neurologic diseases have a MSD long before there is any need for speech therapy. What many affected people need, at a certain point in time, is an understanding of the meaning of their MSD as it relates to its underlying localization and cause, and its possible medical management. Therefore, not infrequently, an experienced clinician can answer questions about a MSD with diagnostic statements in medical record reports such as:

- *'Mixed spastic-flaccid dysarthria, strongly suggestive of mixed bilateral upper and lower motor neuron involvement of the bulbar speech muscles. This pattern and course of speech difficulty is not incompatible with a diagnosis of ALS/MND. It would not be compatible with a diagnosis of myasthenia gravis'.*
- *'Mixed hypokinetic-ataxic dysarthria, in which the ataxic component is strongly suggestive of cerebellar dysfunction – this would be very unusual in Parkinson's disease alone'.*
- *'Strongly suspect this is a hyperkinetic dysarthria due to jaw and lingual dystonia, and not due to an underlying psychological disturbance'.*

[1] I have used this quotation for the same illustrative purpose elsewhere (Duffy 2005b, p. 23).

16.4 **How did we get good at doing this?**

Although efforts to describe and classify speech characteristics associated with a variety of neurologic diseases extend at least to the nineteenth century (Duffy 2007), the firm roots of our current skills arguably emerged about 40 years ago when Darley, Aronson, and Brown published their now classic dysarthria studies (Darley et al., 1969 a, b) whose perceptual method of classifying the dysarthrias is now often referred to as the Mayo System. Their studies established the links between auditory-perceptual characteristics of speech and the presumed lesions and pathophysiology of LMNs, UMNs, the cerebellum, the basal ganglia, or some combination of them. AOS – with its localization to the left hemisphere – was included in their 1975 book, *Motor Speech Disorders* (Darely et al., 1975), as an additional major subcategory of MSDs.

The Mayo system approach to classifying MSDs – with some modifications and additions over the years – has provided a vocabulary for concise description and communication in clinical work and research. It also has provided a conceptual framework for acoustic and physiologic studies that have improved our understanding of the disorders and further refined how we evaluate and think about them clinically (Duffy and Kent 2001).

For the past several decades, research has generated descriptive data that capture the relatively homogeneous, but sometimes very heterogeneous salient speech characteristics of the MSDs that can be associated with a number of neurological diseases. Table 16.1 lists a number of the diseases for which there have been at least some interpretable descriptions of deviant auditory-perceptual speech characteristics; for several of them, accompanying acoustic or physiological analyses are also available. As a result of these studies, it is possible for clinicians to make statements about the degree to which particular speech characteristics – or constellation of speech characteristics, or particular MSD types – are or are not compatible with suspected (or unknown) neurologic localization or diagnosis. They put medical speech pathologists in a position to help modify, narrow, or expand neurologic diagnostic efforts. This is no small matter for people whose speech disorders are the prominent or sole manifestation of a neurologic disease, especially when the causal pathology is not apparent on standard neuroimaging.

Table 16.1 Examples of neurologic conditions for which auditory-perceptual speech characteristics of associated MSDs have been described (sometimes also with acoustic and physiologic analyses)

Amyotrophic lateral sclerosis (ALS)	Paraneoplastic cerebellar degeneration
Cerebral palsy	Parkinson's disease
Cervical spinal cord injury	Progressive multifocal leukoencephalopathy
Corticobasal degeneration	Progressive supranuclear palsy
Essential voice tremor	Shy-Drager syndrome
Freidreich's ataxia	Spasmodic dysphonia
Meige syndrome	Spasmodic torticollis
Multiple sclerosis	Stroke
Multiple system atrophy	Traumatic brain injury
Olivopontocerebellar atrophy	Vocal fold paralysis
	Wilson's disease

16.4.1 Some recent examples

A few recent studies further illustrate the value of adequate clinical perceptual descriptions and diagnoses of specific MSDs as they relate to neurologic localization and diagnosis.

Paslawski et al. (2005) described – retrospectively in 28 patients, and prospectively in five patients – speech findings in patients with paraneoplastic cerebellar degeneration (PCD), an autoimmune disease that reflects a non-metastatic remote effect of cancer in which the neurological syndrome can precede discovery of the primary cancer by weeks or even years. The diagnosis can be confirmed through detection of Purkinje cell antibodies (known as PCA-1) in serum or spinal fluid. PCD usually presents with the subacute development of ataxia and visual and speech disturbances. Although dysarthria can be the first manifestation of PCD, the features and type of dysarthria had not been well-characterized. The study found that ataxic dysarthria was the most common MSD, but an accompanying spastic component was recognized frequently enough to justify a conclusion that ataxic or mixed ataxic-spastic dysarthria are the most common MSDs associated with PCD. The fairly frequent presence of a spastic component was initially bothersome because PCD has been thought of as a cerebellar condition, but it is now clear that it can be associated with other clinical signs that suggest brainstem involvement (e.g., Dalmau et al., 2007); thus, brainstem involvement could well explain the finding of a spastic component in a number of the patients studied. The value of this study, in the context of this chapter, is that its observations permit clinicians to make statements about the compatibility of a dysarthria type(s) when PCD is suspected, or to raise the possibility of PCD when an ataxic or mixed ataxic-spastic dysarthria develops subacutely without obvious explanation, especially if it is the only sign of disease. Although this study did not establish that PCD could involve non-cerebellar structures, its findings are confirmatory of that conclusion. Thus, the findings also illustrate the potential for motor speech diagnoses to raise questions about involvement of structures and pathways not commonly thought to be involved in certain neurologic diseases.

Three additional recent studies provide support for the importance of distinguishing AOS from aphasia and the dysarthrias (Duffy 2006; Duffy et al., 2007; Josephs et al., 2006). In a retrospective study, Duffy (2006) documented the speech characteristics and associated demographic and neurological findings for 80 patients with neurodegenerative AOS as the only communication problem, or at least more severe than any accompanying aphasia. This condition is likely buried in the literature on primary progressive aphasia (PPA) because many investigators seem not to recognize the distinction between aphasia and AOS, or do not believe the distinction is important (see Duffy [2005a] and McNeil, Robin and Schmidt [2009] for summaries of the perceptual distinctions between AOS and aphasia). An important finding of the study was that when a more specific neurologic diagnosis emerged, it was most often tied to diseases with prominent motor impairments, such as PSP, CBD, or even ALS. Now, when clinicians encounter patients with such a presentation, an explicit statement can be made in diagnostic reports to referring neurologists that a predominant progressive AOS tends to be associated with neurologic diagnoses of CBD, PSP, or ALS. Relatedly, Duffy et al. (2007) subsequently described in detail the speech characteristics of the seven individuals in Duffy's (2006) study who received clinical diagnoses of ALS. Although mixed spastic-flaccid dysarthria is the classic MSD associated with ALS, and spastic or mixed spastic-flaccid dysarthria was also present in their subjects, the authors concluded that clinicians need to be aware that AOS can occur in ALS, although it is rare. More important, the observations suggest that ALS should be a diagnostic consideration when AOS is a prominent sign of undiagnosed progressive neurologic disease.

The third study addresses the degree to which clinical neurologic diagnoses of neurodegenerative diseases (e.g., Alzheimer's disease, Pick's disease, PSP, CBD) can predict pathology at autopsy;

such predictions clearly are less than perfect (Petersen 2003). Under an assumption that diagnoses of progressive AOS and PPA might be predictive of post-mortem diagnoses, Josephs et al. (2006) correlated speech-language diagnoses for 17 patients with their pathological diagnoses, including biochemistry. Eleven of the 17 patients had evidence of AOS. Six did not have AOS, but rather had PPA. In all patients with AOS, regardless of whether the AOS was less or more severe than aphasia, the pathology was characterized by underlying tau biochemistry, commonly called tauopathies. Five of the six cases without AOS did not have a tauopathy, but rather had pathology consistent with frontotemporal lobar degeneration with ubiquitin-only-immunoreactive changes (FTLD-U). In seven of the 11 patients with AOS, the AOS was more prominent than any non-fluent aphasia that was present. Five of those seven had a pathologic diagnosis of PSP, one had CBD, and one had Pick's disease. In the three patients who had AOS and non-fluent aphasia of about equal severity, the pathology was CBD. Five of the six patients who were aphasic but not apraxic had FTLD-U; the remaining patient had CBD. Taken together, these findings indicate that the presence of a predominant AOS, or AOS of about equal severity to a non-fluent aphasia, predicted PSP or CBD pathology in 90% of the patients, and tau biochemistry in 100%. PSP or CBD, and thus tauopathy, was possible when AOS was not present, but only in 17%. These results obviously need replication, but they raise the possibility that the accurate identification of AOS, as a problem separable from aphasia, not only tends to predict clinical neurologic diagnoses, but also underlying pathology and biochemistry. This is a powerful argument for explicitly distinguishing AOS from aphasia, something neurology has been slow to recognize or accept.

16.5 How can we do better?

What can future research do to advance clinical diagnostic practice, and what can be done to improve how researchers and clinicians communicate with each other? The following suggestions are not particularly theoretically motivated, but achieving them should help us to better understand MSDs. They mostly reflect practical needs and goals. Several of the suggestions made here, and others that go beyond diagnostic issues, have been discussed elsewhere (Duffy 2007).

16.5.1 Continue to link MSDs to neurologic diagnoses

There are a substantial number of neurologic diseases in which MSDs can occur whose speech characteristics have not been described with sufficient specificity to be clinically useful or that could help focus acoustic or physiologic studies. A few examples include spinal muscle atrophies; muscular dystrophies; polymyositis; primary lateral sclerosis; a variety of hereditary spinocerebellar ataxias; normal pressure hydrocephalus; hypoxic encephalopathy; systemic lupus erythematosis. Thorough descriptions of the MSDs associated with such diseases will expand clinicians' ability to address the compatibility of MSD diagnoses with them. It is conceivable that sufficiently large epidemiologic studies of MSDs will permit the development of probabilities for certain neurologic diagnoses when MSD type and the history are known, something that may be of particularly high neurologic diagnostic value when speech is a prominent presenting complaint.

16.5.2 Make acoustic, physiologic, and neuroimaging studies more informative to clinical practice

Movement away from compartmentalized investigations of different levels of the speech system, or the use of single methods by disciplines working independently, toward multilevel, multimethod, and multidisciplinary studies, hold promise for a better integrated and clinically relevant understanding of MSDs (Kent 2000). Weismer's (2006) recommendation that consortiums be developed to collect data on large numbers of people with MSDs using standardized tasks and common equipment and measurement approaches, selected on the basis of an integrated theory of speech production, likely would speed up and refine the description, classification, and understanding of MSDs. Clinical practice would be a major beneficiary if such efforts were planned with an eye toward eventual translation to clinical diagnostic and management practice.

Some have expressed the hope that 'the speech scientist and clinician of the future will have ready access to tools that meld perceptual judgment and instrumental analysis into a reliable and informative summary' (Duffy and Kent 2001, p.284). This is a lofty goal but one worth pursuing. Duffy (2007) has suggested that, for acoustic and physiologic analyses to become part of standard clinical diagnostic practice, they should be able to reliably and quantitatively confirm or improve on the sensitivity or specificity of clinical differential diagnosis of MSDs beyond that which can now be achieved through auditory-perceptual evaluation alone. Even if those diagnostic ends cannot be achieved, acoustic and physiological methods would have a greater presence in clinical practice if they can efficiently detect and quantify changes in intelligibility or speech efficiency, or provide feedback during therapy more effectively or efficiently than non-instrumental feedback.

16.5.3 **Refine classification**

The Mayo system's accuracy in localizing lesions has never been explicitly cross-validated. It has certainly been indirectly supported in numerous studies but more rigorous, blinded assessment of its localization value is necessary. Such cross-validation also might lead to refinements in the classification system, at least as it relates to localization (Duffy and Kent 2001, p.280).

The Mayo system has undergone some refinement over the years. Recently, questions have been raised about whether subtypes of some of the major dysarthria types exist, beyond dividing flaccid dysarthrias according to the specific nerves involved, and hyperkinetic dysarthrias according to the specific underlying movement disorder (e.g., tremor, dystonia) (Duffy 2005a). For example, some authors have raised the possibility of subtypes of ataxic and hypokinetic dysarthria (Boutsen et al., 1997; Duffy 2007; Kent et al., 1998). We also need to determine what, if anything, distinguishes the dysarthria resulting from unilateral versus bilateral UMN lesions. Issues like these clearly have implications for diagnostic specificity in clinical practice.

16.5.4 **Improve training**

Clinical descriptions and diagnoses must be reliable. We clearly need more systematic efforts to train reliability of auditory-perceptual judgments of speech and diagnostic conclusions drawn from them. In doing so, it will help to pay attention to what experienced clinicians actually do in clinical practice, which almost certainly has more to do with pattern recognition than exhaustive linear analytic ratings of the 38 dimensions that were used by Darley, Aronson, and Brown for their research purposes (Duffy and Kent, 2001; Kent et al., 1998).

16.5.5 **Improve communication among researchers and clinicians**

In an editorial discussion of focal dementia syndromes Petersen (2003) said, 'Because no single dimension – imaging, neuropathology, genetics, biochemistry – is likely to provide the absolute answer, *it remains incumbent on the clinician to classify persons with these disorders as accurately as possible[emphasis mine]* to allow for diagnostic, treatment, counselling, and prognostic advice for patients and families' (p.422). We should ask no less of clinicians who work with people with MSDs.

Perhaps less obvious, we need to communicate more precisely about speech abnormalities in acoustic, physiologic, and neuroimaging research. This seems self-evident, but scrutiny of the literature suggests it is not. For example, in a recent systematic review of the literature on treatment for AOS, less than 20% of 59 publications provided information sufficient for a reasonable degree of confidence about the diagnosis of AOS (Wambaugh et al., 2006). In my own cursory survey of 50 recent data-based articles focusing on dysarthrias in primary speech-language journals, about one-in-five articles described neither dysarthria type nor the abnormal speech characteristics; this problem is greatly amplified in primary neurology journals. For example, numerous sophisticated neuroimaging studies have not, in my opinion, done much to advance our understanding of dysarthria because they have failed to describe the dysarthria, leaving readers knowing a lot about where the lesion was but very little about the speech problem itself. A notable and exemplary exception is that of Urban et al. (2006), a localization study of stroke-induced dysarthria that provided detailed description of deviant auditory-perceptual speech characteristics and their relationship to MRI findings. The specificity of the speech description and neuroimaging components of the study have clear implications for both neurologists and speech-language pathologists.

Only by including adequate description of the perceptual features of MSDs in the literature that studies them can we hope to translate laboratory findings into clinical practice in diagnostically meaningful ways. A case can be made that, with few exceptions, studies of any MSD should contain a characterization of the salient auditory-perceptual characteristics of speech. This seems essential even if, and perhaps especially if, the central thrust of a study is acoustic or physiological or neuroimaging. Simply saying subjects are dysarthric or apraxic should not suffice. Clinicians who want to know how the results of research on MSDs might influence their practice should not be left wondering what the subjects of a research report sounded like – neither should researchers. To neglect such characterization is to obscure appreciation of what is being studied and restrict our ability to understand and generalize findings.

A partial solution to this problem of communication would be to develop a published consensus about what constitutes a diagnosis of a particular dysarthria type, a kind of Diagnostic and Statistical Manual for MSDs. Such guidelines could improve consistency across studies and provide a shorthand for conveying to reviewers and readers the salient characteristics of study subjects. For those who would disagree with the criteria, their very explicitness would help focus debate and promote research to justify modifications.

Finally, and returning to diagnostic practice issues, clinical practice and training might do well to adopt a dictum that no clinical evaluation report should end without a statement about the speech-language diagnosis, even if the statement is that a specific diagnosis cannot be made. This also seems self-evident, but clinical experience suggests that this often is not the case. Even clinical reports that contain considerable acoustic and physiologic data often are nearly devoid of conclusions about the nature of the speech deficit. Routinely drawing diagnostic conclusions about the nature of a deficit, its localization, and its compatibility with neurologic diagnosis implicitly recognizes that while therapy is a crucial part of a clinician's work, it alone does not define it. More important, it potentially improves medical diagnosis and care, and our efforts at behavioural treatment and management.

References

Boutsen FR, Bakker, K, and Duffy, JR (1997). Subgroups in ataxic dysarthria. *Journal of Medical Speech-Language Pathology, 5*, 27–36.

Dalmau J, Gonzalez RG, and Lerwill MF (2007). Case 4-2007: A 56-year-old woman with rapidly progressive vertigo and ataxia. *New England Journal of Medicine*, 356, 612–620.

Darley FL, Aronson AE, and Brown JR (1969a). Differential diagnostic patterns of dysarthria. *Journal of Speech and Hearing Research, 12*, 246–269.

Darley FL, Aronson AE, and Brown JR (1969b). Clusters of deviant speech dimensions in the dysarthrias. *Journal of Speech and Hearing Research, 12,* 462–496.

Darley FL, Aronson AE, and Brown JR (1975). *Motor Speech Disorders.* Philadelphia: W.B. Saunders.

Duffy JR (2007). Motor speech disorders: History, current practice, future trends and goals. In G Weismer (Ed.) *Motor Speech Disorders.* San Diego: Plural Publishing Inc., 7–56.

Duffy JR (2005a). *Motor Speech Disorders: Substrates, Differential Diagnosis, and Management* (2nd edn) St. Louis, MO: Elsevier Mosby.

Duffy JR (2005b). Pearls of wisdom – Darley, Aronson, and Brown and the classification of the dysarthrias. *Perspectives on neurophysiology and neurogenic speech and language disorders,* 15 (3), 22–27.

Duffy JR (2006). Apraxia of speech in degenerative neurologic disease. *Aphasiology,* 20 (6), 511–527.

Duffy JR and Kent RD (2001). Darley's contributions to the understanding, differential diagnosis, and scientific study of the dysarthrias. *Aphasiology,* 15, 275–289.

Duffy JR, Peach RK, and Strand EA (2007). Progressive apraxia of speech as a sign of motor neuron disease. *American Journal of Speech-Language Pathology,* 16, 198–208.

Josephs KA, Duffy JR, Strand EA, et al. (2006). Clinicopathological and imaging correlates of progressive aphasia and apraxia of speech. *Brain,* 129, 1385–1398.

Kent RD (2000). Research on speech motor control and its disorders: a review and prospective. *Journal of Communication Disorders, 33,* 391–428.

Kent RD, Kent JF, Duffy JR, and Weismer G (1998). The dysarthrias: Speech-voice profiles, related dysfunctions, and neuropathology. *Journal of Medical Speech-Language Pathology, 6,* 165–211.

McNeil MR, Robin DA, and Schmidt RA (2009). Apraxia of speech. In MR McNeil (Ed.) *Clinical Management of Sensorimotor Speech Disorders* (2nd edn) New York: Thieme, 249–268.

Paslawski T, Duffy JR, and Vernino S (2005). Speech and language findings associated with paraneoplastic cerebellar degeneration. *American Journal of Speech-Language Pathology,* 14, 200–207.

Petersen RC (2003). Focal dementia syndromes: in search of the gold standard (editorial). *Annals of Neurology,* 49, 421–422.

Urban PP, Rolke R, Wicht S, et al. (2006). Left-hemisphere dominance for articulation: A prospective study on acute ischaemic dysarthria at different localizations. *Brain,* 129, 767–777.

Wambaugh JL, Duffy JR, McNeil MR, Robin DR, and Rogers MA (2006). Treatment guidelines for acquired apraxia of speech: a synthesis and evaluation of the evidence, *Journal of Medical Speech-Language Pathology,* 14, xv–xxxiii.

Weismer G (2006). Philosophy of research in motor speech disorders. *Clinical Linguistics and Phonetics, 20,* 315–349.

Chapter 17

Laryngeal articulatory coupling in three speech disorders

Christopher Dromey

Abstract

Laryngeal and articulatory actions are carefully coordinated in normal speech. This chapter focuses on data from three speech disorders to illustrate articulatory changes that arise when the larynx is the nominal target of treatment. In each case, articulatory acoustic or kinematic data were collected to determine whether clinical efforts directed at phonation would have measurable effects on articulator movement. The finding of treatment effects spreading beyond the target of the larynx has important implications for our understanding of disordered speech motor control as well as for intervention strategies in these populations. Lip kinematics in seven speakers with spasmodic dysphonia were recorded before and after Botox injection of the vocal folds. Bilabial coordination indexes were more aberrant when spasm severity was greatest, moving towards control speaker values after voice treatment. Pre/post treatment recordings from 111 women with muscle tension dysphonia were analyzed for evidence of articulatory changes. Although treatment focused on the larynx, increases in vowel space and diphthong formant transitions suggest that increased articulatory dynamics accompanied the voice improvements. Lip kinematic data from 10 speakers with Parkinson disease (PD) revealed increased amplitudes and velocities, along with more consistent trajectories over multiple repetitions for loud speech. Acoustic recordings from a speaker with PD were analyzed for F2 diphthong transitions, which revealed evidence of increased articulatory excursions following intensive voice treatment, even though no therapy exercises involved articulation. The data from these speakers reveal altered vocal tract behavior when the larynx is the primary target of therapy.

17.1 Coordination in speech production

Because talking requires that the lungs, the larynx, and the articulators work together in sometimes complex ways, the notion of coordination is inherently interesting to speech scientists. Even the simplest contrasts, such as voiced–voiceless distinctions, involve great precision in the relative timing of an articulatory movement and the onset of vocal fold vibration. The features of linguistic or affective prosody are woven into the segmental sound stream to enhance meaning or signal the speaker's emotional state. This requires that a speaker orchestrate adjustments to the output of the lungs and the configuration of the vocal folds with segmental articulatory behaviour that can span entire utterances.

Although the mechanisms of coordination by the central nervous system cannot be viewed directly, a number of studies have demonstrated functional linkages across structures and systems by measuring speech activity at the periphery. These have included acoustic, electromyographic, and kinematic investigations of normal speech production. Abbs (1989) observed that in an effort to understand speech, some investigators have conveniently divided its production into the subsystems of respiration, phonation, and articulation. He points out, however, that such divisions 'are not justified by their neural control or biomechanics' (p. 163). When a person speaks, activity is choreographed at multiple levels, and is also influenced by input from the periphery (Abbs and Connor 1991). For example, perturbation studies have shown that when the movement of the lips is disrupted during articulation, not only do the nearby articulators modify their trajectories; there are also changes in laryngeal behaviour, revealing a system-wide response to the disturbance (Folkins and Zimmermann 1982; Van Lieshout et al., 1997).

Our understanding of coordination has been further advanced through studies of disordered speech. Knowledge of the site of lesion has allowed comparisons with normal speech activity in a way that has clarified the contributions to speech motor control of a variety of neural structures and systems. Speech discoordination and timing irregularity have been reported in ataxic dysarthria, where cerebellar damage leads to a loss of fine motor regulation (Kent et al., 1999). However, other sites of lesion do not always appear to have a direct impact on the way the articulators work together. A recent study found that for dysarthric speakers with Parkinson disease (PD) or amyotrophic lateral sclerosis (ALS), coordination was not seriously impaired, at least for the speech tasks under investigation (Weismer et al., 2003). Instead, articulatory undershoot appeared to play a larger role in their speech disorder. Whether or not a particular neurological deficit results in a breakdown in movement coordination, it is nevertheless important to recognize the way the different parts of the speech mechanism work together. Several studies of normal speech have shown that respiratory or vocal effort changes can influence activity further 'downstream' (Dromey 1995; Dromey and Ramig 1998a, b). These reports suggested that volitional changes to vocal loudness or rate are 'global' in their effect. This is, they necessarily involve adjustments to respiratory, laryngeal, and articulatory behaviour without the speaker attending individually to each component. Because clinical speech intervention requires effort from both the patient and the clinician, it is relevant to know more about the clinical potential for a spreading of treatment effects. If a single target for treatment can be selected which is known to provide multiple benefits, therapy can become more efficient and also possibly more effective. The focus of this chapter is on the changes in supraglottic behaviour that occur when the voice is the primary target during treatment.

17.2 **Disorders of speech**

One way of classifying disordered communication would be to identify the deficit as involving primarily the source or the filter. For example, vocal nodules impair the quality of phonation, but are not typically associated with abnormal articulation. In contrast, consonant production is often disturbed following glossectomy surgery, but the voice is usually unaffected. This convenient dichotomy allows clinicians to categorize cases as voice problems or speech disturbances. In many cases, however, both source and filter are impacted by the same aetiology. Degenerative neurological illnesses can be the cause of dysarthrias which are characterized by both laryngeal deficits and consonant imprecision. One dysarthria subtype, along with two types of dysphonia will be considered in the following pages. Hypokinetic dysarthria is known to affect many aspects of speech production, although voice-related issues are recognized as being prominent in this population (Ackermann and Ziegler 1991; Adams 1996; Critchley 1981). This particular disorder is included here because a current mainstream treatment focuses directly on vocal effort, with no clinical attention being directed to the disordered articulation. The other two conditions – spasmodic dysphonia and muscle tension dysphonia (MTD) – have been traditionally diagnosed and treated as voice problems, and little consideration is usually given to articulatory function. In each of these disorders the voice is the primary intervention target, yet recent work has revealed evidence of a spreading of treatment effects beyond the larynx.

17.2.1 **Hypokinetic dysarthria**

Most individuals with PD will experience some degree of disordered communication as a consequence of their condition. Reduced vocal intensity, flattened prosody, and imprecise consonant articulation are key features of this type of dysarthria (Adams 1996; Gentil and Pollak 1995). Studies of speech changes in response to drug treatment have been equivocal (Nakano et al., 1973; Poluha et al., 1998; Sanabria et al., 2001), and the often dramatic improvements in limb and axial function accompanying deep brain stimulation have not been matched by equivalent changes in voice or speech activity (Dromey et al., 2000). Consequently, patients with hypokinetic dysarthria secondary to PD must consider behavioural means for improving the quality and effectiveness of their communication.

The Lee Silverman Voice Treatment (LSVT) has been documented to result in meaningful improvements in speech performance, lasting as long as 12–24 months after therapy (Ramig et al., 2004; Sapir et al., 2002; Ramig et al., 1995; Smith et al., 1995; Ramig and Dromey 1996; Ramig et al., 1995; Ramig et al., 1996). This intensive therapy approach involves vigorous drills of loud phonation in vowel prolongation, pitch elevation exercises, functional phrases, and other conversational tasks. The patient is encouraged to breathe in deeply and to 'be loud' in all of the tasks. No attention is directed towards articulation or prosody, either directly through drill work, or indirectly through rate adjustments. However, there is evidence of beneficial changes in both prosody and supraglottal articulation, even though these are not directly targeted as part of the therapy. A case study of an individual with PD, which involved spectrographic analysis of articulatory performance, showed that formant transitions during diphthongs increased in extent and rate following intensive treatment targeting loudness (Dromey et al., 1995). These articulatory improvements were in addition to the benefits of increased vocal intensity and fundamental frequency variability in reading and conversation. A recent acoustic study of 15 speakers with PD revealed an increase in the area of the acoustic vowel triangle following loud speech treatment (Sapir et al., 2007). In both studies, a focus on increased speech effort resulted in acoustically measurable changes in articulation.

The findings from these acoustic investigations have been reinforced by those from studies of lip movements during speech. A kinematic study which evaluated the simulated treatment of loud speech compared with increased articulatory effort revealed that while both approaches resulted in larger lip movements, the loud speech intervention resulted in less variable movements across repetitions and smoother kinematic trajectories (Dromey 2000). This finding was reinforced in a subsequent study comparing rate and loudness changes in speakers with PD (Kleinow et al., 2001). The single treatment goal of increased loudness makes it simple for the patient to focus on the task – one which is already familiar from a lifetime of speaking. In contrast, having the patient concentrate on moving the individual articulators more deliberately is a novel and more complex requirement, and would involve more careful attention to the movements themselves. This is important for patients with PD, who have been shown to have difficulty in tasks which demand attention to more than a single goal (Ho et al., 2002). A key factor in providing treatment in this population is the selection of the most appropriate goal. Working intensively on the target of loudness appears to affect not only the hypophonic voice, but also articulation and even facial expressivity (Spielman et al., 2003). To date there are no published accounts to suggest that the opposite would be true – i.e., that vocal function would improve in response to the focal treatment of lip movement or facial expression, even though all are affected by PD. Rosenbek and LaPointe described over two decades ago their approach to treating loudness. They recommended a focus on stronger respiratory drive, increased laryngeal adduction, and a deliberately wider mouth opening to improve communication in speakers with loudness deficits (Rosenbek and LaPointe 1985). The more recent studies outlined above suggest that a deliberate focus on larger jaw movements is unnecessary, and that these larger movements will occur spontaneously as vocal effort increases. Because vocal weakness is a prominent sign of hypokinetic dysarthria (Logemann et al., 1978), it makes sense to address it directly in therapy, particularly given the evidence of improvement in other aspects of communication. Thus, while the larynx is nominally the target for this intensive treatment, the clinician appears in fact to be influencing the whole speech mechanism because of the natural control linkages between the contributing components of respiration, phonation, and articulation. The deliberate scaling of loudness naturally involves adjustments to the scaling of activity in the respiratory system and the supraglottic vocal tract, making LSVT more of a speech treatment than a purely vocal intervention.

17.2.2 **Spasmodic dysphonia**

Adductor spasmodic dysphonia (SD) is generally viewed as a focal dystonia of the larynx (Miller and Woodson 1991). Because of the strained-strangled quality of the voice during adductory spasms, clinicians sometimes confuse it with muscle tension dysphonia, with which it shares a number of perceptual features. In some cases the two can even be present in the same individual (Barkmeier et al., 2001). Accurate diagnosis usually requires that an experienced otolaryngology/speech pathology team work together to assess laryngeal function during respiration, vowel prolongation, and a variety of speech tasks. For most individuals the spasms only occur during speech, and they may become less frequent or disappear entirely for whispering or singing (Ludlow 1995). Traditional voice therapy has proven ineffective in reducing the severity of SD symptoms (Miller and Woodson 1991). The most effective treatment currently available involves the injection of botulinum toxin (BT) into the thyroarytenoid muscle, either unilaterally or bilaterally (Fisher et al., 1996; Jankovic and Brin 1991). The effects of this treatment, however, are temporary, and patients must return for repeated injections every few months in order to maintain the desired voice quality. A more permanent solution is to sever the branch of the recurrent laryngeal nerve which activates the thyroarytenoid, and replace its innervation with a branch from the ansa cervicalis. This selective denervation/re-innervation procedure maintains muscle tone in the thyroarytenoid while bypassing the circuitry which carries the disordered neural commands which lead to spasms (Berke et al., 1999). This procedure is not in widespread use, however, and may not be suitable for all patients with SD.

Even though SD is diagnosed and treated by professionals who specialize in voice disorders, a number of studies have suggested that this condition affects more than just the larynx. Cannito (1989) reasoned that the proposed extrapyramidal source of the spasms in SD may affect the steadiness of the vocal tract, even though Aronson and colleagues (Aronson et al., 1968) had distinguished SD from the dysarthrias because 'patients with spastic dysphonia do not have articulation defects as an integral part of their disorder' (p. 210). These authors did note, however, that 'the rate and fluency of articulation were profoundly influenced by the occurrence of spasm' (p. 210), and that articulation would occasionally cease until the spasm had subsided.

Cannito (1989) noted that the coordination of laryngeal and supraglottic activity could underlie such findings, and was careful to exclude the direct influence of laryngeal spasms by using an electrolarynx as the sound source in his study. He found that individuals with SD had higher levels of unsteadiness in the second formant than controls, which he attributed to the influence of their dystonia on the supraglottic vocal tract, which represented 'an extralaryngeal locus of motor abnormality' (p. 259). Taken together, these studies suggest that both the laryngeal spasms' influence on fluent speech production and also disease-related vocal tract unsteadiness may combine in some way to make SD more than purely a voice disorder.

Cannito and his colleagues conducted a number of further studies, which demonstrated that hand movements in individuals with SD are sometimes slower than controls (Cannito and Kondraske 1990), and that articulation during syllable repetition can be slow and fragmented, surprisingly even during whispering (Cannito et al., 1994). They took this as evidence of a co-occurring articulatory disturbance in SD. A question remains as to whether these articulatory abnormalities are influenced by the presence of spasms, or whether they would qualify SD as a type of motor speech disorder, since it appears to involve more than just the larynx. One study (Cannito et al., 1997) found that speakers with SD were perceptually rated as being much less fluent than controls. Their speech was perceived as being slower and more effortful, and the authors noted that there have been reports of improved speech fluency following treatment. A valuable contribution of this paper was the suggestion that fluency analysis could help provide a clearer clinical picture of SD than a narrow focus on sustained vowel phonation and other larynx-centred measures. A follow-up study (Cannito et al., 2004) of changes after BT treatment in 42 patients revealed improvements in both voice and fluency measures, particularly for younger or more severely affected individuals. The parallel improvements in both speech fluency and voice measures suggest that spasm severity may be associated with the degree of speech impairment. These results appear consistent with the hypothesis that the natural coupling of laryngeal and articulatory behaviour may account for at least a portion of the disturbed articulatory behaviour in SD.

In an effort to more directly measure articulatory behaviour in SD, as well as its link to phonatory activity, two studies were undertaken in our laboratory. The first study (Tingley and Dromey 2000) revealed differences between speakers with SD and controls in their lip trajectories. Where the normal movement would involve a single velocity peak during an opening or closing gesture, a speaker with severe SD exhibited multiple velocity peaks, reflecting unsteadiness in the regulation of lip movement (Fig. 17.1). This abnormal movement pattern coincided with the audible occurrence of a vocal spasm, which interrupted the fluent production of the utterance. In the whispered condition, the number of velocity peaks decreased towards the normal value, suggesting that the absence of a perceptible vocal spasm was associated with an improvement in lip movement control. Another measure – the continuous correlation function – reflected similar improvements for this speaker when he whispered. This measure was calculated by computing a Pearson correlation between the displacements of the upper and lower lips over a 50-point window that was moved along the recording of the utterance. In theory, the two lips move apart or approach each other approximately 180° of out phase for a series of bilabial stops and vowels. This would be reflected in a correlation coefficient approaching −1 during these gestures. In this study, the speaker with severe SD showed fluctuations in the continuous correlation function that spanned almost the entire range between −1 and 1 in the voiced speech condition (Fig. 17.2). When he whispered, the correlation function remained closer to the theoretical out-of-phase pattern. Again, the implication is that a reduction in the severity of the dysphonia is linked to more normal lip movement patterns. However, since whispered speech did not lead to entirely normal lip movements, it was speculated that either a concomitant articulatory disturbance was

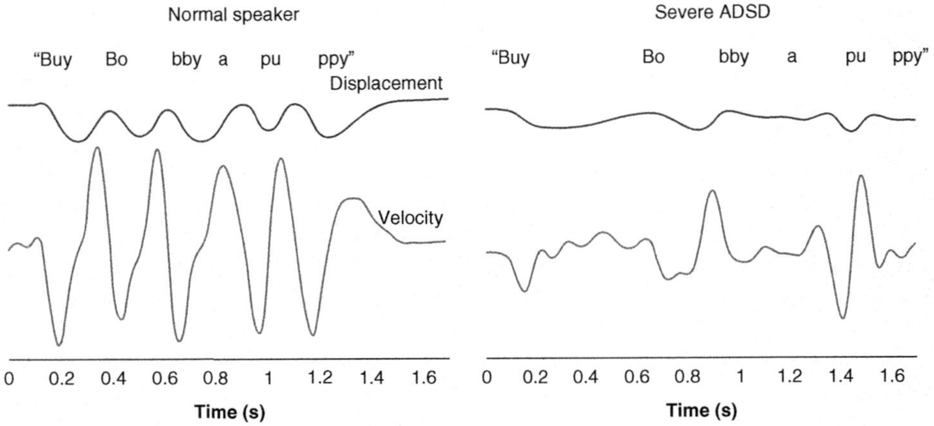

Fig. 17.1 Lower lip displacement and velocity records for a normal speaker (left) and a speaker with severe adductor SD (right) during voiced speech showing multiple velocity peaks for the disordered speaker. Amplitude is displayed in arbitrary units, and individual tokens are shown.

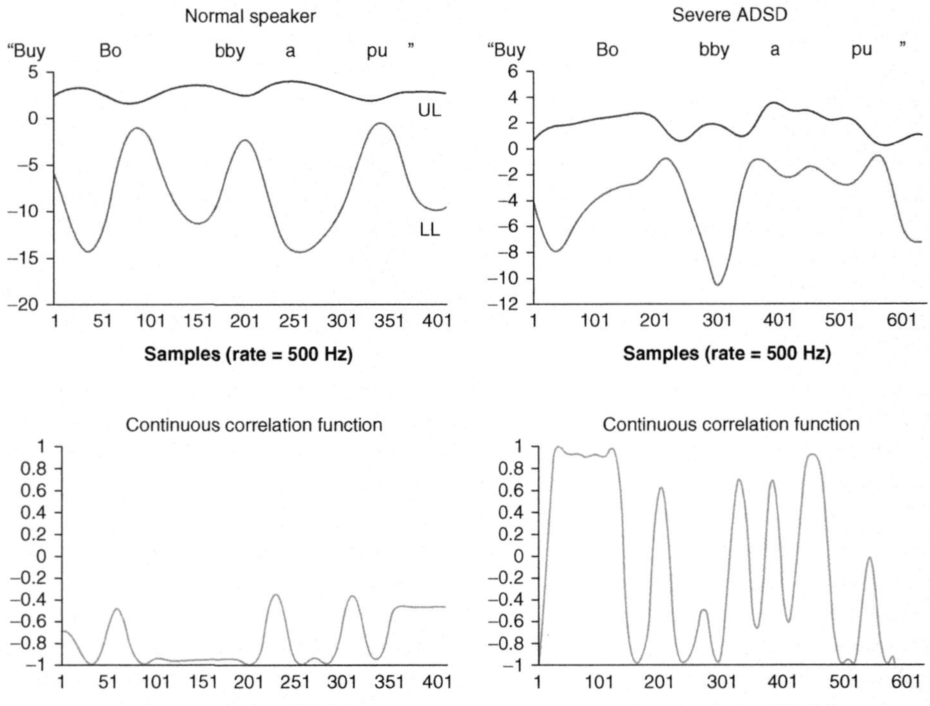

Fig. 17.2 Continuous correlation function (CCF) for a normal speaker (left) and a speaker with severe adductor SD (right) during voiced speech. Amplitude is displayed in arbitrary units, and individual tokens are shown. UL = upper lip, LL = lower lip.

Source: Reprinted with permission from Journal of Medical Speech – Language Pathology (Tingley & Dromley, 2000)

responsible at least in part for the lip findings, or that compensatory behaviours on the part of the speaker carried over from voiced speech into whispering (Tingley and Dromey 2000).

We undertook an additional study of seven individuals with SD in order to learn more about any changes in lip movements which might accompany successful treatment of the voice with BT. On the basis of the findings of Cannito's group (Cannito et al., 1997, 2004), it appeared reasonable to anticipate changes in articulatory behaviour for voices that were smoother after treatment. Aerodynamic data from our speakers showed a decrease in laryngeal resistance, and listener ratings indicated that the voice quality improved following treatment. The data analysis methods employed in this study (Dromey et al., 2007) were similar to those used in our previous experiment (Tingley and Dromey 2000). Speakers with SD showed abnormalities in their lip movements prior to BT injection, which became more normal after treatment. This was true for qualitative features of the movement waveforms as well as for measures such as the continuous correlation function and the count of velocity peaks. Examination of the signals from which the correlations were calculated revealed that at times prior to BT injection, the lips were both moving in the same direction for parts of the utterance. Following treatment these movements became far more like those from the control speakers. However, the articulatory movements did not move entirely into the normal control range. This may in part be due to the fact that perceptual ratings of the voice still remained worse than for the controls, even though they showed dramatic improvement following BT injection. Another explanation, which would be consistent with several previous studies (Cannito 1989; Cannito et al., 1991, 1994), is that there may be a degree of articulatory disturbance in this population which is independent of the vocal spasms. These deficits may be linked to the neuropathology that causes the dystonia, which manifests itself more widely than in the vocal folds alone.

In light of these findings, it could be speculated that the abnormal kinematic features detected in speakers who experience vocal spasms are traceable to several sources. One would be a concomitant disorder of vocal tract control that arises from the same source as the dystonic spasms of the larynx. A second source of movement disturbance appears to be the natural coordinative connection between laryngeal and articulatory function. The coupling of the activity of the larynx with the movements of the lips has been documented in studies of normal speech production (Gracco and Löfqvist 1994; Munhall et al., 1994; McClean and Tasko 2002). There is no reason to expect that such coupling would be absent in a disordered speaker. In the individual with SD, it may be that as the larynx 'stumbles' during a vocal spasm, the articulators are constrained to hesitate also, and cannot continue with their planned trajectories because the larynx has not completed its task. In other words, if the actions of the larynx and the supraglottic vocal tract are orchestrated in speech production, a hesitation at one level halts the entire performance, rather than allowing the contributions of the different structures to proceed independently of each other. Van Lieshout and colleagues reported equivalent 'linked' delays in the activity of the respiratory, laryngeal, and articulatory systems of a speaker who stuttered, in that a block at the laryngeal level influenced the activity of the other speech subsystems (Van Lieshout et al., 1997). In the present study, a linkage between laryngeal and articulatory activity may explain why multiple velocity peaks arise in what should be smooth and simple opening and closing gestures of the lips. The slower speech articulation that has been documented to accompany vocal spasms may rely on different regulation mechanisms, possibly involving feedback monitoring, which can result in unsteady articulatory behaviour (Adams et al., 1993). A third source of articulatory disturbance could be linked to compensatory strategies undertaken by the speaker. When a spasm occurs, the speaker may invoke adjustments – either consciously or not – to move ahead with speech even though the larynx is making such forward progress difficult. The relief offered by BT injection may lessen, although not entirely remove, the need for such compensation.

17.2.3 **Muscle tension dysphonia**

Muscle tension dysphonia is a commonly presenting condition in most voice clinics. The voice quality may be severely disordered, in spite of a structurally normal larynx and the absence of any organic illness (Schalen and Andersson 1992; Sama et al., 2001). Its perceptual features may include tight, strangled phonation or a breathy, whispered quality. Some individuals' voices fluctuate between these extremes. The dysphonia is attributed to excessive tension in the intrinsic and extrinsic muscles of the larynx. Several causes have been suggested for this condition, some of which may co-exist. These may include psychological stress or other personality factors (Aronson 1990; Butcher 1995), maladaptive compensatory behaviours (Koufman and Blalock 1982), or other types of voice misuse (Morrison et al., 1983; Morrison and Rammage 1993).

As is the case with SD, MTD is a usually diagnosed by an experienced speech pathology and otolaryngology team. Disordered articulation is not a characteristic of this condition, and it is not viewed as a motor speech disorder. Nonetheless, extralaryngeal tension is a common feature of MTD, and many individuals experience tightness or pain that can extend upward in the neck as far as the ears. Boone and McFarlane (2000) noted that 'we see too many people with vocal hyperfunction who appear to speak through clenched teeth, with very little mandibular or labial movement'. (p. 177). These authors have suggested exaggerated movements of the jaw and tongue as a potential means for indirectly lowering the tension in and around the larynx.

Although MTD may spontaneously fluctuate in severity, it is generally necessary to provide clinical treatment to achieve lasting improvements in quality. A number of interventions are aimed at reducing laryngeal tension, depending on the presentation of the dysphonia as excessively breathy or pressed. One treatment technique that has been documented to result in substantial long-term improvements in voice quality in these individuals is circumlaryngeal massage (Roy and Leeper 1993; Roy et al., 1996, 1997; Roy and Bless 1998). The larynx in MTD is often elevated, accompanied by tightness of the surrounding musculature. When this tension, which is detectable as a palpable tightness of the surface of the neck upon clinical examination, is reduced through carefully targeted massage, and the larynx is repositioned lower in the neck, voice quality can dramatically improve. Indeed, severely dysphonic speakers who visit the clinic for an initial evaluation may in many cases leave the extended session with a normal sounding voice once circumlaryngeal massage has been applied. This dramatic improvement is attributed to a reduction of excessive tension and rebalancing of muscle tone in the hyolaryngeal region.

Because the hyoid has muscle attachments to the tongue and jaw above it, we speculated that the same excessive hyolaryngeal tension which results in dysphonia might also impact articulatory movements. It was recognized that abnormal articulation has not been reported for MTD. Nevertheless, there may be a subtle impact on articulation that is not sufficiently severe to reach clinically perceptible levels. Therefore, we undertook an acoustic study to learn whether there was evidence of changed articulation following successful voice treatment in MTD (Dromey et al., 2008). This work involved an analysis of an existing clinical database of acoustic recordings, and thus aerodynamic and other physiologic measures were not available. Over 100 speakers were included, all of whom improved perceptually in their voice quality following circumlaryngeal massage. When they read a passage there was a decrease in the total time taken, and the proportion of time spent speaking versus pausing increased, suggesting that speech became more fluent or continuous with the improved voice quality. Measures of formant transitions during diphthongs revealed evidence of increased movements of the articulators as a side effect of the voice treatment. The second formant slope became steeper during diphthong production through an increase in the extent of the movement, rather than a change in its timing.

Although the precise mechanisms responsible for these articulatory changes cannot be identified from acoustic recordings, it could be speculated that either neural or biomechanical factors played a role. One explanation would be that the massage applied to the hyolaryngeal region was successful not only in lowering the larynx in the neck and reducing the extralaryngeal tension, but also that it affected the level of tension in the muscles attaching to the hyoid from above. It was speculated on the basis of the acoustic findings that the reduced tightness at the base of the tongue may have allowed it to move more freely during speech, thus generating larger formant movements during diphthongs. Clearly, physiologic measures would be needed to test this speculative mechanism. It would, however, be consistent with the suggestions of others (Higgins et al., 1998; McClean and Tasko 2002) that laryngeal-articulatory coupling may involve this type of biomechanical linkage. Thus, the reduced tension in one area (in this case, in and around the larynx) may contribute to improved activity in both regions. An alternative explanation would be that the massage influenced the level of neural activation of the muscles of the neck, lowering their tension. Some authors have suggested that a parallel neural drive to both articulatory and laryngeal muscles may be mediated via cortical coactivation or brainstem reflexes (Cookman and Verdolini 1999). Thus, a successful lowering of the activation of the laryngeal muscles in these speakers may have been accompanied by decreased nervous system drive to the articulators. In spite of the limitations inherent in an acoustic study, where no direct physiologic measures were available, this work has shown that a treatment aimed directly at the larynx can influence supraglottic vocal tract activity.

17.3 **Theoretical and clinical considerations**

In each of the disorders discussed in this chapter, a treatment was applied to target disordered phonation. Yet all three conditions showed evidence of a change in articulatory behaviour. This suggests that there was a spreading of treatment effects beyond the larynx. This is not entirely unexpected in the case of PD, where the treatment required that the speaker employ a much higher level of effort in producing speech. The notion of a coordinated global upscaling of effort across the entire speech mechanism in disordered speakers is consistent with reports of similar phenomena in people with normal speech (Dromey and Ramig 1998a; Schulman 1989). Less predictable, however, were the changes in lip movement associated with BT treatment of the vocal folds in SD. In this case, the patient is a passive recipient of the intervention by the physician, which contrasts markedly with the level of involvement required of the speaker with PD who engages in high effort speech therapy. The changes in SD articulation appear at least in part to be attributable to the coupling of laryngeal activity with articulatory behaviour, such that a disturbance to phonation from a spasm prevents the smooth progress of articulatory movements. From a functional standpoint, it would serve little purpose to allow the supraglottic vocal tract to continue producing articulatory movements in the absence of the contribution of the laryngeal sound source. In light of this observation, it would appear that the larynx may play an important regulatory role in the coordination of speech production across the entire system. The findings from the speakers with MTD have shown that targeting the larynx can yield changes in articulator movements, possibly via biomechanical or even neural linkages. Although the clinician is ostensibly targeting only the voice, there may be an unintended positive impact on neighbouring structures.

The implication of these observations is that a clinician needs to be mindful of the potential for carry-over to aspects of speech production which are not directly targeted in treatment. Although only three specific disorders were considered here, there may be other conditions in which treating laryngeal behaviour helps alleviate problems in other parts of the speech mechanism.

References

Abbs, J. H. (1989). Motor coordination for functional human behaviors: Perspectives from a speech motor data base. In S.A.Wallace (Ed.), *Perspectives on the Coordination of Movement* (pp. 157–183). North-Holland: Elsevier Science Publishers B.V.

Abbs, J. H. and Connor, N. P. (1991). Motorsensory mechanisms of speech motor timing and coordination. *Journal of Phonetics, 19,* 333–342.

Ackermann, H. and Ziegler, W. (1991). Articulatory deficits in parkinsonian dysarthria: An acoustic analysis. *Journal of Neurology, Neurosurgery and Psychiatry, 54,* 1093–1098.

Adams, S. G. (1996). Hypokinetic dysarthria in Parkinson's disease. In M.R. McNeil (Ed.), *Clinical Management of Sensorimotor Speech Disorders* (pp. 259–282). New York: Thieme.

Adams, S. G., Weismer, G., and Kent, R. D. (1993). Speaking rate and speech movement velocity profiles. *Journal of Speech and Hearing Research, 36,* 41–54.

Aronson, A. E. (1990). *Clinical voice disorders: An interdisciplinary approach.* (3rd edn) New York, NY: Thieme.

Aronson, A. E., Brown, J. R., Litin, E. M., and Pearson, J. S. (1968). Spastic dysphonia. I. Voice, neurologic, and psychiatric aspects. *Journal of Speech and Hearing Disorders, 33,* 203–218.

Barkmeier, J. M., Case, J. L., and Ludlow, C. L. (2001). Identification of symptoms for spasmodic dysphonia and vocal tremor: A comparison of expert and nonexpert judges. *Journal of Communication Disorders, 34,* 21–37.

Berke, G. S., Blackwell, K. E., Gerratt, B. R., Verneil, A., Jackson, K.S. et al. (1999). Selective laryngeal adductor denervation-reinnervation: A new surgical treatment for adductor spasmodic dysphonia. *Annals of Otology, Rhinology and Laryngology, 108,* 227–231.

Boone, D. R. and McFarlane, S. C. (2000). *The Voice and Voice Therapy.* (6th edn) Boston: Allyn and Bacon.

Butcher, P. (1995). Psychological processes in psychogenic voice disorder. *European Journal of Disorders of Communication, 30,* 467–474.

Cannito, M. P. (1989). Vocal tract steadiness in spasmodic dysphonia. In K.M. Yorkston and D. R. Beukelman (Eds.), *Recent Advances in Clinical Dysarthria* (pp. 243–262). Boston: Little, Brown and Co.

Cannito, M. P., Burch, A. R., Watts, C., Rappold, P. W., Hood, S. B., and Sherrard, K. (1997). Disfluency in spasmodic dysphonia: A multivariate analysis. *Journal of Speech, Language, and Hearing Research, 40,* 627–641.

Cannito, M. P., Ege, P., Ahmed, F., and Wagner, S. (1994). Diadochokinesis for complex trisyllables in individuals with spasmodic dysphonia and nondisabled subjects. In J.A. Till, K. M. Yorkston, and D. R. Beukelman (Eds.), *Motor Speech Disorders: Advances in Assessment and Treatment* (pp. 91–100). Baltimore: P.H. Brooks Pub. Co.

Cannito, M. P. and Kondraske, G. V. (1990). Rapid manual abilities in spasmodic dysphonic and normal female subjects. *Journal of Speech and Hearing Research, 33,* 123–133.

Cannito, M. P., Kondraske, G. V., and Johns, D. F. (1991). Oral-facial sensorimotor function in spasmodic dysphonia. In C.A. Moore, K. M. Yorkston, and D. R. Beukelman (Eds.), *Dysarthria and Apraxia of Speech: Perspectives on Management* (pp. 205–225). Baltimore: Paul H. Brookes.

Cannito, M. P., Woodson, G. E., Murry, T., and Bender, B. (2004). Perceptual analyses of spasmodic dysphonia before and after treatment. *Archives of Otolaryngology – Head and Neck Surgery, 130,* 1393–1399.

Cookman, S. and Verdolini, K. (1999). Interrelation of mandibular laryngeal functions. *Journal of Voice, 13,* 11–24.

Critchley, E. M. (1981). Speech disorders of Parkinsonism: A review. *Journal of Neurology, Neurosurgery and Psychiatry, 44,* 751–758.

Dromey, C. (1995). *Global and Component-Specific Modifications of Speech: A Multi-Level Study.* Unpublished dissertation. University of Colorado-Boulder.

Dromey, C. (2000). Articulatory kinematics in patients with Parkinson disease using different speech treatment approaches. *Journal of Medical Speech-Language Pathology, 8*, 155–161.

Dromey, C., Kumar, R., Lang, A., and Lozano, A. (2000). An investigation of the effects of subthalamic nucleus stimulation on acoustic measures of voice. *Movement Disorders, 15*, 1132–1138.

Dromey, C., Nissen, S., Roy, N., and Merrill, R. M. (2008). Articulatory changes following treatment of muscle tension dysphonia: Preliminary acoustic evidence. *Journal of Speech, Language, and Hearing Research, 51*, 196–208.

Dromey, C. and Ramig, L. (1998a). Intentional changes in sound pressure level and rate: Their impact on measures of respiration, phonation and articulation. *Journal of Speech, Language and Hearing Research, 41*, 1003–1018.

Dromey, C. and Ramig, L. (1998b). The effect of lung volume on selected phonatory and articulatory variables. *Journal of Speech, Language and Hearing Research, 41*, 491–502.

Dromey, C., Ramig, L. O., and Johnson, A. B. (1995). Phonatory and articulatory changes associated with increased vocal intensity in Parkinson disease: a case study. *Journal of Speech and Hearing Research, 38*, 751–764.

Dromey, C., Reese, A., and Howey, S. (2007). Lip kinematics in spasmodic dysphonia before and after treatment with botulinum toxin. *Journal of Medical Speech-Language Pathology, 15*, 263–277.

Fisher, K. V., Scherer, R. C., Guo, C. G., and Owen, A. S. (1996). Longitudinal phonatory characteristics after botulinum toxin type A injection. *Journal of Speech and Hearing Research, 39*, 968–980.

Folkins, J. W. and Zimmermann, G. N. (1982). Lip and jaw interaction during speech: Responses to perturbation of lower-lip movement prior to bilabial closure. *Journal of the Acoustical Society of America, 71*, 1225–1233.

Gentil, M. and Pollak, P. (1995). Some aspects of Parkinsonian dysarthria. *Journal of Medical Speech-Language Pathology, 3*, 221–237.

Gracco, V. L. and Löfqvist, A. (1994). Speech motor coordination and control: Evidence from lip, jaw, and laryngeal movements. *Journal of Neuroscience, 14*, 6585–6597.

Higgins, M. B., Netsell, R., and Schulte, L. (1998). Vowel-related differences in laryngeal articulatory and phonatory function. *Journal of Speech, Language, and Hearing Research, 41*, 712–724.

Ho, A., Iansek, R., and Bradshaw, J. L. (2002). The effect of a concurrent task on Parkinsonian speech. *Journal of Clinical and Experimental Neuropsychology, 24*, 36–47.

Jankovic, J. and Brin, M. F. (1991). Therapeutic uses of botulinum toxin. *The New England Journal of Medicine, 324*, 1186–1194.

Kent, R. D., Weismer, G., Kent, J. F., Vorperian, H. K., and Duffy, J. R. (1999). Acoustic studies of dysarthric speech: Methods, progress and potential. *Journal of Communication Disorders, 32*, 141–186.

Kleinow, J., Smith, A., and Ramig, L. O. (2001). Speech motor stability in IPD: Effects of rate and loudness manipulations. *Journal of Speech, Language, and Hearing Research, 44*, 1041–1051.

Koufman, J. A. and Blalock, P. D. (1982). Classification and approach to patients with functional voice disorders. *Annals of Otology, Rhinology, and Laryngology, 91*, 372–377.

Logemann, J. A., Fisher, H. B., Boshes, B., and Blonsky, E. R. (1978). Frequency and cooccurrence of vocal tract dysfunctions in the speech of a large sample of Parkinson patients. *Journal of Speech and Hearing Disorders, 43*, 47–57.

Ludlow, C. L. (1995). Pathophysiology of the spasmodic dysphonias. In F. Bell-Berti and L. J. Raphael (Eds.), *Producing speech: Contemporary issues for Katherine Safford Harris* (pp. 291–308). New York: American Institute of Physics.

McClean, M. D. and Tasko, S. M. (2002). Association of orofacial with laryngeal and respiratory motor output during speech. *Experimental Brain Research, 146*, 481–489.

Miller, R. H. and Woodson, G. E. (1991). Treatment options in spasmodic dysphonia. *Otolaryngologic Clinics of North America, 24*, 1227–1237.

Morrison, M. D. and Rammage, L. A. (1993). Muscle misuse voice disorders: Description and classification. *Acta Oto-Laryngologica, 113*, 428–434.

Morrison, M. D., Rammage, L. A., Gilles, M. B., Pullan, C. B., and Nichol, H. (1983). Muscular tension dysphonia. *Journal of Otolaryngology, 12*, 302–306.

Munhall, K. G., Lofqvist, A., and Kelso, J. A. S. (1994). Lip-larynx coordination in speech: Effects of mechanical perturbations to the lower lip. *Journal of the Acoustical Society of America, 95*, 3605–3616.

Nakano, K. K., Zubick, H., and Tyler, H. R. (1973). Speech defects of Parkinsonian patients. Effects of levodopa therapy on speech intelligibility. *Neurology, 23*, 865–870.

Poluha, P. C., Teulings, H. L., and Brookshire, R. H. (1998). Handwriting and speech changes across the levodopa cycle in Parkinson's disease. *Acta Psychologica, 100*, 71–84.

Ramig, L. O., Countryman, S., O'Brien, C., Hoehn, M., and Thompson, L. (1996). Intensive speech treatment for patients with Parkinson's disease: short-and long-term comparison of two techniques. *Neurology, 47*, 1496–1504.

Ramig, L. O., Countryman, S., Thompson, L. L., and Horii, Y. (1995). Comparison of two forms of intensive speech treatment for Parkinson disease. *Journal of Speech and Hearing Research, 38*, 1232–1251.

Ramig, L. O. and Dromey, C. (1996). Aerodynamic mechanisms underlying treatment-related changes in vocal intensity in patients with Parkinson disease. *Journal of Speech and Hearing Research, 39*, 798–807.

Ramig, L. O., Fox, C., and Sapir, S. (2004). Parkinson's disease: Speech and voice disorders and their treatment with the Lee Silverman Voice Treatment. *Seminars in Speech and Language, 25*, 169–180.

Rosenbek, J. C. and LaPointe, L. L. (1985). The dysarthrias: Description, diagnosis, and treatment. In D.F. Johns (Ed.), *Clinical Management of Neurogenic Communication Disorders* (pp. 97–152). Boston: Little, Brown.

Roy, N. and Bless, D. M. (1998). Manual circumlaryngeal techniques in the assessment and treatment of voice disorders. *Current Opinion in Otolaryngology Head and Neck Surgery, 6*, 151–155.

Roy, N., Bless, D. M., Heisey, D., and Ford, C. N. (1997). Manual circumlaryngeal therapy for functional dysphonia: An evaluation of short- and long-term treatment outcomes. *Journal of Voice, 11*, 321–331.

Roy, N., Ford, C. N., and Bless, D. M. (1996). Muscle tension dysphonia and spasmodic dysphonia: The role of manual laryngeal tension reduction in diagnosis and management. *Annals of Otology Rhinology and Laryngology, 105*, 851–856.

Roy, N. and Leeper, H. A. (1993). Effects of the manual laryngeal musculoskeletal tension reduction technique as a treatment for functional voice disorders – perceptual and acoustic measures. *Journal of Voice, 7*, 242–249.

Sama, A., Carding, P. N., and Price, S. (2001). The clinical features of functional dysphonia. *Laryngoscope, 111*, 458–463.

Sanabria, J., Ruiz, P. G., Gutierrez, R., Marquez, F., Escobar, P., Gentil, M. et al. (2001). The effect of levodopa on vocal function in Parkinson's disease. *Clinical Neuropharmacology, 24*, 99–102.

Sapir, S., Ramig, L. O., Hoyt, P., Countryman, S., O'Brien, C., and Hoehn, M. (2002). Speech loudness and quality 12 months after intensive voice treatment (LSVT) for Parkinson's disease: A comparison with an alternative speech treatment. *Folia Phoniatrica et Logopaedica, 54*, 296–303.

Sapir, S., Spielman, J. L., Ramig, L. O., Story, B. H., and Fox, C. (2007). Effects of intensive voice treatment (the Lee Silverman Voice Treatment [LSVT]) on vowel articulation in dysarthric individuals with idiopathic Parkinson disease: acoustic and perceptual findings. *Journal of Speech, Language, and Hearing Research, 50*, 899–912.

Schalen, L. and Andersson, K. (1992). Differential diagnosis and treatment of psychogenic voice disorder. *Clinical Otolaryngology, 17*, 225–230.

Schulman, R. (1989). Articulatory dynamics of loud and normal speech. *Journal of the Acoustical Society of America, 85*, 295–312.

Smith, M. E., Ramig, L. O., Dromey, C., Perez, K. S., and Samandari, R. (1995). Intensive voice treatment in Parkinson disease: Laryngostroboscopic findings. *Journal of Voice, 9*, 453–459.

Spielman, J. L., Borod, J. C., and Ramig, L. O. (2003). The effects of intensive voice treatment on facial expressiveness in Parkinson disease: preliminary data. *Cognitive and Behavioral Neurology, 16*, 177–188.

Tingley, S. and Dromey, C. (2000). Phonatory-articulatory relationships: Do speakers with spasmodic dysphonia show aberrant lip kinematic profiles? *Journal of Medical Speech-Language Pathology*, *8*, 249–252.

van Lieshout, P. H. H. M., Peters, H. F. M., and Bakker, A. J. (1997). En route to a speech motor test: A first halt. In W.Hulstijn, H. F. M. Peters, and P. H. H. M. van Lieshout (Eds.), *Speech Production: Motor Control, Brain Research and Fluency Disorders* (pp. 463–471). Amsterdam: Elsevier.

Weismer, G., Yunusova, Y., and Westbury, J. R. (2003). Interarticulator coordination in dysarthria: An x-ray microbeam study. *Journal of Speech, Language, and Hearing Research*, *46*, 1247–1261.

Chapter 18

Electrical stimulation of deep brain structures and speech

Elina Tripoliti and Patricia Limousin

Abstract

Since the beginnings of stereotactic surgery and electrical stimulation of deep brain structures the role of basal ganglia in speech motor control has triggered a multidisciplinary debate. Deep brain stimulation (DBS) is an effective treatment of the motor symptoms of Parkinson's disease (PD). It involves the implantation of two electrodes either in the ventro-intermediate nucleus (Vim) of the thalamus, or the globus pallidus internum (Gpi) or the subthalamic nucleus (STN), depending on the symptomatology. Speech changes can be an intriguing side effect in all the above targets.

Bilateral thalamic stimulation induces speech impairment in the majority of patients. Speech difficulties following DBS in the Gpi have been infrequently reported. Speech outcome is variable following DBS in the STN with improvement noted in some acoustic measures and oro-motor non-speech tasks but deterioration of speech intelligibility in the majority of patients. Factors affecting speech response following STN-DBS are partly surgical, i.e. current spread and contact location. There is the need for further research into ways speech is affected by deep brain stimulation in order to maximize the benefits of the treatment.

18.1 Introduction

Fluent articulation is a complex motor skill that involves the coordinated use of approximately 100 muscles, such that speech sounds are produced at a rate of 15 per second (Levelt 1989). Dysfunction in the basal ganglia can affect the smooth coordination of these muscles in the majority of patients with Parkinson's disease (PD) (Darley et al., 1975; Logemann et al., 1978). However, there is a wide variability in the perceptual and acoustic manifestation of hypokinetic dysarthria associated with PD (Rosen et al., 2005) and a lack of strong relationship with limb motor disability (Kent and Kim 2003; Metter and Hanson 1986). There is also a variable response of speech to medical and surgical treatment (De Letter et al., 2005; Goberman and Blomgren 2003; Pinto et al., 2004a). Thus, there is still a fundamental dissociation between the obvious disruption of motor speech production by the dysfunction of basal ganglia and the lack of significant beneficial effects from either medical or surgical therapies that improve other motor symptoms. The aim of this chapter is to describe the effects of deep brain stimulation in the thalamus and basal ganglia on speech in PD.

18.2 The basal ganglia and thalamus

The basal ganglia are traditionally seen as composed of four major nuclei: the neostriatum, the globus pallidus (GP), the substantia nigra (SN), and the subthalamic nucleus (STN). The neostriatum is divided by the internal capsule into the caudate nucleus and putamen. The GP consists of two major parts, the external segment (GPe) and the internal segment (GPi). The SN consists of two major subnuclei, the pars compacta (SNc) and the pars reticulata (SNr) (Tepper et al., 2007). In a broader sense it has been argued that basal ganglia are part of a loop that supports thalamocortical interactions and thus cortical function (Wilson 2004) (Fig. 18.1).

18.3 Deep brain stimulation for Parkinson's disease

Deep brain stimulation in the modern era involves the application of electrical current mainly in the STN or GPi or the ventro-intermediate nucleus (Vim) of the thalamus. Patients are implanted bilaterally with quadripolar electrodes with four platinum iridium cylindrical contacts (Fig. 18.2). The electrodes most commonly used are model 3389 of Medtronic (Medtronic Neurological Division, Minneapolis) with the following dimensions for each contact: 1.27 mm diameter, 1.5 mm in length, centre-to-centre separation 2 mm. Electrodes are connected to a pulse generator, implanted under general anaesthesia. Postoperative management aims to adjust the stimulation in order to determine which of the four contacts is the most effective on each side. Electrical parameters of stimulation are relatively similar for both Gpi and STN (Limousin and Martinez-Torres 2008). The frequency, in order to be effective, must be higher than 100 Hz with 130 Hz the most frequently used. Voltage is usually set between 2V and 4V. Patients implanted with DBS need a long-term follow-up by a specialist team (Limousin and Martinez-Torres 2008) in order to adjust stimulation and medication and to treat side effects.

Early studies described the acute speech effect of electrical stimulation, mainly in the thalamus, from the brief application of electrical current during lesioning procedures. Recent studies describe the effect of chronic electrical stimulation in the thalamus, the GPi, and the STN. Speech deterioration can be a side effect of these procedures, limiting the benefits from the alleviation of motor symptoms. Speech deterioration can also be an underreported side effect (Hariz 2003; Hariz and Fodstad 2002, 'The Deep –Brain Stimulation for Parkinson's Disease Study Group', 2001).

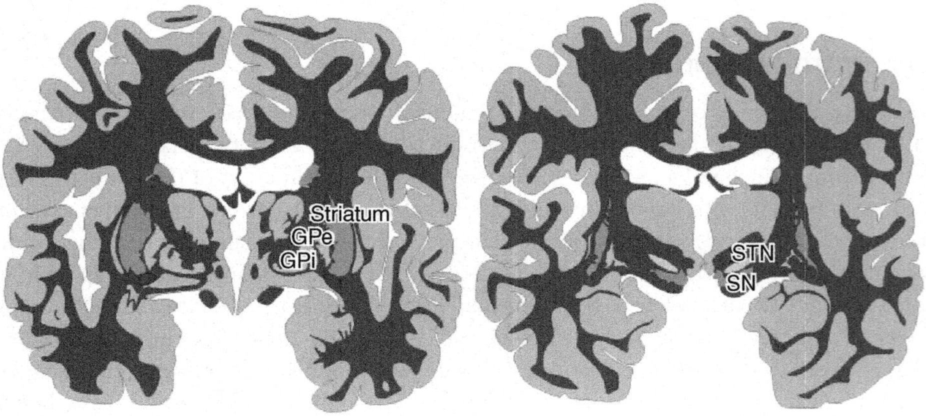

Fig. 18.1 Basal ganglia coronal sections. Gpi: Globus Pallidus Internum, Gpe: globus Pallidus externum, STN: Subthalamic nucleus, SN: Substantia nigra.

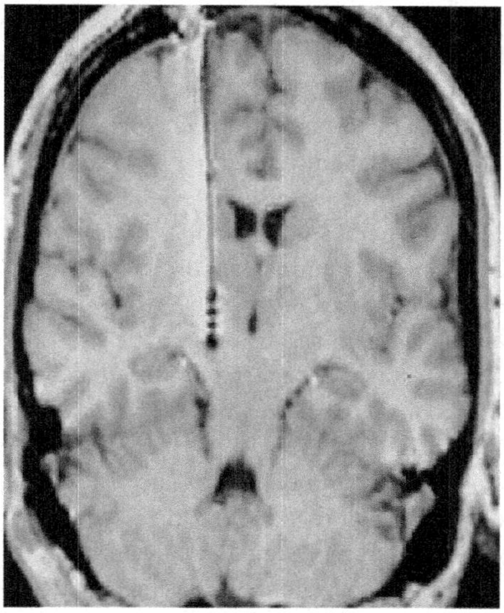

Fig. 18.2 DBS electrode implanted showing the four contact tips.

Thus investigating speech effects of deep brain stimulation is challenging and demands a multidisciplinary approach.

18.3.1 Early studies on electrical stimulation of deep brain structures and its effects on speech and language

In 1908 Sir Victor Horsley (1857–1914) and Robert Henri Clarke (1850–1926) developed the stereotactic instruments and applied electricity to study cerebellar structures and functions in monkeys (Horsley and Clarke 1908). In 1947 Spiegel and Wycis became the first to apply Clarke's idea for human stereotaxis by performing a thalamotomy in a depressed man (Spiegel et al., 1947). Stimulation of deep cerebral structures was used initially to guide lesioning procedures in the early years of surgical treatment of PD. This development of basal ganglia lesioning procedures gave rise to an interest in the role of thalamus and basal ganglia on speech. Very early in the course of stereotactic neurosurgery it was observed that 'improvement in speech should not be the prime goal in selecting patients for surgical treatment of parkinsonism. Rather patients should be selected on a basis of the degree of incapacitation due to rigidity and tremor. They should be informed that whereas 70% of patients obtain material alleviation of tremor and rigidity following operation on the GP, less than 20% experience a similar degree of improvement in speech' (Buck and Cooper 1956, p.122). Guiot and colleagues (1961) were the first to describe speech phenomena in the course of stereotactic procedures, in each of the three areas – thalamus, internal capsule, pallidum – traversed by the needle for stimulation, before destroying the selected region. The point stimulated was situated in the ventrolateral nucleus of the thalamus near the thalamocapsular boundary. They described two distinct speech modifications, one was total arrest and the other was speech acceleration, coupled with 'progressive weakening of the voice and an enunciation which ends in a kind of incomprehensible jumbling of several figures or the last figure uttered' (p.367). The cause of these speech phenomena was hypothesized to be a diffusion of the current mainly in the internal capsule. Furthermore, they noted that 'stimulation by a volley of impulses can excite a number of positive responses which vary according to individual patients and of which the origin may be quite remote from the point stimulated'

(Guiot et al., 1961, p.367). Van Buren (1975) and Hassler and colleagues (1960) described similar observations from stimulation in the head of the caudate nucleus, the pallidum and the frontal limb of the internal capsule.

In 1969, Samra and colleagues (1969) reported their experience from the surgical treatment of 6,000 individuals who underwent thalamic surgery for the relief of parkinsonian tremor and rigidity. Their language and speech were routinely evaluated before and after surgery. Speech overall deteriorated in 35% of unilateral and 75% of bilateral surgeries. However, it was not clear why some patients developed language and speech difficulties and others did not. The surgical target was the ventrolateral nucleus of the thalamus in all cases. Results from the correlation of the site of the lesion in 27 brains of deceased parkinsonian patients – out of the initial 6,000 – and all language and speech deficits that might have resulted from thalamic surgery showed that partial involvement of the STN, the red nucleus or even the internal capsule could be tolerated, provided that the pyramidal tract remained intact. Deficits in sentence formulation seemed related to left thalamic unilateral surgery; there was no definite relationship between postoperative speech deficits and either the site or the size of the lesion. Samra and colleagues (1969) concluded that 'the motor processes associated with speech –mainly rate and rhythm of articulation – might be related more directly and exclusively to motor cortex-ventrolateral thalamus modulation than to thalamic influences in general' (pp. 538–539). Bell (1968) on the other hand could not find any relationship between the pre- and postoperative speech deficits in Parkinson's dysarthria and concluded that the speech deterioration following thalamic surgery was due to lesions in the internal capsule.

Schaltenbrand (1975) summarized his observations from thalamic stimulation using a bipolar electrode on the tip of a stereotactic needle and stimulation of 32 Hz, 8 volts, and 10–20 μsec pulse width. He described mainly silencing and slowing of speech with thalamic stimulation, monosyllabic yells and exclamations, some stammering, repetition of syllables and words and 'compulsory speech'. He concluded that the function of the thalamus could not be that of initiating speech but of releasing and silencing preformed patterns, therefore of timing. He warned against the production of large lesions in this area because the effects on speech could be lasting.

In the earlier studies, neurosurgeons were predominantly involved with peri-operative observations and descriptions of long-term results of their operations on speech. Cooper and his colleagues (1968) founded the multidisciplinary approach to management of surgical patients with emphasis on vocational rehabilitation. The aim of the two-to-four-weeks postoperative rehabilitation was restoring vocational function. Most parkinsonian patients who underwent surgery were given speech therapy. The postoperative techniques were directed towards the difficulties of voice volume. 'Since difficulties in volume are paramount we emphasize strengthening of the voice. One of these methods is essentially a *'boosting'* technique and involves various means of using the entire body to support the tone of voice' (Cooper et al., 1968, p.1215). In order to ensure generalization, family and friends of the patient were 'instructed not to respond to the patient unless he speaks with sufficient volume. This is sometimes tedious and frustrating task but experience has shown that only constant attention to his own voice and constant awareness of his difficulties can produce the desired results.' (p.1215). The programme involved techniques for rate control through reading and singing, but mainly free conversation in groups of 6–8 and individual sessions. The intensity and the voice focus of these techniques remind one of the Lee Silverman Voice Treatment (LSVT) (Ramig et al., 2001).

In summary, the debate on the role of the thalamus in speech production started with the interest of the pioneers of stereotactic neurosurgery on the overall effects of their treatments. The exact role of the thalamus in speech deterioration following surgery for the alleviation of parkinsonian rigidity and tremor was disputed due to the variability and high occurrence of speech deficits.

The role of and the involvement of the internal capsule in the postoperative speech problems was also a topic of debate.

18.3.2 Recent studies on electrical stimulation of deep brain structures and its effects on speech

After the introduction of L-dopa in the late 1960s, stereotactic surgery for PD went to a world-wide hibernation (Hariz 2003). Following the initial satisfactory response to levodopa many patients developed motor fluctuations that were difficult to control. The patients alternated between a state of severe parkinsonism (the 'off medication' period) and a state of improved mobility (the 'on medication' state) when movement was often impaired by dyskinesias. In 1991, Benabid and colleagues (1991) published the long-term results of thalamic DBS with emphasis on its reversibility and adaptability compared to destructive lesions. It appeared that thalamic stimulation was effective mainly for tremor and therefore only useful to a small proportion of people with PD (Limousin et al., 1998). Dysarthria was reported in up to 20% of patients after bilateral thalamic DBS (Limousin et al., 1999). Advances in the knowledge of basal ganglia pathophysiology and neurosurgical procedures led to the development of high-frequency stimulation in the GPi (Siegfried and Lippitz 1994) and the STN (Limousin et al., 1995, 1998) as a treatment of choice for the majority of parkinsonian signs.

18.3.2.1 Gpi-DBS and speech

Speech difficulties following GPi-DBS have been infrequently reported. Initially, Gross and colleagues (1997) reported improvement in speech following one year GPi stimulation in six patients as measured by the Unified Parkinson's Disease Rating Scale-motor part III (Fahn et al. 1987). Only one item (18) from the UPDRS-III motor scale measures speech intelligibility, using a five-point scale ranging from zero for normal speech to four for unintelligible speech (for comments on the reliability of UPDRS-III as a speech measure see Section 18.4, Methodological issues). Ghika and colleagues (1998) reported dysarthria as a side effect that was controlled by modulation of stimulation. However, they did not give any more details of the nature of this modulation. Speech intelligibility deterioration, as measured by the UPDRS-III, item 18, has been reported in other studies (Lyons et al., 2002; Krause et al., 2001).

Solomon and colleagues (2000) examined the effects of pallidal stimulation on aerodynamic and intelligibility data. They measured airflow and air pressure during slow syllable repetitions and speech intelligibility before surgery on and off medication and 6 months and 12 months after. The results showed a variable response with respect to speech intelligibility. Speech improved in one patient, through the alleviation of painful oromandibular dyskinesias, and deteriorated in the other two. They also concluded that it was laryngeal rather than respiratory dysfunction that contributed to the speech impairment. Maruska and colleagues (2000) described the changes in speech intelligibility of four patients on and off medication and on and off stimulation. Stimulation and medication were beneficial to speech intelligibility. Increase of intelligibility was coupled with a decrease in the numbers of errors and an increase in speaking rate and loudness.

18.3.2.2 STN-DBS and speech

Studies on the effects of STN-DBS on speech, using clinical scales, have shown a variable response to stimulation (Limousin et al., 1998). Hariz and colleagues (2000) illustrated the barrier speech deterioration can become towards fully utilizing the motor benefits from the procedure. They described a patient following one year of STN stimulation with good motor effects, but with worsening of pre-operative dysphonia and drooling. They concluded that 'improvement in motor function may not be sufficient alone to improve the overall disability of a patient in whom cognitive decline and speech problems are present preoperatively' (p.138). In recent reports of long-term follow-up, using the UPDRS-III scale, dysarthria has been reported as a common stimulation-induced side effect of STN-DBS with a prevalence ranging from 4% to 17% (Deuschl et al., 2006). Speech was the only function that did not improve following five years STN stimulation (Krack et al., 2003), with some patients reporting unequivocal worsening of speech over time and after surgery, and displaying a progression of speech difficulties that was not modifiable with adjustment of medication and stimulation (Kleiner-Fisman et al., 2004).

Other studies, using electrophysiological measures of speech, showed a marked improvement of non-speech oral motor tasks with STN-DBS. Gentil and colleagues (1999) studied the oral force control of ten selected patients using load sensitive devices to measure the compression forces generated by the upper and lower lip and tongue. STN stimulation improved speech as measured with the UPDRS-III speech item 18, and increased the maximal strength, accuracy, and precision of the articulatory organs. The same group reported beneficial effects of stimulation on acoustical data of 26 PD patients. They found longer duration of sustained vowels, shorter duration of sentences, more variable fundamental frequency in sentences and more fundamental frequency stability in vowels. Relative intensity was unchanged (Gentil et al., 2001, 2003). These studies were on selected patients and selected non-speech motor tasks with no reference to speech intelligibility. They also compared the off with the on stimulation conditions without reference to the pre-operative state. However, not all studies reported similar results; discrepancies in the outcome are further discussed in Section 18.4, Methodological issues.

Dromey and colleagues (2000) measured the STN stimulation effects on acoustical variables of speech in seven patients compared to their pre-operative state. They found modest but significant increases in vocal intensity and in fundamental frequency variability in the on-medication condition. They also noted that these changes did not have a substantial impact on functional communication and that the subjective UPDRS-III speech rating was not directly associated with the acoustic measures. Rousseaux and colleagues (2004) were the first to assess speech intelligibility and compared the obtained intelligibility scores with perceptual indices of voice and articulatory quality in seven patients. Intelligibility in spontaneous speech and in read sentences did not show any significant change in any of the stimulation and medication conditions, but it did have the tendency to drop more at the stimulation-on/medication-on condition. Two out of seven patients, who also exhibited increased facial and trunk dyskinesias, had a definite worsening of dysarthria at the stimulation-on/medication-on condition. Their speech was characterized by slowness, hypophonia, aprosody, and difficulties in articulation. At a group level the non-significant decrease in speech intelligibility was neither associated with oro-motor difficulties, nor with the pre-operative speech level or surgical parameters.

One study so far has compared speech changes through disease progression over one year of medical (pharmacological) treatment and one year of surgical treatment with bilateral STN-DBS (Tripoliti et al., 2006). Sixteen patients were randomized in two groups. Eight patients received surgical treatment with bilateral STN DBS and eight continued to receive medical (pharmacological) treatment. Patients were assessed one week before randomization, both on and off medication. The same assessment was repeated one year later on and off medication and on and off stimulation for the surgical group. Speech intelligibility was assessed using the Assessment of Intelligibility of the Dysarthric Speech (AIDS) (Yorkston and Beukelman 1981), which includes a 60-second monologue about a topic of the speakers' choice and sustained phonation. Movement was assessed using the UPDRS-III. Sound Pressure Level (SPL) was calculated for sustained phonation and Long Term Average Spectra (LTAS) means were used for the analysis of the read sentences and the monologue samples. Sentence intelligibility data for both groups did not change significantly following surgical or medical treatment over one year, when on medication and on stimulation. The surgical group presented with a wide variability. Speech intelligibility decreased by 40% in two out of eight patients while the rest decreased insignificantly. In accordance with previous reports (Gentil et al., 2001), SPL for sustained phonation was significantly higher for the surgical group compared to their pre-operative measures. For the medical group SPL decreased over one year but not significantly. LTAS means were significantly higher for the connected speech tasks of the surgical group compared to the medical group. However the relationship between this acoustic measure and perceptual judgment is still not clear. The study confirmed the contradiction of loud voice with reduced speech intelligibility in the surgical group. Their speech could be described as hypernasal with continuous voicing of hyperfunctional quality and reduced lip and tongue movement. The location of the stimulating electrodes of the two patients who deteriorated was similar to that of the six other patients as was the improvement in their motor UPDRS-III scores.

Four case studies reported by Pinto and colleagues (2005) illustrated similar variability. Response to STN stimulation varied from improvement with medication and stimulation to deterioration with increased voltage intensity. Furthermore, they noted that 'motor speech subcomponents can improve like other limp motor aspect but that complex coordination of all speech anatomical substrates is not responsive to STN stimulation' (p.1507). They concluded that diffusion of the current outside the target may be responsible for speech deterioration.

Laterality of stimulation and its effects on speech have been investigated. Santens and colleagues (2003) analysed the effects of left and right STN separately on different perceptual aspects of speech in seven patients. All patients reported subjective decrease of speech intelligibility following bilateral STN stimulation. There was a significant deterioration of prosody, articulation, and intelligibility when stimulating the left STN compared to the right STN alone. Wang and colleagues (2006) investigated the effect of unilateral STN- DBS on speech in 20 PD patients, 10 operated on the left STN and 10 on the right. They presented the results on articulatory accuracy and syllable rate for diadochokinetic tasks. Left STN stimulation decreased articulatory accuracy and speaking rate.

One case report (Burghaus et al., 2006) so far described a PD patient treated with bilateral STN-DBS and with severe deterioration of his childhood stuttering under effective stimulation. Positron emission tomography (PET) of regional cerebral blood flow (rCBF) in stimulation on and off conditions showed overactivation of cerebral and cerebellar motor systems, which is in line with other studies on brain activation during stuttering. The abnormal rCBF pattern was increased in the stimulation – on condition and was associated with a marked worsening of stuttering.

Putzer and colleagues (2008) studied the effect of STN-DBS in nine consecutive patients on and off stimulation with no pre-operative data. They collected electroglottograph data together with acoustic recording of syllable repetition /pa/ta/ka/ as fast as possible. They observed a varied response in both the phonation and supraglottal system of speech. No data on speech intelligibility were given. Klostermann and colleagues (2007) investigated the effect of STN-DBS on acoustic measures of speech and speech intelligibility in 19 selective patients, on medication and on and off stimulation. They concluded that speech intelligibility declined, despite an improvement in glottic tremor, increased sustained phonation time and increased rate of reading. They hypothesized that this discrepancy was due to the nature of the voice measures and the difficulty in measuring prosodic changes of connected speech. Similarly, D'alatri and colleagues (2008) assessed 12 selected patients 2–5 years post-bilateral STN DBS in all medication and stimulation conditions. They analysed sustained phonation, one set of sentences for intonation and diadochokinesis for rate control. Perceptual speech evaluation was conducted using the UPDRS-III speech item. They found the same discrepancy of improvement in acoustic parameters related to glottal vibration and voice tremor, and lack of effect on speech intelligibility.

In PD dysarthria increased loudness is associated with increased speech intelligibility (Rosen et al., 2006; Tjaden and Wilding 2004). The lack of change in loudness and spectral measures with decreased speech intelligibility observed in the above studies, could point towards a perceptually different dysarthria type associated with STN stimulation. A larger sample of consecutive patients with controls and appropriate choice of tasks and analysis is needed for a more precise description.

18.3.2.3. Comparison of Gpi and STN effects on speech

The effects on speech of STN and GPi stimulation have been compared in three studies using the UPDRS-III motor scale, speech item 18. In a multicentre study of bilateral DBS with four-years follow-up Rodriguez-Oroz and colleagues (2005) reported that speech and postural stability showed significant worsening for both the GPi and the STN group, but more commonly for the STN group. Volkman and colleagues (2001) compared one-year results of bilateral DBS of the STN and the GPi and found equal improvement in the motor symptoms apart from a significant worsening of speech and swallowing tasks only in the STN patients. A recent large multicentre study on adverse events following deep brain stimulation (Hariz et al., 2008) compared adverse events following 4 years of STN versus Gpi stimulation. They reported 9 out of 49 patients with STN DBS to have speech problems compared to 1 out of 20 with Gpi DBS, again showing worse results for STN.

18.4 **Methodological issues**

Sampling and protocol selection can partly account for the variability in speech results following DBS.

18.4.1 **Sampling**

The earlier studies are especially restricted since sample sizes were typically small, ranging from 10 consecutive patients (Van Buren 1975), to 125 out of the 6,000 total number of operated patients for the Samra report (Samra et al., 1969). Most of the later studies on the speech effects of GPi and STN DBS used small samples of selected patients (Pinto et al., 2004a) and compared off- and on-stimulation at a variety of postoperative timings and no pre-operative data were given. Moreover, most studies lack a large control sample to compare speech changes induced by neurosurgical interventions to those induced by the disease process and pharmacological intervention over time (Rousseaux, et al., 2004; Tripoliti et al., 2006).

18.4.2 **Protocol**

The choice of a speech protocol that adequately reflects the complexity of speech and all of its components – the respiratory, phonatory, and articulatory systems – and can represent the changes in functional communication is an ongoing debate (Weismer 2006; Ziegler 2003). In the earlier studies speech changes were described perceptually during stimulation (Bell 1968; Schaltenbrand 1975; Van Buren 1975). Perhaps the most comprehensive speech scale for the speech examination of pre- and postoperative parkinsonian patients was developed already in the 50-ies by Buck and Cooper (1956). Areas of assessment included oral musculature, 'integrated activity of the articulators' (through repetition of sentences and reading of passages containing labial and alveolar sounds), observations on phonation (four-point scale), observations on language ability, speech involvement (five-point scale rating speech intelligibility), physical involvement for the activities of daily living, and structural-parkinsonian symptoms (i.e. tremor, rigidity, akinesia).

Despite the fact that in later studies the main speech tasks remained the same, namely counting, diadochokinesis, reading of set sentences and conversation, they utilized a wider variability of acoustical and electrophysiological measures. Use of perceptual scales was limited to speech intelligibility scales and to UPDRS-III, speech item 18. UPDRS-III has poor inter-rater reliability for speech and facial expression (Richards et al., 1994). The use of a single item, a five-point scale range from 0, no impairment to 4, unintelligible, for an overall estimation of speech intelligibility, has been criticized as insufficient for rating speech changes following neurosurgical interventions, due to the limitations in span of the scale and aspects of speech assessed (Pinto et al., 2005a). So far, there have not been any studies that evaluated the changes in conversational speech, despite the fact that patients tend to report increased communication difficulties following neurosurgery.

18.5 Factors affecting speech response following DBS

18.5.1 Electrical parameters

Speech motor outcome following STN-DBS could be dependent on both clinical, and surgical and implant characteristics specific to individual patients. Clinical factors, such as speech impairment before surgery, speech response to medication and to disease process have not been examined systematically for their effect on speech after surgery.

Electrical parameters of stimulation, such as frequency (in Hz) and amplitude (in Volts) of stimulation have been implicated in speech deterioration.

Krack and colleagues (2002, 2003) have reported speech deterioration with increased electrical parameters such as frequency and voltage amplitude of stimulation.

Tornqvist and colleagues (2005) compared the differential effects on speech intelligibility of 11 different parameter settings with varying amplitude and frequency of stimulation on 10 patients. They found that the greatest impairment of speech was induced following either a 25% increase in amplitude or in the frequencies 185 Hz and 130 Hz compared to 70 Hz. However, they did not report the concomitant effects on movement. Tommasi and colleagues (2007) analysed the pyramidal tract side effects (PTSEs) induced by increased voltage of stimulation. They also studied the relationship between the voltage threshold for the PTSEs and the distance from the centre of the used contact to the medial border of the pyramidal tract as measured on MRI in 14 patients treated with bilateral STN DBS (i.e. for 28 electrodes). They differentiated between stimulus-dependent involuntary contractions of speech muscles (jaw and lip muscles) and dysarthria assessed by (a) the subjective effort to speak reported by the patient and the objective observation by the physician of the qualitative speech changes time-locked to the stimulus, (b) the worsening of speech disturbances in parallel with the voltage increase and (c) the reproducibility of these effects. Results showed increased contractions in the forehead, eyebrow, eyelid, cheek, lip, and chin with progressive increase in voltage. Contractions of the lower face were opposite to the stimulation site for all the electrodes and bilateral for the upper face. Furthermore, dysarthria was observed upon stimulation of 7 out of 28 electrodes and was characterized by hypophonic, slurred speech, rapid fatiguing, and hesitation with frequent, long pauses. However, dysarthria was rarely involved as the initial PTSE, which was instead mainly located in the face. They also found a linear correlation between the distance from the chronically used contact and the medial pyramidal tract border and the voltage threshold for motor contractions. This confirmed their hypothesis that the observed motor contractions were induced by spread of current to the pyramidal tract. However, they reported no correlation between the motor contractions of the face observed as early signs of PTSE's in the majority of the electrodes and dysarthria, observed in a small number of patients and with increased stimulation voltage.

Tripoliti and colleagues (2008) studied the role of the location of the stimulated contact and the role of the voltage amplitude in speech and motor function. Fourteen patients were recruited consecutively, each following 6–12 months of bilateral STN-DBS. A neurosurgeon independently assessed the anatomical position of each contact in relation to the visualized STN. The contact closest to the centre of the STN (henceforth 'inside') and that furthest of the STN ('outside') were thus identified. Low voltage was defined as 2V and high voltage as 4V. Patients were studied after overnight withdrawal from their antiparkinsonian medication. Six conditions were studied in a random order: inside the nucleus at 2V; inside the nucleus at 4V; outside the nucleus at 2V; outside the nucleus at 4V; as well as DBS on at usual clinical parameters and DBS off. Both assessors and the patients were blinded with respect to the stimulation condition. The speech assessment consisted of three tasks: sustained vowel phonation, the sentence part of Assessment of Intelligibility for the Dysarthric Speech (AIDS, Yorkston 1981) and a 60-seconds monologue about a topic of the speaker's choice. Movement was assessed using the UPDRS-III. For speech recording and analysis the Computerised Speech Lab (CSL, Kay Pentax, 4150) was used. The files from the AIDS sentences were rated blindly. For the acoustical analysis of intensity of sustained phonation, reading and monologue the mean vocal SPL dB was calculated from the speech recording of each condition.

The findings showed that high voltage had a significantly worsening effect on speech intelligibility in comparison to low voltage, irrespective of contact location. The mean speech intelligibility score for the 'inside-high' condition was 53.4%, 'outside-high' 53.4%, 'inside-low' 72%, and 'outside-low' 69.2%. Detailed examination of individual patients' data revealed two distinct subgroups of patients. One group was not much affected by the stimulation, while the other showed a higher than average deterioration of speech with increased amplitude. Patients whose speech was less affected had electrodes positioned more posteriorily in the STN area, whereas patients showing marked deterioration had electrodes positioned more medially or anteriomedially to the STN. In terms of acoustic measures, intensity (SPL dB) for sustained phonation, a one-minute monologue and read sentences did not change significantly with contact location or voltage amplitude. High voltage had a significantly more beneficial effect on motor scores (as assessed by UPDRS-III) than low voltage. Additionally contacts inside the STN had a significantly more beneficial effect on movement than contacts outside the STN.

It was demonstrated in this study that speech intelligibility could deteriorate with high voltage for contacts both inside and outside the STN. Deterioration in speech intelligibility was not linked to a significant deterioration of vocal loudness. High voltage stimulation of contacts inside the STN could have a beneficial effect on motor scores (as assessed by UPDRS-III) and at the same time induce a significant deterioration of speech intelligibility. The degree to which speech intelligibility was affected by high voltage stimulation was variable between patients.

Several hypotheses could explain the worsening effect of high voltage STN stimulation on speech. STN could have a different role or a different somatotopy for speech and body control. Another hypothesis is that the current could spread to other pathways in the area.

18.5.2 **Somatotopy of the STN for speech and limb motor control**

The role of the site of stimulation within the STN area and its relationship to limb motor control has also been investigated. Yelnik and colleagues (2003) described the dorsolateral part as more effective for improvement in limb motor control. More recently, Herzog and colleagues (2004) and Plaha and colleagues (2006) described the caudal zona incerta, dorsal/dorsomedial to the STN as optimal stimulation sites for improvement in limb movement.

With respect to speech, reports from stimulation in contacts dorsomedial or medial to the STN have resulted in reversible, hypophonic, and slurred speech, unlike those in caudal zona incerta and the one inside the STN, which did not induce dysarthria as a side effect (Plaha et al., 2006). Similarly, stimulation in the prelemniscal radiation caused dysarthria despite improvement in tremor and rigidity (Velasco et al., 2001). Paek and colleagues (2008) investigated the clinical outcome from bilateral STN DBS in 53 patients. The electrode position was divided into 6 types, according to its relationship to the STN and the red nucleus. Most off-medication on-stimulation UPDRS-III scores improved regardless of the type of electrode position. However speech improved only in the patients whose electrodes were correctly positioned within the STN as opposed to the red nucleus or the area between the STN and the red nucleus. It is possible that the stimulation could affect oral and limb neural control from different somatotopic zones within the STN. Information on the somatotopy of the STN with respect to oral musculature is limited. In the monkey (Macaca Mulatta), neurons in the dorsolateral part of the STN and the SN have been identified to be particularly active during oral movements for feeding (DeLong et al.,1983; Mora et al., 1977). Mora and colleagues (1977) also reported mouth movements being elicited by electrical stimulation applied in the STN area. Also in the monkey, representation of the face was found to be in the most lateral zone of the STN (Wichmann et al.,1994). However, these reports may not be relevant to the effects of STN stimulation in humans in general, and on speech in particular. For example, in a study of PD patients, Rodriguez-Oroz and her colleagues (Rodriguez-Oroz et al., 2001, 2004) found neurons corresponding to the oromandibular musculature in the middle of the STN and ventral to the neurons corresponding to the arm and leg.

Using Positron Emission Tomography (PET), Pinto (2004b) investigated the brain activation changes resulting from STN stimulation during speech. Speech production in PD patients off stimulation was associated with underactivation of the orofacial primary motor cortex (M1) and cerebellum and overactivation of the supplementary motor area (SMA), superior premotor cortex and the dorsolateral prefrontal cortex (DLPFC). These abnormal activations were restored with STN stimulation and correlated with improvement in tongue force control and UPDRS-III speech item 18 scores. In contrast, STN stimulation during a hand joystick movement restored abnormal overactivation of primary motor and lateral premotor cortex and underactivation in the SMA, the superior premotor cortex, and the DLPFC (Limousin et al., 1997). Thus, it is possible that these different pathways compete for speech and limb motor control and that they are affected differently by STN stimulation.

18.5.3 **Mechanisms of stimulation and effects on speech**

Although the clinical benefits of DBS have been well documented, fundamental questions remain about the therapeutic mechanism of action (Fodstad and Hariz 2007; McIntyre et al., 2003). The electric field generated by DBS electrodes is capable of directly activating a large volume of tissue. Simulation studies show that the stimulating effect can spread outside the borders of the STN and can result in activation of Zona Incerta, fields of Forel (H2) and Internal Capsule (Astrom et al., 2008; McIntyre et al., 2004).

This diffusion hypothesis was first proposed by Guiot and colleagues (1961) and has recently been advocated by Krack and colleagues (2002). It concerns the 'spread of current to the more laterally located corticobulbar tract' (p. S194). However, if the effects on speech were caused by the spread of current to the internal capsule and the corticobulbar pathways for laryngeal motor control, we would expect a significant change on sustained phonation and other acoustical parameters of connected speech, which was not observed. Spread in other pathways, namely the pallidofugal and the cerebellothalamic fibres, could also affect speech. According to Plaha and colleagues (2006), due to the length from the tip of the DBS lead to the uppermost contact and the axis of implant, there could be one or possibly two contacts lying either dorsal or dorsomedial to the STN in the region of the pallidofugal fibres and the rostral ZI, areas for which speech difficulties have been reported before. However, diffusion of the current in the cerebello-thalamo-cortical fibres is equally likely, especially from patients with medially placed contacts (Mattias et al., 2008; Tripoliti et al., 2008). At this point, we still lack the perceptual and imaging information that is necessary to assign the spread to one pathway or another. We also require a better knowledge of the actual position of the DBS electrodes, so that we could aim to provide a more refined stimulation, including a more focal distribution of the electrical fields and a better selection of stimulation parameters (Paek et al., 2008).

18.6 **Summary**

Since the beginning of the stereotactic surgery and electrical stimulation of deep brain structures, the role of basal ganglia in speech motor control has triggered a multidisciplinary debate. Bilateral thalamic stimulation induced speech impairment in the majority of patients, whereas speech difficulties following Gpi DBS have been infrequently reported. With respect to STN DBS, speech outcome has been shown to be variable, with improvement noted in some acoustic measures and oro-motor non-speech tasks but deterioration of intelligibility in the majority of patients. Electrical current spread and contact location have been investigated as possible factors contributing to this variability.

Speech remains a challenge in need of further multidisciplinary investigations in order to maximize the effects of DBS in movement and improve the quality of life of operated patients with PD. As Guiot and colleagues (1961) have commented, 'in spite of the difficulty of the interpretation, the phenomena of arrest and acceleration of the speech under the influence of deep cerebral stimulation are in themselves sufficiently curious to justify the description which we have tried to give' (p 368).

References

Astrom M., Zrinzo LU., Tisch S., Tripoliti E., Hariz MI., and Wardell K., (2008), 'Method for patient-specific finite element modeling and simulation of deep brain stimulation', *Med Biol Eng Comput, vol, 47, pp. 21–28.*

D'Alatri L., Paludetti G., Contarino FM., Galla S., Marchese MR., and Bentivoglio AR. (2008), 'Effects of bilateral subthalamic nucleus stimulation and medication on parkinsonian speech impairment', *J Voice, vol, 22(3), pp.365–72.*

The Deep Brain Stimulation for Parkinson's Disease Study Group. 'Deep-brain stimulation of the subthalamic nucleus or the pars interna of the globus pallidus in Parkinson's disease', *N Engl J Med, 2001, vol, 345(13), pp. 956–963.*

Bell, DS. (1968), 'Speech functions of the thalamus inferred from the effects of thalamotomy', *Brain, vol, 91(4), pp. 619–638.*

Benabid, AL., Pollak, P., Gervason, C., Hoffmann, D., Gao, DM., Hommel, M., Perret, J. E., and de, R. J. (1991), 'Long-term suppression of tremor by chronic stimulation of the ventral intermediate thalamic nucleus', *Lancet, vol, 337(8738), pp. 403–406.*

Bergman, H., Wichmann, T., and DeLong, MR. (1990), 'Reversal of experimental parkinsonism by lesions of the subthalamic nucleus', *Science., vol, 249(4975), pp. 1436–1438.*

Buck, JF. and Cooper, IS. (1956), 'Speech problems in parkinsonian patients undergoing anterior choroidal artery occlusion or chemopallidectomy', *J Am Geriatr Soc, vol, 4(12), pp. 1285–1290.*

Burghaus L., Hilker R., Thiel A., Galdikis N., Lehnhardt FG., Zaro-Weber O., Sturm V., and Heiss W-D. (2006), 'Deep brain stimulation of the subthalamic nucleus reversibly deteriorates stuttering in advanced Parkinson's Disease', *J Neural Transmission, vol, 113(5), pp. 625–631.*

Cooper, I. S., Riklan, M., Stellar, S., Waltz, JM., Levita, E., Ribera, VA., and Zimmerman, J. (1968), 'A multidisciplinary investigation of neurosurgical rehabilitation in bilateral parkinsonism', *J Am Geriatr Soc, vol, 16(11), pp. 1177–1306.*

Darley, FL., Aronson, AE., and Brown, JR. (1975), *Motor Speech Disorders*, W.B. Saunders Company. Philadelphia, London, Toronto.

De Letter, M., Santens, P., and Van Borsel, J. (2005), 'The effects of levodopa on word intelligibility in Parkinson's disease', *J Commun Disord, vol, 38(3), pp. 187–196.*

DeLong, MR., Crutcher, MD., and Georgopoulos, AP. (1983), 'Relations between movement and single cell discharge in the substantia nigra of the behaving monkey', *J.Neurosci, vol, 3(8), pp. 1599–1606.*

Deuschl, G., Herzog, J., Kleiner-Fisman, G., Kubu, C., Lozano, AM., Lyons, KE., Rodriguez-Oroz, MC., Tamma, F., Troster, AI., Vitek, JL., Volkmann, J., and Voon, V. (2006), 'Deep brain stimulation: Postoperative issues', *Mov Disord, vol, 21(S14), pp. S219–S237.*

Dromey, C. (2003), 'Spectral measures and perceptual ratings of hypokinetic dysarthria', *Journal of Medical Speech and Language Pathology, vol, 11, pp. 85–94.*

Dromey, C., Kumar, R., Lang, A. E., and Lozano, A. M. (2000), 'An investigation of the effects of subthalamic nucleus stimulation on acoustic measures of voice', *Mov Disord, vol, 15(6), pp. 1132–1138.*

Fahn S., Elton RL., UPDRS Program Members. Unified Parkinson's Disease rating scale. In: Fahn S., Marsden CD., Goldstein M., Calne DB, eds. *Recent developments in Parkinson's Disease*, Vol 2. Florham Park, NJ: Macmillan Healthcare Information; 1987. *pp. 153–163, 293–304.*

Fodstad, H. and Hariz, M.(2007), 'Electricity in the treatment of nervous system disease', *Acta Neurochir Suppl, vol, 97(Pt 1), pp. 11–19.*

Gentil, M., Chauvin, P., Pinto, S., Pollak, P., and Benabid, AL. (2001), 'Effect of bilateral stimulation of the subthalamic nucleus on parkinsonian voice', *Brain Lang, vol, 78(2), pp. 233–240.*

Gentil, M., Garcia-Ruiz, P., Pollak, P., and Benabid, AL. (1999), 'Effect of stimulation of the subthalamic nucleus on oral control of patients with parkinsonism', *J Neurol Neurosurg Psychiatry, vol, 67(3), pp. 329–333.*

Gentil, M., Pinto, S., Pollak, P., and Benabid, AL. (2003), 'Effect of bilateral stimulation of the subthalamic nucleus on parkinsonian dysarthria', *Brain Lang, vol, 85(2), pp. 190–196.*

Ghika, J., Villemure, JG., Fankhauser, H., Favre, J., Assal, G., and Ghika-Schmid, F. (1998), 'Efficiency and safety of bilateral contemporaneous pallidal stimulation (deep brain stimulation) in levodopa-responsive patients with Parkinson's disease with severe motor fluctuations: a 2-year follow-up review', *J Neurosurg, vol, 89(5), pp. 713–718.*

Goberman, AM. and Blomgren, M. (2003), 'Parkinsonian speech disfluencies: effects of L-dopa-related fluctuations', *J Fluency Disord, vol, 28(1), pp. 55–70.*

Gross, C., Rougier, A., Guehl, D., Boraud, T., Julien, J., and Bioulac, B. (1997), 'High-frequency stimulation of the globus pallidus internalis in Parkinson's disease: a study of seven cases', *J Neurosurg, vol, 87(4), pp. 491–498.*

Guiot, G., Hertzog, E., Rondot, P., and Molina, P. (1961), 'Arrest or acceleration of speech evoked by thalamic stimulation in the course of stereotaxic procedures for Parkinsonism', *Brain, vol, 84(363–79), pp. 363–379.*

Hariz, MI. (2003), 'From functional neurosurgery to 'interventional' neurology: survey of publications on thalamotomy, pallidotomy, and deep brain stimulation for Parkinson's disease from 1966 to 2001', *Mov Disord, vol, 18(8), pp. 845–853.*

Hariz, MI. and Fodstad, H. (2002), 'Deep brain stimulation in Parkinson's disease', *N Engl J Med, vol, 346(6), pp. 452–453.*

Hariz, MI., Johansson, F., Shamsgovara, P., Johansson, E., Hariz, GM., and Fagerlund, M. (2000), 'Bilateral subthalamic nucleus stimulation in a parkinsonian patient with preoperative deficits in speech and cognition: persistent improvement in mobility but increased dependency: a case study', *Mov Disord, vol, 15(1), pp. 136–139.*

Hariz, MI., Rehncrona, S., Quinn, NP., Speelman, JD., Wensig, C., and the Multicenter Advanced Parkinson's Disease Deep Brain Stimulation Group (2008), 'Multicenter study on deep brain stimulation in Parkinson's Disease: an independent assessment of reported adverse events at 4 years', *Mov Disord, vol 23(3), pp. 416–421.*

Hassler, R., Riechert, T., Mundinger, F., Umbach, W., and Gangleberger, JA. (1960), 'Physiological observations in stereotaxic operations in extrapyramidal motor disturbances', *Brain, vol, 83(337–350), pp. 337–350.*

Herzog, J., Fietzek, U., Hamel, W., Morsnowski, A., Steigerwald, F., Schrader, B., Weinert, D., Pfister, G., Muller, D., Mehdorn, HM., Deuschl, G., and Volkmann, J. (2004), 'Most effective stimulation site in subthalamic deep brain stimulation for Parkinson's disease', *Mov Disord, vol, 19(9), pp. 1050–1054.*

Horsley, VICT. and Clarke, RH. (1908), 'The structure and functions of the cerebellum examined by a new method', *Brain, vol, 31(1), pp. 45–124.*

Kent, RD. and Kim, YJ. (2003), 'Toward an acoustic typology of motor speech disorders', *Clin Linguist Phon, vol, 17(6), pp. 427–445.*

Kleiner-Fisman, G., Fisman, DN., Zamir, O., Dostrovsky, JO., Sime, E., Saint-Cyr, JA., Lozano, AM., and Lang, AE. (2004), 'Subthalamic nucleus deep brain stimulation for parkinson's disease after successful pallidotomy: clinical and electrophysiological observations', *Mov Disord, vol, 19(10), pp. 1209–1214.*

Klostermann, F., Ehlen, F., Vesper, J., Nubel, K., Gross, M., Manzinzik, F., Curio, G., andSappok, T. (2008), Effects of subthalamic nucleus deep brain stimulation on dysarthrophonia in Parkinson's Disease. *J Neurol Neurosurg Phychiatr, vol 79(5), pp. 522–529.*

Krack, P., Batir, A., Van Blercom, N., Chabardes, S., Fraix, V., Ardouin, C., Koudsie, A., Limousin, PD., Benazzouz, A., LeBas, JF., Benabid, AL., and Pollak, P. (2003), 'Five-year follow-up of bilateral stimulation of the subthalamic nucleus in advanced Parkinson's disease', *N Engl J Med, vol, 349(20), pp. 1925–1934.*

Krack, P., Fraix, V., Mendes, A., Benabid, A. L., and Pollak, P. (2002), 'Postoperative management of subthalamic nucleus stimulation for Parkinson's disease', *Mov Disord, vol, 17 Suppl 3:S188–97.*

Krack, P., Pollak, P., Limousin, P., Hoffmann, D., Xie, J., Benazzouz, A., and Benabid, AL. (1998), 'Subthalamic nucleus or internal pallidal stimulation in young onset Parkinson's disease', *Brain, vol, 121 (Pt 3), pp. 451–457.*

Krause, M., Fogel, W., Heck, A., Hacke, W., Bonsanto, M., Trenkwalder, C., and Tronnier, V. (2001), 'Deep brain stimulation for the treatment of Parkinson's disease: subthalamic nucleus versus globus pallidus internus', *J Neurol Neurosurg Psychiatry, vol, 70(4), pp. 464–470.*

Levelt, WJM. (1989), *Speaking: from intention to articulation.* MIT Press.

Limousin, P., Greene, J., Pollak, P., Rothwell, J., Benabid, AL., and Frackowiak, R. (1997), 'Changes in cerebral activity pattern due to subthalamic nucleus or internal pallidum stimulation in Parkinson's disease', *Ann Neurol, vol, 42(3), pp. 283–291.*

Limousin, P., Krack, P., Pollak, P., Benazzouz, A., Ardouin, C., Hoffmann, D., and Benabid, AL. (1998), 'Electrical stimulation of the subthalamic nucleus in advanced Parkinson's disease', *N Engl J Med, vol, 339(16), pp. 1105–1111.*

Limousin, P., Pollak, P., Benazzouz, A., Hoffmann, D., Le Bas, JF., Broussolle, E., Perret, JE., and Benabid, AL. (1995), 'Effect of parkinsonian signs and symptoms of bilateral subthalamic nucleus stimulation', *Lancet, vol, 345(8942), pp. 91–95.*

Limousin P. and Martinez-Torres I., (2008), 'Deep brain stimulation for Parkinson's disease', *Neurotherapeutics, vol, 5(2), pp.309–319.*

Logemann, J.A., Fisher, HB., Boshes, B., and Blonsky, ER. (1978), 'Frequency and cooccurrence of vocal tract dysfunctions in the speech of a large sample of Parkinson patients', *J Speech Hear Disord, vol, 43(1), pp. 47–57.*

Lyons, KE., Wilkinson, SB., Troster, AI., and Pahwa, R. (2002), 'Long-term efficacy of globus pallidus stimulation for the treatment of Parkinson's disease', *Stereotact Funct Neurosurg, vol, 79(3–4), pp. 214–220.*

Maruska, KG., Smit, AB., Koller, WC., and Garcia, JM. (2000), 'Sentence production in Parkinson's Disease treated with deep brain stimulation and medication', *J Med Speech Lang Pathol,vol, 8[4], pp. 265–270.*

McIntyre, CC., Savasta, M., Walter, BL., and Vitek, JL. (2004), 'How does deep brain stimulation work? Present understanding and future questions', *J Clin Neurophysiol, vol, 21(1), pp. 40–50.*

Metter, EJ. and Hanson, WR. (1986), 'Clinical and acoustical variability in hypokinetic dysarthria', *J Commun Disord, vol, 19(5), pp. 347–366.*

Mora, F., Mogenson, GJ., and Rolls, ET. (1977), 'Activity of neurons in the region of the substantia nigra during feeding in the monkey', *Brain Res, vol, 133(2), pp. 267–276.*

Paek SH., Han JH., Lee JY., and Kim CK., (2008), 'Electrode position determined by fused images of preoperative and postoperative MRI and surgical outcome after subthalamic nucleus deep brain stimulation', *Neurosurgery, vol, 63(5)pp.925–936.*

Pinto, S., Gentil, M., Fraix, V., Benabid, A. L., and Pollak, P. (2003), 'Bilateral subthalamic stimulation effects on oral force control in Parkinson's disease', *J Neurol, vol, 250(2), pp. 179–187.*

Pinto, S., Gentil, M., Krack, P., Sauleau, P., Fraix, V., Benabid, A. L., and Pollak, P. (2005), 'Changes induced by levodopa and subthalamic nucleus stimulation on parkinsonian speech', *Mov Disord, vol, 20(11), pp. 1507–1515.*

Pinto, S., Ozsancak, C., Tripoliti, E., Thobois, S., Limousin-Dowsey, P., and Auzou, P. (2004a), 'Treatments for dysarthria in Parkinson's disease', *Lancet Neurol, vol, 3(9), pp. 547–556.*

Pinto, S., Thobois, S., Costes, N., Le Bars, D., Benabid, AL., Broussolle, E., Pollak, P., and Gentil, M. (2004b), 'Subthalamic nucleus stimulation and dysarthria in Parkinson's disease: a PET study', *Brain, vol, 127(Pt 3), pp. 602–615.*

Plaha, P., Ben-Shlomo, Y., Patel, NK., and Gill, SS. (2006), 'Stimulation of the caudal zona incerta is superior to stimulation of the subthalamic nucleus in improving contralateral parkinsonism', *Brain, vol, 129(Pt 7), pp. 1732–1747.*

Putzer M., Barry Wj., Moringlane JR., (2008), 'Effect of bilateral stimulation of the subthalamic nucleus on different speech subsystems in patients with Parkinson's disease', *Clinical Linguistics and Phonetics, vol, 22(12): 957–978.*

Ramig, LO., Sapir, S., Fox, C., and Countryman, S. (2001), 'Changes in vocal loudness following intensive voice treatment (LSVT) in individuals with Parkinson's disease: a comparison with untreated patients and normal age-matched controls', *Mov Disord, vol, 16(1), pp. 79–83.*

Richards M., Marder K., Cote L., Mayeux R. (1994), 'Interrater reliability of the Unified Parkinson's disease Rating Scale motor examination'. *Mov Disord, vol 9 (1), pp. 89–91.*

Riecker, A., Ackermann, H., Wildgruber, D., Dogil, G., and Grodd, W. (2000), 'Opposite hemispheric lateralization effects during speaking and singing at motor cortex, insula and cerebellum', *Neuroreport, vol, 11(9), pp. 1997–2000.*

Rodriguez-Oroz, MC., Obeso, JA., Lang, AE., Houeto, JL., Pollak, P., Rehncrona, S., Kulisevsky, J., Albanese, A., Volkmann, J., Hariz, MI., Quinn, NP., Speelman, JD., Guridi, J., Zamarbide, I., Gironell, A., Molet, J., Pascual-Sedano, B., Pidoux, B., Bonnet, AM., Agid, Y., Xie, J., Benabid, AL., Lozano, AM., Saint-Cyr, J., Romito, L., Contarino, MF., Scerrati, M., Fraix, V., and Van, BN. (2005), 'Bilateral deep brain stimulation in Parkinson's disease: a multicentre study with 4 years follow-up', *Brain, vol, 128(Pt 10), pp. 2240–2249.*

Rodriguez-Oroz, MC., Rodriguez, M., Guridi, J., Mewes, K., Chockkman, V., Vitek, J., DeLong, M. R., and Obeso, J. A. (2001), 'The subthalamic nucleus in Parkinson's disease: somatotopic organization and physiological characteristics', *Brain, vol, 124(Pt 9), pp. 1777–1790.*

Rodriguez-Oroz, MC., Zamarbide, I., Guridi, J., Palmero, MR., and Obeso, JA. (2004), 'Efficacy of deep brain stimulation of the subthalamic nucleus in Parkinson's disease 4 years after surgery: double blind and open label evaluation', *J Neurol Neurosurg Psychiatry, vol, 75(10), pp. 1382–1385.*

Rosen, KM., Kent, RD., Delaney, AL., and Duffy, JR. (2006), 'Parametric quantitative acoustic analysis of conversation produced by speakers with dysarthria and healthy speakers', *J Speech Lang Hear Res, vol, 49(2), pp. 395–411.*

Rosen, KM., Kent, RD., and Duffy, JR. (2005), 'Task-based profile of vocal intensity decline in Parkinson's disease', *Folia Phoniatr Logop, vol, 57(1), pp. 28–37.*

Rousseaux, M., Krystkowiak, P., Kozlowski, O., Ozsancak, C., Blond, S., and Destee, A. (2004), 'Effects of subthalamic nucleus stimulation on parkinsonian dysarthria and speech intelligibility', *J Neurol, vol, 251(3), pp. 327–334.*

Samra, K., Riklan, M., Levita, E., Zimmerman, J., Waltz, JM., Bergmann, L., and Cooper, IS. (1969), 'Language and speech correlates of anatomically verified lesions in thalamic surgery for parkinsonism', *J Speech Hear Res, vol, 12(3), pp. 510–540.*

Santens, P., De Letter, M., Van Borsel, J., De Reuck, J., and Caemaert, J. (2003), 'Lateralized effects of subthalamic nucleus stimulation on different aspects of speech in Parkinson's disease', *Brain Lang, vol, 87(2), pp. 253–258.*

Schaltenbrand, G. (1975), 'The effects on speech and language of stereotactical stimulation in thalamus and corpus callosum', *Brain Lang, vol, 2(1), pp. 70–77.*

Siegfried, J. and Lippitz, B. (1994), 'Bilateral chronic electrostimulation of ventroposterolateral pallidum: a new therapeutic approach for alleviating all parkinsonian symptoms', *Neurosurgery, vol, 35(6), pp. 1126–1129.*

Solomon, NP., McKee, AS., Larson, KJ., Nawrocki, MD., Tuite, PJ., Eriksen, S., Low, WC., and Maxwell, RE. (2000), 'Effects of pallidal stimulationon speech in three men with severe Parkinson's Disease', *Ame J Speech Lang Pathol, 9, 241–256.*

Spiegel, EA., Wycis, HT., Marks, M., and Lee, AJ. (1947), 'Stereotaxic apparatus for operations on the human brain', *Science, vol, 106(2754), pp. 349–350.*

Tepper, JM., Abercrombie, ED., and Bolam, JP. (2007), 'Basal ganglia macrocircuits', *Prog Brain Res, vol, 160(3–7), pp. 3–7.*

Tjaden, K. and Wilding, GE. (2004), 'Rate and loudness manipulations in dysarthria: acoustic and perceptual findings', *J Speech Lang Hear Res, vol, 47(4), pp. 766–783.*

Tommasi, G., Krack, P., Fraix, V., LeBas, JF., Chabardes, S., Benabid, AL., and Pollak, P. (2007), 'Pyramidal tract side effects induced by deep brain stimulation of the subthalamic nucleus', *J Neurol Neurosurg Psychiatry, vol, 79, pp. 813–819.*

Tornqvist, AL., Schalen, L., and Rehncrona, S. (2005), 'Effects of different electrical parameter settings on the intelligibility of speech in patients with Parkinson's disease treated with subthalamic deep brain stimulation', *Mov Disord, vol, 20(4), pp. 416–423.*

Tripoliti, E., Limousin, P., Tisch, S., Borrell, E., and Hariz, MI. (2006), 'Speech in Parkinson's Disease following subthalamic nucleus deep brain stimulation: preliminary results', *J Med Speech Lang Pathol, vol 14(4), pp. 309–315.*

Tripoliti, E., Zinzro, L., Borrell, E., Frost, E., Tisch, S., Martinez, I., Hariz, M., and Limousin, P. (2008), 'Effect of contact location and voltage amplitude on speech and movement in bilateral Subthalamic nucleus deep brain stimulation', *Mov Disord, vol, 23, (16), pp. 2377–2383.*

Van Buren, JM. (1975), 'The question of thalamic participation in speech mechanisms', *Brain Lang., vol, 2(1), pp. 31–44.*

Velasco, F., Jimenez, F., Perez, ML., Carrillo-Ruiz, JD., Velasco, AL., Ceballos, J., and Velasco, M. (2001), 'Electrical stimulation of the prelemniscal radiation in the treatment of Parkinson's disease: an old target revised with new techniques', *Neurosurgery, vol, 49(2), pp. 293–306.*

Volkmann, J., Allert, N., Voges, J., Weiss, PH., Freund, HJ., and Sturm, V. (2001), 'Safety and efficacy of pallidal or subthalamic nucleus stimulation in advanced PD', *Neurology, vol, 56(4), pp. 548–551.*

Wang, EQ., Metman, LV., Bakay, RAE., Arzbaecher, J., Bernard, B., and Corcos, D. (2006), 'Hemisphere-specific effects on subthalamic nucleus deep brain stimulation on speaking rate and articulatory accuracy of syllable repetitions in Parkinson's Disease', *J Med Speech Lang Pathol, vol,14(4), 323–333.* Weismer, G. (2006), 'Philosophy of research in motor speech disorders', *Clin Linguist Phon, vol, 20, no. 5, pp. 315–349.*

Wichmann, T., Bergman, H., and DeLong, MR. 1994, 'The primate subthalamic nucleus. I. Functional properties in intact animals', *J Neurophysiol, vol, 72(2), pp. 494–506.*

Wilson, J. (2004), 'The basal ganglia'. In: *The Synaptic Organisation of the Brain*, Oxford University Press, Oxford, *pp. 361–414.*

Yelnik, J., Damier, P., Demeret, S., Gervais, D., Bardinet, E., Bejjani, BP., Francois, C., Houeto, JL., Arnule, I., Dormont, D., Galanaud, D., Pidoux, B., Cornu, P., and Agid, Y. (2003), 'Localization of stimulating electrodes in patients with Parkinson disease by using a three-dimensional atlas-magnetic resonance imaging coregistration method', *J Neurosurg, vol, 99(1), pp. 89–99.*

Yorkston, KM. and Beukelman, DR. (1981), 'Communication efficiency of dysarthric speakers as measured by sentence intelligibility and speaking rate', *J Speech Hear Disord, vol, 46(3), pp. 296–301.*

Ziegler, W. (2002), 'Psycholinguistic and motor theories of apraxia of speech', *Semin Speech Lang, vol, 23(4), pp. 231–244.*

Ziegler, W. (2003), 'Speech motor control is task-specific: Evidence from dysarthria and apraxia of speech', *Aphasiology, vol, 17(1), pp. 3–36.*

Section 6

Methods

Chapter 19

Recent advances in the physiological assessment of articulation: introducing 3D technology

Bruce E. Murdoch

Abstract

Recent years have seen the development and introduction of a range of new physiological instruments for investigating various aspects of articulatory function. Included among these techniques are electromagnetic articulography (EMA), electropalatography (EPG) and pressure-sensing EPG. The aim of this chapter is to describe and evaluate these techniques, highlighting their relative advantages, disadvantages, and specific applications in assessing articulation in normal and disordered speakers. Emphasis will be given to those instruments that enable researchers and clinicians to examine articulatory functions in three dimensions, such as 3D EPG and 3D EMA (AG500). In addition, the development and application of pressure-sensing EPG will also be outlined. Each of these physiological techniques will be described in terms of their component hardware and underlying principles of operation. Problems encountered in the development and application of each instrument will be highlighted, including difficulties with calibration, accuracy of data, transducer limitations, and so on. Research findings reported to date based on each of the above physiological instruments will be reviewed and the results summarized. Future development and potential application of 3D technologies in the rehabilitation of motor speech disorders by way of 3D physiological biofeedback will be highlighted.

19.1 Introduction

Recent years have been witness to a quantum increase in the use of physiological instrumentation in the investigation and management of motor speech disorders. The so-called 'physiological approach' to the assessment and treatment of motor speech impairments as espoused by Hardy (1967), Netsell (1986), and Murdoch (1996) evolved from the concept that assessment of the individual motor subsystems of the speech production mechanism (articulatory, velopharyngeal, laryngeal, and respiratory subsystems) was crucial in defining the underlying speech pathophysiology and consequently for enabling the development of optimal treatment programmes (Abbs and DePaul 1989; Murdoch 1996). Although it has, therefore, been recognized for some time that closer linking of the treatment of motor speech disorders to an understanding of the pathophysiology of the speech production system is likely to produce greater treatment efficacy, the success of the physiological approach has been hampered by a lack of appropriate physiological techniques. In particular, the unavailability, until recently, of instruments capable of recording, in a safe and non-invasive manner, the dynamics of articulatory movements during speech production, has greatly restricted the application of the physiological approach to the remediation of articulatory impairments seen in motor speech disorders associated with a wide range of neurological disorders.

The importance of assessing articulatory dynamics in speakers with motor speech disorders was emphasized by Hirose (1986) who stated that 'since dysarthric speech is the end product of the pathological dynamics of the articulators, its perceptual characteristics must depend on the motor characteristics of the articulators. Therefore, the analysis of the motor patterns of the articulators in dysarthric subjects seems to be a more direct approach to disclose the nature of dysarthric speech' (p. 62). Other researchers have also acknowledged the importance of dynamic physiological assessments from a speech physiology and clinical perspective (Coelho et al., 1994; Duffy 2005; McHenry et al., 1994). An obstacle to directly studying articulatory dynamics in the past, however, has been the methodological difficulties encountered in viewing and tracking movements of the articulators and, in particular, movements of the tongue, due to its confinement within the oral cavity.

Advances in technology have seen the introduction of several physiological instruments capable of assessing articulatory dynamics in a non-invasive and safe manner. Notable among these instruments are the electropalatograph (EPG), capable of recording in real time tongue to palate contacts during speech, and electromagnetic articulography (EMA) which is able to record real time movements of the tongue, lips and jaw during speech production. Although both EPG and EMA have made significant contributions to our understanding of the nature of articulatory breakdown in motor speech disorders, their application in both the assessment and treatment of these conditions has been limited by the two-dimensional (2D) nature of their outputs. For instance, traditional EPG outputs provide only 2D representations of tongue to palate contacts and consequently do not provide any indication of the influence of palatal geometry on tongue to palate contacts during speech. Likewise, the EMA systems in predominant use worldwide provide information regarding movement of the articulators in the midsagittal plane. Given that articulatory movements, and in particular tongue movements, are three-dimensional (3D) actions, in order to more accurately assess the functioning of the tongue and other articulators during speech, instruments capable of providing 3D representations of the articulators are needed. The aim of the current chapter is to provide an update of the progress in development of new techniques to quantify articulatory function, with emphasis on 3D technologies to highlight the relative advantage/disadvantages of each method. Some of the problems encountered in the development and application of new technologies for assessing the dynamics of articulation, including 3D techniques, will be outlined. Specifically three new instrumental techniques will be described and discussed, including: 3D EPG, pressure-sensing palatography (PPG), and 3D EMA.

19.2 3D Electropalatography

Electropalatography records the location and timing of tongue contacts against the hard palate during speech (Hardcastle 1996) and has proven a useful tool in both the assessment and treatment of articulatory disorders. Although several different EPG systems are available commercially, the system in most common use in laboratories and clinics worldwide is the Reading EPG-3. This latter instrument involves the use of an individually moulded artificial acrylic palate that contains an array of 62 touch sensitive miniature electrodes. The artificial palate is placed inside the mouth over the hard palate (see Fig. 19.1). A hand-held or body electrode is used to pass a small sinusoidal signal through the client's body. When the tongue contacts the electrodes on the artificial palate, a circuit is completed and an electrical signal is transmitted from the palate via lead-out wires to an external processing unit, which displays the location and pattern of contact on a computer screen, either in real time or over time, as a series of EPG frames or tongue to palate contact diagrams (see Fig. 19.2).

Traditional 2D EPG is a well-established technique being used in many speech science laboratories and clinics (Hardcastle 1996) for both the assessment and treatment of speech disordered populations, including individuals with motor speech disorders (Goozée et al., 1999, 2000; Hartelius et al., 2005; McAuliffe et al., 2007; Murdoch et al., 2000), structural abnormalities such as cleft palate, hearing impairment, and children with developmental speech disorders (Hardcastle 1996). Despite this, traditional 2D EPG is limited by the nature of its display. The classic 2D tongue to palate diagrams (see Fig. 19.2) that represent the output of the system fail to demonstrate either the unique anatomical characteristics of the individual palates or the relative spacing between the touch sensitive electrodes. Given that it is well accepted that palatal shape varies widely from individual to individual (some individuals have narrow, high-arched palates while other have broad, flat palates) and that shape influences tongue to palate contacts during speech (Goozée et al., 2003; Hiki and Itoh 1986), this failure may cause the data derived from traditional 2D EPG to be misinterpreted, especially when comparisons of the amount, location, and pattern of contacts are to be made among different speakers (e.g., narrow, high-arched palates are associated with an increased number of tongue-to-palate contacts due to closer proximity of the touch sensitive electrodes).

In an attempt to provide a solution to the limitations of traditional 2D EPG, researchers at the Motor Speech Research Centre, University of Queensland, have recently developed a 3D EPG system aimed at improving graphic representation of tongue-to-palate contacts by way of computer-generated, interactive 3D palatal models (Goozée et al., 2003). Although this latter system utilizes the same hardware and artificial acrylic palates as the traditional 2D Reading EPG-3, it provides researchers and clinicians the ability to visualize 3D images of their client's tongue-to-palate contacts during speech. Specifically, the 3D system utilizes 3D laser scanning of the EPG

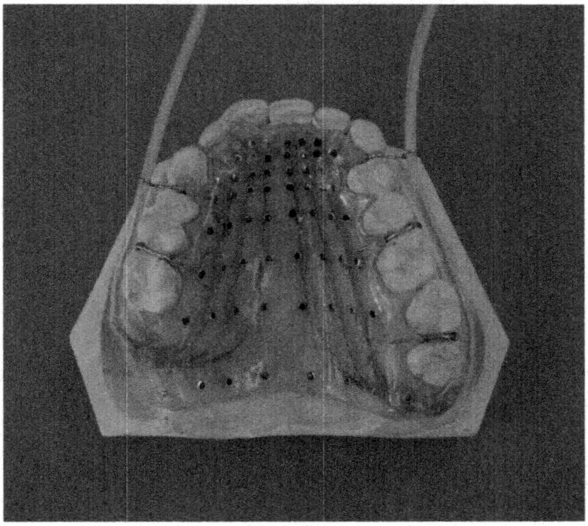

Fig. 19.1 Artificial acrylic EPG palate with 62 touch sensitive electrodes.

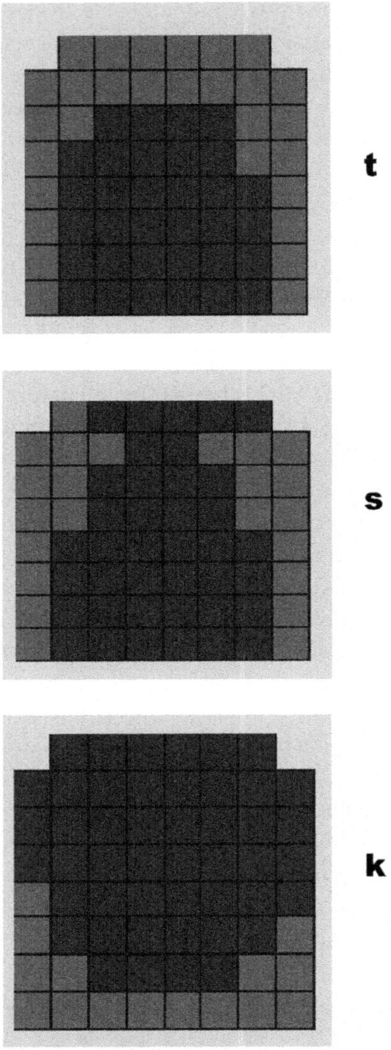

Fig. 19.2 Typical EPG tongue to palate contact diagrams for the sounds /t/, /s/ and /k/ (Lighter grey areas reflect contact areas).

palates combined with a custom-developed software package to enable simultaneous integration and display of the spatial geometry of the palate with details of tongue contact. Briefly, the dental cast of the client's hard palate required for moulding and manufacturing of the artificial palate is scanned using a portable Polhemus Fast Scan hand-held laser profile scanner connected to a personal computer. The scanner scores 3D coordinates from the surface of the cast using a projected laser line and cameras mounted at an angle to the laser line to create a 3D mesh representation of the palate (see Fig. 19.3). These coordinates are then uploaded into a custom-written software package (3D EPG viewer) to render a 3D image of the individual's palate which includes virtual sensors representative of the touch sensitive electrodes in the artificial palate and which change colour according to the position and timing of tongue contacts with the artificial palate (see Fig. 19.4).

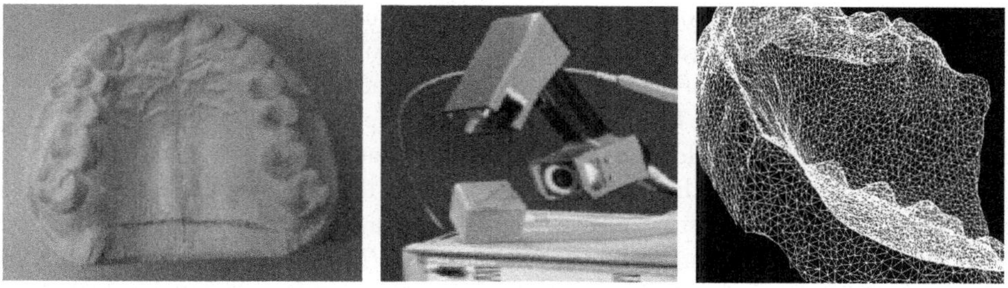

Fig. 19.3 Laser scanning of the palatal cast to create a 3D mesh image.

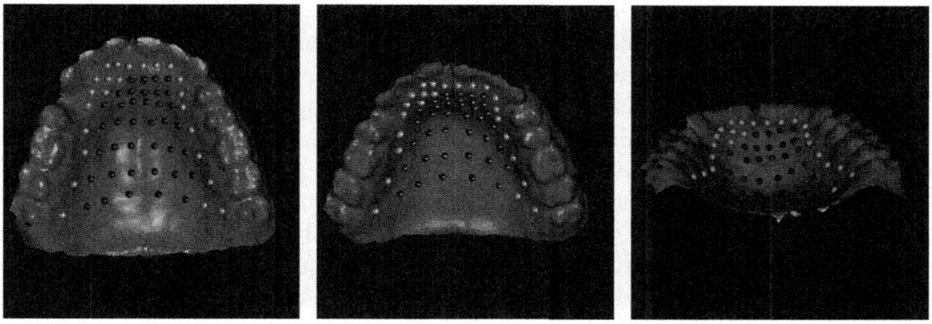

Fig. 19.4 3D image of the palate with virtual sensors showing tongue to palate contact.

Goozée et al. (2003) compared the effect of 2D versus 3D presentation on the interpretation of deviant EPG tongue to palate contact patterns by a panel of experienced speech/language pathologists. They reported that, based on presentation of the 2D diagrams, the panel of clinicians only provided a neurologically based explanation for the deviant contact patterns recorded from a group of dysarthric patients post-traumatic brain injury, neglecting the possible influence of palatal geometry. In contrast, when provided with the 3D outputs, the panel provided both anatomically based as well as neurologically based explanations for the observed discrepancies in the EPG contact patterns. These findings highlight the potential for 2D EPG diagrams to be misinterpreted leading to the application of inappropriate therapy procedures. Clearly the findings of Goozée et al. (2003) demonstrate that the 3D EPG system was superior to the traditional 2D EPG in that it provided clinicians with a better basis on which to make judgements as to the potential factors that contribute to the discrepant EPG contact patterns in their clients, thereby enabling development of more appropriate treatment strategies.

19.3 **Pressure-sensing palatography**

As outlined above, EPG allows the timing, location, and patterns of tongue contacts against the hard palate to be examined during speech and, in doing so, provides important insights into the physiological disturbances that may underlie an individual's motor speech disorder. Indeed, both timing and spatial disturbances in tongue-to-palate contacts have been described in EPG studies of dysarthric speakers (Goldstein et al., 1994; Goozée et al., 1999, 2003; Hardcastle et al., 1985; Hartelius et al., 2005; Morgan Barry 1993; Murdoch et al., 2000). The disturbances identified were posited to be responsible for, or at least to have contributed to, some of the deviant features perceived, including consonant imprecision and disturbances in speech intelligibility and rate.

Aberrant EPG findings, like those reported in the various studies of dysarthric speech, lead to the question of 'what physiological mechanism/s are responsible for those spatial and/or timing tongue-to-palate contact disturbances?' Answers to such questions would help to further specify treatment goals and guide the development of even more effective physiologically based treatment approaches. One possible mechanism underlying spatial and time disturbances might be aberrations in the pressure with which the tongue contacts the hard palate. Indeed, disturbances in the control of tongue pressure and tongue weakness have been commonly identified using static physiological measures in individuals with dysarthria (McNeil et al., 1990; Theodoros et al., 1995). Unfortunately, no instruments are currently commercially available to directly measure the dynamic tongue pressures generated during actual speech production. Consequently, the next step in the evolution of EPG is to extend its capabilities to dynamic pressure sensing. A device that records the spatial, timing, and pressure features of tongue contacts against the hard palate during speech would extend the capabilities of researchers and clinicians in determining the physiological bases of tongue dysfunction in a variety of speech disorders.

Although the development of a device to measure dynamic lingual pressures represents the new frontier in EPG, the concept of measuring tongue-to-palate pressure during speech production is by no means a new one. In the 1960s and early 1970s a series of primarily phonetic-based studies were carried out to examine lingual pressures exerted during articulation in normal and alternate conditions (e.g., different rates of speech, intensity levels) and to investigate issues such as the usefulness of lingual pressure measures in physiologically differentiating speech sounds (McGlone and Proffit 1967; McGlone et al., 1967; Proffit and McGlone 1975; Proffit et al., 1965). These studies were often limited, however, in regards to the instrumentation and the recording and analysis procedures employed with typically only one to three relatively bulky strain gauge pressures transducers, either embedded in an artificial palate or attached to the teeth, being used to record tongue pressures with little or no rationale provided regarding choice of sensor position. Pursued by only a small number of researchers, primarily McGlone and Proffit, this line of research appeared to be abandoned before the 1980s.

Recently, there has been a resurgence in interest regarding tongue-to-palate pressures, with instruments being developed by researchers in Japan and in the USA (Wakumoto et al., 1999; Yokoyama et al., 2001), in Germany (Müller et al., 2002), in France (Jeannin et al., 2008), and by researchers at the Motor Speech Research Centre, University of Queensland, Australia (Murdoch et al., 2004) for examining tongue pressures exerted against the palate during speech and/or swallowing. The development and features of the Australian prototype PPG are briefly outlined below. For a full description of the instrument, including calibration procedures, the reader is referred to Murdoch et al. (2004). A requisite for devising the Australian dynamic tongue-to-palate pressure-sensing instrument was that, in addition to measuring pressure, it would incorporate the important dynamic features and capabilities of the successful Reading EPG-3 system. That is, it would also be able to provide information regarding the timing and spatial characteristics of tongue contacts during speech. The pressure-sensing systems used in the 1960s and 1970s were limited in this regard due to a small number (typically only one to three) of relatively bulky pressure transducers being employed, resulting in inadequate coverage of sensors across the palate. To meet this criterion, an innovative sensor design was required to allow relatively small contact areas and pressures during potentially long contact times to be sampled during speech. In addition, the thickness of the sensor needed to be relatively thin, in line with dimensions of the acrylic palates that form the essential element of current EPG systems. Minimizing the thickness of the pressure-sensing palate would be expected, in turn, to minimize the impact of the palate on speech. Such capabilities would allow spatial and timing features of tongue-to-palate contacts to be measured in line with current EPG systems, together with pressure.

Following evaluation of a range of sensing techniques, Hall effect transistors (HETs) (Allegro Microsystems) were selected as the best option for the pressure sensors, with other technologies failing critical design parameters. HETs take advantage of the Lorentz force phenomenon and operate as conductors within magnetic fields, such that when they are placed in a magnetic field a voltage is induced. When the magnetic field is static, a constant voltage output is recorded from the HET. When the magnetic field density changes (e.g., a magnet moving in relation to the HET), dynamic changes in voltage output are recorded, the output voltage being proportional to the magnetic field density. For the HET to act as a pressure sensor, a magnet mounted to a deflection mechanism (e.g., cantilever beam) was required to be incorporated into the design. Figure 19.5 shows a sketch of the design and assembly of the sensor elements used in the prototype PPG. When the tongue presses against the HET sensor, the deflection mechanism and magnet move in relation to the HET, changing the magnetic field density and, in turn, the output voltage of the HET. This voltage can then be converted into an applied pressure using appropriate calibration curves and a dedicated Matlab programme to acquire and display these signals in real time, with the pressure of each sensor being depicted on a 3D palate model. The deflection mechanism selected for use in the device was a cantilever beam while the magnet selected was a neodymium (NEO29090) magnet.

In the initial prototype PPG, five pressure sensors (three in the alveolar region and two in the velar region) were embedded in an acrylic palate specifically moulded to an individual's hard palate using a replica cast, as per current EPG palates. A photograph of the prototype PPG is presented in Fig. 19.6.

On the basis of the findings of trials performed on both normal (Goozée et al., in press; Murdoch et al., 2004) and dysarthric speakers (Goozée et al., in press), it is evident that, although at the prototype stage, PPG represents the new generation of EPG, being capable of recording dynamic tongue-to-palate pressures with minimal to no interference to speech detected perceptually. Further, PPG has been shown to be sufficiently sensitive to detect tongue pressure differences between different consonants and was reported to be able to register lingual pressures for all of the alveolar consonants examined by Murdoch et al. (2004). Despite this, as is expected in the case of instruments at the prototype stage of development, further refinements and improvements to the instrument are needed. For instance, the restricted number of pressure sensors in the prototype PPG has been reported to cause some problems in the optimal positioning of the pressure sensor to detect consonant lingual pressures (Murdoch et al., 2004). This problem, however, is expected to be largely overcome by increasing the number of pressure sensors in the palate

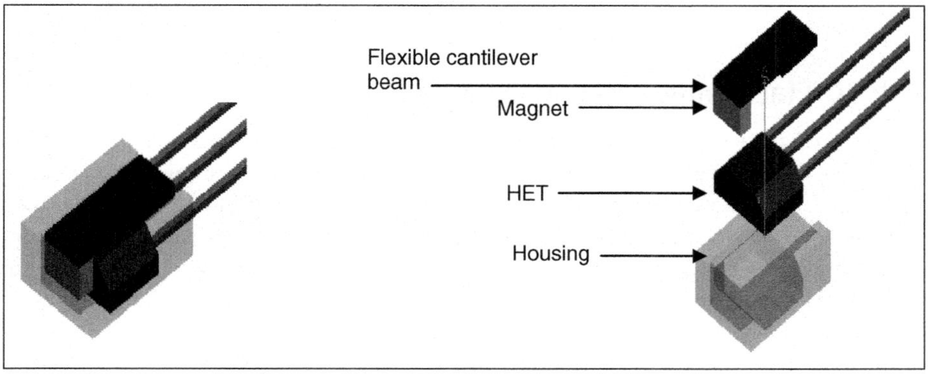

Fig. 19.5 Sketch of Hall effect pressure sensor unit used in prototype pressure sensing palate.

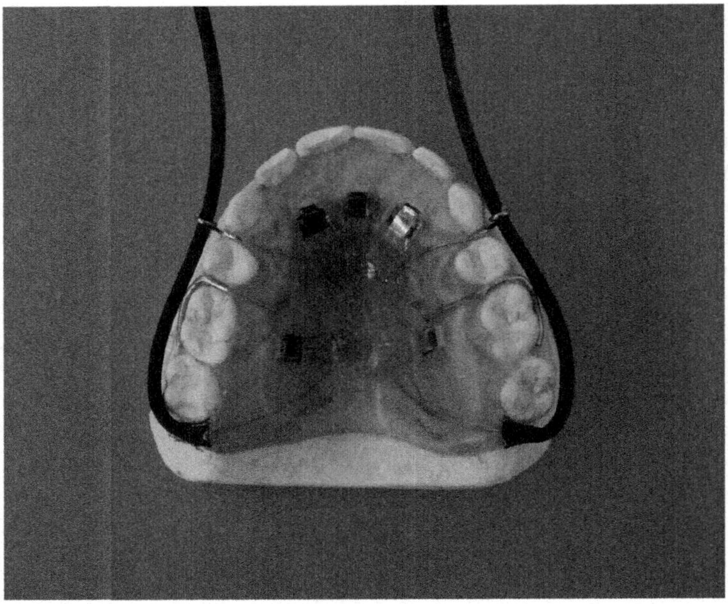

Fig. 19.6 Photograph of prototype pressure-sensing palate, with five embedded pressure sensors (three in anterior region and two posterior).

thereby increasing sensor coverage across the palate. Further refinements of the prototype PPG are also currently in progress including optimization of the artificial palate using future polymer concepts with the intended goal of producing a flexible palate substructure that can be reused and moulded to a person's hard palate. In addition, investigations are currently underway to replace the bulk magnet with a magnetic film attached to the cantilever beam thereby enabling reduction in the size of each sensor and an increase in the number of sensors embedded in the artificial palate. An upgraded data analysis programme for the PPG is currently being written to allow for 3D pressure field displays for use in real time biofeedback applications.

Overall, despite the need for further development and refinement, the PPG has already proven to be a useful addition to the battery of instruments currently available to assess tongue function during speech. PPG has the potential to extend the capabilities of researchers and clinicians in determining the physiological bases of tongue dysfunction in a variety of speech disorders thereby enabling more specific treatment goals to be devised that target the underlying physiological disturbance/s.

19.4 **3D Electromagnetic articulography**

Electromagnetic articulography is a technique for tracking articulatory movements during speech using alternating electromagnetic fields. Specifically, the movements of miniature receiver coils, which can be fixed to various articulators, including the tongue, upper and lower lips, jaw and velum, are detected and recorded over time. In the case of 2D EMA systems currently in most frequent use, these movements are recorded along the midsagittal plane (Hasegawa-Johnson 1998; Kaburagi and Honda 1997, 2002; Schönle et al., 1987; Wakamiya et al., 2003). The first commercially available 2D EMA system, the AG100, was developed by Carstens Medizinelektronik in 1988. Since that time, an upgraded 2D EMA, the AG200, has also been released. In both the AG100 and AG200 2D EMA systems transmitter coils, housed in an assembly that fits around a person's head and positioned in the midsagittal plane, generate alternating magnetic fields at different frequencies, which in turn induce alternating signals in a set of miniature receiver coils (see Fig. 19.7). The distance between a single receiver coil and a transmitter coil can be determined by the magnitude (or relative strength) of the alternating electrical signal induced in the receiver coil, as it will be inversely proportioned to the cube of the distance from the transmitter coil (Perkell et al., 1992; Schönle et al., 1987), provided the transmitter and receiver coil axes are in parallel alignment. The alternating signal induced in a receiver coil placed within the magnetic fields generated by the transmitter coils is comprised of signal components of differing frequencies that match the frequencies of the transmitter coils. By separating the signal components at each receiver coil and determining the distance between the receiver coil and each transmitter coil using the magnitude of each signal component, the location (x-y coordinates) of the receiver coil within the 2D representation of articulator movements along the midsagittal parameters can be computed, including the velocity, acceleration/deceleration, displacement and duration of articulatory movements. To date 2D EMA has been used to study articulatory kinematics in a range of normal and disordered speakers including: children (Murdoch and Goozée 2003) and adults (Kuruvilla et al., 2007) with dysarthria subsequent to traumatic brain injury; adults with dysarthria post-stroke (Chen et al., 2008); and speech disordered children exhibiting differentiated and undifferentiated lingual gestures (Goozée et al., 2007a). The technique has also been used to investigate lingual kinematic strategies used to increase speech rate in younger and older adults (Goozée et al., 2007b). For a recent review of the use of 2D EMA see Van Lieshout (2006).

Despite the ability of 2D EMA systems to identify aberrant articulatory kinematics in speakers with motor speech disorders associated with a variety of neurological conditions, the greatest limitation of 2D EMA is its restriction to tracking movements in the midsagittal plane. A major consequence of this limitation is that 2D EMA is not able to monitor substantial lateral deviations of the tongue and jaw from the midline (e.g., as occurs in flaccid dysarthria associated with unilateral lesioning of the XIIth cranial nerve) without error. To overcome this limitation, Carstens Medizinelektronik has more recently developed the AG500 EMA which is capable of tracking articulatory movements in three dimensions. The 3D EMA involves six transmitter coils housed within a plastic box-like helmet (see Fig. 19.8). Importantly, unlike the 2D EMA systems, the 3D EMA helmet does not restrict movement of the individual undergoing assessment which facilitates the use of the instrument with children (who are more prone to movement than adults) and persons with movement disorders (e.g., Parkinson's disease, Huntington's disease, etc.).

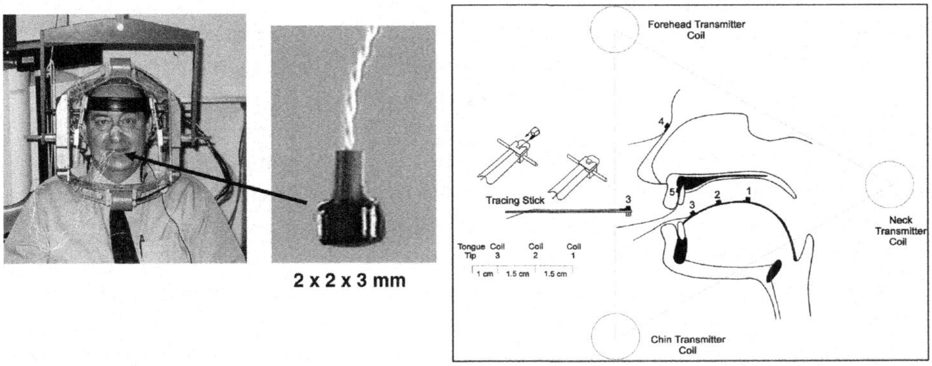

Fig. 19.7 2D electromagnetic articulograph showing the helmet and transmitter coils, miniature receiver coil and typical placements for receiver coils on the articulators in the midsagittal plane.

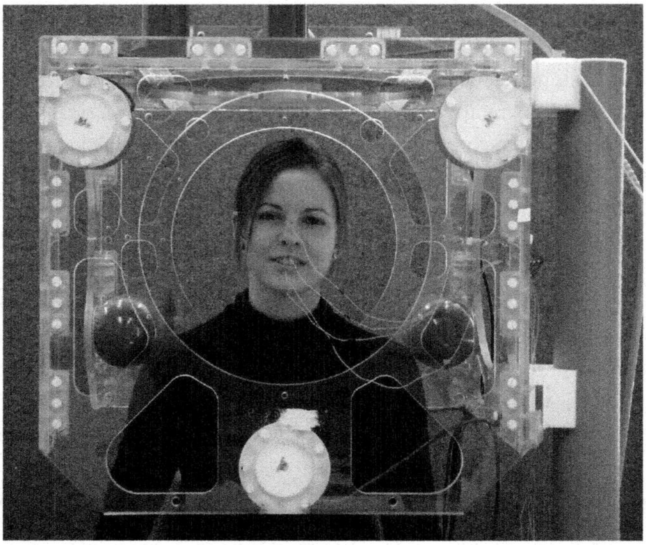

Fig. 19.8 3D electromagnetic articulograph (AG500).

Importantly, the 3D EMA system allows not only full spatial recording of sensor movement, but also measurement of the sensor orientation. Consequently, unlike 2D EMA, lateral tongue and jaw movements provide a source of information rather than error. Given that the AG500 can track articulatory movements in 3D raises the possibility that movement signals (e.g., tongue movement) acquired by the AG500 may be able to be translated into visual representations (e.g., of tongue movement) that could be utilized in biofeedback therapy for the treatment of a range of articulatory disorders as has been tested with 2D EMA (Katz et al., 1999, 2007a, b). Prior to the use of the AG500 in this type of application, however, a number of inherent limitations need to be overcome.

In practical terms, one of the most hindering aspects of the AG500 system in its original form was its inability to display the trajectory data in real time or at least at the end of each sweep. This was a direct consequence of the computational complexity in solving the positional coordination from the sensor coil amplitudes. Without immediate feedback of sensor trajectory the researcher/clinician/operator is unable to ascertain problems that may arise with coil placement and their connectivity to the participant's body. If one or more sweeps are invalidated due to a loose sensor, for example, this could jeopardise the complete assessment thus requiring the assessment to be repeated. In the case of participants with serious neurological deficits, such a repeat may not be practical or desirable. Fortunately, a recent upgrade of the AG500 system has eliminated this problem, with real time display of the trajectory data now possible.

A second limitation of the AG500 relates to complexity of the calibration procedure. There are six variables pertaining to the calibration of each sensor coil and it is important that each of these fall within a given range of values in order to obtain accurate trajectory measures from the system. Although in the author's laboratory a Matlab programme has been written to assist this evaluation, in practice it has been the author's experience that it remains difficult to get all 12 sensors to fully comply. Problems with the AG500 calibration system, called the Circal, were also raised by Zierdt (2007) who stated that a basic calibration problem exists in that the Circal neglects sensor orientation outside of the x-y plane. To test the spatial accuracy of the AG500 system, the Circal is rotated through 360°. Ideally, the positional data should prescribe a perfect circle in the x-y

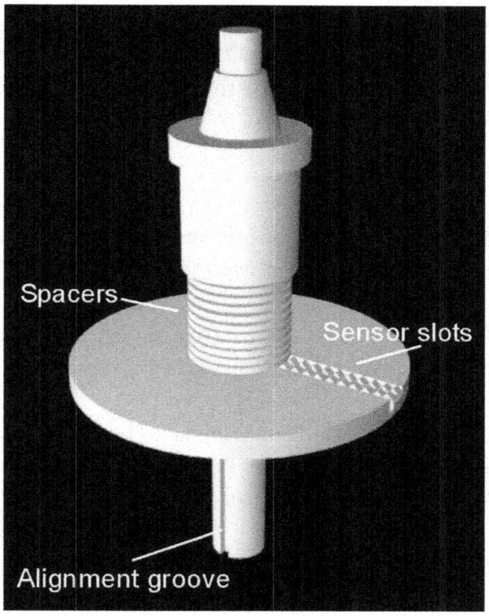

Fig. 19.9 New Circal device for the AG500.

plane and remain static in the vertical plane. In practice this is often not true, with distortions regularly appearing along these test circumferences, indicating limitations with either the calibration/reconstruction algorithms or possibly the structure of the magnetic field itself. In an attempt to correct these distortions, researchers at the Motor Speech Research Centre, University of Queensland, have designed and produced a new Circal device (see Fig. 19.9) that allows measurements to be taken both radially and vertically, thus enabling a complete 3D description of the distortion across the whole measurement field of the AG500 and thereby allowing for calculation of appropriate corrections.

Once issues relating to calibration are overcome, the 3D EMA has the potential to provide, for the first time, the opportunity to quantify lingual, jaw and lip movements during speech in three dimensions. In this way, 3D EMA will provide a greater understanding of the physiology of articulatory function in normal speech as well as the pathophysiology of articulatory breakdown in speech disorders associated with neurological diseases, orofacial abnormalities (e.g., cleft palate), etc. Further 3D EMA would appear to offer an unprecedented opportunity to develop 3D visual models of the tongue for use in physiological biofeedback programmes for the treatment of a range of articulatory disorders. The AG500 EMA system therefore has potential to be used not only as a research tool but also clinically as a biofeedback device.

19.5 **Conclusion**

Articulation of speech is a highly complex and relatively poorly understood process that is dependent on the precise and coordinated movements of the tongue, lips, and jaw. For most of our history, with the possible exception of studies based on x-ray microbeam and ultrasound techniques, the secrets of tongue function in speech remained hidden within the confines of the oral cavity due to a lack of appropriate instrumentation. Only relatively recently have tools and instruments in the form of 2D technologies such as 2D EPG and 2D EMA provided a means of visualizing, in a limited way, the functioning of the tongue and other articulators during speech.

The 3D technologies outlined above, when fully developed, have the potential to provide unprecedented opportunities to quantify normal and disordered articulatory function from a more realistic 3D perspective with direct benefits for the development of more efficacious treatment approaches for a wide range of speech disorders.

References

Abbs JH and DePaul R (1989). Assessment of dysarthria: the critical prerequisite to treatment. In MM Leahy, ed. *Disorders of Communication: The Science of Intervention*, pp. 206–227. Taylor & Francis, London.

Chen Y-T, Murdoch BE and Goozée JV (2008). Electromagnetic articulographic assessment of tongue function in dysarthric and nondysarthric speakers following stroke. *Journal of Medical Speech-Language Pathology*, *16*, 22–32.

Coelho CA, Gracco VL, Fourakis M, Rossetti M and Oshima K (1994). Application of instrumental techniques in the assessment of dysarthria. A case study. In JA Till, KM Yorkston and DR Beukelman, eds. *Motor Speech Disorders: Advances in Assessment and Treatment*, pp. 103–118. Paul H Brooks, Baltimore.

Duffy JR (2005). *Motor Speech Disorders: Substrates, Differential Diagnosis and Management.* Mosby, St Louis.

Goldstein P, Ziegler W, Vogel M and Hoole P (1994). Combined palatal-lift and EPG-feedback therapy in *dysarthria*: a case study. *Clinical Linguistics and Phonetics*, 8, 201–218.

Goozée JV, LaPointe LL and Murdoch BE (2003). Effects of speaking rate on EMA-derived lingual kinematics: a *preliminary* investigation. *Clinical Linguistics and Phonetics*, 17, 375–381.

Goozée JV, Murdoch BE, Ozanne A, Cheng Y, Hill A and Gibbon F (2007a). Lingual kinematics and coordination in speech-*disordered* children exhibiting differentiated versus undifferentiated lingual gestures, 42, 1–22.

Goozée JV, Murdoch BE and Theodoros, DG (1999). Electropalatographic assessment of articulatory timing *characteristics* in dysarthria following traumatic brain injury. *Journal of Medical Speech-Language Pathology*, 7, 209–222.

Goozée JV, Murdoch BE, Theodoros DG and Stokes PD (2000). Kinematic analysis of tongue movements in *dysarthria* following traumatic brain injury using electromagnetic articulography. *Brain Injury*, 14, 153–174.

Goozée JV, Stephenson DK, Murdoch BE, Darnell RE and LaPointe LL (2007b). Lingual kinematic strategies used to increase speech rate: comparison between younger and older adults. *Clinical Linguistics and Phonetics*, 19, 319–334.

Goozée JV, Seow N, Scott D, Murdoch BE, Meyers I and Veidt M (in press) Investigating tongue-to-palate pressures during speech in dysarthria following traumatic brain injury. *Clinical Linguistics and Phonetics.*

Hardcastle WJ (1996). Current developments in instrumentation for studying supraglottal structures. In MJ Ball and M Duckworth, eds. *Advances in Clinical Phonetics*, pp. 27–49. John Benjamins, Amsterdam.

Hardcastle WJ, Morgan Barry RA and Clark CJ (1985). Articulatory and voicing characteristics of adult dysarthric and verbal dyspraxic speakers: an instrumental study. *British Journal of Disorders of Communication*, 20, 249–270.

Hardy JC (1967). Suggestions for physiological research in dysarthria. *Cortex*, 3, 128–156.

Hartelius L, Theodoros DG and Murdoch BE (2005). Use of electropalatography in the treatment of disordered articulation following traumatic brain injury: a case study. *Journal of Medical Speech-Language Pathology*, 13, 189–204.

Hasegawa-Johnson M (1998). Electromagnetic exposure safety of the Carstens Articulograph AG100. *Journal of the* Acoustical *Society of America*, 104, 2529–2532.

Hiki S and Itoh H (1986). Influence of palate shape on lingual articulation. *Speech Communication*, 5, 141–158.

Hirose H (1986). Pathophysiology of motor speech disorders (dysarthria). *Folia Phoniatrica et Logopaedica*, 88, 61–88.

Jeannin, C, Perrier, P, Payan, Y, Dittmar, A and Grosgogeat, B (2008). Tongue pressure recordings during speech using complete denture. *Materials Science and Engineering C*, *28*(5), 835–841.

Kaburagi T and Honda M (1997). Calibration methods of voltage-to-distance function for an electromagnetic articulometer (EMA) system. *Journal of the Acoustical Society of America*, 101, 2391–2394.

Kaburagi T and Honda M (2002). Electromagnetic articulograph based on a nonparametric representation of the magnetic field. *Journal of the Acoustical Society of America*, 111, 1414–1421.

Katz, WF, Bharadwaj, SV and Carstens, B (1999). Electromagnetic articulography treatment for an adult with Broca's aphasia and apraxia of speech. *Journal of Speech Language and Hearing Research*, 42(6), 1355–1366.

Katz, WF., Carter, GC and Levitt, JS (2007a). Treating buccofacial apraxia using augmented kinematic feedback. *Aphasiology*, 21(12), 1230–1247.

Katz, WF, Garst, DM, Carter, GS, McNeil, MR, Fossett, TR, Doyle, PJ, et al. (2007b). Treatment of an individual with aphasia and apraxia of speech using EMA visually-augmented feedback. *Brain and Language*, 103(1–2), 213–214.

Kuruvilla M, Murdoch BE and Goozée JV (2007). Electromagnetic articulography assessment of articulatory function in adults with dysarthria following traumatic brain injury. *Brain Injury*, 21, 601–613.

McAuliffe MJ, Ward EC and Murdoch BE (2007). Intra-participant variability in Parkinson's disease: an electropalatographic examination of articulation. *Advances in Speech Language Pathology*, 9, 13–19.

McGlone RE and Proffit WR (1967). Lingual pressures associated with speaker consistency and syllable varisations. *Phonetics*, 17, 178–183.

McGlone RE, Proffit WR and Christiansen RL (1967). Lingual pressures associated with alveolar consonants. *Journal of Speech and Hearing Research*, 10, 606–615.

McHenry MA, Minton JT and Wilson RL (1994). Increasing the efficiency of articulatory force testing of *adults* with traumatic brain injury. In JA Till, KM Yorkston and DR Beukelman, eds. *Motor Speech Disorders: Advances in Assessment and Treatment*. Paul H Brookes, Baltimore.

McNeil MR, Weismer G, Adams S and Mulligan M (1990). Oral structure nonspeech motor control in normal, dysarthric *and* apraxic speakers: isometric force and static position control. *Journal of Speech and Hearing Research*, 33, 255–268.

Morgan Barry R (1993). Measuring segmental timing in pathological speech using electropalatography. *Clinical Linguistics and Phonetics*, 7, 275–283.

Müller R, Rose A, Hohlfeld O, Blechschmidt R, Schuster G and Werthschutzky R (2002). Telemetric pressure measurement system for orthodontic application. *Sensors and Systems*, International Conference, 24–27 June, St Petersburg, Russia.

Murdoch BE (1996). Physiological rehabilitation of disordered speech following closed head injury. In BP Uzzell and *HH* Stonnington, eds. *Recovery After Traumatic Brain Injury*, pp. 163–184. Lawrence Erlbaum, New Jersey.

Murdoch BE, Gardiner F and Theodoros DG (2000). Electropalatographic assessment of articulatory dysfunction in multiple sclerosis: a case study. *Journal of Medical Speech-Language Pathology*, 8, 359–364.

Murdoch BE and Goozée JV (2003). EMA analysis of tongue function in children with dysarthria following traumatic brain injury. *Brain Injury*, 17, 79–93.

Murdoch BE, Goozée JV, Veidt M, Scott D and Meyers IA (2004). Introducing the pressure-sensing palatograph: the next frontier in electropalatography. *Clinical Linguistics and Phonetics*, 18, 433–445.

Netsell R (1986). *A Neurologic View of the Dysarthrias.* College-Hill Press, San Diego.

Perkell JS, Cohen MH, Svirsky MA, Matthies ML, Garabieta I and Jackson MTT (1992). Electromagnetic midsagittal articulometer systems for transducing speech articulatory movements. *Journal of the Acoustical Society of America,* 92, 3078–3096.

Proffit WR and McGlone RE (1975). Tongue-lip pressures during speech of Australian aborigines. *Phonetica,* 32, 200–220.

Proffit WR, Palmer JM and Kydd WL (1965). Evaluation of tongue pressures during speech. *Folia Phoniatrica et Logopaedica,* 17, 115–128.

Schönle PW, Grabe K, Wenig P, Hohne J, Schrader J and Conrad B (1987). Electromagnetic articulography: use of alternating magnetic fields for tracking movements of multiple points inside and outside the vocal tract. *Brain and Language,* 31, 26–35.

Theodoros DG, Murdoch BE and Stokes P (1995). A physiological analysis of articulatory dysfunction in dysarthric speakers following severe closed head injury. *Brain Injury,* 9, 237–254.

Van Lieshout, PHHM (2006). La utilización de la articulografia mediosagital electromagnética en la investigación sobre movilidad oral [The use of Electro-Magnetic Midsagittal Articulography in oral motor research]. In E. Padrós-Serrat (Ed.), *Bases diagnósticas terapéuticas y posturales del funcionalismo craneofacial* (pp. 1140–1156). Madrid: Ripano.

Wakamiya K, Kaburagi T, Honda M and Sawada M (2003). An investigation on the measurement accuracy of the three-dimensional electromagnetic articulograph. *Journal of the Acoustical Society of America,* 114, 302–307.

Wakumoto M, Masaki S, Honda K, Kusakawa N and Ohue T (1999). Integration of three-dimensional and pressure sensitive palatography for speech production study. *Journal of the Acoustical Society of America,* 105, 1355.

Yokoyama M, Sonies BC, Michiwaki Y and Michi K (2001). Effects of age, gender and race on lingua-palatal pressure during swallows of varing firmness. *Paper presented at Dysphagia Research Society Annual Meeting, October, Albuquerque, NM.*

Zierdt A (2007). EMA and the crux of calibration. *Proceedings of the International Congress on Phonetic* Sciences *(ICPhS XVI), Saarbrücken,* pp. 593–596.

Chapter 20

Five-dimensional articulography

Phil Hoole and Andreas Zierdt

Abstract

Current developments in the use of five-dimensional electromagnetic articulography for speech research are reviewed. Obvious advantages are the higher information density per sensor (three Cartesian coordinates, two spherical coordinates) compared to traditional 2D EMMA systems, and removal of the necessity to constrain the subject's head. The drawbacks are equally related to this higher dimensional space: position calculation involves solving a non-linear optimization problem. In some cases, unstable solutions are encountered, resulting in mistrackings.

On the positive side, we illustrate how the higher information density allows particularly succinct and robust characterizations of tongue configuration. Discussion also focuses on monitoring of head movement. This is crucial for accurate recovery of articulator movements themselves, but is also intrinsically interesting as part of speech motor activity. In addition to improving the naturalness of the speaking situation, the freedom of head movement also means that subjects tolerate longer recording sessions. This can facilitate new experimental paradigms.

Regarding drawbacks (and ways around them), instabilities in position calculation are illustrated and it is shown how a first estimate of the measured positions can be used as a starting point for a more robust estimate, taking the continuity of speech movements into account. Diagnostics for assessing the reliability of the final solution are outlined. While work remains to be done to ensure the same accuracy over the whole 5D-measurement space, it is concluded that the system already offers unparalleled scope for large-scale acquisition of flesh-point data.

20.1 Introduction

Electromagnetic midsagittal articulography (EMMA) systems have now been in routine use for phonetic research for some 15 years. With the increasing availability of so-called three-dimensional (3D) systems (in the form of the commercially available AG500 system [Carstens Medizinelektronik] and the Aurora system [NDI]) it seems now an opportune time to take stock of some of the specific advantages of this latest generation system, but also of the additional complexity in processing the data. Both of these aspects are encapsulated in the fact that a system such as the AG500 is better regarded as a **five**-dimensional (5D) system. On the one hand, the amount of information provided by each sensor is substantially increased compared to the old 2D systems, consisting now of three Cartesian coordinates (x, y, and z) and two angular coordinates (azimuth and elevation). Within the overall context of flesh-point measurement systems, this gives such an electromagnetic system some very useful advantages, practical examples of which will be presented in the first section below. On the other hand, deriving this 5D information for each sensor from the raw data (consisting of the signal induced by six transmitter coils) consists of a search for an optimal solution in a correspondingly high-dimensional space. As Kaburagi et al. (2005, p.440) have remarked, 'a complicated non-linear problem must be solved'. Some of the difficulties that typically need to be grappled with are illustrated in the second part of the chapter.

20.2 Benefits of high-dimensional sensor data

In this section, we will first recap by way of background the main differences between the new 5D systems and old 2D systems. Secondly, we will illustrate the use of the angular coordinates that are new to the 5D system from two points of view: (1) capturing phonetically relevant aspects of tongue shape; (2) potentially increasing the robustness of the data. Thirdly, we will discuss issues related to the monitoring of head movement. The fact that the higher dimensionality of the data means that the subject's head no longer has to be constrained is perhaps the simplest but nonetheless quite possibly the most useful advantage of moving beyond measurements in two dimensions.

20.2.1 Background to EMA and EMMA

In a traditional two-dimensional (2D) EMMA system the movements of sensors attached to structures on the midsagittal plane of the subject (e.g., upper and lower lip, jaw, three or four locations on the tongue) can be tracked at sampling rates of typically at least 200Hz.[1] For best accuracy, the main axis of the sensor coils must remain aligned in parallel with the main axis of the transmitter coils. In other words, the midsagittal plane of the subject must be kept in alignment with the measurement plane of the system. This makes it necessary to have a firm attachment between the head of the subject and the helmet holding the three transmitters. The three-transmitter design makes it possible to compensate to a certain extent for movements off the measurement plane, and for misalignment of the sensors, but such changes in lateral position or in alignment cannot actually be directly measured (see e.g., Hoole and Nguyen [1999] for more background).

In the newer 5D systems exactly the same sensors can be used, but by using more transmitters, namely six, it is possible to recover the theoretical maximum information yield of such a sensor. This consists of the three positional coordinates (x, y, z) and two angular coordinates. The latter coordinates in effect define in a spherical coordinate system the direction in which the sensor is pointing. The coordinates are often referred to as azimuth, which is angular position in the xy-plane (normally the axial or transversal plane of a human subject), and elevation, which is angular displacement out of the xy-plane. For the kind of sensors currently in use in the AG500 system (and previous 2D EMMA systems) there is a further rotational degree of freedom of the sensors which cannot be captured: The system is 'blind' to rotations about the main axis of the sensor, since this does not cause any change in the electromagnetic induction.

In a 2D EMMA system, there is essentially no choice in terms of orientation when attaching sensors to the tongue: As just mentioned, the main axis of the sensor must be parallel to the

[1] The sampling rate for the AG500 system is currently fixed at 200Hz, but it may be possible to increase it in future. The sampling rate of the Aurora system was initially much lower (see Kröger et al., 2008), but has increased in more recent revisions.

transmitter coils. In a 5D EMA system there are different possibilities: If the main axis of the sensor is aligned parallel to the midline of the tongue (essentially at right-angles to the orientation used in the 2D system), then the elevation component of the angular coordinates in effect represents the angle of a tangent to the midline contour of the tongue at the sensor location, and is thus the angular component most closely related to the midline shape of the tongue. This information will be used for the detailed example in Section 20.2.2 below.

20.2.2 **Use of angular coordinates**

In this section, we illustrate the use of the angular coordinates derived for each sensor to provide phonetically useful information, since this new feature of the system has not yet found wide usage in analysis of speech movements. By way of example, we will use some data on consonantal articulation in Moroccan Arabic (see e.g., Zeroual et al., 2007). In Arabic, the so-called emphatic consonants form an interesting feature of the consonantal system. The emphatic consonants are traditionally regarded as being distinguished from the non-emphatic counterparts by pharyngealization, i.e., a secondary articulation involving retraction of the tongue root. However, it has been suggested that there are also characteristic differences at the front part of the tongue, with the emphatic (coronal) consonants being apical and the non-emphatic counterparts laminal.

Figure 20.1 shows data for ten consonant categories as spoken by one speaker (seven repetitions per category, all spoken intervocalically between low vowels). The labels used in the figures are as follows: lower-case 't, d, s' label the non-emphatic consonants and upper-case 'T, D, S' their emphatic counterparts. In addition a nasal, a lateral, a flap and a postalveolar fricative are shown, labelled 'n, l, r, sh', respectively.

The top left panel of the figure shows a traditional mid-sagittal view of the tongue-tip. Mostly there is quite a clear separation of the categories, but there is some overlap between non-emphatic /s/ and emphatic /S/, and emphatic /T/ overlaps not only emphatic /D/ but also non-emphatic /d/.

In the top right panel of Fig. 20.1 we have plotted the elevation component of the angular coordinates for two sensors: that from the tongue-tip on the y-axis, that from the tongue-back (the rearmost tongue sensor in this experiment) on the x-axis. As an aid to interpretation the four corners of the schematic plot at the bottom right of the figure show the orientation of these two tongue sensors at the extreme values of the x and y axes, corresponding to the orientation of the sensors that would be seen by an observer viewing tongue configuration in the sagittal plane (as outlined in the previous section, these orientation vectors here represent a tangent to the midline contour of the tongue at the sensor locations). Thus low values on the y-axis indicate that the tongue-tip is oriented more or less horizontally, while high values indicate that the tongue-tip is angled up, presumably corresponding to a more apical configuration of the tongue. It is interesting to note that the separation between the consonant categories is even more clear-cut in this representation than in the previous Cartesian representation of the tongue-tip: for example, the distinction between emphatic /S/ and non-emphatic /s/ is clearer, and also between non-emphatic /d/ and emphatic /T/, as well as between /n/ and other consonants. Thus, these two angular parameters appear to give a very succinct characterization of important features of the tongue shape.

Many variations on this general approach are conceivable, although they cannot be presented here: For example, if sensors are mounted at right-angles to the midline of the tongue and not only on the midline itself but also lateral to it, then angular information could help to reconstruct the tongue shape in the coronal plane.

A further attractive feature of the angular coordinates is that – at least in some experimental situations – they represent very robust information. Let us imagine a worst-case scenario in which all reference sensors used to compensate for head-movement failed. This situation is simulated in the bottom left panel of Fig. 20.1 for the traditional sagittal Cartesian coordinates of the tongue-tip.

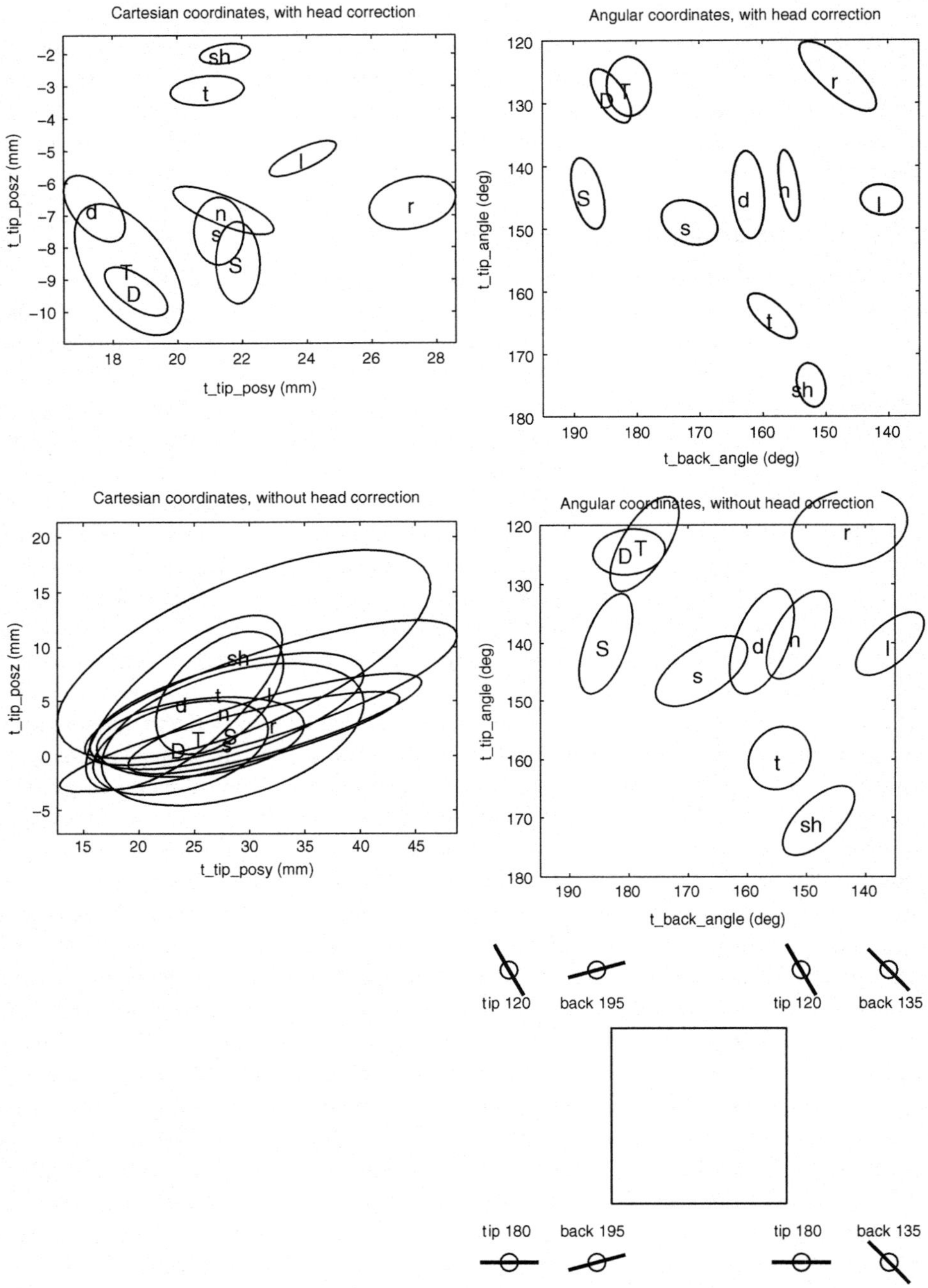

Fig. 20.1 Left column: Traditional sagittal view of position of tongue-tip for articulation of Moroccan Arabic consonants in /aCa/ context. See text for explanation of category labels. Anterior is to the left. Right column: Representation of tongue configuration using orientation of the tip and back sensors in the mid-sagittal plane. Top row: Tongue data after compensation for head movement. Second row: Data without compensation for head movement. Bottom right panel: Schematic illustration of tongue sensor orientations in the sagittal plane, corresponding to the extreme positions on the x and y axes in the two panels above.

Clearly, any regularities in the data have essentially disappeared. This is not surprising: even in a simple lab-speech experiment with the subject sitting quietly in a chair reading prompts from a computer screen then a few centimetres of head translation is likely to occur over the course of the session. This will essentially swamp any linguistic distinctions, which – as can be seen in the top left panel – will normally play out over a range of no more than 1 cm.

On the other hand, in this kind of setup changes in the orientation of the head are likely to be quite small, or at least small relative to the linguistically induced range of orientations which here amounts to about 50 degrees for both sensors. Accordingly, the bottom right panel of the figure shows the same angular data as in the top right panel, but without head-movement correction. It will readily be observed that the separation between the consonant categories is still very clear-cut. While many subjects may change the orientation of their head more than this subject (who rarely exceeded 5°, as indicated by the fact that it was possible to keep the same axis scaling for top and bottom panels on the right), it can still be expected that the robustness of the orientation information will exceed that of the translational information, if thought of as the ratio of linguistically induced changes to posturally induced changes.

This has admittedly been chosen as an extreme example; nevertheless, the next section will show that it is certainly realistic to expect – if not complete failure – then at least some variability in the quality of head-movement correction.

20.2.3 **Monitoring head movement**

In this subsection, we will use monitoring of head movement as a topic to firstly drive home the point about the high information density per sensor, going on to point out some practical issues in correcting for head movement. We will then give an example of where head movement can represent linguistically relevant behaviour in its own right. Finally, we will briefly point out interesting experimental paradigms that become much more feasible when the subject no longer needs to be physically attached to the transmitter assembly.

20.2.3.1 Capturing the degrees of freedom of head movement

In a 2D EMMA system, compensating for head movement involves capturing translation and rotation in the sagittal plane, i.e., two translations and one rotation, typically using sensors mounted on the upper incisors and the bridge of the nose. In the new system, head movement is not restricted, so the requirement is to capture the full six degrees of freedom that characterize rigid-body motion, consisting of three translations and three rotations. In analogy to a ship or aircraft the three rotational components of the head considered as a rigid body can be defined as,

(1) pitch: rotation about an axis perpendicular to the sagittal plane, i.e., about an axis parallel to the lateral axis (the main component of nodding movements to indicate 'yes')

(2) roll: rotation about an axis perpendicular to the coronal plane, i.e., about an axis parallel to the anterior-posterior axis (inclining the head towards the shoulder)

(3) yaw: rotation about an axis perpendicular to the transversal plane, i.e., about an axis parallel to the vertical axis (the main component of shaking movements to indicate 'no').

It is instructive to consider how many sensors are necessary to capture all six degrees of freedom. One might assume that because more degrees of freedom need to be captured than in a midsagittal EMMA system then more sensors must also be required. In fact, this is not the case (though an important caveat will be introduced shortly): Two sensors are in principle sufficient to completely capture head movement; but this depends crucially on the additional angular information provided by each sensor. Consider the typical setup in a 2D EMMA system mentioned above, i.e., with reference sensors attached to upper incisors and nose. Clearly, if each sensor only provided

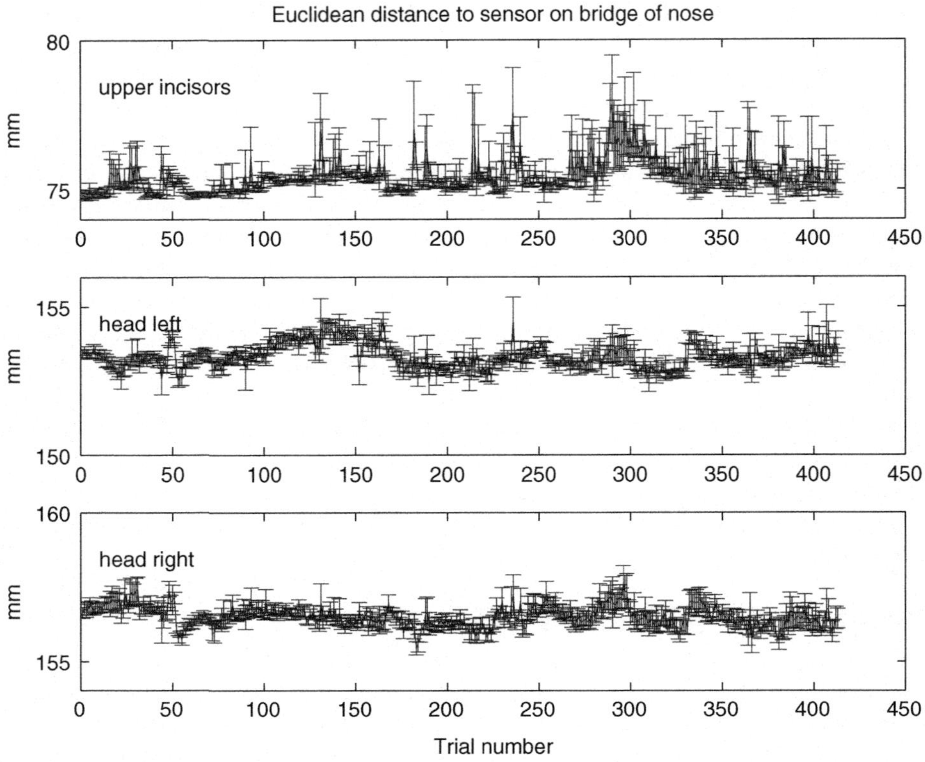

Fig. 20.2 Euclidean distances between pairs of reference sensors.

Cartesian coordinates (x, y, z) then some kinds of head movement would not be recoverable with only two sensors, in particular if the head were to rotate about an axis parallel to the line joining the two sensors. In terms of the definitions given above, this would roughly correspond to yaw.[2]

However, if the main axis of the sensors is mounted at right angles to the line joining the two sensors then the missing degrees information on yaw will be captured in the changes in the angular coordinates of the sensors.

In practice, just using this minimum of two sensors is probably not advisable. Quite apart from the possibility of sensors failing or becoming detached during the experiment it has emerged from experience with many experiments where we typically use four reference sensors (usually sensors mounted just behind each ear in addition to the two traditional EMMA ones) that often the quality of the coordinate data from the different sensors is not equally good. This can be found, for example, from examining the Euclidean distances between all pairs of reference sensors (the distance between any pair of sensors should of course be constant as they are regarded as being

[2] Another way of looking at this is as follows: the total number of coordinates for two purely Cartesian 3D sensors is 6, but when attached to a rigid body this is insufficient to recover the 6 degrees of freedom, since the distance between the sensors is fixed. Thus, in effect one degree of freedom of the two sensors is lost. 5D sensors with 3 Cartesian and 2 angular coordinates provide enough information to make up for this loss. Additional note: For the NDI Aurora system more complex six-degrees-of-freedom sensors are available for special purposes, such as head movement correction. Of course, a lot then depends on this sensor operating reliably.

attached to a rigid body). To illustrate this, Fig. 20.2 shows the mean and standard deviation per trial of the distance between a reference sensor on the bridge of the nose and three other reference sensors over the course of a session consisting of about 400 trials. Clearly, the upper incisor sensor is much less stable than the other two. However, since more than the bare minimum number of reference sensors has been recorded in this case then one could afford to leave out the least reliable one from the head-correction procedure.

20.2.3.2 Relations between head movement and linguistic behaviour: a topic in its own right

Head movement can, of course, itself form part of communicative behaviour and be worth examining in its own right, rather than just being regarded as extraneous movement that needs to be factored out of the measurement of articulatory movement (see e.g., Munhall et al., 2004).

In this section, we use material from a recent study of the articulatory correlates of tone production in Mandarin Chinese as an example for this kind of investigation (see Hoole and Hu 2004). The main thrust of this investigation was to look for different patterns of tongue movement related to the four tones of Mandarin. For this, data was acquired with the AG500. Since head movement had to be monitored anyway the opportunity was taken to examine this as well for any evidence of regularities related to tone production because there is some evidence in the literature that limited tonal perception is possible based on visual information alone (e.g., Burnham et al., 2001; see also Mixdorff and Charnvivit 2004). This raises the question of what visual information actually could be involved here, and head movement is certainly a candidate (see e.g., Munhall et al., 2004 and Yehia et al., 2002 for some evidence that F0 can be quite well predicted from head-motion parameters – at least on an utterance-by-utterance basis).

In a corpus of isolated words spoken by one speaker we found a consistent difference in head position for tone 3 (the low dipping tone) compared to the other tones, particularly compared to tone 2 (the high rising tone): the position of the head tended to be lower and more posterior for tone 3. This is illustrated in Fig. 20.3.

Of course, it is scarcely reasonable to expect that speakers adopt a specific *position* of the head for the different tones (as extracted here at the midpoint of the vowel), or to expect that head movement somehow mimics F0 movement. Thus, it is perhaps of more interest that the overall pattern of movement tended to separate tone 3 from the other tones: Velocity of head movement in the forward and upward direction tended to be higher for tone 3. Velocity patterns are attractive in the context of visible behaviour of this kind because they may be communicatively more robust than subtle differences in position (cf. Keating et al., 2003). Currently we do not know whether these results will generalize to other speakers and other speaking styles. But we find it perfectly plausible that precisely when a speaker is aiming at a very clear style of speech then characteristic patterns of visible behaviour may be coherently integrated with articulatory and phonatory behaviour (see also Craig et al., 2008). And the simple methodological point to be made here is that even these tentative results show that with this kind of measurement system a widening of the perspective on speech-related motor behaviour is worthwhile.

20.2.3.3 Potential for new experimental paradigms

Freedom of head movement, by increasing the subject's comfort, quite simply means that longer experiments are possible. We have successfully run sessions in which over 1,000 utterances were recorded, and in which the net speaking time (i.e., leaving out pauses between utterances) amounts to about 50 minutes. Clearly, this can provide a more solid statistical foundation for almost any kind of experiment. In addition, it makes paradigms much more feasible in which there may be a rather low ratio of 'interesting' material to total recorded material, for example,

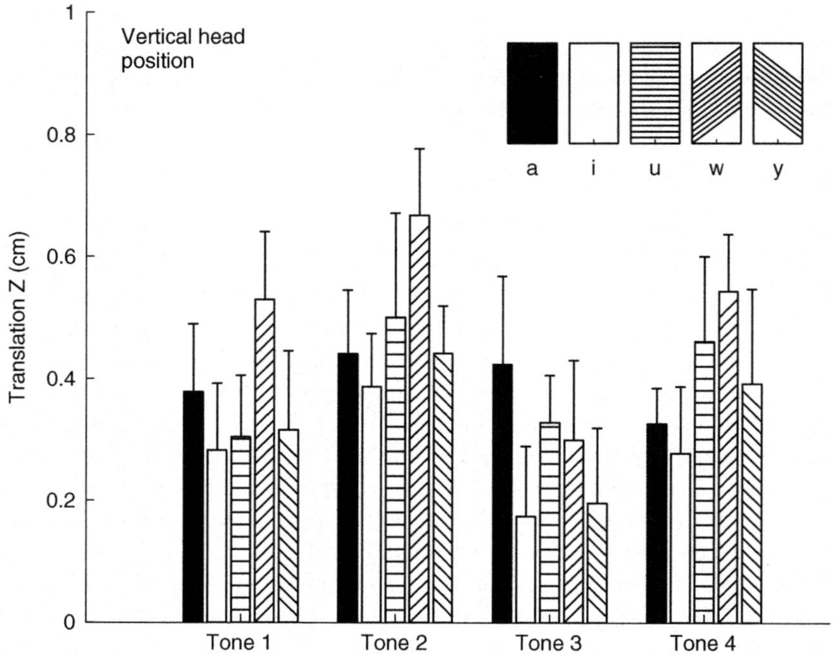

Fig. 20.3 Mean vertical position (in cm) of head at midpoint of vowel ('w' symbolizes a back unrounded vowel) for the four tones of Mandarin (12 repetitions). Before averaging, data were normalized by subtracting the mean of each block of repetitions. Error bars indicate standard deviation. Differences between Tone 3 and Tone 2 significant at $p < 0.01$.

in experiments to elicit speech errors, and in recordings based on spontaneous speech. A further area that could be mentioned here is that of speech technology: the amount of data that can now be acquired is starting to get within the ballpark of what is typically required of training data in applications of this kind (e.g., Ling et al., 2008). Regarding spontaneous speech paradigms, being recorded with a device such as the AG500 will, of course, always be very much a laboratory situation for the subject. Nevertheless, freedom of head movement is certainly an important contributor to utterance naturalness in unscripted speech situations (we have, for example, started to work with a map-task [Anderson et al., 1991], in which one dialogue partner gives directions for a route to follow to the other partner).

Given that an EMA system represents a considerable investment for most labs it appears worthwhile to be alert to possibilities for expanding the range of applications of such a system and we conclude this section with one brief example of further directions that diversification could take.

The example shows that sensors (with a certain amount of circumspection) can be quite easily attached to the eyelids, allowing the time instants of blinks to be detected. In the example in Fig. 20.4 the trace labelled 'T5 raw' is the signal from the eyelid sensor time-aligned with the audio trace. The sharp peaks represent blinks occurring about 0.5 s before the onset of the utterance and roughly at the location of the stressed first syllable in 'relatively' at about 1.75s on the time axis. For an application of this kind, where one may just be interested in the temporal location of a sharply defined event it is probably not even necessary to calculate the sensor positions. The trace

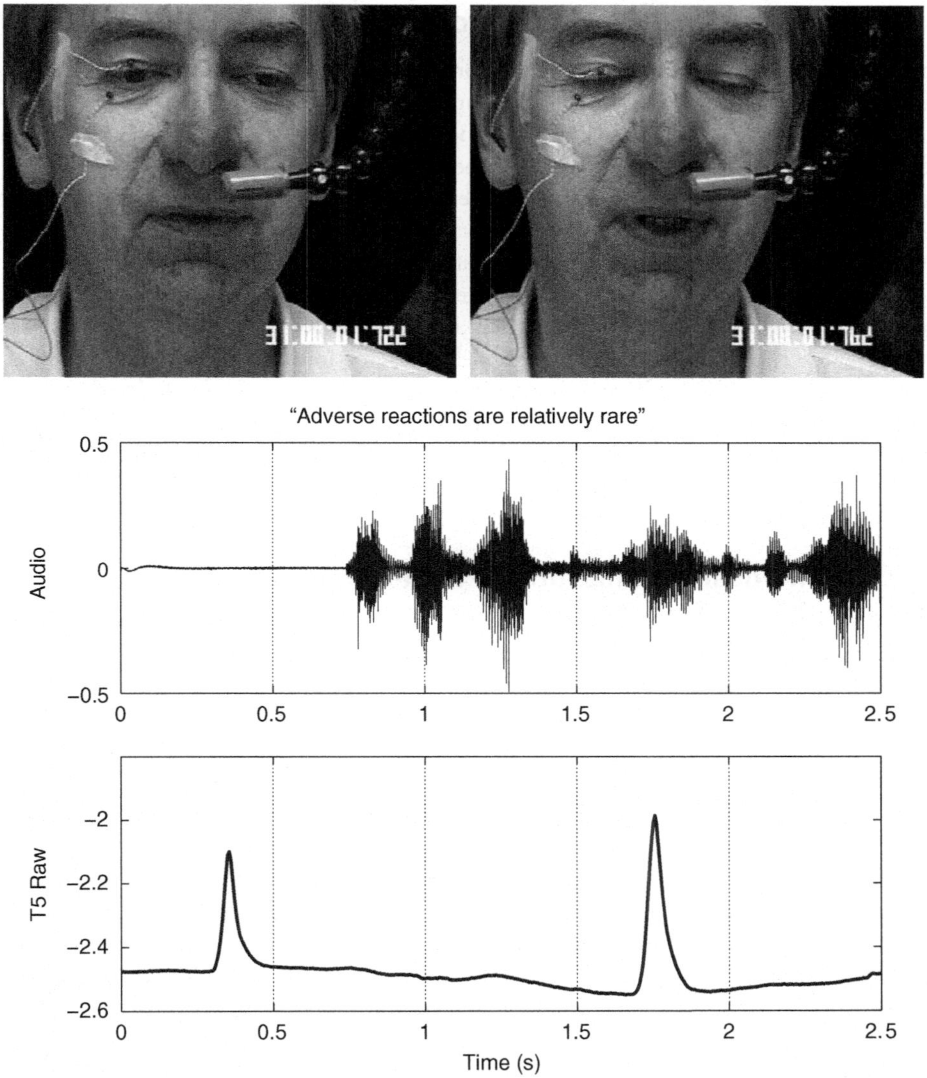

Fig. 20.4 Using an EMA sensor to capture blinking movements. Two consecutive frames from synchronized video. The second frame is located at about the peak of the second blink event at around 1.75s.

used in the figure simply shows the raw signal induced in the sensor, chosen with respect to the transmitter that gave the strongest modulation of the signal for blink events. Another point in this figure that may be of methodological interest is that our experimental setup allows us to synchronize video filming (at 25 frames or 50 fields per second) with the EMA data acquisition. The last four digits in the bottom right corner of the two video stills are generated by a video timer (FORA VTG53) that is triggered by the synchronization signal from the AG500 hardware to start counting at the onset of each EMA trial. They thus indicate the location in seconds of the images with respect to the time traces in the two panels below.

20.3 **Position calculation as a problem in non-linear optimization**[3]

In a 2D EMMA system, calculation of the sensor positions (x and y) just requires applying a simple geometrically based formula to the raw input signals from the three transmitters. The down side to the high dimensionality of the information provided by each sensor in the new system is that a closed-form solution deriving the three sensor positions and two sensor orientations directly from the raw input of the six transmitters is not available, but rather requires a search in a correspondingly high-dimensional space. Essentially, one is searching (for each sensor, at each time instant) for the set of positions and orientations that when plugged into the equation for the electromagnetic field will generate the actually measured signal from each of the six transmitters to within some appropriate tolerance criterion. In this sense, position calculation is a member of the large category of inverse problems, i.e., model parameters must be estimated from the observed data. Because of the presence of non-linear terms in the field equation, we are faced with a non-linear optimization problem. In this section we will first of all use a 'toy' example to give a general appreciation of the kinds of difficulties that can arise in such procedures, and then go on to consider two specific problem areas that have been encountered quite frequently in practical work with large amounts of EMA data and show some potential solutions.

20.3.1 **Non-linear optimization: a toy example to illustrate the basic scenario**

For the example in this section, we will use the following conventions:

x Position
f(x) A non-linear function of x (e.g., the magnetic field model)
y Measured sensor signal

To determine x, solve f(x) − y = 0

The reason for referring to it as a 'toy' problem is that for illustrative purposes the solution search evolves in one dimension, whereas in practice we have a search space of much higher dimensionality to contend with (also neither of the non-linear functions used here as examples are identical to the magnetic field function, but they are realistic enough to illustrate important features).

The basic procedure is illustrated in the left panel of Fig. 20.5. This procedure for finding a solution is based on Newton's method. In practice, we currently generally use the Levenberg-Marquardt approach implemented in Matlab's optimization toolbox since this has generally proven to be more robust, but this makes no difference to the illustration of some basic concepts and difficulties. The search begins at some start value for x (labelled x_0 in the figure). Here $x = 0$ is used, but this is simply the choice that may be made if one has no prior information to go on. As will become apparent below, the choice of start position can be crucial. At the start position, the algorithm makes an estimate of the zero-crossing of the function using the gradient of the function at the start position. The corresponding x location (x_1) is then used to re-estimate the zero-crossing and the procedure iterates until some termination criterion is reached.[4] The right

[3] Discussion in this section is based on our experience with the Carstens AG500 system. The situation with the NDI Aurora system is substantially different since, as far as we are aware, the user has access only to the final sensor coordinate values, and not to the raw signals. It seems that the system sometimes outputs missing data, presumably, when the result of the position calculation is considered unreliable (see Kröger et al., 2008). Recovery of missing data by means of additional off-line processing does not appear to be possible.

[4] The termination criterion may be just based on the number of iterations, but typically also involves some threshold for improvement in the residual from one iteration to the next (or of change in the calculated position).

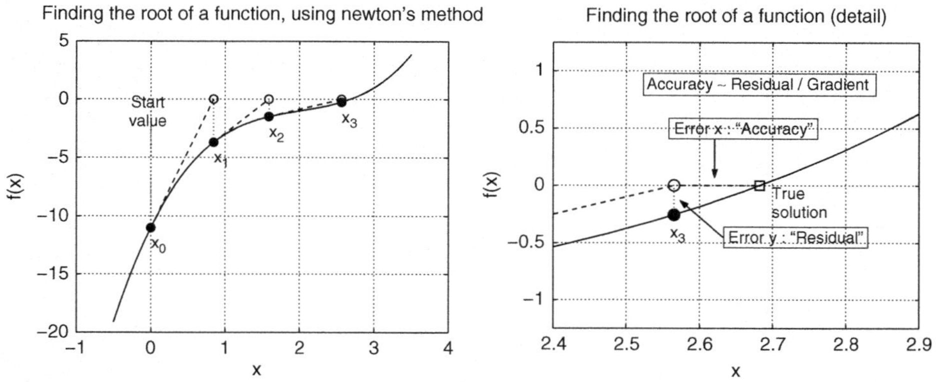

Fig. 20.5 Left panel: Illustration of a few iterations towards a solution using the Newton procedure. Right panel: Zoomed view of the true solution and the calculated solution.

part of the figure zooms in on the situation at termination which is assumed to occur here at x_3. The accuracy of the solution (e.g., positional accuracy in mm) can then be defined as the horizontal distance along the x-axis between the x-value at termination and the true solution at the function zero-crossing. Although accuracy is intuitively the measure one is interested in it can in practice never be known, except in special calibration setups. What is known is the measure referred to here as the residual, i.e., the value of the function f(x) at the termination value of x (i.e., the amount by which the function deviates from the ideal value of zero). In the specific case of the EMA system the position and orientation calculation for each sensor results in a residual with respect to the signal from each of the six transmitters. The root mean square (RMS) over these six values is what the optimization procedure aims to minimize. This is by no means the only way of formulating the optimization problem (e.g., one could imagine minimizing the worst residual) but none of the alternatives examined to date have proved obviously superior. Another important point illustrated in the right panel of Fig. 20.5 is the relationship between accuracy and the residual: this depends on the *gradient* of the function in the vicinity of the solution. Thus, different parts of a recording where the position calculation results in similar RMS residuals may not be equally accurate. In particular, even low RMS values can have relatively high inaccuracy if the gradient at the solution is shallow. This needs to be kept in mind, since the RMS value is the principal quality criterion available to the user.

The previous illustration illustrates the ideal case where the algorithm will converge quickly on a good approximation to the true solution. A more difficult situation is illustrated in the next example (Fig. 20.6). Here, the iteration step starting at x3 fails to get closer to the true solution; rather, x_4 ends up back close to x_2. The algorithm may then become stuck in this region. The right panel of the figure again zooms in on the true and calculated solution. This illustrates from a different perspective the fact that the value of the residual can be quite small, but may nevertheless be associated with poor accuracy. This example also makes clear that the choice of start position can have a major effect on the result. For any given true solution, it is possible to define a convergence region, i.e., the region within which the algorithm is bound to converge on the solution. For start positions outside the convergence region it can be a matter of chance whether one of the iteration steps manages to jump into the convergence region, or whether the iterations become locked into a highly erroneous region where the algorithm then terminates because the residual fails to improve noticeably from one iteration to the next.

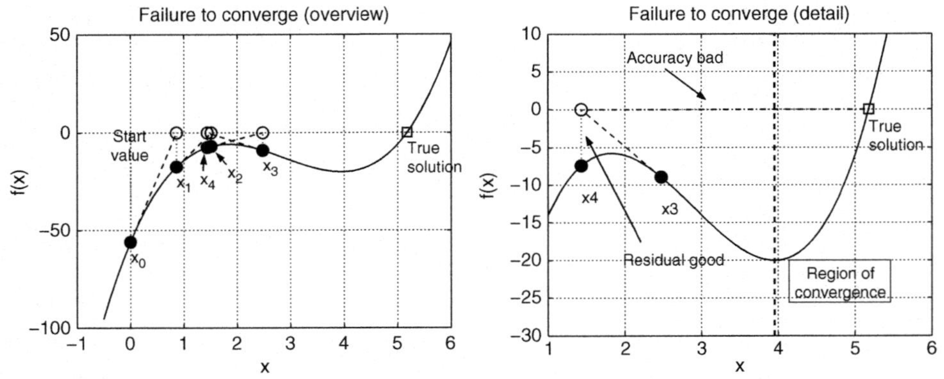

Fig. 20.6 Left panel: Example of failure to converge on true solution. Right panel: Zoomed view of the true and erroneous solution.

What strategies can be followed to choose the start position? First of all, for bootstrapping the procedure we have found the following approach useful: Within each trial for which positions are to be calculated it is possible to determine a sample that is likely to give a robust solution by examining the gradients of the function. Calculation can then proceed forward and backward in time from this location. In addition, in many speech experiments it is possible to have a rough idea in advance of the positions and orientations of the sensors. In particular, a ballpark idea of the orientations appears to be very advantageous and is actually easier to specify than the positions, since they are less dependent on where the subject happens to sit within the transmitter assembly. This start-position (which will normally only be used for the first calculated sample in a trial) can then be refined by calculating a few trials from a whole experiment, and – assuming a reasonable proportion of the data looks reliable – then using the average position from these trials as start position for the bulk of the trials. Once position calculation for a particular trial has been initiated then the default procedure is to use the position of the sample just calculated as the start position for calculation of the next sample. Clearly, this will in most cases give a start position that is fairly close to the solution, but in the light of the above remarks it should be immediately apparent that there are two potential pit-falls: Firstly, if the articulator is moving fast and the convergence region is small, then the position of sample n may be outside the convergence region of sample n+1; secondly, if an erroneous position has been latched onto, then the solution may became stuck in this region for some period of time, particularly if the sensor is not moving very much. There may then be a sudden jump in the data when the raw signals have changed sufficiently for the true solution to be located in a more robust region of the search space.

There are various additional strategies with respect to the start-positions for getting round these difficulties,[5] but none are foolproof, and since current versions of the optimization procedures do not incorporate any continuity constraints on the calculated speech movements, the user is always likely to be confronted with discontinuities that clearly indicate an error in the position calculation.

[5] For example, if a sensor on the tongue is occasionally susceptible to these pitfalls but also has a large proportion of reliable data then it is possible by means of multiple linear regression to use data of other sensors on the tongue to generate a prediction of the reliable data, and then extend the prediction to all sample points of the unstable sensor. This prediction will probably be within a few millimetres of the correct solution and so can act as a good starting point.

The purpose of the next section will be to show how some typical problems of this kind can be handled. One point that is hopefully readily apprehensible from the above discussion is that any distortion or noise in the measured signals will increase the likelihood of problematic situations. In any realistic measurement situation it is highly improbable that the true solution actually corresponds to all-zero residuals in the raw measured signals, simply because the real-life signals will not be perfectly modelled by the magnetic-field equations. However, because we have a slightly overdetermined system (six transmitter signals to determine 5 degrees of freedom in the sensors) there is a good chance that overall the minimization of the RMS will give a result close to the true solution even if this RMS value is indeed greater than zero. However, the stronger any disturbances are, and the more the RMS value even for the true solution departs from zero, then the greater are the chances that a substantially different solution with similar or even lower RMS exists somewhere in the search space.

20.3.2 Some realistic problems in position calculation

20.3.2.1 Reducing instabilities by adjusting the raw signal amplitudes

Figure 20.7 illustrates a category of problem that we have commonly encountered in our data. In the recording session from which the example is taken the middle of three sensors on the tongue occasionally appeared to give unstable results. The top left panel in the figure shows movement in the lateral dimension over time for one trial (similar behaviour was observed in the vertical and anterior-posterior dimensions). Just before 1s on the time axis there is a very sharp to-and-fro movement of over 5 mm that is very untypical for speech movements of this sensor.

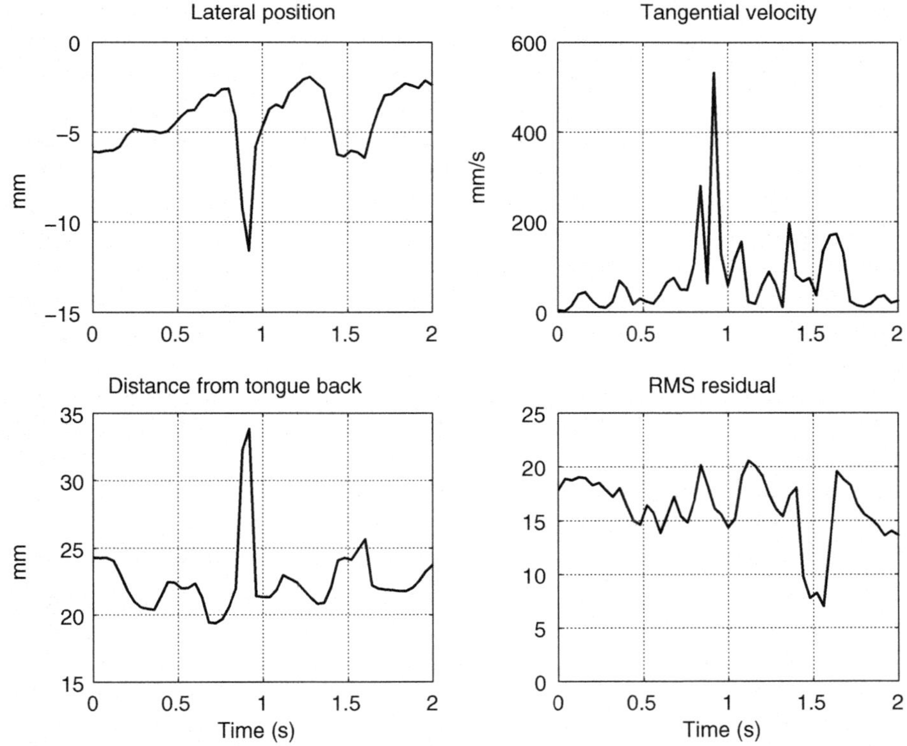

Fig. 20.7 Example of unstable solution of the position calculation.

Correspondingly, the tangential velocity (top right panel) goes up to about 500 mm/s whereas velocities for this sensor would typically not be expected to be much above 200 mm/s. As further evidence of unstable behaviour, the bottom left panel shows the distance of the middle tongue sensor from the back tongue sensor. This shows a large fluctuation of about 10 mm at the same location in time. Overall, it appears very likely that over a period of about 1/10 s the position calculation algorithm has failed to converge on the correct solution. Here this has been presented in terms of eye-balling the data for plausibility, but normally this would be backed up by statistical analysis of the behaviour of the sensor over the course of the recording session.

The bottom right panel shows the RMS residual value; this shows no unusual features in the vicinity of the potential instability, but it is overall quite high (the units of the RMS signal are arbitrary since they are simply related to the units of the AD-convertor that digitized the raw modulated sensor signal, so the statement 'quite high' is just based on what experience has shown to be typical for our system).

The following procedure aims to adjust the raw measured amplitudes so that overall lower RMS values result, in the hope that this will leave less scope for the optimization procedure to veer off towards aberrant solutions. The point of departure for expecting this to have some chance of success is the remark made above that the set of equations is somewhat overdetermined, so in basically stable situations the algorithm will converge on a good solution even if the accompanying minimum RMS residual value is not particularly low, due for example to the sensor picking up spurious signals of some kind or the electromagnetic inductance being slightly different when sensors are attached to the subject compared to the situation when the sensors were calibrated. If these sources of distortion to the signal were purely random noise then nothing more could be done, but if they showed a systematic pattern, i.e., were predictable from the location of the sensor in the measurement field then they could be compensated for, by adjusting the raw amplitudes of each transmitter accordingly. The position calculations can then be repeated based on the adjusted amplitudes. For stable solutions the adjustment can be expected to change the result very little, since one is essentially plugging into the input of the position calculation the amplitudes generated by the magnetic field equations for the solution found in the first pass. However, for unstable solutions the adjustment can be expected to help tilt the balance in favour of a situation in which the lowest RMS value found during the search procedure actually corresponds to a good solution.

Figure 20.8 shows the residual values for one specific transmitter (Transmitter 3 of the mid-tongue sensor) as a function of all transmitter signals for this sensor. It will be observed that the residual has quite a strong linear relation with respect to several transmitters' signals. Essentially we then use multiple linear regression to predict the residual of each signal from all transmitter signals (it is important when calculating the regression coefficients to eliminate data for which the calculated positions are unreliable, since the residuals of this data would act as a source of noise in the regression analysis).[6]

The result of recalculating the specific example here after adjusting the amplitudes by the predicted component of the residual is shown in Fig. 20.9 where the original values (dashed lines) and the corresponding values for the new solution (solid lines) are overlaid. It will be seen that in

[6] In a preliminary version of this adjustment procedure, we simply predicted the residual of each transmitter from the signal of the corresponding transmitter. This is tantamount to adjusting the gain factor for the corresponding sensor-transmitter pair. But if, as seems likely, disturbances in the signal depend more on position of the sensor in the measurement space than just on the strength of the induced signal, then the overall state of the system can be taken better into account by using all transmitter signals in the prediction.

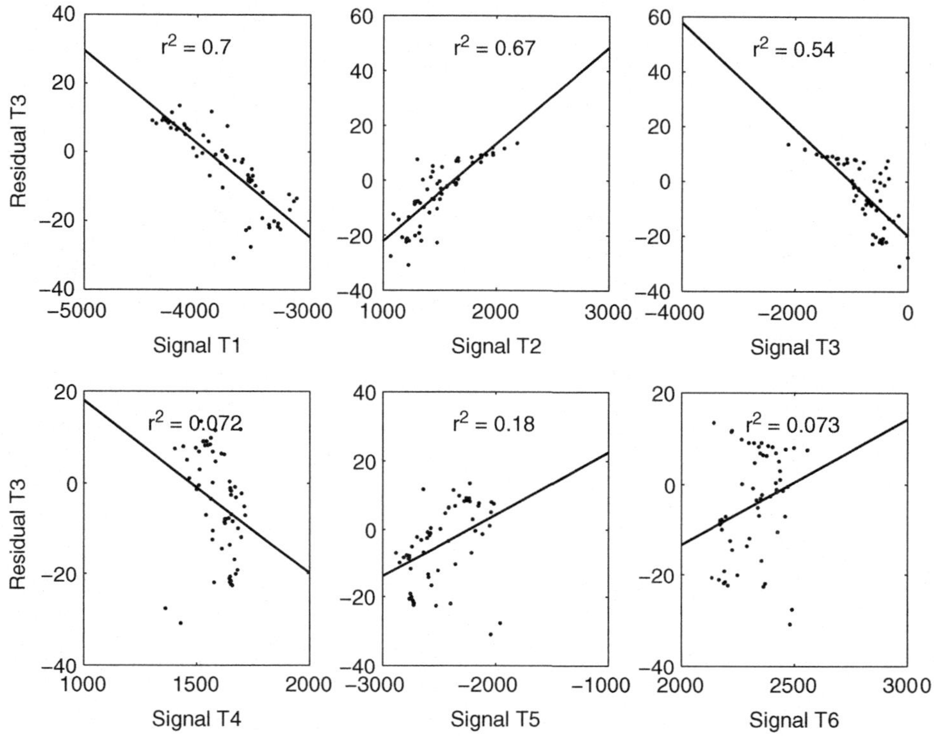

Fig. 20.8 Residual for transmitter 3 plotted as a function of all six transmitter signals.

the panels for position, velocity, and distance from the tongue-back sensor the extreme values in the region of the potential instability have disappeared, but that in other parts of the trial the changes are very small. The substantial decline in the RMS value in the bottom right panel indicates that a large proportion of the original RMS value was systematic and predictable.

20.3.2.2 Reducing instabilities by estimating positions from predicted velocities

The procedures presented in the previous section have proved invaluable in many experiments for reducing the proportion of unstable data. However, some problems may well remain after amplitude correction, Fig. 20.10 showing a case in point. The dashed lines represent the situation at this stage in the processing. A clear discontinuity is still to be observed in the position and velocity trace (again, the lateral dimension has been chosen for illustrative purposes). In this figure the raw data for this sensor (with respect to the six transmitters) has been included as the bottom left panel in order to emphasize that the raw data itself is clearly continuous, i.e., there has not been some low-level measurement error that can explain the present problem. As in the previous section, the 'repair' procedure in the present section has as its first pre-requisite that a reasonable proportion of the calculated positions are basically reliable, and that it is possible to eliminate from the calculations those data points that are likely to be unreliable. The other point of departure is as follows: When the full 5D measurement space is considered then position and orientation of the sensors is a strongly non-linear function of the raw amplitudes induced in the sensors. However, in the short trials typical of many speech experiments (e.g., a few seconds) the sensors will only move through a very small proportion of the total measurement space.

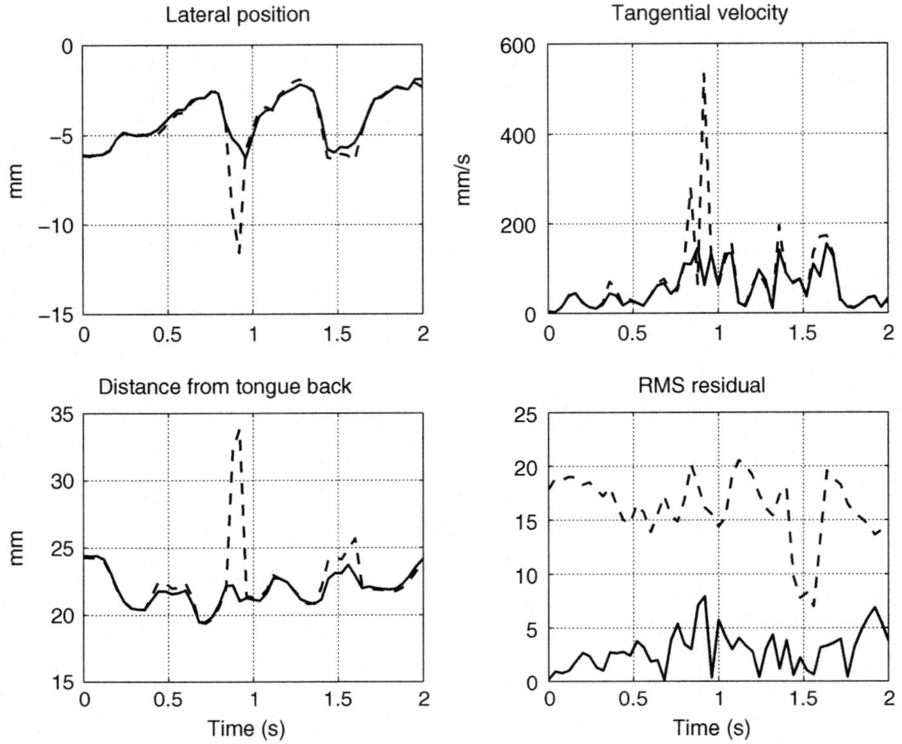

Fig. 20.9 Results for re-calculated positions based on adjustment of raw amplitude data overlaid on the original data (dashed lines: original data; solid lines: re-calculated data).

Therefore, for short stretches of data the relationship between output (position, orientation) and input (induced signals) may be locally linear. This offers the possibility of shortcutting the position calculation based on the non-linear optimization procedure, by using the data where position calculation has been successful to obtain by multiple linear regression a mapping directly from raw amplitude data to the positions. This mapping can then be applied to those data points where the normal position calculation has obviously produced aberrant results. In practice, we obtained better results by predicting sensor velocities from the first derivatives of the raw data. Following integration, the estimated positions in the unstable regions are patched into the data tracks in such a way as to be continuous with the immediately preceding and following stable regions.

The result of this procedure, i.e., the re-estimated data, is given by the solid lines in Fig. 20.10 (overlaid on the original data given by the dashed lines). Clearly, there have been substantial changes in the region of the assumed instability, with the re-calculated version certainly appearing superficially more plausible. The bottom right panel offers a more formal way of assessing whether the re-estimation procedure has produced acceptable results. This overlays the RMS residual of the original position calculation with the corresponding trace for the re-estimated positions. For any set of re-estimated positions (i.e., not just those based on the present procedure) it is absolutely essential to generate the amplitudes predicted for those positions by the field equations and subtract these amplitudes from the measured ones in order to have access to corresponding residual values. These re-estimation procedures may themselves fail, for example, if the identification of reliable and unreliable data was deficient. This may not be immediately obvious if the output is smooth, but if the re-estimated solution is associated with a drastic

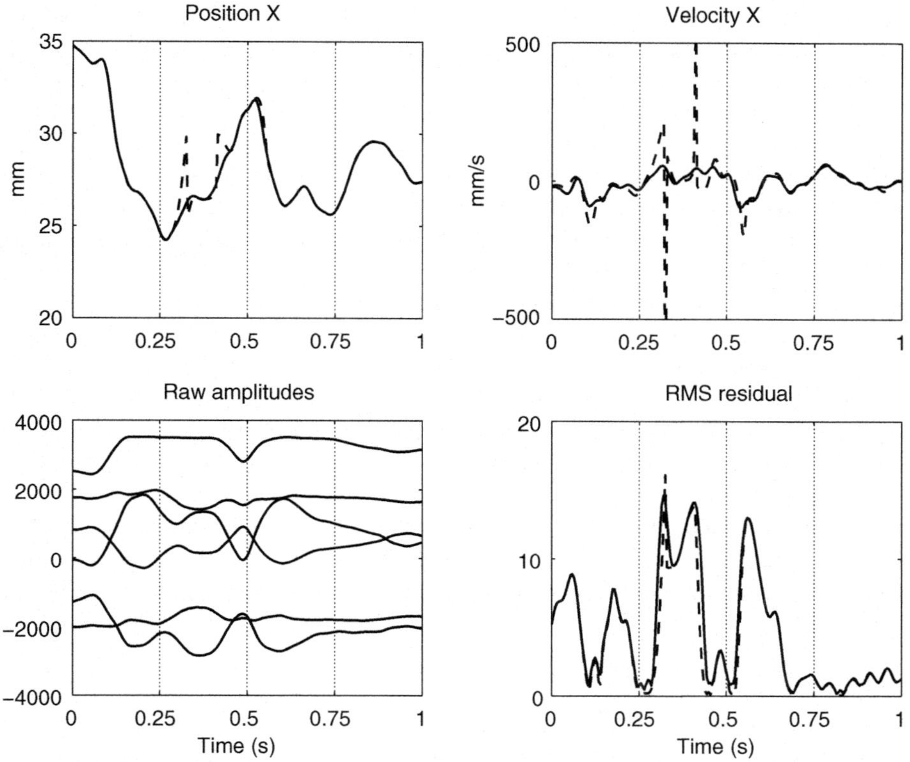

Fig. 20.10 Example of discontinuity in position and velocity data (top panels, dashed lines). Raw data (corresponding to the six transmitters) in the bottom left panel. Data re-estimated by velocity prediction shown in solid lines overlaid on the original data (all panels except bottom left).

increase in the residual values then it must be rejected as unrealistic. In the present case the re-estimation can be regarded as successful because the overlaid traces are almost impossible to distinguish in the figure. This demonstrates with a practical example the point made above with the 'toy' example that solutions with very similar RMS values but widely separated in space can indeed exist. As long as the optimization procedure itself does not incorporate continuity constraints to weight different solutions that may appear equally attractive in terms of RMS then the application of post-hoc procedures of the type outlined here will probably continue to be necessary.

20.4 **Conclusion**

The aim of the present chapter has not been to give an exhaustive review of the state of the art in articulographic measurement procedures, but rather to focus on areas where both the benefit and the bane of the current generation of electromagnetic systems become particularly apparent (for further methodological discussion of current EMA systems see e.g., Zierdt [2007], Yunusova et al., [2009], Kroos [2008], Yunusova et al., [2008]).

On the plus side, due to the high information density per sensor it is apparent that this technique has the potential to provide data for a wide range of both traditional and innovative experimental paradigms, with the increase in subject comfort particularly useful for large-scale recordings.

On the minus side, the user must be prepared to devote considerable effort to assessing the stability of the results of the position-calculation algorithm, and to exploring means of improving the stability of questionable data. Fortunately, the latter usually only constitutes a small proportion of the total amount of data from typical experiments (in our experience perhaps about 10%). But handling this data usually dominates the time required to process a dataset. With regard to the 'repair' procedures outlined above it is worth emphasizing the following points in this concluding section: (1) They depend on a fair proportion of data being basically accurate, and (2) They depend on being able to specify plausible ranges for velocity and inter-sensor distances in speech movements.

In other words, the problems with which we are typically confronted in the current state of the system would be much more intractable if we wanted to measure unconstrained movement of sensors that are not linked among themselves (at least loosely) by being attached to biological tissue. For example, the tongue-tip and tongue-dorsum are sufficiently independent of one another for it to be interesting to study their coordination. But the range of positions they can adopt relative to one another is much more constrained than, for example, the index fingers of the left and right hand.

Nonetheless, it would, of course, ultimately be desirable and more elegant to avoid 'repair' procedures altogether (i.e., procedures that 'patch' after the event), by building more sophisticated constraints a priori into the optimization problem itself. This will be an interesting task for future developments.

References

Anderson A, Bader M, Bard E, Boyle E, Doherty GM, Garrod S, Isard S, Kowtko J, McAllister J, Miller J, Sotillo C, Thompson HS and Weinert R (1991). The HCRC Map TaskCorpus. *Language and Speech*, **34**, 351–366.

Burnham D, Lau S, Tam H and Schoknecht C (2001). Visual discrimination of Cantonese tone by tonal but non-Cantonese speakers, and by non-tonal language speakers. *Proceedings of AVSP 2001*, pp. 155–160.

Craig MS, Van Lieshout PHHM and Wong W (2008). A linear model of acoustic-to-facial mapping: model parameters, data set size and generalization across speakers. *Journal of the Acoustical Society of America*, **124**(5), 3183–3190.

Hoole P and Nguyen N (1999). Electromagnetic articulography in coarticulation research. In WH Hardcastle and N Hewlett, eds. *Coarticulation: Theory, Data and Techniques*, pp. 260–269. Cambridge University Press.

Hoole P and Hu F (2004). Tone-vowel interaction in standard Chinese. *Proceedings of the International Symposium on Tonal Aspects of Languages: Emphasis on Tone Languages, Beijing*, pp. 89–92.

Kaburagi T, Wakamiya K and Honda M (2005). Three-dimensional electromagnetic articulography: a measurement principle. *Journal of the Acoustical Society of America*, **118** (1), 428–443.

Keating P, Baroni M, Mattys S, Scarborough R, Alwan A, Auer E and Bernstein L (2003). Optical phonetics and visual perception of lexical and phrasal stress in English. *Proceedings of the 15th International Congress of Phonetic Sciences, Barcelona*, pp. 2071–2074.

Kröger B, Pouplier M and Tiede M (2008). An evaluation of the aurora system as a flesh-point tracking tool for speech production research. *Journal of Speech Language and Hearing Research*, **51**(4), 914–921.

Kroos C (2008). Measurement accuracy in 3D electromagnetic articulography (Carstens AG500). In R Sock, S Fuchs and Y Laprie, eds. *Proceedings of the Eighth International Seminar on Speech Production, Strasbourg, 2008*, pp. 61–64.

Ling ZH, Richmond K, Yamagishi J and Wang RH (2008). Articulatory control of HMM-based parametric speech synthesis driven by phonetic knowledge. *Proceedings of the Interspeech Brisbane, 2008*, pp. 573–576.

Mixdorff H and Charnvivit P (2004). Visual cues in Thai tone recognition. *Proceedings of the International Symposium on Tonal Aspects of Languages: Emphasis on Tone Languages, Beijing*, pp. 143–146.

Munhall KG, Jones JA, Callan DE, Kuratate T and Vatikiotis-Bateson E (2004). Visual prosody and speech intelligibility: head movement improves auditory speech perception. *Psychological Science: A Journal of the American Psychological Society /APS*, **15**(2), 133–137.

Yehia H, Kuratate T and Vatikiotis-Bateson E (2002). Linking facial animation, head motion and speech acoustics. *Journal of Phonetics*, **30**(3), 555–568.

Yunusova Y, Stanley J and Green JR (2008). Distinguishing place of consonant articulation using the aurora system. ASA meeting Paris Summer 2008. Paper 4pSCb35. *Journal of the Acoustical Society of America*, **123** (5, Pt. 2), p. 3739.

Yunusova Y, Green J and Mefferd A (2009). Accuracy assessment for AG500, electromagnetic articulograph. *Journal of Speech Language and Hearing Research*, **52**, 547–555.

Zeroual C, Hoole P, Fuchs S and Esling JH. (2007). EMA study of the coronal emphatic and non-emphatic plosive consonants of Moroccan Arabic. *Proceedings of the 16th International Congress of Phonetic Sciences, Saarbrücken*, pp. 397–400.

Zierdt, A. (2007). EMA and the crux of calibration. *Proceedings of the 16th International Congress of Phonetic Sciences, Saarbrücken*, pp. 593–596.

Chapter 21

2D and 3D ultrasound imaging of the tongue in normal and disordered speech

Tim Bressmann

Abstract

The chapter discusses the applicability and usefulness of ultrasound imaging for speech science. Basic technical aspects of acquiring two-dimensional brightness mode (B-mode) images of the tongue are explained together with techniques of image measurement. The use of static 3D ultrasound imaging for the analysis of tongue surfaces is described and current 4D ultrasound imaging tools are discussed. The applicability of ultrasound imaging in clinical speech research is demonstrated with summaries of two recent studies of partial glossectomy speakers. In the first study, B-mode ultrasound imaging was used to demonstrate compensatory post-operative increases of tongue velocity and height in ten patients with lateral partial glossectomies. In the second study, static 3D ultrasound imaging was used with twelve partial glossectomees to demonstrate that a lateral partial tongue resection leads to a reduction of the midsagittal groove of the tongue surface in sustained speech sounds. The chapter concludes with a case presentation of a patient with a hypoglossal nerve paralysis related to post-polio syndrome.

21.1 Introduction

Ultrasound imaging is currently gaining popularity as a research tool for speech scientists and speech-language pathologists who are interested in tongue movement (see for example a recent special issue of *Clinical Linguistics and Phonetics*, Volume 19, issue 6–7, 2005). The appeal of ultrasound lies in the simple and direct way of visualizing internal structures in the human body. The tongue can be conveniently visualized by placing the transducer on the neck of the research subject. Since the data acquisition is relatively easy, potentially 'difficult' subjects such as children and patients can be studied. The image of the tongue is provided in real-time. The image is reasonably intuitive and may be used to provide biofeedback to a patient. Besides the ease of data acquisition, the advantages of ultrasound imaging lie in low costs and excellent bio-safety. A medical ultrasound machine provides extremely low radiation levels and the radiation effects of ultrasound do not accumulate, so that examinations may be repeated (Epstein 2005). This is an advantage over x-ray based imaging methods such as videofluoroscopy. Over the last ten years, technological innovation and competition between manufacturers have lead to lower prices for ultrasound machines. This has made ultrasound accessible for many speech science laboratories.

21.2 Basic of ultrasound imaging

Ultrasound works based on the pulse-echo principle. When an acoustic pulse hits an object with suitable conductivity, it puts the object into oscillation and elicits echoes. The echoes can be recorded and analysed. They provide information about the echogeneity and structure of the object. Ultrasound functions like the echo sounder that is used on a ship to determine the depth of the water under the keel. A click is sounded and travels towards the bottom of the sea. Since the velocity of sound in water is known, the time difference between the click and its echo can be used to calculate the depth of the water. The quality of the echo can reveal more details. An echo that is attenuated or scattered can indicate the presence of plankton or schools of fish between the ship and the bottom of the sea.

In medical ultrasound machines, piezoelectric crystals are used to generate sound waves in the megahertz (MHz) range. The piezoelectric crystals are set into oscillation by an electrical current and emit an ultrasound sound wave. When the current is switched off, the crystals are set into receiving mode for the echoes. By repeating this process hundreds of times per second, a two-dimensional (2D) image can be reconstructed. Ultrasound machines in North America deliver a video frame rate of 29.97 frames per second, which corresponds to the National Television Standard Committee (NTSC) standard for video equipment. European machines use the PAL standard with 25 frames per second. Both standards are reasonably fast to capture tongue movement in speech. However, quick articulatory gestures such as lingual plosives or trills cannot always be accurately displayed. The spatial accuracy of medical ultrasound machines is typically within 1 mm. It is important to keep these limitations in mind when planning a speech study with ultrasound imaging.

21.2.1 Ultrasound equipment

Many different manufacturers make ultrasound machines. For speech research, the low-end machines will generally be sufficient. Figure 21.1 shows an ultrasound machine. Regardless of the model, all ultrasound machines have similar image control features. These include image size, focus, contrast, and brightness. More important than the bells and whistles of the particular ultrasound machine is the choice of the transducer. The arrangement of the crystals in a linear or a curved array, the view-angle and the frequency of the transducer will determine what can be seen in the image. For speech research, curved array transducers are preferable for imaging the tongue because the convex curved array allows obtaining a maximum view angle with a minimal footprint. Examples for such transducers are endocavity and intercostal transducers. Another important feature is the transducer frequency. Medical ultrasound transducers normally use frequencies between 3 MHz and 10 MHz. The image depth and the image clarity are in an inverse relationship in ultrasound imaging. Higher frequency transducers (7.5–10 MHz) generate clearer and more detailed images. However, the shorter sound waves are more quickly attenuated by the tissue, so the penetration depth is limited. The tongue is comparatively large and requires an image depth of at least 10 cm. A lower frequency transducer in the range of 3–7 MHz will provide the best compromise between image depth and detail.

21.2.2 The B-mode image

An ultrasound echo can be displayed in different ways. The current standard of medical ultrasound imaging is the brightness mode (B-mode) display. In this mode, the machine records multiple concentric (in a curved array) or parallel scanlines (in a linear array). This way, multiple scan lines can be obtained and a 2D image can be generated. The echo amplitudes are displayed as shades of grey. Echogenic structures are displayed in lighter shades and areas with lower echoes

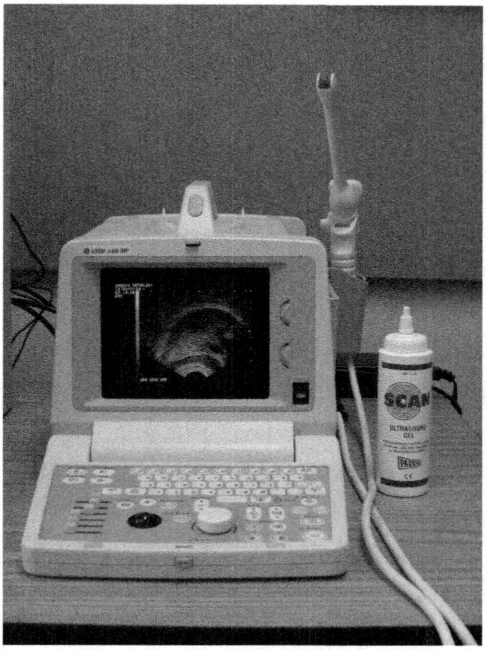

Fig. 21.1 An ultrasound machine with an endocavity transducer and ultrasound gel.

or higher signal attenuation are displayed in darker shades. The experimenter can observe a 2D section of an anatomical structure in real-time.

When an ultrasound pulse travels through an organ, it hits different layers of tissue that have different densities and different degrees of conductivity. Transition areas between different tissues (for instance, the transition from fat to muscle) cause refraction and particularly strong echoes. Therefore, the ultrasound image accentuates the anatomical borders of different organs, which facilitates the viewing and interpretation of the image. Bone and air pose specific limitations for ultrasound imaging. The higher density of the bone and the curvature of the bone surface lead to a deflection and attenuation of the sound wave. The ultrasound image stops at the periosteum so that the bone can only be visualized as a shadow (i.e., an area with no echoes). Air poses a different problem for the reflection of ultrasound waves. When the ultrasound pulse enters into air, the density of the air is too low to transmit an echo back to the transducer, and the signal is lost. Air-filled cavities therefore appear as shadows, too. This limitation is particularly pertinent for speech researchers because the vocal tract is filled with air. For example, the tip of the tongue can usually not be displayed in an ultrasound image because of the air pocket underneath the anterior tongue. The tongue tip can be visualized when the sublingual space is filled with water but this would not be conducive for phonetic experiments.

The tongue can be displayed in the sagittal or the coronal view. The sagittal image displays the anterior–posterior and ventral–cranial movement of the tongue in speech and swallowing. The coronal image displays the intrinsic deformation of the tongue. In particular, this view allows observing the midsagittal groove of the tongue (Fig. 21.2).

21.2.3 **Acquiring and analysing ultrasound data**

Ultrasound images of the tongue look clear and intuitive, which appeals to researchers and research subjects alike. The ultrasound image of the tongue is acquired by holding the transducer

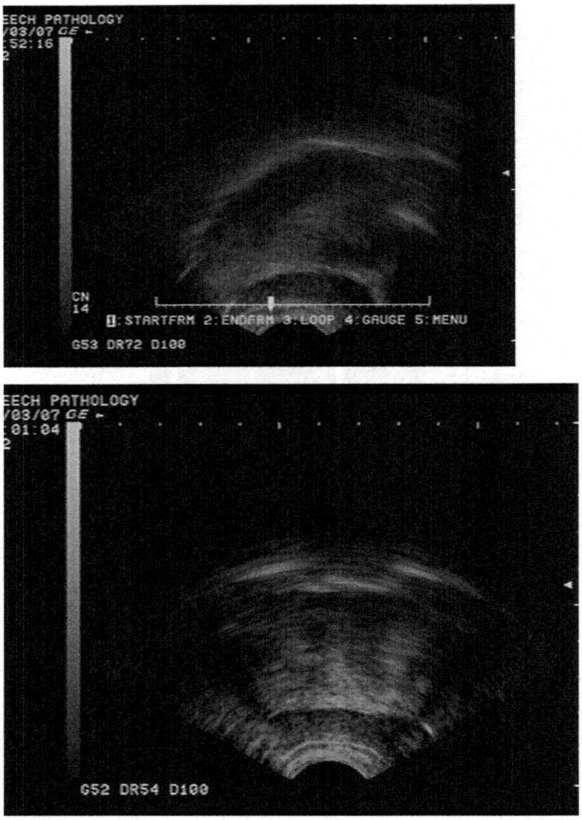

Fig. 21.2 Ultrasound contours of the tongue during speech production. (a) Sagittal view of the tongue. The anterior tongue is towards the right of the image. The tongue tip is raised for the production of /l/. (b) Coronal view of the posterior dorsum of the tongue, demonstrating midsagittal concavity during the production of /i:/.

against the neck of the research participant. However, if data are acquired for research purposes, the procedure is often considerably more involved. It is important to reduce movement of the transducer and the subject's head. Stabilizing the subject's head requires special contraptions such as headrests for the back of the head (Davidson 2006; Stone et al., 1988), headrests for the forehead (Bressmann et al., 2005a; Peng et al., 2000), or head fixation with a halo (Stone and Davies 1995). To ensure coupling when the mandible moves, a stand-off pad can be used (Peng et al., 1994). Figure 21.3 shows a system with an adjustable halo that was developed in our laboratory at the University of Toronto. Whalen et al. (2005) argue that head fixation is inherently unnatural and should be avoided. The authors suggest a method of recording the head and transducer movement using an optical motion tracker.

Most ultrasound machines have an internal image cache that allows freezing a short image sequence and performing simple on-screen measurements such as distance and area measurements. It is also possible to use the motion mode (M-mode) of the ultrasound machine to make vertical distance measurements of tongue movement (Saigusa et al., 2006). However, speech researchers usually have more complex needs for measurement, so they will prefer to record the video image from the ultrasound machine together with the sound to digital video or computer

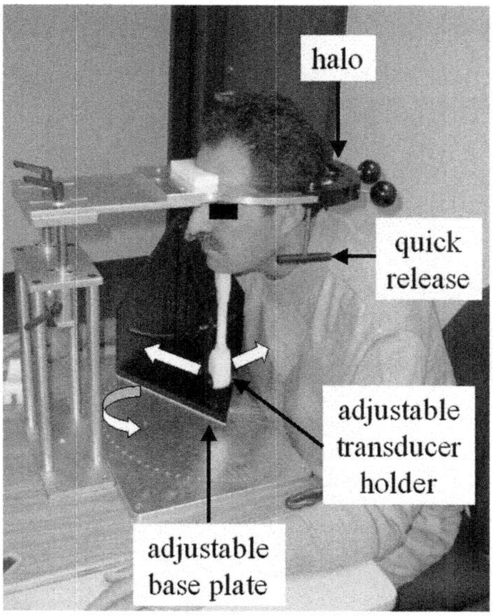

Fig. 21.3 A research participant in the CHASE 2 head anchor. This device has an adjustable halo that allows to stabilizing the research subjects head. The transducer holder is mounted on a swivelling base plate. This allows to position the transducer in a coronal or sagittal scanning position without changing the coupling spot on the participant's neck. In a coronal scanning position, as shown in the image here, the transducer holder can be pivoted backwards and forwards to obtain coronal images from different segments of the tongue.

hard disk. The resulting digital file can then be edited and analysed in a computer. Every second of film corresponds to 30 frames in NTSC machines or 25 frames in PAL machines.

It is possible to track the movement of selected points on the tongue by attaching pellets to the tongue (Kaburagi and Honda 1994). However, it is more common to trace and measure the tongue surface along its length. The researchers at the Vocal Tract Visualization Laboratory at the University of Maryland, have developed a software for the analysis and display of tongue surfaces (Akgul et al., 1999; Li et al., 2005a, b; Unser and Stone 1992). Other programmes have been developed at Queen Margaret University College in Edinburgh (Wrench et al., 2004), and the University of British Columbia in Vancouver (Gick and Rahemtulla 2004). These programmes use automatic movement trackers with spline algorithms. Splines are mathematical functions that are used for fitting curves. A spline is fit to the shape of the tongue by defining a given number of points along the length of the tongue. Since the tongue surface is the point where the ultrasound signal crosses from the tissue into the air of the oral cavity, the ultrasound machine registers a refraction as the pulse passes from one medium into the other. This refraction shows as an energy peak in the B-mode image. The spline latches onto this peak and follows it through the image sequence. However, this automatic tracking of the tongue surface motion is a particularly tricky machine vision problem. On closer inspection, ultrasound images are often quite fuzzy, unclear, and distorted by artefacts. Therefore, the spline algorithm often cannot distinguish meaningful components of the image from noise and the motion tracking may go askew (Iskarous 2005). Trained human observers will draw on their Gestalt perception, which allows them to perceive a pattern of elements as a unified whole. Since it is difficult to emulate this pattern perception in a computer programme, even well-designed spline algorithms will often produce erroneous measurements. Image artefacts or quick movements of the tongue, such as a sudden change from a

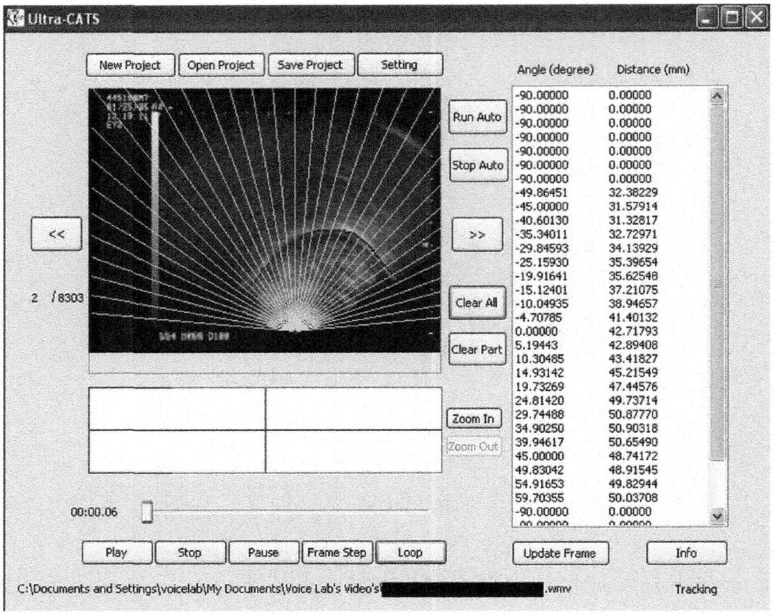

Fig. 21.4 Screenshot of the Ultra-CATS software.

high to a low vowel, may throw off the spline. As a result, the automatic motion trackers will often require copious amounts of hand-correction. It is therefore a reasonable alternative to make all measurements by hand (and eye). The ultrasound films can be measured by tracing the outline of the tongue on the ultrasound image. This approach is more laborious but reduces the time needed for correction. An example of a semi-automatic image analysis software for hand-tracing is the Ultrasonographic Contour Analyzer for Tongue Surfaces (Ultra-CATS; Bressmann et al., 2005a; see Fig. 21.4). The Ultra-CATS software can be downloaded from the FlintBox website for scientific software (www.flintbox.org).

21.2.4 **Applications of B-mode ultrasound imaging in speech research**

Ultrasound has been applied to the study of speech movements since the 1970s. Minifie et al. (1971) and Watkin and Zagzebski (1973) were among the first to demonstrate the usefulness of the technique for imaging the tongue. Since the B-mode ultrasound image can display the tongue as a continuous line, researchers have used the technique in particular to study tongue shapes for vowels (Angerstein 1994; Chiang et al., 2003; Morrish et al., 1984; Shawker and Sonies 1984; Stone et al., 1987, 1988; Wein et al., 1990). Ultrasound can also be used to assess temporal aspects of speech motor control (Keller 1987; Keller and Ostry 1983; Munhall 1985; Ostry et al., 1983; Parush and Ostry 1993). A particular benefit of ultrasound imaging is the ability to display the tongue in the coronal plane (Hamlet et al., 1988; Stone 1990).

There have also been a number of studies using ultrasound for the assessment of swallowing function (Blissett et al., 2007; Casas et al., 2003; Chi-Fishman et al., 1998; De Wijk et al., 2006; Fuhrmann and Diedrich 1994; Neuschäfer-Rube et al., 1997; Peng et al., 2000; Soder and Miller 2002; Shawker et al., 1984, 1983; Sonies et al., 1988, 1984; Stone and Shawker 1986). The method has proven to be useful for the assessment of children (Yang et al., 1997) and even for babies

(Bosma et al., 1990; Miller and Kang 2007). Swallowing and speech have been studied in pathological populations such as patients with cerebral palsies (Casas et al., 1994, 1995; Kenny et al., 1989; Sonies and Dalakas 1991), strokes (Wein et al., 1988a, 1991, 1993), geriatric patients (Sonies et al., 1984), glossectomy (Bressmann et al., 2005b, c, 2007; Schliephake et al., 1998), tongue splitting (Bressmann 2006), and malocclusions (Cheng et al., 2002; Kikyo et al., 1999; Peng et al., 2004, 2003).

Since the tongue shape can be displayed in real-time on the screen, ultrasound is a useful tool for biofeedback in speech therapy of patient groups such as deaf speakers as well as patients with dysarthrias or articulation errors. Shawker and Sonies (1985) described the use of ultrasound biofeedback for the speech therapy of a deaf individual. Recently, researchers at the University of British Columbia have begun to investigate the usefulness of ultrasonographic biofeedback in different patient groups (Adler-Bock et al., 2007; Bernhardt et al., 2003, 2005a, b; Bacsfalvi et al., 2007).

21.2.5 **Static 3D ultrasound imaging of the tongue**

B-mode ultrasound can display a 2D image of the tongue, but the lingual muscular architecture is complex and 3D (Hiiemae and Palmer 2003; Stone 1990). In many instances, it cannot be assumed that the tongue is symmetrical. For example, in patients with partial tongue resections (glossectomies) or strokes, the tongue may exhibit significant asymmetries. It is therefore necessary to develop imaging techniques that capture the 3D structure and function of the tongue.

It is relatively easy to acquire a static tongue surface. If a speaker produces a sustained speech sound, the tongue will be in a relatively constant position and shape. It is possible to sustain not only vowels (such as /a:/), but also frictives (such as /s/), liquids (such as /l/), and nasals (such as /n/). Since a standard B-mode ultrasound transducer can only produce a 2D image, the transducer must be moved along the length of the tongue. If the path of the transducer is known or if the movement of the transducer is tracked, it is possible to reconstruct the 3D volume of the tongue. Watkin and Rubin (1989) were the first to create 3D reconstructions of the tongue surface based on a small set of coronal scans at pre-defined positions. The resulting tongue surfaces were quite coarse. Stone and Lundberg (1996) used a head fixation system with an adjustable, motorized transducer holder to acquire up to 60 slices per sustained speech sound. The resulting 3D tongue surfaces were visually pleasing and anatomically detailed. Lundberg and Stone (1999) discussed how the data acquisition procedure could be simplified by reducing the number of slices. Figure 21.5 shows a 3D surface reconstruction based on multiple coronal slices. Bressmann et al. (2005b, c) used a B-mode ultrasound transducer in combination with a 3D motion sensor. This free-hand scanning system allowed to acquire tongue volume data and to reconstruct 3D tongue surfaces. Figure 21.6 shows a tomographic multi-planar view of a 3D ultrasound volume. The volume shown is based on a voxel cloud. The high density of the data points allows the observer to reconstruct a visually pleasing, photo-realistic volume. However, the software used to generate such data is usually tailored towards medical imaging applications. As such, it does not lend itself very well to the measurement of tongue surfaces for speech science purposes. The data in Fig. 21.5 were generated by mechanically swivelling the transducer to different pre-defined view-angles in 5° intervals. In the end, it is often easier to analyse a sequence of B-mode images than to extract quantitative tongue surface data from 3D voxel clouds, as in Fig. 21.6.

Based on the 3D tongue surface data, one can appreciate the intrinsic deformation of the tongue. It is also possible to derive quantitative measures that describe the shape of the tongue surface. For example, the degree of midsagittal grooving along the length of the tongue can be expressed as a number. This can be done by calculating the average of the left and right lateral free

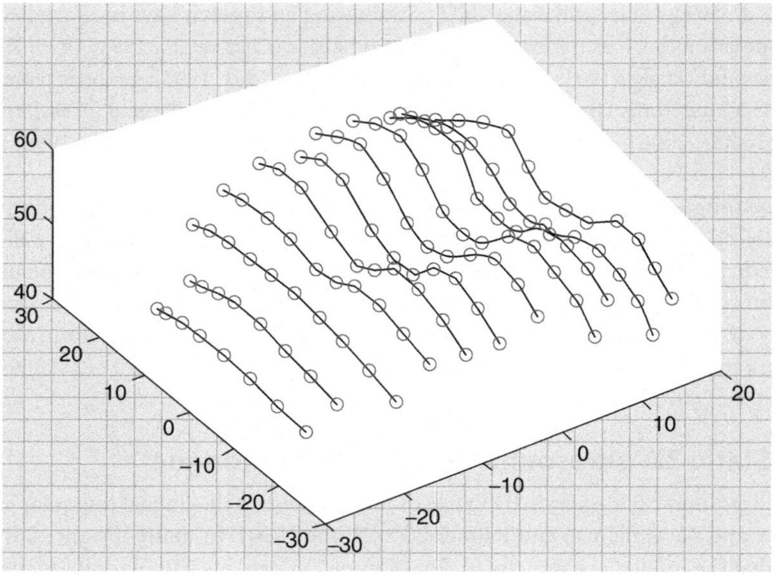

Fig. 21.5 Three-dimensional reconstruction of the tongue surface during a sustained /n/. The anterior tongue is towards the left of the graph. The midsagittal genioglossus furrow is clearly visible towards the centre and right of the graph.

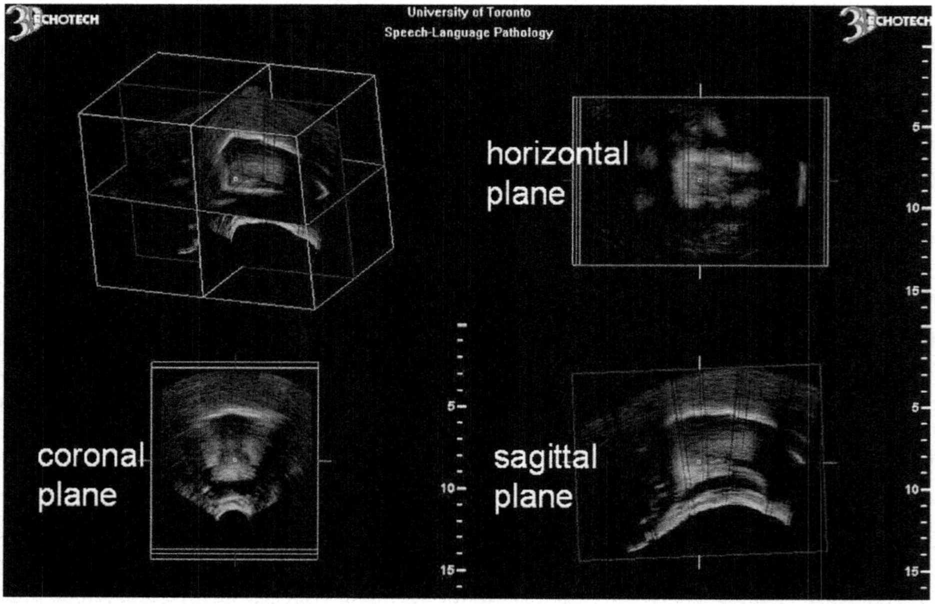

Fig. 21.6 Tomographic view of a three-dimensional ultrasound volume of a sustained /l/, spoken by a normal male adult participant.

margins of the tongue and then subtracting the height of the midsagittal plane. The resulting score will be positive for a concave and negative for a convex tongue surface. In a similar fashion, the degree of asymmetry between the right and left lateral free margin of the tongue can be quantified (Bressmann et al., 2005b, c).

21.2.6 **Dynamic 3D ultrasound imaging of the tongue**

The current generation of B-mode ultrasound machines can visualize the 2D shape and motion of the tongue. It is also possible to reconstruct 3D volumes from a sequence of 2D scans. Obviously, it would be even more interesting if we could obtain moving 3D tongue surfaces. However, there is currently no satisfactory technical solution for this challenge.

Yang and Stone (2002) reconstructed 3D tongue motion from multiple 2D coronal ultrasound scans. The speaker was put into a head stabilizer and the transducer was moved to different pre-set coronal scan positions. The speaker repeated the same sentence multiple times in each scan position. A dynamic programming algorithm was then used to identify different acoustic events in the audio in order to time-align the different image sequences. The data were reassembled into a moving 3D surface. However, the high number of repetitions necessary for the data collection requires a highly compliant research subject. The method is not appropriate for routine patient examinations.

Flowers et al. (2005) expanded on the methodology by Yang and Stone (2002). In this study, tongue movement data were collected in four coronal planes in 10° intervals. The participants were three male and three female normal speakers. A patient with a partial lateral glossectomy also took part in the study. A digital metronome was used to pace the participants' speech. The participants read a stanza from a poem to the metronome beat. The study revealed that the centre of the tongue travelled at a greater speed than the lateral free margins. This greater speed in the centre of the tongue was interpreted as a consequence of the activity of the midsagittal genioglossus furrow. Figure 21.7 illustrates how a moving tongue surface can be reconstructed from multiple coronal scans. The figure shows a sequence of tongue surfaces from a female speaker speaking the sentence 'Have a merry Christmas and happy new year'.

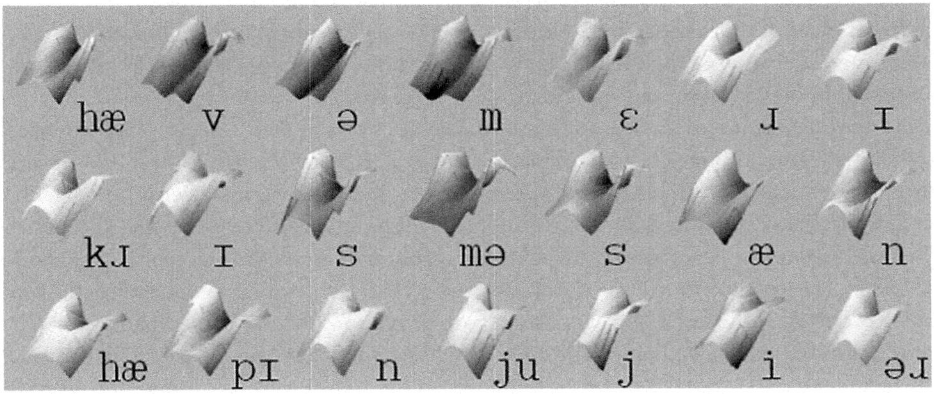

Fig. 21.7 A sequence of reconstructed 3D tongue surfaces based on multiple coronal ultrasound recordings of metronome-paced speech. The anterior tongue is towards the bottom-left of the tongue surface graphs. The posterior tongue and the genioglossus furrow are visible towards the upper right corner of the graphs. The speaker is reciting the sentence 'Have a merry Christmas and happy new year'.

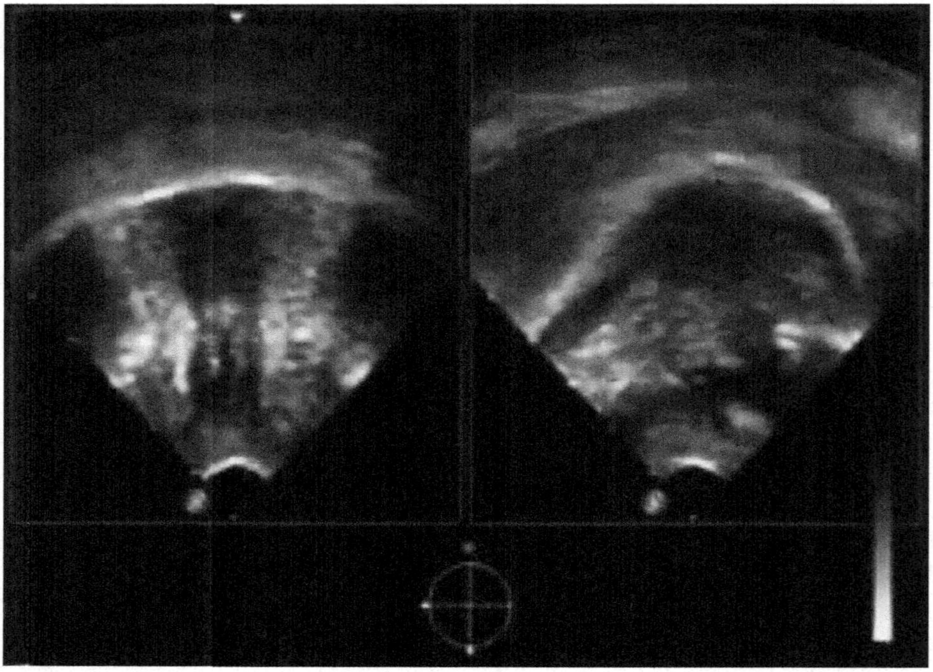

Fig. 21.8 A parallel display of coronal (left) and midsagittal (right) tongue movement in a normal adult female speaker, acquired with a Philips X3-1 matrix transducer. The speaker is producing an /e/.

Over the last decade, so-called 4D ultrasound machines have become commercially available (the fourth dimension is time). Since the tongue is a rather large anatomical structure, most current 4D ultrasound machines can only acquire 5–8 volumes per second, which is too slow for most speech tasks. These machines use transducers that are a combination of array and sector scanners. The piezoelectric crystals are arranged in a line, and a motor swings this array back and forth a number of times per second. Since the array is constantly in motion, it can only capture data from one section of the tongue at any point in time. During speech tasks, this will can to distortions in the reconstructed volumes.

The newest generation of ultrasound transducers uses crystal matrix arrays. The piezoelectric crystals in these arrays are not arranged in a line but in a 2D rectangle. While these transducers are currently very expensive, the scanning speed of the crystal matrix transducer is no longer hampered by mechanical elements such as a motor. Chi-Fishman (2005) reported mixed experiences when she used a first prototype crystal matrix transducer to study the oral phase in swallowing. Processing lags resulted in volume distortions and a relatively poor temporal and spatial resolution. Nevertheless, the technology continues to improve and the first crystal matrix transducers are now commercially available. The company Philips markets the X3-1 matrix transducer, which contains 2400 crystal elements (as opposed to the 100–300 crystals found in conventional transducers). This crystal matrix allows the examiner to acquire two scan planes in real-time (Fig. 21.8). For the first time, the sagittal movement and the intrinsic deformation of the tongue in the coronal plane can be studied at the same time.

The Philips X3-1 transducer can also capture volumetric data of tongue movement at an acquisition speed of around 10 Hz. Figure 21.9 shows a screenshot of the Philips QLab software with

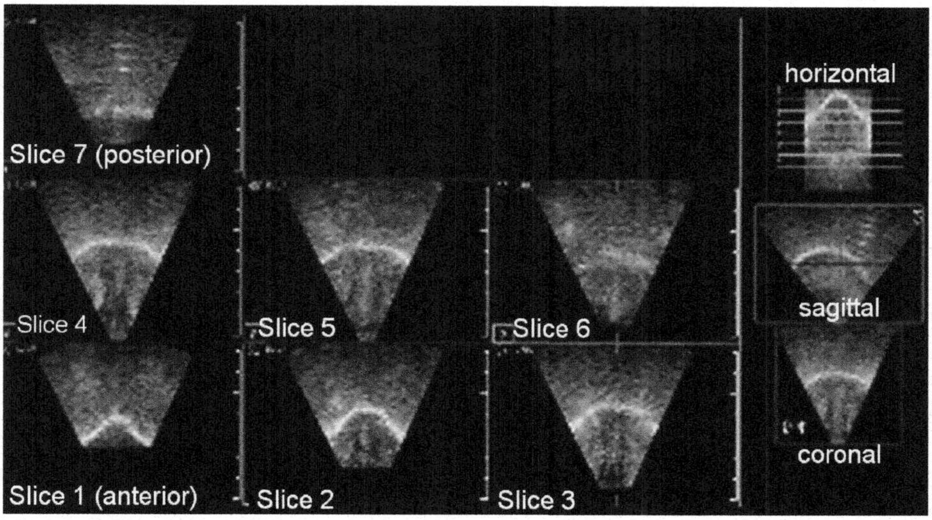

Fig. 21.9 Real-time volume acquisition with the Philips X3-1 matrix transducer. The transducer captures the moving volume of the tongue with a scanning frequency of 10 Hz. The volume can then be displayed in multiple parallel planes, in this case seven coronal planes. The right panel shows a tomographic view of the same volume.

seven parallel coronal slices of the tongue. The crystal matrix transducer technology clearly holds great promise for future generations of ultrasound machines.

21.3 Analysis of tongue movement in partial glossectomees, using ultrasound imaging

In the remainder of this chapter, the results of recent ultrasound research related to tongue movement and speech in patients with partial tongue resections (glossectomies) will be discussed. The main treatment approach for cancer of the tongue or floor of the mouth is surgery, often followed with a course of adjuvant radiation therapy. A partial tongue resection and reconstruction significantly interferes with the patient's ability to speak and interact socially. In turn, these limitations will negatively affect quality of life (Rogers 2001).

Ultrasound imaging is a particularly useful technique for the analysis of glossectomy speech and tongue movement. First, the technique is patient friendly and non-invasive. This is important because glossectomy patients undergo a life-altering surgery and onerous medical examinations and treatments. Great care must be taken not to make additional scientific experiments with these patients overly burdensome. Secondly, ultrasound allows visualizing different aspects of the tongue shape and tongue movement. The investigator can glean varied information about the effects of the lingual ablation and reconstruction on the function of a complex, 3D muscular hydrostat (Smith and Kier 1989; Stone 1990).

It is difficult to predict the exact functional consequences of a glossectomy surgery on the speech of a patient (Bressmann et al., 2004; Mackenzie-Beck et al., 1998). The speech outcomes depend on a complex combination of tumour site, defect volume, and reconstructive technique (McConnel et al., 1998; Nicoletti et al., 2004; Pauloski et al., 1998). The literature on glossectomy speech suggests that a loss of lingual tissue will interfere with the normal movement of the tongue and result in a reduced range of movement (Nicoletti et al., 2004; Pauloski et al., 1998).

This reduction in lingual movement is in turn thought to be responsible for the speech distortions (Korpijaakko-Huuhka et al., 1999).

21.3.1 **Dynamic B-mode imaging of tongue movement in glossectomy speech**

Rastadmehr et al. (2008) used B-mode ultrasound imaging to investigate midsagittal tongue movement in patients with lateral lingual resections before and after the glossectomy surgery. It was expected that the patients would show decreased lingual velocity following the resection, based on the assumption that scar tissue would tether the tongue and restrict function (Rentschler and Mann 1980). Ten patients with lateral lingual carcinomas took part in this study. Six normal speakers comprised the comparison group. The glossectomy patients were seen a few days before and two months after the surgery, when wound healing was complete and swelling had receded. None of the patients had yet undergone radiation therapy.

The participants' tongue movement was recorded in the midsagittal plane. The research setup was similar to the setup shown in Fig. 21.4. The participants read the first four sentences of the Grandfather Passage (Van Riper 1963): 'You wished to know all about my grandfather. Well, he is nearly ninety-three years old. He dresses himself in an ancient black frock coat, usually minus several buttons. Yet, he still thinks as swiftly as ever.' Reading a passage with a variety of phonemes was chosen as a task that was reasonably similar to natural speech (Weismer 2006). The tongue movement was captured with digital video and analysed using the Ultra-CATS software (Fig. 21.4). The data from the Ultra-CATS measurements were used to calculate the velocity of the midsagittal tongue. The tongue height in each ultrasound frame was subtracted from the tongue height in the next frame. In order to calculate the average velocity, the absolute values of the height differences were added up and divided by the total time of the movie sequence.

Previous research had postulated that a glossectomy operation would decrease the speed of movement of the tongue (Korpijaakko-Huuhka et al., 1999). Contrary to this expectation, the glossectomy patients significantly increased the speed of their midsagittal tongue movement in the postoperative speaking condition. This effect was seen in all patients, regardless of the technique of defect reconstruction. The analysis of the mean reading time for the passage demonstrated that the increase in velocity was not related to a faster speaking rate.

At first glance, it may seem counter-intuitive that a lateral lingual ablation should lead to an increase in midsagittal movement speed. However, recent findings from hemiparetic stroke patients demonstrates hyperfunctional compensation strategies on the unaffected side of the body (Higginson et al., 2006; Krakauer, 2006; Roby-Brami et al., 2003). A recent imaging study in a group of glossectomy patients indicated increased activity in the parietal lobes and the cerebellum that was interpreted as evidence of active compensatory adaptation to the structural defects (Mosier et al., 2005). Such compensatory processes may explain the observed increased speed of midsagittal tongue movement. In order to compensate for the lateral resection, the patients were speaking with more effort, resulting in higher velocity of movement. It would be interesting to find out in further research whether the increase in speed leads to a reduction in accuracy. The identification of such compensatory mechanisms may have implications for speech therapy.

21.3.2 **Static 3D ultrasound imaging of the tongue surface in speakers with partial glossectomy**

In another recent study, Bressmann et al. (2007) used static 3D ultrasound to assess and compare the pre- and postoperative tongue surfaces of glossectomy patients with partial lateral tongue resections. The goal was to describe the biomechanical consequences of different reconstructive techniques (free flaps vs. local closures). Twelve patients with partial lateral glossectomies participated in this study. Five patients were reconstructed with radial forearm flaps, in which a skin and muscle transplant is harvested on the inside of the forearm and grafted into the defect site. The flap tissue closes the defect and replaces the bulk and mass of the resected tissue. Seven patients had local defect closures. In this procedure, the surgeon simply sutures the wound margins to close the defect. Twelve normal speakers served as non-matched controls. An ultrasound machine with a 3D electromagnetic motion sensor was used for the data acquisition. A special 3D rendering software was used for the visualization of the ultrasound volumes. The subjects sustained three repetitions of nine phonemes (/a/, /i/, /u/, /s/,/ʃ/, /r/, /l/, /n/, /ŋ/). These sounds represented typical lingual gestures for English speech sounds. For every volume, screenshots from three sagittal slices were imported into a graphics programme and measured. Figure 21.6 displays such a 3D tongue volume. The glossectomy patients were also recorded with a computerized speech test (sentence level speech). To assess speech acceptability, sound clips from these recordings were presented to three listeners.

The resulting 3D tongue surface data were entered into a principal component analysis. The results confirmed previous research which found that many lingual postures can be explained by two mathematical components: A protrusion-retraction dimension related to the posterior tongue and an elevation-lowering dimension at the dorsum of the tongue (Bressmann et al., 2005b; Harshman et al., 1977; Hoole 1999). These two principal components were identified in the normal speakers and in all patients before the surgery. The patients with local closure demonstrated the same pattern after the operation. The patients with flap closure exhibited an altered pattern with a new third component on the operated side. This new component extended to the midline of the tongue, indicating that a free flap forms an adynamical segment that does not move in sync with the rest of the tongue.

To assess the intrinsic deformation of the tongue, a concavity measure was calculated, based on the height difference between the lateral free margins and the midsagittal plane of the tongue. The patients with flap closure showed a more pronounced decrease in midsagittal grooving than the patients with local closure. The listener ratings demonstrated that the patients with the local closure and the flaps had comparable preoperative speech acceptability. Speech acceptability deteriorated significantly in both groups after the surgery but the patients with flap reconstructions had significantly poorer results than the patients with the local defect closure. A correlation analysis showed that the flatter a patient's midsagittal groove following a lateral glossectomy, the poorer his or her speech acceptability.

The study demonstrated that the resection and reconstruction of the lateral tongue affects the intrinsic deformation of the tongue. This is an important finding because midsagittal grooving is a complex and non-volitional aspect of tongue movement. An inability to groove the tongue properly can lead to audible and stigmatizing speech sound distortions.

21.4 **Use of B-Mode and 3D ultrasound imaging in a case of post-polio syndrome**

Ultrasound imaging is a useful tool for the imaging of tongue function not only in structurally related speech disorders but also in neurogenic disorders of speech motor control. The term post-polio syndrome describes the late manifestations that occur in patients three to four decades after an initial occurrence of acute poliomyelitis. The syndrome comprises neurologic symptoms such as weakness, muscle atrophy, dysphagia, dysphonia, and, in advanced stages, respiratory failure. The patients also experience musculoskeletal manifestations such muscle and joint pain, spinal spondylosis, scoliosis, and peripheral nerve compression (Jubelt 2004). Among the first severe

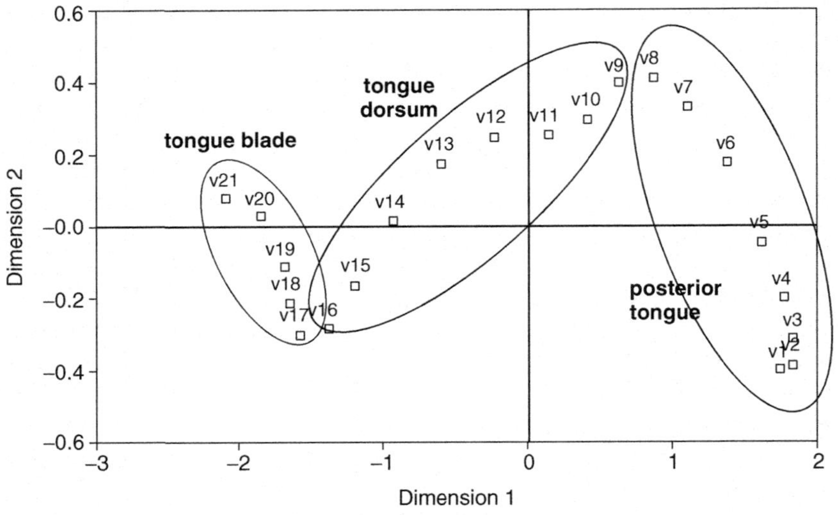

Fig. 21.10 Multidimensional scaling plot of five repetitions of /ana/, spoken by a normal speaker.

signs noted by many patients are dysphonia, velopharyngeal dysfunction, and dysphagia (Sonies 1996; Sonies and Dalakas 1991).

Mrs. Page (name changed) had originally contracted polio in the 1950s. Almost 50 years later, the post-polio complications arose. At the time of the examination, the patient reported that her symptoms had been stable for a year. In the patient's orofacial examination, severely reduced lingual movement range and strength (XIIth cranial nerve) were noted. The velar elevation was significantly reduced (Xth cranial nerve). There was weakness of the right perioral branch of the VIIth cranial nerve, which resulted in poor control of saliva. The patient presented with a rough and strained voice quality with compensatory falsetto and intermittent diplophonia. Mrs. Page had severe hypernasality with audible nasal emissions (without nasal turbulence), and her vowels and consonant sounds were poorly differentiated. As a result, her speech intelligibility was very poor. A sentence intelligibility test was evaluated off-line by a single phonetically untrained listener. Out of 80 words in 20 sentences, the listener was able to identify 5 words correctly (6.25%).

Mrs. Page underwent a 2D midsagittal ultrasound recording that consisted of individual consonants in VCV contexts as well as a short reading passage. As discussed in Section 3.2 above, normal movement of the tongue can be described in terms of a three-component model (Bressmann et al., 2005b; Harshman et al., 1977; Hoole 1999). It was noted that the movement of Mrs. Page's tongue was limited mostly to protrusion and retraction. Tongue blade control and especially dorsum height and position control were severely reduced.

Figure 21.10 displays tongue movement data from a typical normal female speaker during five repetitions of the VCV /ana/ in a multidimensional scaling plot. The multidimensional scaling procedure converts the data points from a data matrix into Euclidian distances and plots these distances in a 2D space. The figure shows how the measurement points on the 2D plot paralleled the most salient features of the tongue movement in this speaker: tongue blade elevation for /n/, and tongue dorsum and root retraction for /a/.

Figure 21.11 depicts the corresponding multidimensional scaling plot for Mrs. Page's tongue for five repetitions of /ana/. The ultrasound recording showed that there was very little differentiated tongue movement. The tongue was protruded and elevated. However, neither the tongue

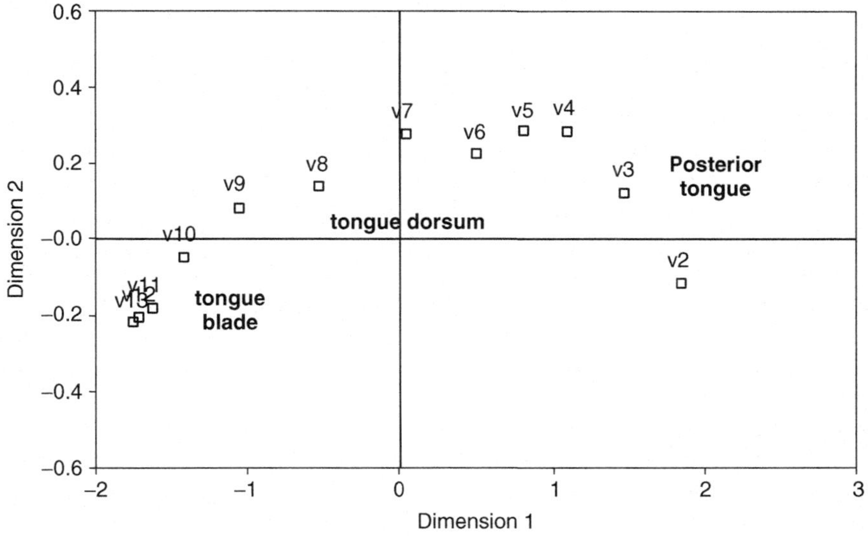

Fig. 21.11 Multidimensional scaling plot of five repetitions of /ana/, spoken by Mrs. Page.

blade elevation for /n/ nor the lingual retraction for /a/ could be observed. The results from the multidimensional scaling confirmed this observation.

Mrs. Page also underwent a 3D ultrasound recording that consisted of different sustained vowel and consonant sounds. The data from the 3D ultrasound further confirmed that Mrs. Page mainly moved her tongue by protruding and retracting it. She had lost most of the fine motor control in her tongue blade and dorsum, including the ability to groove her tongue.

21.5 Conclusions

Ultrasound offers exciting new possibilities for speech scientists and Speech-Language Pathologists. Patients and research participants generally tolerate ultrasound examinations very well. The real-time visualization on the screen is often interesting and motivating for research subjects. One of the most interesting aspects of ultrasound imaging is that it lends itself to 3D visualization of the tongue. Currently, it is probably the most cost-effective instrumentation for the acquisition of 3D tongue shapes. An exciting new prospect for speech researchers is the crystal matrix transducer technology that is just becoming available. It is to be expected that over the next decade, ultrasound imaging of the tongue will become a more common and widespread technology in speech science laboratoriess and clinical settings. The technology will significantly add to our understanding of mechanisms of speech motor control and the 3D shape and function of the tongue.

Acknowledgements

The author gratefully acknowledges the invaluable contributions of the following people (in alphabetical order) to the research described here: Elizabeth Ackloo, Yarixa Barillas, Kevin Cannons, Brent Carmichael, Michelle Ciccia, Marisa Fenos, Rebecca Fleming, Heather Flowers, Jiayun (Jenny) Gu, Catherine Hau, Chiang-Le Heng, Jonathan C. Irish, Bill Johnson, Gajanan (Kiran) Kulkarni, Orchid Rastadmehr, Theresia Stahl, Ihab Suwwan, Parveen Thind, Catherine Uy, and Willy Wong. Funding for this research was provided by the Canadian Institutes for Health Research (grant fund # MOP 62960).

References

Adler-Bock M, Bernhardt BM, Gick B, and Bacsfalvi P (2007). The use of ultrasound in remediation of North American English /r/ in 2 adolescents. *American Journal of Speech-Language Pathology*, **16**, 128–139.

Akgul YS, Kambhamettu C, and Stone M (1999). Automatic extraction and tracking of the tongue contours. *IEEE Transactions on Medical Imaging*, **18**, 1035–1045.

Angerstein W (1994). Ultraschallgestützter Untersuchungsgang zur Beurteilung der Zungenbeweglichkeit. *Sprache Stimme Gehör*, **18**, 80–84.

Bacsfalvi P, Bernhardt BM, and Gick B (2007). Electropalatography and ultrasound in vowel remediation for adolescents with hearing impairment. *Advances in Speech Language Pathology*, **9**, 36–45.

Bernhardt B, Gick B, Bacsfalvi P, and Ashdown J (2003). Speech habilitation of hard of hearing adolescents using electropalatography and ultrasound as evaluated by trained listeners. *Clinical Linguistics and Phonetics*, **17**, 199–216.

Bernhardt B, Bacsfalvi P, Gick B, Radanov B, and Williams R (2005a) Exploring the use of electropalatography and ultrasound in speech habilitation. *Journal of Speech-Language Pathology and Audiology*, **29**, 169–182.

Bernhardt B, Gick B, Bacsfalvi P, and Adler-Bock M (2005b). Ultrasound in speech therapy with adolescents and adults. *Clinical Linguistics and Phonetics*, **19**, 605–617.

Blissett A, Prinz JF, Wulfert F, Taylor AJ, and Hort J (2007). Effect of bolus size on chewing, swallowing, oral soft tissue and tongue movement. *Journal of Oral Rehabilitation*, **34** (8), 572–582.

Bosma JF, Hepburn LG, Josell SD and Baker K (1990). Ultrasound demonstration of tongue motions during suckle feeding. *Developmental Medicine and Child Neurology*, **32**, 223–229.

Bressmann T, Sader R, Whitehill TL, and Samman N (2004). Consonant intelligibility and tongue motility in patients with partial glossectomy. *Journal of Oral and Maxillofacial Surgery*, **62**, 298–303.

Bressmann T, Heng CL, and Irish JC (2005a). Applications of 2D and 3D ultrasound imaging in speech-language pathology. *Journal of Speech-Language Pathology and Audiology*, **29**, 158–168.

Bressmann T, Uy C, and Irish JC (2005b). Analysing normal and partial glossectomee tongues using ultrasound. *Clinical Linguistics and Phonetics*, **19**, 35–52.

Bressmann T, Thind P, Uy C, Bollig C, Gilbert RW, and Irish JC (2005c). Quantitative three-dimensional ultrasound analysis of tongue protrusion, grooving and symmetry: data from 12 normal speakers and a partial glossectomee. *Clinical Linguistics and Phonetics*, **19**, 573–588.

Bressmann T (2006). Speech adaptation to a self-inflicted cosmetic tongue split: perceptual and ultrasonographic analysis. *Clinical Linguistics and Phonetics*, **20**, 205–210.

Bressmann T, Ackloo E, Heng CL and Irish JC (2007). Quantitative three-dimensional ultrasound imaging of partially resected tongues. *Otolaryngology – Head and Neck Surgery*, **136**, 799–805.

Casas MJ, Kenny DJ, and Macmillan RE (2003). Buccal and lingual activity during mastication and swallowing in typical adults. *Journal of Oral Rehabilitation*, **30**, 9–16.

Casas MJ, Kenny DJ, and McPherson KA (1994). Swallowing/ventilation interactions during oral swallow in normal children and children with cerebral palsy. *Dysphagia*, **9**, 40–46.

Casas MJ, McPherson KA, and Kenny DJ (1995). Durational aspects of oral swallow in neurologically normal children and children with cerebral palsy: an ultrasound investigation. *Dysphagia*, **10**, 155–159.

Cheng CF, Peng CL, Chiou HY, and Tsai CY (2002). Dentofacial morphology and tongue function during swallowing. *American Journal of Orthodontics and Dentofacial Orthopedics*, **122**, 491–499.

Chi-Fishman G (2005). Quantitative lingual, pharyngeal and laryngeal ultrasonography in swallowing research: a technical review. *Clinical Linguistics and Phonetics*, **19**, 589–604.

Chi-Fishman G, Stone M, and McCall GN (1998). Lingual action in normal sequential swallowing. *Journal of Speech, Language, and Hearing Research*, **41**, 771–785.

Chiang YC, Lee FP, Peng CL, and Lin CT (2003). Measurement of tongue movement during vowels production with computer-assisted B-mode and M-mode ultrasonography. *Otolaryngology – Head and Neck Surgery*, **128**, 805–814.

Davidson L (2006). Comparing tongue shapes from ultrasound imaging using smoothing spline analysis of variance. *Journal of the Acoustical Society of America*, **120**, 407–415.

Epstein MA (2005). Ultrasound and the IRB. *Clinical Linguistics and Phonetics*, **19**, 567–572.

Flowers H, Bressmann T, Carmichael B, Heng CL, and Wong W (2005). Reconstructing 3D tongue movement trajectories from multiplanar paced ultrasound scans. *Canadian Acoustics*, **33**, 50–51.

Fuhrmann RA and Diedrich PR (1994). B-mode ultrasound scanning of the tongue during swallowing. *Dentomaxillofacial Radiology*, **23**, 211–215.

Gick B and Rahemtulla S (2004). *Recent developments in quantitative analysis of ultrasound tongue data.* Paper presented at the meeting of the Second Ultrasound Roundtable, Vancouver, BC.

Gu J, Bressmann T, Cannons K, and Wong W (2004). *The Ultrasonographic Contour Analyzer for Tongue Surfaces (Ultra-CATS).* Toronto: University of Toronto.

Hamlet SL, Stone M, and Shawker TH (1988). Posterior tongue grooving in deglutition and speech: preliminary observation. *Dysphagia*, **3**, 65–68.

Harshman R, Ladefoged P, and Goldstein L (1977). Factor analysis of tongue shapes. *Journal of the Acoustical Society of America*, **62**, 693–713.

Higginson JS, Zajac FE, Neptune RR, Kautz SA, and Delp SL (2006). Muscle contributions to support during gait in an individual with post-stroke hemiparesis. *Journal of Biomechanics*, **39**, 1769–1777.

Hiiemae KM and Palmer JB (2003). Tongue movements in feeding and speech. *Critical Reviews in Oral Biology and Medicine*, **14**, 413–429.

Hoole P (1999). On the lingual organization of the German vowel system. *Journal of the Acoustical Society of America*, **106**, 1020–1032.

Iskarous K (2005). Detecting the edge of the tongue: a tutorial. *Clinical Linguistics and Phonetics*, **19**, 555–565.

Jubelt B (2004). Post-polio syndrome. *Current Treatment Options in Neurology*, **6** (2), 87–93.

Kaburagi T and Honda M (1994). An ultrasonic method for monitoring tongue shape and the position of a fixed point on the tongue surface. *Journal of the Acoustical Society of America*, **95**, 2268–2270.

Keller E (1987). Mesures ultrasoniques des mouvements du dos de la langue en production de la parole: Aspects cliniques. *Folia Phoniatrica*, **39**, 51–60.

Keller E and Ostry DJ (1983). Computerized measurement of tongue dorsum movements with pulsed-echo ultrasound. *Journal of the Acoustical Society of America*, **73**, 1309–1315.

Kenny DJ, Casas MJ, and McPherson KA (1989). Correlation of ultrasound imaging of oral swallow with ventilatory alterations in cerebral palsied and normal children: preliminary observations. *Dysphagia*, **4**, 112–117.

Korpijaakko-Huuhka AM, Söderholm AL, and Lehtihalmes M (1999). Long-lasting speech and oral motor deficiencies following oral cancer surgery: a retrospective study. *Logopedics Phoniatrics Vocology*, **24**, 97–106.

Krakauer JW (2006). Motor learning: its relevance to stroke recovery and neurorehabilitation. *Current Opinion in Neurology*, **19**, 84–90.

Li M, Kambhamettu C, and Stone M (2005a). Automatic contour tracking in ultrasound images. *Clinical Linguistics and Phonetics*, **19**, 545–554.

—— (2005b). Tongue motion averaging from contour sequences. *Clinical Linguistics and Phonetics*, **19**, 515–528.

Lundberg A and Stone M (1999). Three-dimensional tongue surface reconstruction: practical considerations for ultrasound data. *Journal of the Acoustical Society of America*, **106**, 2858–2867.

Mackenzie-Beck J, Wrench A, Jackson M, et al. (1998). Surgical mapping and phonetic analysis in intra-oral cancer. In: Ziegler W, Deger K, eds. *Clinical Phonetics and Linguistics*, pp. 481–92. Whurr, London.

McConnel FM, Pauloski BR, Logemann JA, et al. (1998). Functional results of primary closure vs. flaps in oropharyngeal reconstruction: a prospective study of speech and swallowing. *Archivs of Otolaryngolology – Head and Neck Surgery*, **124**, 625–630.

Miller JL and Kang SM (2007). Preliminary ultrasound observation of lingual movement patterns during nutritive versus non-nutritive sucking in a premature infant. *Dysphagia*, **22**, 150–160.

Minifie FD, Kelsey CA, Zagzebskija JA, and King TW (1971). Ultrasonic scans of the dorsal surface of the tongue. *Journal of the Acoustical Society of America*, **49**, 1857–1860.

Morrish KA, Stone M, Sonies BC, Kurtz D, and Shawker T (1984). Characterization of tongue shape. *Ultrasonic Imaging*, **6**, 37–47.

Mosier K, Liu WC, Behin B, et al. (2005). Cortical adaptation following partial glossectomy with primary closure: implications for reconstruction of the oral tongue. *Annals of Otology, Rhinology and Laryngolology*, **114**, 681–687.

Munhall KG (1985). An examination of intra-articulator relative timing. *Journal of the Acoustical Society of America*, **78**, 1548–1553.

Neuschäfer-Rube C, Wein BB, Angerstein W, Klajman S, and Fischer-Wein G (1997). Sektorbezogene Grauwertanalyse videosonographisch aufgezeichneter Zungenbewegungen beim Schlucken. *HNO*, **45**, 556–562.

Nicoletti G, Soutar DS, Jackson MS, Wrench AA, Robertson G, and Robertson C (2004). Objective assessment of speech after surgical treatment for oral cancer: experience from 196 selected cases. *Journal of the American Society of Plastic Surgeons*, **113**,114–25.

Ostry DJ, Keller E, and Parush A (1983). Similarities in the control of the speech articulators and the limbs: kinematics of tongue dorsum movement in speech. *Journal of Experimental Psychology: Human Perception and Performance*, **9**, 622–636.

Parush A and Ostry DJ (1993). Lower pharyngeal wall coarticulation in VCV syllables. *Journal of the Acoustical Society of America*, **94**, 715–722.

Pauloski BR, Logemann JA, and Colangelo LA (1998). Surgical variables affecting speech in treated patients with oral and oropharyngeal cancer. *Laryngoscope*, **108**, 908–16.

Peng CL, Jost-Brinkmann PG, Miethke RR, and Che-Tong L (2000). Ultrasonographic measurement of tongue movement during swallowing. *Journal of Ultrasound in Medicine*, **19**, 15–20.

Peng CL, Jost-Brinkmann PG, Yoshida N, Miethke RR, and Lin CT (2003). Differential diagnosis between infantile and mature swallowing with ultrasonography. *European Journal of Orthodontics*, **25**, 451–456.

Peng CL, Jost-Brinkmann PG, Yoshida N, Chou HH, and Lin CT (2004). Comparison of tongue functions between mature and tongue-thrust swallowing – An ultrasound investigation. *American Journal of Orthodontics and Dentofacial Orthopedics*, **125**, 562–570.

Rastadmehr O, Bressmann T, Smyth R, and Irish JC (2008). Increased midsagittal tongue velocity indicates articulatory compensation in patients with lateral partial glossectomies. *Head and Neck*, **30**, 718–726.

Rentschler GJ and Mann MB (1980). The effects of glossectomy on intelligibility of speech and oral perceptual discrimination. *Journal of Oral and Maxillofacial Surgery*, **38**, 348–354.

Roby-Brami A, Feydy A, Combeaud M, Biryukova EV, Bussel B, and Levin MF (2003). Motor compensation and recovery for reaching in stroke patients. *Acta Neurologica Scandinavica*, **107**, 369–381.

Rogers SN (2001). Surgical principles and techniques for functional rehabilitation after oral cavity and oropharyngeal oncologic surgery. *Current Opinion in Otolaryngolology – Head and Neck Surgery*, **9**, 114–119.

Saigusa H, Saigusa M, Aino I, Iwasaki C, Li L, and Niimi S (2006). M-mode color Doppler ultrasonic imaging of vertical tongue movement during articulatory movement. *Journal of Voice*, **20**, 38–45.

Schliephake H, Schmelzeisen R, Schönweiler R, Schneller T, and Altenbernd C (1998). Speech, deglutition and life quality after intraoral tumour resection. A prospective study. *International Journal of Oral and Maxillofacial Surgery*, **27**, 99–105.

Shawker TH and Sonies BC (1984). Tongue movement during speech: a real-time ultrasound evaluation. *Journal of Clinical Ultrasound*, **12**, 125–133.

Shawker TH and Sonies BC (1985). Ultrasound biofeedback for speech training. Instrumentation and preliminary results. *Investigative Radiology*, **20**, 90–93.

Shawker TH, Sonies B, Stone M, and Baum BJ (1983). Real-time ultrasound visualization of tongue movement during swallowing. *Journal of Clinical Ultrasound*, **11**, 485–490.

Shawker TH, Sonies BC, and Stone M (1984). Soft tissue anatomy of the tongue and floor of the mouth: an ultrasound demonstration. *Brain and Language*, **21**, 335–350.

Smith KK and Kier WM (1989). Trunks, tongues, and tentacles: moving with skeletons of muscle. *American Scientist*, **77**, 28–35.

Soder N and Miller N (2002). Using ultrasound to investigate intrapersonal variability in durational aspects of tongue movement during swallowing. *Dysphagia*, **17**, 288–297.

Sonies BC (1996). Dysphagia and post-polio syndrome: past, present, and future. *Seminars in Neurology*, **16**, 365–370.

Sonies BC, Baum BJ, and Shawker TH (1984). Tongue motion in elderly adults: initial in situ observations. *Journal of Gerontology*, **39**, 279–283.

Sonies BC and Dalakas MC (1991). Dysphagia in patients with the post-polio syndrome. *New England Journal of Medicine*, **324**, 1162–1167.

Sonies BC, Parent LJ, Morrish K, and Baum BJ (1988). Durational aspects of the oral-pharyngeal phase of swallow in normal adults. *Dysphagia*, **3**, 1–10.

Stone M and Shawker TH (1986). An ultrasound examination of tongue movement during swallowing. *Dysphagia*, **1**, 78–83.

Stone M, Morrish K, Sonies BC, and Shawker TH (1987). Tongue curvature: a model of shape during vowel production. *Folia Phoniatrica*, **39**, 302–315.

Stone M, Shawker TH, Talbot TL, and Rich AH (1988). Cross-sectional tongue shape during the production of vowels. *Journal of the Acoustical Society of America*, **83**, 1586–1596.

Stone M (1990). A three-dimensional model of tongue movement based on ultrasound and x-ray microbeam data. *Journal of the Acoustical Society of America*, **87**, 2207–2217.

Stone M and Davis EP (1995). A head and transducer support system for making ultrasound images of tongue/jaw movement. *Journal of the Acoustical Society of America*, **98**, 3107–3112.

Stone M and Lundberg A (1996). Three-dimensional tongue surface shapes of English consonants and vowels. *Journal of the Acoustical Society of America*, **99**, 3728–3737.

Stone M (2005). A guide to analysing tongue motion from ultrasound images. *Clinical Linguistics and Phonetics*, **19**, 455–501.

Unser M and Stone M (1992). Automated detection of the tongue surface in sequences of ultrasound images. *Journal of the Acoustical Society of Canada*, **91**, 3001–3007.

Van Riper C (1963). *Speech correction: Principles and Methods, 4th edition.* Prentice-Hall, Englewood Cliffs.

Watkin KL and Rubin JM (1989). Pseudo-three-dimensional reconstruction of ultrasonic images of the tongue. *Journal of the Acoustical Society of America*, **85**, 496–499.

Watkin KL and Zagzebski JA (1973). On line ultrasonic technique for monitoring tongue displacements. *Journal of the Acoustical Society of America*, **54**, 544–547.

Wein B, Angerstein W, and Klajman S (1993). Suchbewegungen der Zunge bei einer Sprechapraxie: Darstellung mittels Ultraschall und Pseudo-3D-Abbildung. *Nervenarzt*, **64**, 143–145.

Wein B, Bockler R, Huber W, Klajman S, and Willmes K (1990). Computersonographische Darstellung von Zungenformen bei der Bildung der langen Vokale des Deutschen. *Ultraschall in der Medizin*, **11**, 100–103.

Wein B, Bockler R and Klajman S (1991). Temporal reconstruction of sonographic imaging of disturbed tongue movements. *Dysphagia*, **6**, 135–139.

Wein B, Klajman S, Huber W, and Doring WH (1988a). Ultraschalluntersuchung von Koordinationsstörungen der Zungenbewegung beim Schlucken. *Nervenarzt*, **59**, 154–158.

Weismer G (2006). Philosophy of research in motor speech disorders. *Clinical Linguists and Phonetics*, **20**, 315–349.

Whalen DH, Iskarous K, Tiede MK, Ostry DJ, Lehnert-LeHouillier H, Vatikiotis-Bateson E, and Hailey DS (2005). The Haskins optically corrected ultrasound system (HOCUS). *Journal of Speech, Language and Hearing Research*, **48**, 543–553.

de Wijk RA, Wulfert F, and Prinz JF (2006). Oral processing assessed by M-mode ultrasound imaging varies with food attribute. *Physiology and Behavior*, **89**, 15–21.

Wrench A (2004 April). *QMUC Matching, merging and means: Spline productivity tools for ultrasound analysis.* Paper presented at the meeting of the Second Ultrasound Roundtable, Vancouver, BC.

Yang CS and Stone M (2002). Dynamic programming method for temporal registration of three-dimensional tongue surface motion from multiple utterances. *Speech Communication*, **38**, 199–207.

Yang WT, Loveday EJ, Metreweli C, and Sullivan PB (1997). Ultrasound assessment of swallowing in malnourished disabled children. *British Journal of Radiology*, **70**, 992–994.

Index

Locators for headings which also have subheadings refer to general aspects of that topic only
Locators in **bold** refer to major content
Locators in *italic* refer to figures/diagrams

The manufacturer's authorised representative in the EU for product safety is Oxford University Press España S.A. of El Parque Empresarial San Fernando de Henares, Avenida de Castilla, 2 - 28830 Madrid (www.oup.es/en or product.safety@oup.com). OUP España S.A. also acts as importer into Spain of products made by the manufacturer.
Printed and bound by CPI Group (UK) Ltd, Croydon, CR0 4YY
05/10/2026
02227970-0005